Role of the Gut Flora
in Toxicity and Cancer

Role of the Gut Flora
in Toxicity and Cancer

Edited by

I.R. Rowland

BIBRA, Carshalton, UK

1988

ACADEMIC PRESS
Harcourt Brace Jovanovich, Publishers
London   San Diego   New York
Boston   Sydney   Tokyo   Toronto

ACADEMIC PRESS LIMITED
24–28 Oval Road
London NW1 7DX

U.S. Edition published by
ACADEMIC PRESS INC.
San Diego. CA 92101

British Library Cataloguing in Publication Data
Rowland, Ian
  Role of the gut flora in toxicity and cancer.
  I. Title
  612'.33

ISBN 0–12–599920–8

Typeset by Photo·graphics, Honiton, Devon
and printed in Great Britain by St Edmundsbury Press Limited,
Bury St. Edmunds, Suffolk

Contributors

H. ADLERCREUTZ *Department of Clinical Chemistry, University of Helsinki, Meilahti Hospital, SF–00290, Helsinki, Finland*

J.P. BROWN *Zoecon Corporation, 975 California Avenue, Palo Alto, CA 94304, USA**

Ph. CAENEPEEL *The Rega Institute, Katholieke Universiteit Leuven, Minderbroedeersstraat 10, B–3000 Leuven, Belgium*

M.E. COATES *Robens Institute of Industrial and Environmental Health and Safety, University of Surrey, Guildford, Surrey GU2 5XH, UK*

B.S. DRASAR *Department of Medical Microbiology, London School of Hygiene and Tropical Medicine, Keppel Street, London WC1 7HT, UK*

H. EYSSEN *The Rega Institute, Katholieke Universiteit Leuven, Minderbroedersstraat 10, B–3000 Leuven, Belgium*

J.B. HENEGHAN *School of Medicine in New Orleans, Louisiana State University, Medical Center, 1542 Tulane Avenue, New Orleans, LA 70112, USA*

M.J. HILL *Bacterial Metabolism Research Laboratory, PHLS, Centre for Applied Microbiology and Research, Porton Down, Wiltshire, UK*

G.L. LARSEN *Metabolism and Radiation Research Laboratory, Agriculture Research, Science and Education Administration, United States Department of Agriculture, State University Station, Fargo, ND 58105, USA*

R.E. MC CARTHY *Department of Microbiology, University of Illinois, Urbana, Ill. 61801, USA*

* home address 767 Montrose Avenue, Palo Alto, CA 94303, USA.

A.K. MALLETT	*Microbiology Department, British Industrial Biological Research Association, Woodmansterne Road, Carshalton, Surrey SM5 4DS, UK*

A.G. RENWICK	*University of Southampton, Medical and Biological Sciences Building, Bassett Crescent East, Southampton SO9 3TU, UK*

D.E. RICKERT	*Department of General and Biochemical Toxicology, Chemical Industry Institute of Toxicology, PO Box 12137, Research Triangle Park, NC 27709, USA*

I.R. ROWLAND	*Microbiology Department, British Industrial Biological Research Association, Woodmansterne Road, Carshalton, Surrey SM5 4DS, UK*

A.A. SALYERS	*Department of Microbiology, University of Illinois, Urbana, Ill. 61801, USA*

K.D.R. SETCHELL	*Children's Hospital Medical Center, Children's Hospital Research Foundation, Department of Pediatrics, College of Medicine, University of Cincinnati, Elland and Bethesda Avenues, Cincinnati, OH 45229, USA*

S. VENITT	*The Institute of Cancer Research, Royal Cancer Hospital, Clifton Avenue, Sutton, Surrey SM2 5PX, UK*

R. WALKER	*Department of Biochemistry, University of Surrey, Guildford, Surrey GU2 5XH, UK*

O.M. WRONG	*The Rayne Institute, Faculty of Clinical Sciences, University College Hospital Medical School, London WC1E 6JJ, UK*

Preface

The relationship between the gut microflora and its host is the main topic of this book. To a certain extent the two are capable of independent existence — continuous culture studies, in which the flora is maintained outside the host, show that it is possible to maintain the flora without any direct host inputs. Equally, germ-free animals, in which the flora is entirely absent, often survive longer than their conventional flora counterparts. However, when these two entities of flora and host are brought together in the 'conventional flora' animal, the opportunities for benefit and detriment blossom.

In the realms of toxicology the gut microflora is often overlooked as a site of metabolism of foreign compounds, or is used as a 'scapegoat' when investigations of potential mammalian sites of metabolism have drawn blanks. The technical difficulties of culturing organisms from the gut and the stringent conditions needed for metabolism studies with anaerobic bacteria are some of the reasons for neglecting to study the flora. However, as knowledge of the flora has increased and the technical facilities for anaerobic bacteriology have become more widely available, a large body of knowledge regarding foreign compound metabolism has developed. The study, both bacteriological and metabolic, of the gut microflora has been given impetus by the strong circumstantial evidence linking the flora with the aetiology of a number of human cancers, such as those of the large bowel, prostate and breast, which comprise a large proportion of cancer deaths in Western Europe and the USA.

This volume aims to provide a comprehensive and current view of the contribution of the gut flora to foreign compound metabolism in man and laboratory animals. The object has been to relate this bacterial metabolism to toxic events occurring in mammals and to consider the interrelationships of bacterial and mammalian metabolic pathways. The early chapters are intended to 'set the scene' and provide a background to the sections on metabolism of specific groups of compounds which follow.

The succeeding chapters encompass the bacterial metabolism of both xenobiotics and food components and concentrate on those reactions which have actual, or potential toxicological and/or clinical importance. A planned chapter on azo compound metabolism did not materialize, but there are a number of reviews on this subject in the recent literature. The concluding chapters are intended to provide assessments of the role of the gut flora in the aetiology of cancer, in particular from the point of view of the formation of carcinogens, mutagens and promotors within the large bowel.

I am very grateful to all the authors, who gave up so much of their valuable time to contribute to this book.

Ian Rowland

Contents

1

Methodological Considerations for the Study of Bacterial Metabolism

*M. E. COATES, B. S. DRASAR, A. K. MALLETT and
I. R. ROWLAND*

A. Introduction

Because of the prevailing physicochemical conditions in the gut, particularly the low redox potential and low oxygen tension, studies of the gut microflora (whether bacteriological, biochemical or toxicological) require specialized techniques of varying degrees of sophistication and expense. Many of the methods designed for culturing and identifying the component microorganisms of the flora have been extensively reviewed elsewhere and hand-books are available which describe in detail the apparatus, culture media and isolation methods for anaerobic bacteriological studies (Holdeman and Moore, 1975; Mitsuoka *et al.*, 1976; Drasar and Hill, 1974; Brown, 1977; Sutter *et al.*, 1980). The methods used for quantitating these organisms and also for the less fastidious anaerobes and facultative anaerobes are summarized with their advantages and disadvantages in Table 1.1.

This review will concentrate on the techniques, *in vitro* and *in vivo*, that may be used for studying the role of the flora in metabolism and toxicity of chemicals.

B. Studies of Gut Flora Metabolism *in vitro*

1. *Incubation with Gut Contents From Animals and Man*

(a) Obtaining samples. The most widely used approach is to remove the caecum from the animal immediately after death and express the contents into a suitable suspension medium (see below). In humans a freshly collected sample of faeces can be treated in the same way. How

ROLE OF THE GUT FLORA IN TOXICITY AND CANCER
ISBN 0-12-599920-8

Table 1.1 *Determination of bacterial numbers in faeces and gut contents*

Method	Reference	Comments
Direct microscopic count (DMC)	Holdeman and Moore (1975)	Total count of all microorganisms, living and dead
Viable count, aerobic incubation		Variety of selective agars available enabling identification down to family or even genus level. However, aerobic count is generally less than 1% of anaerobic viable count.
Viable count, anaerobic jar methods	Brown (1977) Mitsuoka (1969, 1982)	Counts O_2-tolerant anaerobes; usually 20–50% of DMC can be recovered.
Anaerobic cabinet	Drasar (1967)	Better recovery of anaerobes than anaerobic jar method. Enables dilution, plating, incubating and subculturing to be done in a virtually O_2-free atmosphere.
Roll tubes Plate in bottle	Holdeman and Moore (1975) Mitsuoka (1969, 1982)	Both methods exclude O_2 completely and are used for very fastidious anaerobes. If suitable media are used 90–100% of DMC can be cultured.

representative the faecal flora is of the flora of the colon is debatable (Fernandez *et al.*, 1985) but in most instances it is the only practical means of obtaining a sample of the lower gut flora from the healthy human. Alternative methods of varying degrees of complexity and unpleasantness for the subject have been developed for obtaining samples from the lower ileum and colon, such as nasal tubes and capsules operated by radio control. Such techniques, however, have several disadvantages and do not necessarily provide samples representative of the gut region under study (Drasar and Barrow, 1985). It should also be recognized that the samples obtained from humans or laboratory animals are not uniform and their metabolic activity may be affected by, for example, diet, age and housing conditions.

Ideally the conditions of suspension and incubation of the sample should be such as to mimic, as closely as possible, the conditions within the gut. Thus it is important to transfer quickly the sample to an anaerobic cabinet or to flush the collection vessel with anaerobic gases.

Faecal or gut contents samples may be heterogeneous so thorough mixing of a complete sample is crucial before removing a portion for suspension in medium. Suspensions of gut contents should be kept on ice and used as soon as possible after preparation. The freezing of samples to be used in bacteriological or biochemical assays is not recommended and results in loss of viability and, in the case of reductive enzymes such as azo-, nitro- and nitrate reductase, rapid loss of activity. The activity of hydrolytic enzymes such as β-glucuronidase and urease is usually not decreased by freezing but may actually increase, presumably due to cell lysis allowing greater access of substrates to enzymes (Vince *et al.*, 1976).

(b) Incubation conditions. The conditions for the *in vitro* incubation should be chosen so as to mimic closely the *in vivo* system and to distort as little as possible the balance of organisms in the flora.

The maintenance of anaerobic conditions during incubation is essential to avoid loss of cell viability and concomitant loss of enzyme activity, particularly since certain reductase enzymes are inhibited by the presence of oxygen (Mason and Holtzman, 1975). Some hydrolytic activities are similar under aerobic and anaerobic conditions (e.g. urease, β-glycosidase, β-glucuronidase) over short time periods (20–30 minutes) although it is preferable even here to maintain anaerobiosis so that the incubation conditions reflect those *in vivo* (Rowland *et al.*, 1985). To achieve anaerobic conditions, bubbling oxygen-free nitrogen through the medium appears to be adequate (Scheline, 1968; Erikson and Gustafsson, 1970). These methods are described by Illing (1981), who also compared reductive and hydrolytic activities in rat caecal contents suspended in buffer or two types of growth media. Little difference was observed in bacterial metabolism over 1 hour suggesting that a simple buffer is adequate for metabolic studies with the gut flora. Complex media may indeed complicate the interpretation of an experiment by allowing growth of some or all of the flora during the incubation period, thereby biasing the results, or by encouraging adventitious bacterial metabolism such as production of ammonia and volatile fatty acids with consequent changes in enzyme activities (reviewed by Rowland *et al.*, 1985). The pH of the buffer should be chosen to reflect that of the sample, in the case of rat caecal contents and human faeces approximately pH 6.0–7.6 (Ward *et al.*, 1986; Brown *et al.*, 1974; van Dokkum *et al.*, 1983). Although incubation times of 1–96 hours have been used (see Illing 1981, for review), incubation periods of up to 2 hours are sufficient to determine whether metabolism is occurring for most metabolic studies. Indeed, longer incubation times may yield spurious results due to loss of sensitive organisms and growth of others. Where prolonged incubation is necessary the use of more sophisticated systems such as continuous culture (see below) is likely to yield more representative results.

It is important to bear in mind that unless a suspension of gut contents is fractionated it may contain enzymes from sources other than bacteria such as intestinal mucosal cells and soluble mammalian enzymes. The use of suitable control incubations containing antibiotics can help to discriminate these various enzyme sources.

In view of the complexity of the flora and the difficulties involved in conventional bacteriological approaches to studying the flora of man and laboratory animals, several research groups have monitored faecal or caecal suspensions for the presence of bacterial enzymes known to be important in drug metabolism. This approach has been applied to the study of effects of diet on the gut flora of rats (Reddy *et al.*, 1974; Goldin and Gorbach, 1976) and to comparisons of the gut floras of various laboratory animals and human population groups (Rowland *et al.*, 1983, 1986; Drasar *et al.*, 1986).

2.   *Incubations with Pure Cultures of Gut Organisms*

Incubations with pure cultures of organisms isolated from the gut have been used to identify the bacteria responsible for a particular reaction such as bile acid metabolism (Goddard and Hill, 1973), heavy metal biotransformation (Rowland *et al.*, 1978) and *p*-nitrobenzoic acid reduction (Zachariah and Juchau, 1974). It is important to note however that the activity of an organism may be modified by the presence of other members of the flora and by the environment of the host gut (Cole *et al.*, 1985).

It is difficult to obtain direct evidence that any particular biotransform-ation is mediated by a single species of bacteria present in the gut flora. This problem is well illustrated by consideration of inactivation of digoxin which occurs via reduction by the gut flora of some people.

Eubacterium lentum is the organism known to perform the reaction, but neither the presence of these bacteria nor their concentration in the gut relates simply to digoxin reductions (Dobbin *et al.*, 1983). The problem is comparatively simple now that the bacterial species involved has been identified. However, the extent of possible difficulties can be appreciated when it is realized that the log of the number of *Eu. lentum* per gram of faeces ranges from 3.6 to 11.7 (Finegold *et al.*, 1983). Thus, in some individuals examination of ten colonies of non-sporing anaerobes would ensure isolation while in others as many as one hundred million colonies would have to be studied.

The problem is presented diagrammatically in Fig. 1.1. Thus, the number of species of bacteria isolated is related to the number of bacterial colonies that are isolated and screened. It is seldom possible to screen

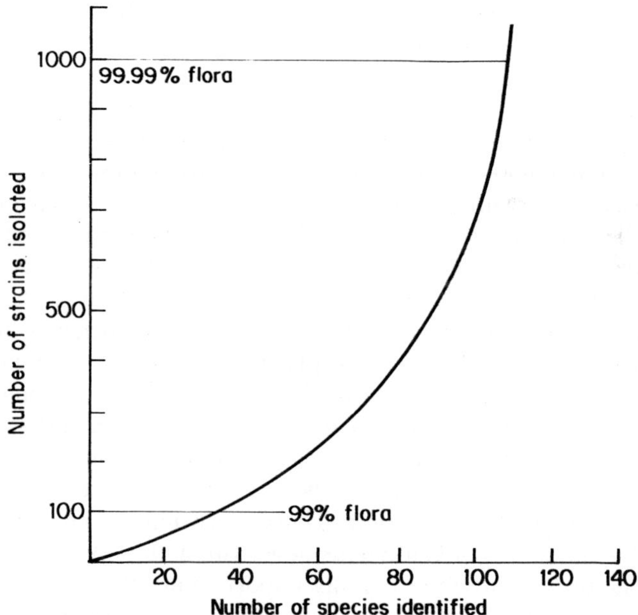

Fig 1.1   The relation of the number of colonies examined to the number of species identified from media inoculated with faecal material.

more than 100 colonies from any sample, even if time and money are not limited; 10 colonies is a more reasonable estimate for most investigators. The isolation and identification of the bacteria responsible for a particular biotransformation is seldom a sensible approach to this problem. Unless a large collection of isolated and named bacterial strains is available for screening it is unlikely that the relevant species will be easily identified. Even if a suitable collection of bacteria is available we have no means of ensuring that it is comprehensive. Attempts to isolate and identify the bacteria responsible for a reaction are likely to be both difficult and unrewarding. Even if an organism able to perform the reaction is isolated an extensive bacteriological investigation would be needed to verify the role of similar organisms in the intestinal ecology.

3. *Incubations with Cell-free Extracts*

Methods have been developed to prepare cell-free extracts of caecal contents or faeces (cecalase, fecalase). Such extracts have been used in particular to study metabolism, to mutagens in the Ames test, of azo dyes and plant glycosides (Brown and Dietrich, 1979).

4. *Application of Continuous Culture Methodology*

In the majority of studies of bacterial metabolism, the intestinal flora has been maintained under simple batch culture conditions, i.e. a closed incubation system, with or without the provision of bacterial nutrients. It should be appreciated, however, that such incubation methods, whilst adequately demonstrating the potential for metabolism of a compound by microbial processes, fall short of the conditions naturally present within the alimentary tract. In particular, abiotic factors (e.g. nutrient availability, the accumulation of waste products, pH, redox potential) may alter over the course of an incubation, particularly for studies extending over a number of hours. One consequence of such changes in incubation conditions may be that certain species of micro-organisms thrive at the expense of other members of the gut flora and result in a distorted picture of bacterial metabolism. In contrast, the gastro-intestinal flora *in situ* exists under conditions of continuous flow, with a more or less constantly available supply of nutrients. Equally important are the dynamics of the gut, since gastric emptying, peristalsis and defaecation constantly remove a portion of the microbial population from a given gut compartment (stomach, intestine and colon, respectively, in the above examples) allowing the residual organisms to multiply until nutrient availability or host physiological processes limit growth.

One method of modelling the dynamic equilibrium naturally present within the gut is through the use of *in vitro* continuous culture methodology by which a bacterial population is maintained near to steady state of growth by the continuous addition of fresh growth medium and continuous removal, at the same rate, of spent culture. Methodology of this type has been applied to the maintenance of mixed bacterial populations comprising the hypochlorhydric stomach (Coutts *et al.*, 1987) and large intestinal floras (Veilleux and Rowland, 1981; Miller and Wolin, 1981; Freter *et al.*, 1983a,b; Knoke and Bernhardt, 1984; Edwards *et al.*, 1985). Examples of these various systems are considered below.

(a) Models of the rodent gut flora.   Veilleux and Rowland (1981) described an anaerobic continuous culture model of the bacterial ecosystem present in the rat large intestine. Various combinations of pH and dilution rate were investigated, the greatest similarity to the native gut flora resulting when a two-stage apparatus with cell recycle was employed. The community structure *in vitro* reflected the bacterial group proportions and species composition present in the faecal inoculum, with a mixed population of anaerobes comprising approximately 90% of the total organisms present.

Subsequent studies showed that the range of hydrolytic bacterial enzyme activities present in the culture closely resembled that of rat caecal contents (Mallett *et al.*, 1983). Quantitative determinations of bacterial biotransformation reactions returned comparable activities for azoreductase, β-glucosidase, nitrate reductase and nitroreductase enzymes *in vitro* or in caecal contents, but β-glucuronidase activity was very low in culture. However, this latter enzyme was induced within the *in vitro* system after addition of a glucuronide substrate (*p*-nitrophenyl-β-D-glucuronide) to give a rate of metabolism indistinguishable from that of the caecal flora. The addition of bile acids (cholic acid, chenodeoxycholic acid) also increased β-glucoside and β-glucuronide hydrolysis *in vitro*. These observations suggested that bacterial metabolism in the gut is regulated by the entry of host products (bile salt, glucuronide conjugates) into the large intestine (Mallett *et al.*, 1983). The bacterial population of the rat gut flora also converted the artificial sweetener cyclamate to cyclohexylamine (Mallett *et al.*, 1985) mimicking the *in vivo* induction of sulphamatase activity in the hindgut flora reported by other workers (Renwick and Williams, 1972; Bickel *et al.*, 1974). No induction of cyclamate metabolism was found in batch culture incubations of rat caecal contents, however, demonstrating a high degree of similarity between the continuous culture ecosystem and the rat caecal microflora (Mallett *et al.*, 1985). Furthermore, the addition of the *bis*-azo dye Brown HT to a culture of rat hindgut micro-organisms resulted in a range of metabolites qualitatively similar to those found in faeces after oral administration of this compound to the rat, while batch culture incubations of rat faeces and Brown HT gave a metabolic profile unrepresentative of that found *in vivo* (Mallett *et al.*, 1986). These observations demonstrate several applications of continuous flow methods to the study of bacterial metabolism of xenobiotic compounds *in vitro*.

A continuous flow culture modelling the bacterial ecosystem of the mouse hindgut was developed by Freter *et al.* (1983a) and, as was noted for the rat intestinal population (Veilleux and Rowland, 1981), a very high degree of similarity in the taxonomic species composition was found when compared to the *in vivo* gut population. The system was used to characterize certain of the mechanisms regulating inter-species relationships within the gut microflora (Freter *et al.*, 1983a,b) and did not address bacterial metabolism of xenobiotic or host derived products by the flora. Nevertheless the system further demonstrated the applicability of continuous flow techniques for the maintenance of bacterial gut microorganisms *ex vivo*.

(b) Studies on the human gut flora. A system allowing the culture of the human large intestinal flora *in vitro* for extended periods (in excess of 81 days) was described by Miller and Wolin (1981), using a single stage, anaerobic culture with freshly voided faeces as the source of inoculum. Nutrients were supplied semi-continuously (every 12 hours) in the form of comminuted fibrous food materials (lettuce, celery, carrot, apple), deoxycholate, urea, casein, vitamins and salts in order to approximate the growth factors available to the flora in the large intestine. Metabolic fidelity of the culture was assessed from the generation of fermentation products (short-chain fatty acids, methane, hydrogen and carbon dioxide) which closely approximate those normally present in human faeces. *Bacteroides, Fusobacterium, Ruminococcus* and *Clostridium* species were isolated from the culture, although the predominant nonsporing anaerobes in the bacterial population were found to alter when the ratio of plant components added to the medium was varied. Thus dietary intake appears to have the potential to modify the species composition of the intestinal microflora. The semi-continuous addition of nutrients was intended to imitate the flow of nutrients into the large intestine during normal eating practices and, despite the simplification inherent in all *in vitro* studies, succeeded in reproducing the fermentative and microbial profiles normally occurring in the human hindgut.

A continuous culture of colonic bacteria, using a defined medium simulating ileal effluent, was described by Edwards *et al.* (1985) for the study of carbohydrate degradation, volatile fatty acid formation and ammonia production by intestinal micro-organisms. The total concentration of volatile fatty acids in the culture approximated that of the faecal inoculum, with acetic and propionic acids predominating.

(c) Human achlorydric stomach flora. The metabolic activities of the microflora colonizing regions of the gastro-intestinal tract additional to the large intestine may generate important toxic products. One such site is stomach contents of individuals exhibiting hypochlorhydria (reduced secretion of gastric acid), with a resultant increase in gastric pH to values of 6–9. The lack of acid conditions allows a specialized flora to develop which may generate genotoxic agents implicated in the genesis of gastric cancer. Coutts *et al.* (1987) devised a method for maintaining the bacteria obtained from the hypochlorhydric stomach under continuous culture conditions. The total numeric population of the culture remained constant over a period of up to 120 days, although the concentration of the component bacterial strains varied. Nitrate reductase and β-glucosidase activities were present in the culture suggesting that the flora was capable of generating carcinogenic aglycones from plant glycosides, or nitrosamines from nitrate and a suitable amine acceptor. Subsequent investigations demonstrated the formation of detectable amounts of a model nitroso compound (*N*-nitrosproline) by the culture, further evidence for the involvement of microbial enzymes in the initiation of stomach cancer (Coutts, Alldrick and Rowland, 1987; unpublished observations).

5. *Expression of Bacterial Enzyme Data*

Many studies of gut flora metabolism involve the expression of the data for enzyme activity in relation to one or more faecal or caecal parameters, such as wet weight, dry weight, total stool output, total caecal weight, unit number of bacteria. The mode of expression of enzyme activity can influence the conclusions drawn. This subject has been discussed in detail elsewhere (Rowland *et al.*, 1985) but the various advantages and disadvantages are summarized in Table 1.2. For studies *in vivo* using laboratory animals the most appropriate modes of expression of data are in terms of total caecal contents, which gives some idea of the total capacity of the gut flora to metabolize a compound and hence permits assessment of possible toxic consequences of changes in activity, and

     M. E. COATES *et al.*

Table 1.2 *Expression of enzymic data*

Method	Remarks — advantages and disadvantages
1. Specific activity per gram wet weight	Data presented in this way may be influenced by water content and dry matter content (e.g. fibre) of the sample. These variables may make inter-animal comparisons difficult, especially in studies of effects of dietary modification.
2. Specific activity per gram dry weight	Eliminates variation due to differences in water content of sample, but results are still liable to interference from inert non-bacterial material.
3. Specific activity per milligram protein	Protein fraction of colon contents contains both bacterial and host-derived material and so does not accurately reflect the bacterial content of gut. An alternative may be the use of the bacterial cell wall marker diaminopimelic acid.
4. Total activity per caecum	This mode of expression of data provides information of biological and toxicological relevance to the host animal and is unaffected by water content or inert material. This method also takes into account changes in caecal size which are brought about by certain dietary treatments.
5. Activity per unit number of bacteria	Gives indication of whether the overall activity of the individual organisms of the flora is altered by treatment and is unaffected by water or dry matter content of sample. Assumes all bacterial cells possess same ability to catalyse reaction.

secondly in terms of unit number of bacteria which provides information on changes in overall activity of the organisms.

In humans, there is little evidence that the volume of colon contents increases in response to diet or antibiotics as it does in rats and mice. It would appear that under conditions where the bulk of the faeces increases the frequency of defaecation increases correspondingly. Consequently it is inappropriate to calculate enzymic data in terms of total faecal weight. Results are usually expressed as activity per gram wet weight or per milligram dry weight.

C. Studies of Gut Flora Metabolism *in vivo*

1. *Comparison of Oral and Parenteral Dosing*

Differences in rates of metabolism, metabolic products or toxic activity when a compound is administered orally or by another route (intravenous or intraperitoneal) can indicate that intestinal enzymes are involved in the metabolism. This technique has been used to good effect in studies of the metabolism and toxicity of azo dyes. For example tartrazine is reduced to its component amines after oral administration but not when given parenterally (Jones *et al.*, 1964), and Brown FK was toxic to rats only after oral dosing (Grasso and Goldberg, 1968). This technique however is of limited use since it does not distinguish metabolism by bacterial and mammalian enzymes. Furthermore, parenteral dosing does not necessarily bypass the gut since many substrates are secreted into the intestine in the bile and then undergo bacterial metabolism.

2. *Antibiotic Treatment*

Animals lacking a gut microflora can be obtained very conveniently by pretreatment with antibiotics. Although the resultant animal cannot be considered truely gnotobiotic or germ-free, the gut flora may remain suppressed for up to three weeks depending on the antibiotics used, although reported experiments have usually lasted less than a week (Table 1.3). By comparison to gnotobiotic animals therefore only relatively short-term experiments are possible, which are usually adequate for metabolic studies but not for long-term toxicity or carcinogenicity assays. Although some workers have used single antibiotics such as lincomycin or ampicillin, better suppression of the flora can be achieved by mixtures (Table 1.3). It is necessary to start antibiotic treatment a few days before, and maintain it throughout the experimental period since the gut is rapidly recolonized (usually within 24 hours; Gingell *et al.*, 1971) when treatment is discontinued. Even with continuous antibiotic treatment, the gut eventually becomes colonized with yeasts or antibiotic resistant bacteria. The use of sterilized diet and drinking water may delay this material repopulation (Rowland *et al.*, 1980).

It is important to be aware that the antibiotics may themselves influence the metabolism and absorption of xenobiotics for example by reacting with, or binding to, the compound or by interfering with the physiology and metabolic processes of the animal (Remmel *et al.*, 1981).

Table 1.3 *Examples of the use of antibiotic treatments for studying xenobiotic metabolism*

Species	Antibiotic regimen	Duration of experiment	Xenobiotic	Reference
Rat	Lincomycin 500 mg/1 DW[a] days 1–7 + 25 mg twice daily, days 1–4	3 days (days 5–7)[b]	Morphine	Walsh and Levine (1975)
Rat	Neomycin in diet 120–600 mg/kg/day Days 1–10	10 days (days 1–10)	Salicylazosulphapyridine	Peppercorn and Goldman (1975)
Rat	Neomycin 100 mg Bacitracin 50 mg, and Tetracycline 50 mg p.o. twice daily, days 1–4	2 days (days 3–4)	p-nitrobenzoic acid protosil, neoprontosil	Zachariah and Juchau (1974) Gingell *et al.* (1971)
Rat	Neomycin 2 mg, Bacitracin 2 mg, and Streptomycin 2 mg per ml DW, days 1–15	11 days (days 4–15)	Methylmercuric chloride	Rowland *et al.* (1980)
Rat	Neomycin 400 mg/kg, Bacitracin 400 mg/kg, and Tetracycline 200 mg/kg p.o. twice daily, days 1–5	3 days (days 3–5)	Warfarin	Remmel *et al.* (1981)
Mouse	Neomycin 3 mg, Bacitracin 3 mg, and Streptomycin 3 mg p.o. daily, days 1–12	6 days (days 7–12)	Methylmercuric chloride	Rowland *et al.* (1984)

[a] DW is drinking water.
[b] After initial exposure to antibiotics.

Although not often done, it is advisable to culture the faecal samples from antibiotic-treated animals during the experiment to assess the degree of suppression of the flora or to check that the *in vitro* metabolism of the test compound by gut contents has been suppressed by antibiotics.

3. *Use of Gnotobiotic Animals*

A gnotobiotic animal (or gnotobiote) is defined as one in which all the life forms are known. It may be germ-free, i.e. free from any detectable microbial associates, or it may be associated with any number of strains of micro-organism the identity of which are known. The gnotobiote thus presents a useful tool in which to investigate the influence of the indigenous microflora on the host. There are however, problems in interpretation of results, which may be equivocal for two main reasons. The first is the host's response to the presence of a microflora, which leads to significant differences in physiology and metabolism between the germ-free animal and its conventional control. The second concerns the behaviour of microbial strains, which may not function characteristically when introduced into an otherwise germ-free gastro-intestinal tract.

4. *Practical Considerations in Experiments with Gnotobiotic Animals*

It is self-evident that all equipment, diets and other items essential to the experiment, as well as the animals themselves, must be microbiologically sterile. Full details of the production and maintenance of gnotobiotes and their applications in biomedical research are given in *Laboratory Animal Handbook No. 9* (1984). The following paragraphs delineate the more important points that must be taken into account when planning experiments with gnotobiotes or considering the implications of the findings.

(a) Animals. Germ-free rats and mice are readily available from commercial producers; other species usually have to be derived by the user. The conventional counterparts may be supplied from a parallel colony maintained in the open laboratory. Alternatively, animals born germ-free may be taken into the conventional environment at weaning and allowed to acquire a microflora. This system has the advantage that littermates can be distributed between the germ-free and conventional experimental treatments. When the young animals are removed from the

germ-free environment they must be immediately exposed to the microflora peculiar to their species to prevent invasion by opportunist pathogens. For this purpose they may be housed on litter soiled by their conventional counterparts, or gavaged with a suspension of indigenous organisms. The dominant strains rapidly become established, but it may take several weeks for the more fastidious components of the flora to become detectable.

(b) Equipment.   It is customary to maintain gnotobiotes in flexible film isolators which, if thoroughly clean, are readily sterilized with peracetic acid vapour. Metal cages, food hoppers and other equipment that may retain traces of animal excreta are more reliably sterilized by autoclaving. For most purposes positive pressure is maintained within the isolator, the ventilating air being sterilized by passage through filters. If carcinogens or other materials likely to create a hazard to the operator are being used the system can be reversed to operate under negative pressure.

(c) Supplies.   Diets are usually sterilized by autoclaving or gamma radiation, the latter method being on the whole less damaging to their nutrient content. As a precaution vitamin supplements are generally increased to compensate for possible losses during sterilization, as well as for the absence of those vitamins normally contributed by microbial synthesis. Because sterilization procedures may cause more subtle unsuspected changes, the sterilized diet must be fed to the conventional controls as well as to the gnotobiotes.

The method of choice for sterilizing xenobiotics depends on their chemical properties. In many instances the effects of heat or, more particularly, radiation are not precisely known, and it is necessary to test the sterilized and unsterilized material in conventional circumstances to ascertain whether any major change has been incurred during the sterilization process. Aqueous and oily solutions of heat-labile substances can be effectively sterilized by filtration. It is unwise to irradiate aqueous solutions since the generation of active radicals from the water can bring about severe oxidative changes in the solute. Some materials can be irradiated without damage in the dry state and dissolved in sterile water inside the isolator.

(d) Experimental procedures.   Most of the common experimental procedures including anaesthesia, dosing and surgery can be satisfactorily performed within an isolator in spite of some restriction of space and movement. Given some ingenuity and patience to adapt the operation and the operator to isolator conditions there is little or no restriction on the type of experiment that can be conducted on gnotobiotes.

(e) Monitoring for sterility.   The validity of an animal's germ-free status depends on the adequacy of the tests used to detect viable micro-organisms in the system. Since the tests are aimed at proving a negative situation it is impossible to contend with absolute certainty that an animal or an isolator is germ-free. The best that can be claimed is that it is free from any organisms capable of growing under the conditions of the test. Tests for virus contamination have been devised, but for most laboratories they are too elaborate and costly for routine use. Details of recommended tests for monitoring sterility have been published by the National Academy of Sciences (1970).

5.   *The Host's Reactions to the Presence of a Microflora*

The mammalian foetus before birth, or the avian embryo before hatching, is microbiologically sterile and its physiological characteristics are those of a germ-free animal or bird. As the neonate acquires its microflora these characteristics are modified, the greatest changes occurring at the sites of major microbial exposure, notably the gastro-intestinal tract.

(a) Reactions in the gastro-intestinal tract.   The small intestinal wall of the conventional animal is thicker than that of its germ-free counterpart. The extra thickness is contributed in part by a greater proportion of lymphoid elements but mainly by an increase in submucosal tissue. The turnover rate of mucosal cells is faster in the conventional animal, and several groups of workers have explored the possibility that the more mature epicytes in the germ-free intestine accumulate higher concentrations of enzymes such as phosphatases and disaccharidases. The specific activity of mucosal enzymes is usually measured in homogenates of the intestine or of tissue scraped from its internal surface, being expressed as units per milligram of tissue or protein. It has been demonstrated that if this procedure is applied to comparisons between germ-free and conventional animals the values may be biased by the difference in mucosal thickness to give a misleadingly lower value for the conventional gut. For this reason total activity of the whole small intestine has been recommended as a more valid parameter (Siddons and Coates, 1972; Whitt and Savage, 1980).

The most dramatic difference in gut morphology between germ-free and conventional rodents is the development of a grossly enlarged caecum in the germ-free state. The anomaly seems to result from the accumulation of substances that are removed from the lower gut of conventional animals by the microflora. These included mucins, which have strong water-retaining properties, and sundry vaso-active peptides that influence muscle tone and local blood flow. The net result is the retention of fluids in the germ-free caecum which, with its contents, may account for up to 30–40% of the total bodyweight of the animal. This renders invalid any comparison of growth rate between germ-free and conventional rodents, and the administration of drugs according to bodyweight becomes problematic. It also presents a hazard in long-term studies, as it is a major cause of death from intestinal volvulus in ageing animals. Caecal enlargement does not occur in the germ-free chicken or dog, and the former has been the model of choice for growth studies. Microbial metabolism alters the physicochemical characteristics of the gut contents to produce a less positive redox potential and a generally lower pH, which could have important effects on the metabolism and disposition of xenobiotics. For example, it was observed that *N*-nitrosation proceeded more readily in conventional than in germ-free rats, as was to be expected from earlier studies *in vitro* by Klubes *et al.* (1972), which indicated a catalytic role for some intestinal bacteria in the *N*-nitrosation reaction. However, as the pH of the stomach of the conventional animals was significantly more acid, thereby favouring the non-enzymic formation of *N*-nitroso compounds, the authors point out that no direct microbial involvement need have occurred (Ward *et al.*, 1986). In this instance although it is clear that the gut micro-organisms facilitate nitrosamine formation, it remains uncertain whether the effect is a result of direct metabolic action, an indirect consequence of the lowering of pH, or a combination of the two.

(b) Association with specific strains of organisms. When it has been established that the gut microflora is involved in a particular biological phenomenon, identification of the responsible component is usually tackled by introducing different isolates into germ-free animals until one is found to reproduce the phenomenon. However, the results of such experiments must be interpreted with some caution since a single strain introduced into a germ-free gastro-intestinal tract may spread beyond the gut and no longer function as it would in the presence of the whole flora. Misleading results may also arise from monoassociation experiments when a metabolic reaction follows a series of steps each performed by a different organism, such as bile acid metabolism. Alternatively, some types of organism, notably the obligate anaerobes, rely on the presence of others to create the conditions on which their viability depends. For instance *Eubacterium* 21408, which has been shown to reduce Δ^5-sterols *in vitro*, required the presence of *Clostridium* $C1_8$ to decrease the redox potential of the gut before performing this reaction *in vivo* (Eyssen *et al.*, 1972). More complex interactions between strains can be inferred from studies on the microbial reduction of bilirubin to urobilins. The only organism

so far known to effect the transformation is *Clostridium ramosum*. Germ-free rats associated with *Escherichia coli* and *Cl. ramosum* show an increase in urobilin excretion compared to animals monoassociated with *Clostridium* alone, although excretion did not attain the values found in conventional rats. The results suggest that there are other as yet unidentified components of the conventional microflora capable of reducing bilirubin, or alternatively, organisms in addition to *E. coli* are needed to establish conditions in the gut for optimal activity of *Cl. ramosum* (Gustafsson, 1982).

The influence of intestinal colonization by the flora may extend to other organs, since Mizutani and Mitsuoka (1979) showed a differing incidence of liver tumours in gnotobiotic mice associated with strains of human and animal micro-organisms. In this context, gnotobiotes associated with human organisms are potentially valuable experimental models (Hazenberg *et al.*, 1981, 1983; Mallett *et al.*, 1987) but the available data are insufficient to assess how nearly they reproduce the host–microflora relationships in man.

6. *General Comments*

Gnotobiotic animals offer an invaluable means of studying microbial metabolism *in vivo*. The technology of maintaining them is relatively simple, although it demands meticulous care to exclude contamination. The germ-free animal represents a 'pure culture' of the animal *per se*. Its physiological and metabolic reactions provide a base-line for comparison, but it should never be considered as a passive receptacle for a microbial burden. Association with one or more microbial strains sets in motion an intricate series of interactions between the host and the organisms and between the organisms themselves. Thus the results of experiments with gnotobiotes cannot always be taken at their face value, and their more subtle implications frequently need further exploration. Nevertheless research with gnotobiotic animals has proved a fertile field in which to study the interrelationships between the host and its microflora, and its potential value in the fields of toxicology and carcinogenesis is beginning to be exploited.

References

Bickel, M. H., Burkard, B., Meier-Strasser, E. and van der Broek-Boot, M. (1974). Enterobacterial formation of cyclohexylamine in rats ingesting cyclamate. *Xenobiotica* **4**, 425–439.

Brown, J. P. (1977). The role of gut bacterial flora in nutrition and health; a review of recent advances in bacteriological techniques, metabolism and factors affecting flora composition. *Crit. Rev. Fd Sci. Nutr.* **8**, 229–336.

Brown, J. P. and Dietrich, P. S. (1979). Mutagenicity of plant flavonols in the salmonella/mammalian microsome test. Activation of flavonol glycosides by mixed glycosidases from rat cecal bacteria and other sources. *Mut. Res.* **66**, 223–240.

Brown, R. L., Gibson, J. A., Sladen, G. E., Hicks, B. and Dawson, A. M. (1974). Effects of lactulose and other laxatives on ileal and colonic pH as measured by a radiotelemetry device. *Gut* **15**, 999–1004.

Cole, C. B., Fuller, R., Mallet, A. K. and Rowland, I. R. (1985). The influence of the host on expression of intestinal microbial enzyme activities involved in metabolism of foreign compounds. *J. appl. Bacteriol.* **58**, 549–553.

Coutts, T. M., Alldrick, A. J. and Rowland, I. R. (1987). Use of continuous culture to study the gastric microflora of a hypochlorhydric patient. *Toxic. in vitro* **1**, 17–21.

Dobbin, J. F., Saha, J. R., Butler, V. P., Neu, H. C. and Lindenbaum, J. (1983). Digoxin inactivating bacteria: identification in human gut flora. *Science* **220**, 325–327.

van Dokkum, W., de Boer, B. C. J., van Faassen, A., Pikaar, N. A. and Hermus, R. J. J. (1983). Diet, faecal pH and colorectal cancer. *Br. J. Cancer* **48**, 109–110.

Drasar, B. S. (1967). The cultivation of anaerobic intestinal bacteria. *J. Path. Bact.* **94**, 417–427.

Drasar, B. S. and Barrow, P. A. (1985). "Intestinal Microbiology. Aspects of Microbiology 10". American Society for Microbiology, Washington.

Drasar, B. S. and Hill, M. J. (1974). "Human Intestinal Flora". Academic Press, London.

Drasar, B. S., Montgomery, F. and Tomkins, A. M. (1986). Faecal flora in three dietary groups in rural Northern Nigeria. *J. Hyg. Camb.* **96**, 59–65.

Edwards, C. A., Duerden, B. I. and Read, N. W. (1985). Metabolism of mixed human colonic bacteria in a continuous culture mimicking the human cecal contents. *Gastroenterol.* **88**, 1903–1909.

Erikson, H. and Gustaffson, J. A. (1970). Steroids in germfree and conventional rats. Sulpho- and glucuronohydrolase activities of caecal contents from conventional rats. *Eur. J. Biochem.* **13**, 198–202.

Eyssen, H., Piessens-Denef, M. and Parmentier, G. (1972). Role of the cecum in maintaining ∇^5-steroid- and fatty acid-reducing activity of the rat intestinal microflora. *J. Nutrition* **102**, 1501–1511.

Finegold, S. M., Sutter, V. L. and Mathiesen, G. E. (1983). Normal indigenous intestinal flora. *In* "Human Intestinal Microflora in Health and Disease", pp. 3–31, (Ed. D. J. Hentges). Academic Press, New York.

Fernandez, F., Kennedy, H., Hill, M. and Truelove, S. (1985). The effect of diet on the bacterial flora of ileostomy fluid. *Microbiol. Aliment. Nutr.* **3**, 47–52.

Freter, R., Stauffer, E., Cleven, D., Holdeman, L. V. and Moore, W.E. C. (1983a). Continuous-flow cultures as *in vitro* models of the ecology of the large intestinal flora. *Infect. Immun.* **39**, 666–675.

Freter, R., Brickner, H., Botney, M., Cleven, D. and Aranki, A. (1983b). Mechanisms that control bacterial populations in continuous-flow culture models of mouse large intestinal flora. *Infect. Immun.* **39**, 676–685.

Gingell, R., Bridges, J. W. and Williams, R. T. (1971). The role of the gut flora in the metabolism of prontosil and neoprontosil in the rat. *Xenobiotica* **1**, 143–156.

Goddard, P. and Hill, M. J. (1973). The dehydrogenation of the steroid nucleus by human gut bacteria. *Biochem. Soc. Trans.* **1**, 1113–1115.

Goldin, B. R. and Gorbach, S. L. (1976). The relationship between diet and rat faecal bacterial enzymes implicated in colon cancer. *J. Natl Cancer Inst.* **57**, 371–375.

Grasso, P. and Goldberg, L. (1968). Problems confronted and lessons learnt in the safety evaluation of Brown FK. *Fd Cosmet. Toxicol.* **6**, 737–747.

Gustafsson, B. E. (1982). The physiological importance of the colonic microflora. *Scand. J. Gastroenterol. Suppl.* **77**, 117–131.

Hazenberg, M. P., Boom, M., Bakker, M. and Merwe, J. P. (1983). Effects of antibiotics on the human intestinal flora in mice. *Antonie van Leeuwenhoek* **49**, 97–109.

Hazenberg, M. P., Bakker, M. and Verschoor-Burggraaf, A. (1981). Effects of the human intestinal flora on germ-free mice. *J. appl. Bacteriol.* **50**, 95–106.

Holdeman, L. V. and Moore, W. E. C. (1975). "Anaerobe Laboratory Manual". (3rd edn). VPI Laboratory, Blacksburg, Va.

Illing, H. P. A. (1981). Techniques for microfloral and associated metabolic studies in relation to the absorption and enterohepatic circulation of drugs. *Xenobiotica* **11**, 815–830.

Jones, R., Ryan, A. J. and Wright, S. E. (1964). The metabolism and excretion of tartrazine in the rat, rabbit and man. *Fd Cosmet. Toxicol.* **2**, 447–452.

Klubes, P., Cerna, I., Rabinowitz, A. D. and Jondorf, W. -R. (1972). Factors affecting dimethylnitrosamine formation from simple precursors by rat intestinal bacteria. *Fd Cosmet. Toxicol.* **10**, 757–767.

Knoke, M. and Bernhardt, H. (1984). Simulation of intestinal biocenosis in continuous flow culture. *Microecol. Ther.* **14**, 127–135.

Laboratory Animal Handbook No. 9. (1984). "The Germ-free Animal in Biomedical Research" (Eds M. E. Coates and B. E. Gustafsson), Laboratory Animals Ltd., London.

Mallett, A. K., Bearne, C. A. and Rowland, I. R. (1983). Metabolic activity and enzyme induction in rat fecal microflora maintained in continuous culture. *Appl. environ. Microbiol.* **46**, 591–595.

Mallett, A. K., Bearne, C. A. and Rowland, I. R. (1986). The use of continuous flow systems for studying the metabolic activity of the hindgut microflora *in vitro*. *Fd Chem. Toxicol.* **24**, 743–747.

Mallett, A. K., Bearne, C. A., Rowland, I. R., Farthing, M. J. G., Cole, C. B. and Fuller, R. (1987). The use of rats associated with a human faecal flora as a model for studying the effects of diet on the human gut microflora. *J. appl. Bacteriol.* **63**, 39–45.

Mallett, A. K., Rowland, I. R., Bearne, C. A., Purchase, R. and Gangolli, S.D. (1985). Metabolic adaptation of rat faecal microflora to cyclamate *in vitro*. *Fd Chem. Toxicol.* **23**, 1029–1034.

Mason, R. P. and Holtzman, J. L. (1975). The role of catalytic superoxide formation in the O_2 inhibition of nitroreductase. *Biochem. Biophys. Res. Commun.* **67**, 1267.

Miller, T. L. and Wolin, W. J. (1981). Fermentation by the human large intestine microbial community in an *in vitro* semi continuous culture system. *Appl. environ. Microbiol.* **42**, 400–407.

Mitsuoka, T. (1969). An improved method for comprehensive investigation of intestinal flora. *Excerpta Medica Int. Congress Series* No. 213, 422–424.

Mitsuoka, T. (1982). Recent trends in research on intestinal flora. *Bifidobacteria Microflora* **1**, 3–24.

Mitsuoka, T., Ohno, K., Benno, Y., Suzuki, K. and Namba, K. (1976). The fecal flora of man. IV. Communication: comparison of the newly developed method with the old conventional method for the analysis of intestinal flora. *Zbl. Bakt. Hyg. I. Abt. Orig. A.* **234**, 219–233.

Mizutani, T. and Mitsuoka, T. (1979). Effects of intestinal bacteria on the incidence of liver tumors in gnotobiotic C3H/He male mice. *J. Natl Cancer Inst.* **63**, 1365–1370.

National Academy of Sciences (1970). *In* "Gnotobiotes: Standards and Guidelines for the Breeding, Care and Management of Laboratory Animals" pp. 28–39. National Academy of Sciences, Washington, D.C.

Peppercorn, M. A. and Goldman, P. (1975). The role of intestinal bacteria in the metabolism of salicylazosulfapyridine. *J. Pharmacol. Exp. Ther.* **181**, 555–562.

Reddy, B. S., Weisburger, J. H. and Wynder, E. L. (1974). Faecal bacterial B glucuronidase: control by diet. *Science* **183**, 416–417.

Remmel, R. P., Pohl, L. R. and Elmer, G. W. (1981). Influence of the intestinal microflora on the elimination of warfarin in the rat. *Drug. Metab. Disp.* **9**, 410–414.

Renwick, A. G. and Williams, R. T. (1972). The fate of cyclamate in man and other species. *Biochem. J.* **129**, 869–879.

Rowland, I. R., Robinson, R. D. and Doherty, R. A. (1984). Effects of diet on mercury metabolism and excretion in mice given methylmercury: role of gut flora. *Arch. Environ. Hlth.* **39**, 401–408.

Rowland, I. R., Davies, M. J. and Evans, J. G. (1980). Tissue content of mercury in rats given methylmercuric chloride orally: influence of intestinal flora. *Arch. environ. Hlth* **35**, 135–160.

Rowland, I. R., Davies, M. J. and Grasso, P. (1978). Metabolism of methylmercuric chloride by the gasto-intestinal flora of the rat. *Xenobiotica* **8**, 37–43.

Rowland, I. R., Mallett, A. K., Bearne, C. A. and Farthing, M. J. G. (1986). Enzyme activities of the hind gut microflora of laboratory animals and man. *Xenobiotica* **16**, 519–523.

Rowland, I. R., Mallett, A. K. and Wise, A. (1985). The effect of diet on the mammalian gut flora and its metabolic activities. *Crit. Rev. Toxicol.* **16**, 31–103.

Rowland, I. R., Wise, A. and Mallett, A. K. (1983). Metabolic profile of faecal micro-organisms from rats fed indigestable plant cell wall components. *Fd Chem. Toxicol.* **21**, 25–29.

Scheline, R. R. (1968). Metabolism of phenolic acids by the rat intestinal microflora. *Acta Pharmacol. Tox.* **26**, 189–205.

Siddons, R. C. and Coates, M. E. (1972). The influence of the intestinal microflora on disaccharidase activities in the chick. *Br. J. Nutrition* **27**, 101–112.

Sutter, V. L., Citron, D. M. and Finegold, S. M. (1980). Wadsworth Anaerobic Bacteriology Manual (3rd Edn). The C.V. Mosby Company, St. Louis.

Veilleux, B. G. and Rowland, I. R. (1981). Simulation of the rat intestinal ecosytem using a two-stage continuous culture system. *J. Gen. Microbiol.* **123**, 103–115.

Vince, A., Down, P. F., Murison, J., Twig, F. J. and Wrong, O. M. (1976). Generation of ammonia from non-urea sources in a fecal incubation system. *Clin. Sci. Molec. Med.* **51**, 313.

Walsh, C. T. and Levine, R. R. (1975). Studies on the enterohepatic circulation of morphine in the rat. *J. Pharmacol. Exp. Ther.* **195**, 303–310.

Ward, F. W., Coates, M. E. and Walker, R. (1986). Nitrate reduction, gastro-intestinal pH and *N*-nitrosation in gnotobiotic and conventional rats. *Fd Chem. Toxic.* **24**, 17–22.

Whitt, D. D. and Savage, D. C. (1980). Kinetics of changes induced by the indigenous microbiota in the activity levels of alkaline phosphatase and disaccharidases in the small intestinal enterocytes in mice. *Infect. Immunol.* **29**, 144–151.

Zachariah, P. K. and Juchau, M. R. (1974). The role of gut flora in the reduction of aromatic nitro-groups. *Drug Metab. Dispos.* **2**, 74–78.

2

The Bacterial Flora of the Intestine

B. S. DRASAR

A. Introduction

Investigations of the intestinal bacteria have concentrated on studies of the human intestine, although other aspects of gastro-intestinal ecology, particularly the rumen, have not been neglected. Much of the information about the gut bacteria is reviewed and the development of understanding traced in a series of books (Drasar and Hill, 1974; Clarke and Bauchop, 1977; Hentges, 1983; Drasar and Barrow, 1985).

Realization of the importance of the metabolic activities of the flora has been stimulated by studies on malabsorption (Drasar *et al.*, 1966), large bowel cancer (Aries *et al.*, 1969) and drug metabolism. These themes were discussed at a major symposium (Banbury Report, 1981) and in recent books (Hill, 1986a,b). The theme of drug metabolism by intestinal bacteria is a recurrent one and has been reviewed (e.g. Scheline, 1968; Goldman, 1973, 1981; Smith, 1978; Rowland, 1981; Goldin, 1986). However, most of these publications stress the biochemical and toxicological aspects of the problem rather than the bacteriological. This chapter is concerned with the bacteriological aspects of the problem, and presents a comparison of the intestinal floras of man and other animals used in toxicological research.

B. Comparison of the Intestinal Flora of Man and Other Animals

The study of the gut bacteria of man and animals has yielded large amounts of data on the bacteria of individual animal species and elucidated some of the mechanisms that are important in determining the distribution of bacteria in the intestine. However, there are very few studies that compare the bacterial flora present in the intestine of a number of species.

ROLE OF THE GUT FLORA IN TOXICITY AND CANCER
ISBN 0-12-599920-8

As a consequence of this, the relationship of the flora of man to that of other animals, and indeed of the flora of one species of laboratory animal to other animal species, remains uncertain.

The extensive differences that exist between the microfloras of various animal species are in part obscured by the methods used to investigate the problem and by the apparent uniformity imposed on the data as a result of the identification of a limited number of bacterial groups. The major consequence of the cost of such studies is to limit the number of bacterial isolates that can be identified. Thus, many isolates from each sample can be examined or fewer isolates from more samples. This difficulty becomes more apparent if an attempt is made to assign the bacterial strains isolated to particular species. It is conventional to describe the flora in terms of a relatively small number of bacterial genera or groups and to set aside the question of bacterial species.

The numbers of bacteria of a particular group that were present in a sample of intestinal contents are assessed by counting the number of colonies formed when serial dilutions of the sample are inoculated onto or into suitable media. Most of the intestinal bacteria are strict anaerobes so the incubation conditions are of crucial importance. The use of an anaerobic cabinet (Drasar, 1967; Aranki *et al.*, 1969) or pre-reduced anaerobically sterilized media in roll-tubes (Hungate, 1950) has greatly improved our ability to isolate anaerobic bacteria, but many bacterial forms that can be demonstrated microscopically in intestinal contents from several animal species cannot be recognized in culture (Savage, 1977).

The media used in studies of the normal flora have seldom been specifically designed for this purpose. Many are based on those used for the isolation of bacterial pathogens or for the study of the bovine rumen. Furthermore, though there have been major improvements in our ability to identify anaerobic bacteria (Holdeman *et al.*, 1977), many more species remain to be recognized. Indeed it has been estimated that less than 10% of the species in the rodent colon have been described or named (Wilkins, 1981). Thus, in a very real sense the methods that are used in these studies determine the results that are reported.

1. *The Distribution of Bacteria in the Intestine*

The type and distribution of bacteria in the intestine reflects the physiology of the host and the interactions between the bacteria. Many of the data from animal studies were discussed by Savage (1977). The diversity of gut structure and functions and hence of microbial ecologies is illustrated by Morton (1979).

Those studies discussed here were chosen on the basis of (*i*) the animal species examined; particular attention is focused on the studies comparing differing animals and (*ii*) the bacteriological methods used. It will be appreciated that a further problem results from the methods used to obtain gut contents. Animals are usually sacrificed and gut removed. Human intestinal contents have most often been obtained by intubation techniques though operation specimens and guts from road accident victims have been studied. The distribution of bacteria within the gastro-intestinal tract is determined by the animal species, diet, habitat and perhaps geographical location. Some of the more prominent differences between the species are outlined in Fig. 2.1. The apparent simplicity of this diagram conceals other major sources of variation and can at best be regarded as a single 'snapshot' of a series of dynamic systems. It must be noted that the scale has been adjusted to create apparent intestinal equivalence which must result in distortions. The data on man are restricted to studies in North America and Europe. Very different results are obtained in other areas (e.g. Bhat *et al.*, 1972). Major differences in gut bacteria of NCS mice have been related to environment, and such factors have seldom been examined.

To a major extent the factors that control the distribution of the flora in the intestine are unknown. Factors usually cited include gastric acid, coprophagy, local immunity, intestinal motility and diet. However, though

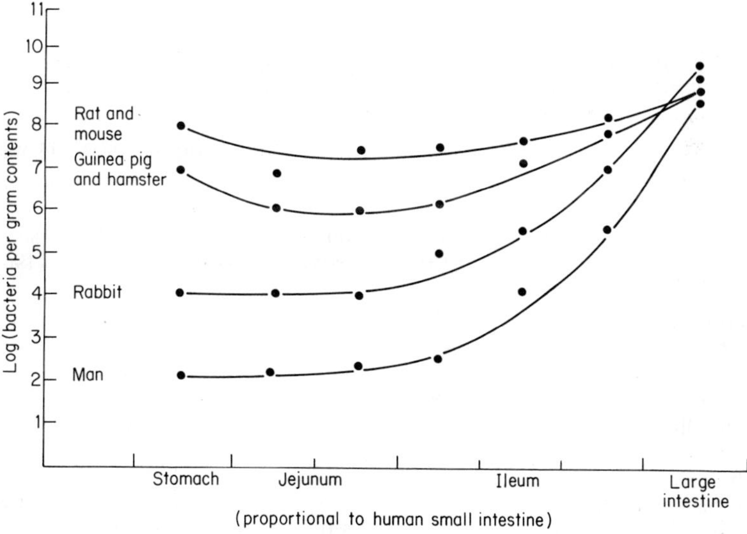

Fig 2.1 The distribution of bacteria in the gastro-intestinal tract of rat, mouse, hamster, man, rabbit and guinea-pig.

general statements may be made, specific analysis of any particular ecological interaction is seldom attempted.

(a) The stomach. The stomach functions as a reservoir that controls the entry of materials into the small intestine. The bacterial content of material entering the small intestine is controlled by antibacterial mechanisms in the stomach. Similarly these same mechanisms alter the bacteriology of stomach contents. The most important of the mechanisms is gastric acid, but differences in acid secretion alone are not adequate to explain the differences in the bacteria isolated from the gastric contents of different species (Tables 2.1 and 2.2). In man changes in gastric acid secretion consequent of gastric surgery, age, disease or anti-secretory drugs may allow colonization of the stomach. Such changes may be of practical importance in terms of an increased susceptibility to gastro-intestinal pathogens and the direct competition between human and bacterial metabolism for nutrients etc. However, such considerations are not important in laboratory animals.

The rabbit seems to be almost as effective as man in reducing the bacterial content of the stomach. Other species of laboratory animals have a high bacterial load in the stomach. The reasons for these differences include coprophagy and diet, which together alter the number of bacteria entering the intestine, but the presence of a permanent self-maintaining flora in the stomach of at least some animals has been established. The most important debate about gastric flora relates to mucosal colonization.

Table 2.1 *Bacterial flora of stomach contents from rat, mouse and hamster (log_{10} bacteria per gram wet weight)*

	Rat		Mouse		Hamster
	Drasar et al. (1970)	Smith (1965)	Drasar et al. (1970)	Smith (1965)	Smith (1965)
Bacteroides	7–9	–	6–7	–	–
Eubacteria	–	–	–	–	–
Peptococcaceae	–	–	–	–	–
Bifidobacteria	7–8	–	7–9	–	–
Lactobacilli	7–9	8.4	8–9	8.4	7.0
Clostridia	2–3	–	–3*	1.7	–
Fusobacteria	–	–	–	–	–
Enterobacteriaceae	3–6	2.0	2–4	2.0	3.3
Streptococci	–	5.0	5–6	6.0	6.5

*Not present in all individuals

Table 2.2 *Bacterial flora of the contents of the stomach from man, rabbit and guinea-pig (log$_{10}$ bacteria per gram wet weight)*

	Man		Rabbit		Guinea-pig	
	Drasar *et al.* (1969)	Mitsuoka (1982)	Drasar *et al.* (1970)	Smith (1965)	Drasar *et al.* (1970)	Smith (1965)
Bacteroides	−3*	−	−6*	4.2	−	−
Eubacteria	−	−	−	−	−	−
Peptococcaceae	−	−	−	−	−	−
Bifidobacteria	−	−	−6*	−	4–6	−
Lactobacilli	−2	−4*	−	−	2–4	7.6
Clostridia	−	−	−	−	−4*	−
Fusobacteria	−	−	−	−	−	−
Enterobacteriaceae	−2*	−	−	−	−2*	−
Streptococci	−5*	−3*	−	−	−	5.0

*Not present in all individuals

The stomach of mice, rats and some other animals has both secreting and non-secreting regions. The mucosa of the non-secreting portion of the stomach is colonized by specific bacteria, often lactobacilli (Savage, 1977), and this flora is maintained independently of the bacterial load in the gastric contents. It is uncertain to what extent such a mucosally associated flora can be found in all species, but even in man some such flora could exist.

(b) The small intestine. The distribution of the bacteria in the small intestine reflects the numbers of bacteria entering from the stomach and the cleansing mechanisms of the small intestine, principally motility. Those animals that have low bacterial loads in the stomach have low bacterial numbers in the proximal small intestine (Tables 2.3 and 2.4). The differences are less in the distal small intestine (Tables 2.5 and 2.6), presumably reflecting the slower rate of transit in these areas and perhaps some bacterial multiplication.

Our understanding of the bacterial flora of the small intestine is complicated by the microscopic observation of a mucosal flora in rodents and the microscopic observation of many more bacteria than can be cultured in the intestinal content from man. The significance of these findings is unknown.

Only intestinal motility is well established as a control mechanism in the small intestine. Bile acids, lysozyme, digestive enzymes and local immunity may also play a role, but this would seem to be in determining

Table 2.3 *Bacterial flora of contents of the proximal small intestine in rat, mouse and hamster (log$_{10}$ bacteria per gram wet weight)*

	Rat		Mouse		Hamster
	Drasar et al. (1970)	Smith (1965)	Drasar et al. (1970)	Smith (1965)	Smith (1965)
Bacteroides	5–6	–	5–8	–	–
Eubacteria	–	–	–	–	–
Peptococcaceae	–	–	–	–	–
Bifidobacteria	5–7	–	6–8	–	–
Lactobacilli	6–7	7.0	7–8	6.3	6.5
Clostridia	–	–	2–3	–	–
Fusobacteria	–	–	–	–	–
Enterobacteriaceae	3–5	–	3–6	1.7	–
Streptococci	4–5	3.0	3–4	5.0	4.5

Table 2.4 *Bacterial flora of the contents of the proximal small intestine of man, rabbit and guinea-pig (log$_{10}$ bacteria per gram wet weight)*

	Man		Rabbit		Guinea-pig	
	Drasar et al. (1969)	Mitsuoka (1982)	Drasar et al. (1970)	Smith (1965)	Drasar et al. (1970)	Smith (1965)
Bacteroides	–3*	–	–5*	3.8	–	–
Eubacteria	–	–	–	–	–	–
Peptococcaceae	–	–	–	–	–	–
Bifidobacteria	–	–	–5*	–	4–5	–
Lactobacilli	–	–2*	–	–	2–5	6.7
Clostridia	–	–	–	–	–3	–
Fusobacteria	–2*	–	–	–	–	–
Enterobacteriaceae	–4*	–2*	–	–	–	–
Streptococci	–6*	–3*	–	–	–2	4.0

*Not present in all individuals

which bacteria survive in the gut, rather than in controlling those able to do so.

(c) The large intestine and faeces. In man the major problem related to studies of the large intestine is that of obtaining samples. Animal studies have concentrated on the flora of the caecum while human studies relate

Table 2.5 *Bacterial flora of contents of the distal small intestine in rat, mouse and hamster (log_{10} bacteria per gram wet weight)*

	Rat		Mouse		Hamster
	Drasar *et al.* (1970)	Smith (1965)	Drasar *et al.* (1970)	Smith (1965)	Smith (1965)
Bacteroides	6–8	–	6–7	–	–
Eubacteria	–	–	–	–	–
Peptococcaceae	–	–	–	–	–
Bifidobacteria	6–8	–	7–8	–	–
Lactobacilli	6–7	8.0	7–8	8.0	6.6
Clostridia	–	–	2–3	–	–
Fusobacteria	–	–	–	–	–
Enterobacteriaceae	3–5	4.5	3–6	4.0	2.0
Streptococci	2–6	5.0	4–7	6.7	5.8

Table 2.6 *Bacterial flora of the contents of the distal small intestine of man, rabbit and guinea-pig (log_{10} bacteria per gram wet weight)*

	Man		Rabbit		Guinea-pig	
	Drasar *et al.* (1969)	Mitsuoka (1982)	Drasar *et al.* (1970)	Smith (1965)	Drasar *et al.* (1970)	Smith (1965)
Bacteroides	5–7	2.5	4–7	6.7	–6	–
Eubacteria	–	5	–	–	–	–
Peptococcaceae	–	–	–	–	–	–
Bifidobacteria	5–7	7	5–7	–	4–6	–
Lactobacilli	3–6	7	–	–	2–3	8.7
Clostridia	–	–	2–4	–	2–4	–
Fusobacteria	–	–				
Enterobacteriaceae	3–4	3	–2*	–	3–5	–
Streptococci	–	6	–2*	–	–	5.9

*Not present in all individuals

to operation specimens such as excised appendices (Tables 2.7 and 2.8).

The large intestine is the most heavily colonized region of the intestine. The major metabolic impacts of the flora in normal animals must result from its activities. Bacteria–bacteria interactions are the most important factors controlling the flora. Attempts have been made to explain the composition and activities of the flora in terms of a continuous culture

Table 2.7 *Bacterial flora of contents of the large intestine from rat, mouse and hamster (log$_{10}$ bacteria per gram wet weight)*

	Rat		Mouse		Hamster	
	Drasar *et al.* (1970)	Smith (1965)	Drasar *et al.* (1970)	Smith (1965)	Smith (1965)	Lusk *et al.* (1978)
Bacteroides	7–9	8.2	9–10	9.4	7.8	8.4
Eubacteria	–	–	–	–	–	–
Peptococcaceae	–	–	–	–	–	–
Bifidobacteria	8–9	–	8–9	–	–	–
Lactobacilli	8–9	8.4	8–9	8.8	7.9	–
Clostridia	–6*	2.0	–3*	–	–	6.8
Fusobacteria	–	–	–	–	–	–
Enterobacteriaceae	5–7	5.2	4–6	5.4	2.4	5.0
Streptococci	5–7	6.0	6.8	6.0	7.8	3.1

*Not present in all individuals

Table 2.8 *Bacterial flora of contents of the large intestine from man, rabbit and guinea-pig (log$_{10}$ bacteria per gram wet weight)*

	Man		Rabbit		Guinea-pig	
	Seeliger and Werner (1962)	Gorbach *et al.* (1967)	Drasar *et al.* (1970)	Smith (1965)	Drasar *et al.* (1970)	Smith (1965)
Bacteroides	8.5*	7.9	8–9	8.5	6–8	7.8
Eubacteria	–	–	–	–	–	–
Peptococcaceae	–	–	–	–	–	–
Bifidobacteria	6.6	5.2	4–5	–	8–9	–
Lactobacilli	6.4	2.8	–	–	3–4	9.0
Clostridia	–	–	–4	–	2–3	–
Fusobacteria	8.3*	–	–	–	–	–
Enterobacteriaceae	6.9	6.2	–	–	–	–
Streptococci	7.0	2.6	–3	4.0	–	6.5

*Not present in all individuals

fermenter (Freter *et al.*, 1983). Provided that these concepts are adapted to include aspects of bacteria–mucosa and bacteria–bacteria adhesion an adequate theoretical treatment can be developed. Metabolic inhibitors produced by the flora, such as volatile fatty acids and H$_2$S, are also significant ecological determinants. Intestinal immunity may play a role in modulating bacteria–mucosa interactions.

Table 2.9 *Bacterial flora of faeces from rat, mouse and hamster ($\log_{10}$ bacteria per gram wet weight)*

	Rat			Mouse			Hamster		
	Drasar *et al.* (1970)	Smith (1965)	Mitsuoka (1982)	Drasar *et al.* (1970)	Smith (1965)	Mitsuoka (1982)	Smith (1965)	Mitsuoka (1982)	Lusk *et al.* (1978)
Bacteroides	7–9	8.4	9.9	8–10	9.4	10.5	7.9	9.9	8.4
Eubacteria	–	–	9.5	–	–	9.1	–	–	–
Peptococcaceae	–	–	9.3	–	–	8.9*	–	9.7	9.9
Bifidobacteria	8–9	–	8.2	8–9	–	7.1*	–	9.0	–
Lactobacilli	8–9	8.6	9.6	8–9	9.0	9.5	8.0	9.7	–
Clostridia	6*	1.7	2.1*	3*	1.7	8.6*	–	–	6.8
Fusobacteria	–	–	9.2	–	–	9.8	–	9.6	–
Enterobacteriaceae	5–7	5.6	5.3	4–6	6.0	4.7	1.7	6.3	5.0
Streptococci	5–7	6.2	8.2	6–8	6.2	5.6	7.0	5.1	3.1

*Not present in all individuals

Unabsorbed food residues play an important role, acting as culture media components in the continuous culture analogy. This may explain why xenobiotics are metabolized by the flora. These chemicals may be regarded as providing new or extending existing ecological niches, thus providing bacteria able to undertake their metabolism with a selective advantage.

Faeces may be regarded as the spent culture medium of the large gut fermenter. It has been studied because it is readily available and provides a source material for the major groups of intestinal bacteria (Tables 2.9, 2.10 and 2.11). The composition of the bacterial flora of faeces resembles that of the large gut and it is assumed that freshly passed faeces can be considered as representative of the large gut flora.

Table 2.10 *Bacterial flora of faeces from rabbits and guinea-pigs (log$_{10}$ bacteria per gram wet weight)*

	Rabbit			Guinea-pig		
	Drasar *et al.* (1970)	Smith (1965)	Mitsuoka (1982)	Drasar *et al.* (1970)	Smith (1965)	Mitsuoka (1982)
Bacteroides	7–9	8.7	9.6	7–9	7.6	8.5
Eubacteria	–	–	5.6	–	–	8.1
Peptococcaceae	–	–	8.3	–	–	9.1
Bifidobacteria	7–9	–	7.8*	8–9	–	8.8
Lactobacilli	3	–	–	3–4	8.8	8.2
Clostridia	–3*	–	2.3*	–3*	–	–
Fusobacteria	–	–	–	–	–	–
Enterobacteriaceae	–3*	–	3.5*	–2*	–	6.4
Streptococci	2–4	4.7	3.6*	–4*	6.0	6.9

*Not present in all individuals

2. *The Intestinal Bacteria*

For many years it was generally accepted that the intestine harboured a very limited range of bacteria. Prominent among these were *Escherichia coli*, *Streptococcus faecalis* and *Clostridium perfringens*. Studies on the faecal flora of man have revealed that these organisms are seldom of

Table 2.11 *Bacterial flora of human faeces as described by various investigators*

| | Log$_{10}$ bacteria per gram wet weight | | Log$_{10}$ bacteria per gram dry weight | | |
	Drasar *et al.* (1976)	Mitsuoka (1982)	Finegold *et al.* (1975)	Moore and Holdeman (1974)	Reddy *et al.* (1975)
Bacteroides	10.2	10.9	11.0	11.0	11.0
Eubacteria	9.5	–	10.1*	11.0	10.8
Peptococcaceae	10.0*	10.2	10.9*	10.6	10.6
Bifidobacteria	10.0	10.0	9.5*	10.7	10.9
Lactobacilli	4.1*	5.8*	6–10*	10.0	5.4
Clostridia	6.0	9.5*	9.5	9.5	–
Fusobacteria	–	–	5.5*	10.6	–
Enterobacteriaceae	7.1	7.8	9.5	9.5	8.4
Streptococci	8.0	7.9	8.5	6.7	7.0

*Not present in all individuals

major importance. It is estimated the human intestine contains some 400–500 species of bacteria. It is likely that the intestines of other animals harbour similar numbers of species. At present it is not known if the same bacterial species are present in all animal species but it is likely that each animal species has a corresponding group of bacteria. Even if the same species are present it is likely that the strains associated with a particular animal species will be unique to that species. Table 2.12 lists those bacterial species that have been isolated from the intestine.

When faced with the complexity of the gut bacteria it is useful to note that several groups must be considered as represented.

(*i*) Contaminants or transient organisms from the environment.
(*ii*) Indigenous bacteria, i.e. bacteria that have colonized the individuals under investigation. These may include bacterial species normal in the study group but not present in all members of the species.
(*iii*) The autochthenous flora: this group of organisms may be considered as having undergone parallel evolution with the host and to represent the true intestinal organisms.

In the context of the current discussion all groups may prove to be important. Thus administration of xenobiotics may allow transient organisms to colonize more permanently and alter the metabolic activity or ecological status of indigenous or autochthenous organisms.

Table 2.12 *Some of the bacterial species isolated from the intestine. From the data of Drasar and Hill (1974), Moore and Holdeman (1974), Holdeman and Moore (1974), Holdeman* et al. *(1976), Finegold et al. (1975, 1977, 1983).*

Bacteroides
Bacteroides amytophilus

Bacteroides assacharolyticus
Bacteroides capillosus
Bacteroides coagulans
Bacteroides distasonis
Bacteroides eggerthii
Bacteroides fragilis
Bacteroides hypermegas

Bacteroides melaninogenicus
s.s. melaninogenicus

Bacteroides multiacidus
Bacteroides oralis
Bacteroides ovatus

Bacteroides pneumonsintes

Bacteroides praeacutus
Bacteroides putredinis
Bacteroides ruminicola
s.s. brevis
Bacteroides rumunicola
s.s. ruminicola
Bacteroides splanchinicus

Bacteroides succinogenes

Bacteroides thetaiotaomicron
Bacteroides uniformis

Bacteroides ureolyticus

Bacteroides vulgatus

Eubacteria

Eubacterium aerofaciens
Eubacterium alactolyticum
Eubacterium biforme
Eubacterium budayi
Eubacterium cellulosolvens
Eubacterium combesii
Eubacterium contortum
Eubacterium cylindroides

Eubacterium dolichum

Eubacterium eligens
Eubacterium formicigenerans

Eubacterium hallii
Eubacterium lentum
Eubacterium limosum

Eubacterium moniliforme
Eubacterium multiforme
Eubacterium nitritogenes
Eubacterium ramulus

Eubacterium rectale
Eubacterium ruminantium

Eubacterium saburream
Eubacterium siraeum

Eubacterium tenue
Eubacterium tortuosum
Eubacterium ventriosum

Peptococcaceae

Peptococcus asaccharolyticus
Peptococcus magnus
Peptococcus prevotii

Peptococcus saccharolyticus
Peptococcus variabilis
Peptostreptococcus anaerobius
Peptostreptococcus micros
Peptostreptococcus parvulus

Peptostreptococcus productus
Ruminococcus albus
Ruminococcus bromii
Ruminococcus flavefaciens

Ruminococcus lactaris
Ruminococcus obeum
Ruminococcus torques

Sarcina ventriculi

Other anaerobic cocci

Acidaminococcus fermentans

Coprococcus cutactus
Coprococcus catus
Coprococcus comes
Gemiger formicilis

Megasphera elsdenii

Table 2.12   *(Continued)*

Streptococcus constallatus

Streptococcus hansenii

Streptococcus intermedius
Streptococcus morbillorium
Veillonella parvula

Bifidobacteria

Bifidobacterium adolescentis
Bifidobacterium angulatum
Bifidobacterium bifidum
Bifidobacterium breve
Bifidobacterium catenulatum
Bifidobacterium cornutum
Bifidobacterium dentium

Bifidobacterium eriksonii

Bifidobacterium infantis
Bifidobacterium longum
Bifidobacterium pseudolongum

Other Gram positive anaerobic rods

Actinomyces naeslundii
Actinomyces odontolyticus

Arachnia propionica
Lachnospira multiporus
Propionobacterium acnes
Propionobacterium avidum
Propionobacterium granulosum
Propionobacterium jensenii

Lactobacillus

Lactobacillus acidophilus
Lactobacillus brevis
Lactobacillus buchneri
Lactobacillus casei
Lactobacillus catenaforme
Lactobacillus crispatus
Lactobacillus fermentum
Lactobacillus helveticus
Lactobacillus lactis
Lactobacillus leichmannii
Lactobacillus minutus
Lactobacillus planareum

Lactobacillus rogosae
Lactobacillus ruminis
Lactobacillus salivarius

Clostridia

Clostridium acetobutylicum
Clostridium aminovalericum
Clostridium aurantibutyricum
Clostridium barati
Clostridium barkeri
Clostridium bejerinkii
Clostridium bifermentans
Clostridium butyricum
Clostridium cadaveris
Clostridium canis
Clostridium celartum
Clostridium cellobioparum
Clostridium chauvoei
Clostridium clostridiiforme
Clostridium cochlearium
Clostridium difficile
Clostridium fallax
Clostridium felsineum
Clostridium ghoni
Clostridium glycolicum
Clostridium haemolyticum
Clostridium indolis
Clostridium innocum
Clostridium irregularis
Clostridium lentoputrescens
Clostridium limosum
Clostridium leptum
Clostridium malenominatum
Clostridium mangenoti
Clostridium nexile
Clostridium oceanicum
Clostridium oroticum
Clostridium paraputrificum
Clostridium pasteurianum
Clostridium perfringens
Clostridium plagarum
Clostridium pseudotetanicum
Clostridium putrefaciens "B"
Clostridium ramosum
Clostridium sartagoformum

Cont'd

Table 2.12 *(Continued)*

Clostridium septicum
Clostridium sordellii
Clostridium sphenoides
Clostridium sporosphaeroides
Clostridium subterminale
Clostridium tertium

Fusobacteria

Fusobacterium gonidiaformans
Fusobacterium mortiferum
Fusobacterium naviforme
Fusobacterium necrogenes
Fusobacterium necrophorum
Fusobacterium nucleatum
Fusobacterium plauti
Fusobacterium prausnitzii
Fusobacterium russi
Fusobacterium symbiosum
Fusobacterium varium

Other Gram negative anaerobic rods

Butyrivibrio fibrisolvens
Desulfotomaculum nigrificans
Desulfotomaculum ruminis
Desulfotomaculum orientis
Desulfomonas pigra

Leptotrichia buccalis
Oscillospira guillermondii
Selenomonas ruminatium
Sucinimonas amylolytica
Succinivibrio dextrinosolvens
Vibrio succinogenes

Enterobacteriaceae

Citrobacter freundii
Enterobacter aerogenes
Enterobacter cloacae
Enterobacter liquefaciens

Escherichia coli
Klebsiella pneumoniae
Proteus mirabilis
Proteus morganii
Proteus vulgaris
Providencia rettgeri

Streptococcus

Streptococcus faecalis
Streptococcus faecium
Streptococcus bovis
Streptococcus agalactiae
Streptococcus anginosus
Streptococcus avium
Streptococcus cremoris
Streptococcus equisimilius
Streptococcus lactis
Streptococcus mitior
Streptococcus mutans
Streptococcus salivarius
Streptococcus sangis
Streptococcus equinus
Streptococcus durans

Other bacteria

Aerococcus viridans
Aeromonas hydrophila
Alkaligines faecalis
Bacillus cereus
Bacillus subtilis
Corynebacterium species
Micrococcus species
Nocardia species
Pediococcus species
Pseudomonas aeruginosa
Pseudomonas species
Staphylococcus aureus
Staphylococcus albus

References

Aranki, A., Syed, S. A. Kenney, E. B. and Freter, R. (1969). Isolation of anaerobic bacteria from human gingiva and mouse caecum by means of a simplified glove box procedure. *Appl. Micro.* **17**, 568–576.
Aries, V., Crowther, J. S., Drasar, B. S., Hill, M. J. and Williams, R. E. O.

(1969). Bacteria and the aetiology of cancer of the large bowel. *Gut* **10**, 334–335.

Banbury Report (1981). "Banbury Report 7, Gastrointestinal Cancer: Endogenous Factors." Cold Spring Harbor Laboratory, Cold Spring Harbor.

Bhat, P., Shantakumari, S., Rajan, D., Mathan, V. I., Kapadia, C. R., Swamabi, C. and Baker, S. J. (1972). Bacterial flora of the gastrointestinal tract in south Indian control subjects and patients with Tropical Sprue. *Gastroenterol,* **62**, 11.

Clarke, R. T. J. and Bauchop, T. (1977). "Microbial Ecology of the Gut." Academic Press, London, New York.

Drasar, B. S. (1967). Cultivation of anaerobic intestinal bacteria. *J. Path. Bact.* **94**, 417–427.

Drasar, B. S. and Barrow, P. A. (1985). "Intestinal Microecology." Van Nostrand Reinhold, Wokingham.

Drasar, B. S. and Hill, M. J. (1974). "Human Intestinal Flora." Academic Press, London.

Drasar, B. S., Hill, M. J. and Shiner, M. (1966). The deconjugation of bile salts by human intestinal bacteria. *Lancet* **i**, 1237–1238.

Drasar, B. S., Hill, M. J. and Williams, R. E. O. (1970). The significance of the gut flora in safety testing of food additives. *In*: "Metabolic Aspects of Food Safety", pp. 245–260. Blackwell Scientific Publishers, Oxford.

Drasar, B. S., Shiner, M. and McLeod, G. M. (1969). The bacterial flora of the gastrointestinal tract in healthy and achlorhydric persons. *Gastroenterol.* **56**, 71–79.

Finegold, S. M., Flora, D. J., Attebery, H. R. and Sutter, L. V. (1975). Faecal bacteriology of colonic polyp patients and control patients. *Cancer Res.* **35**, 3407–3417.

Finegold, S. M., Sutter, V. L. Sugihara, P. T., Edler, H. A., Lehmann, S. M. and Phillips, R. L. (1977). Faecal flora of Seventh Day Adventist populations and control subjects. *Amer. J. Clin. Nutr.* **30**, 1718–1792.

Finegold, S. M., Sutter, V. L. and Mathisen, G. E. (1983). Normal and indigenous intestinal flora. *In*: "Human Intestinal Microflora in Health and Disease", (ed. D. J. Hentges), pp. 3–31. Academic Press, New York.

Freter, R., Stauffer, E., Cleven, D., Holdeman, L. V. and Moore, W. E. C. (1983). Continuous-flow cultures as *in vitro* models of the ecology of the large intestinal flora. *Infection Immunity* **39**, 666–675.

Goldin, B. R. (1986). *In situ* bacterial metabolism and colon mutagens. *Ann. Rev. Microbiol.* **40**, 367–393.

Goldman, P. (1973). Therapeutic implications of the intestinal microflora. *New England J. Med.* **289**, 623–628.

Goldman, P. (1981). The metabolism of xenobiotics by the intestinal flora. *In*: "Banbury Report 7", pp. 25–39. Cold Spring Harbor Laboratory, Cold Spring Harbor, NY.

Gorbach, S. L., Plaut, A. G., Nahas, L. Weinstein, L., Spanknebel, G. and Levitan, R. (1967). Studies of intestinal microflora II. Microorganisms of the small intestine and their relations to oral and faecal flora. *Gastroenterol.* **53**, 856–867.

Hentges, D. J. (1983). "Human Intestinal Microflora in Health and Disease." Academic Press, New York.

Hill, M. J. (1986a). "Microbial Metabolism in the Digestive Tract." CRC Press, Boca Raton.

Hill, M. J. (1986b). "Microbes and Human Carcinogenesis." Arnold, London.

Holdeman, L. V. Cato, E. P. and Moore, W. E. C. (1977). "Anaerobe Laboratory Manual" (4th edn). VPI and SU, Blacksburg.

Holdeman, L. V., Good, I. J. and Moore, W. E. C. (1976). Human faecal flora: variation in bacterial composition within individuals and a possible effect of emotional stress. *Appl. environ. Microbiol.* **31**(3), 359–375.

Holdeman, L. V. and Moore, W. E. C. (1974). New genus, *Coprococcus* twelve new species, and amended descriptions of four previously described species of bacteria from human faeces. *Int. J. Syst. Bact.* **24**, 260–277.

Hungate, R. E. (1950). The anaerobic mesophilic cellulolytic bacteria. *Bacteriol. Rev.* **14**, 1.

Lusk, R. H., Fekety, R., Silva, J., Browne, R. A., Ringler, D. H. and Abrams, G. D. (1978). Clindamycin induced enterocolitis in hamsters. *J. Infect. Dis.* **137**, 464–475.

Mitsuoka, T. (1982). Recent trends in research on intestinal flora. *Bifidobacteria Microflora* **3**, 3–24.

Moore, W. E. C. and Holdeman, L. V. (1974). Human faecal flora: the normal flora of Japanese-Hawaiians. *Appl. Microbiol.* **27**, 961.

Morton, J. (1979). "Guts." Arnold, London.

Reddy, B. S., Weisburger, J. H. and Wynder, E. L. (1975). Effect of high risk and low risk diets for colon carcinogenesis of faecal microflora and steroids of man. *J. Nutr.* **105**, 878–884.

Rowland, I. (1981). The influence of gut microflora on food toxicity *Proc. Nutr. Soc.* **40**, 67–74.

Savage, D. C. (1977). Microbial ecology of the gastrointestinal tract. *Ann. Rev. Microbiol.* **31**, 107–133.

Scheline, R. R. (1968). Drug metabolism by intestinal micro-organisms. *J. Pharmaceut. Sci.* **57**, 2021–2037.

Seeliger, H. P. R. and Werner, H. (1963). Recherches quantitives et qualitatives sur la flore intestinale de l'homme. *Ann. Instit. Pasteur* **105**, 911–936.

Smith, H. W. (1965). Observations on the flora of the alimentary tract of animals and factors affecting its composition. *J. Path. and Bact.* **89**, 95–122.

Smith, R. V. (1978). Metabolism of drugs and other foreign compounds by intestinal micro-organisms. *World Rev. Nutr. Diet* **29**, 60–76.

Wilkins, T. D. (1981). Microbiological considerations in interpretation of data obtained from experimental animals. *In*: "Banbury Report 7", pp. 3–9. Cold Spring Harbor Laboratory, Cold Spring Harbor, NY.

3

Alimentary Tract Physiology: Interactions between the Host and its Microbial Flora

JAMES B. HENEGHAN

A. Introduction

Even though the normal function or physiology of the alimentary tract is subtly altered by its intimate association with the microbial flora, the combined metabolic effects of the gut mucosa and flora on enteric toxins or xenobiotics are significant. The highest populations of resident microbes found in mammals normally occur at each end of the alimentary tract, in the mouth and colon; the other populations range from very few organisms in the stomach to very high in the lower ileum. Thus, elaborate mechanisms have evolved to safeguard the integrity of these host–parasite relationships. In general, most clinicians and microbiologists have centred their attention on intestinal bacteria which are associated with disease. On the other hand, micro-organisms which are useful and helpful in maintaining normal mammalian life and homeostasis have not been the subjects of extensive scientific study. Work with germ-free animals has shown that within their protected environment, the gastro-intestinal tract functions reasonably well and can maintain normal growth and reproduction in a wide variety of animals. However, the total absence of bacteria or the reduction of the usual bacterial communities found in the gastro-intestinal tract are, like smoking, considered hazardous to your health. These host–microbial interrelationships are difficult to investigate and little is known about them. Several recent reviews have discussed the germ-free animal in the study of gastro-intestinal function and disease (Coates and Gustafsson, 1984); nutrient absorption in gnotobiotic animals (Bruckner and Szabo, 1984); the gastro-intestinal microflora in mammalian nutrition (Savage, 1986); and the physiological interactions between the whole bacterial population and the epithelium of the small and large intestines (Gustafsson, 1982). In view of these complexities and the lack of experimental evidence, it is not surprising that our knowledge of the effects of the microbial flora in toxicology and cancer is very limited. The present review attempts to shed some light on, and possibly stimulate some controversy in, the interactions between the mammalian gastro-intestinal tract and its resident microflora in relation to gastro-intestinal cancer and the metabolism and toxicology of xenobiotics. The first step is a brief summary of the effects of the microbial flora on the structure and function of the alimentary tract. Secondly, the parallel phenomena acting within the host to maintain normal alimentary tract function are discussed with special emphasis on the role of intestinal secretion. Then three specific areas of active current research — endocrine function, mucus, and pancreatic enzymes — are considered in detail. Finally, the practicality of these efforts and the directions for future research are summarized.

B. Complexity of the Microbial Ecology

At each level of the intestine, the microbial ecology has demonstrated cross-sectional variations (Gorbach, 1975; Savage, 1977). The microbes that may reside in the lumen and on the surface of food particles or residue may differ from those at the mucosal interface. Along the epithelial surfaces, the tips of villi may provide a different environment from the crypts, and a series of different microhabitats probably exists. Gustafsson and Maunsbach (1971) demonstrated that the crypts of Lieberkuhn harbour bacteria at various distinct levels or depths in pure cultures. On the other hand, the number of strains of bacteria in the plaque-like mucus on the surface is somewhat higher. Within the small intestine are many factors that contribute to the microbial ecology (Heneghan, 1973). The microbial challenge to the mucosal surfaces of the alimentary tract, therefore, varies in both location and time, and, thus, the normal morphology and function of the alimentary tract are influenced by these variations.

C. Alimentary Tract Physiology

Alimentary tract physiology is influenced by a complex interplay between the physiological action and reactions along the entire length of the gastro-intestinal tract, as modified by the metabolic activity of the resident, and possibly transient, microflora. Table 3.1 summarizes these interactions at various sites along the tract, with emphasis on the host's contributions. Quantities mentioned are in the normal range for man.

Table 3.1 *Host – flora interactions on xenobiotics and toxins*

Site	Actions	
	Host	Flora
Oral cavity	Dilution by salivary secretion, 1.5 *l*/day Digestion by α-amylase, ptyalin Absorption limited, 0.2 l/day	Minimal metabolic activity
Stomach	Dilution by gastric juice, 2.0 l/day Hydrolysis by HC1 Absorption if fat soluble Proteolytic and lipolytic enzymes present but not efficient	Possible metabolism by oral and/or ingested flora Little or no metabolism few resident flora
Small intestine Upper 1/3	Dilution by secretions, pancreatic, bile, Brunner's glands, 3.5 l/day Dilution by shed enterocytes, 250 g/day Extensive digestion by amylo-, proteo- and lipo-lytic enzymes Rapid absorption of luminal contents tends to maintain isotonicity Vast absorption of H_2O, 8.5 l/day	Little or no metabolism few resident flora Possible metabolism by oral and/or ingested flora
Middle 1/3	Absorption slightly less than upper 1/3, but can absorb what escapes upper 1/3	Normally low microbial flora but can be increased in pathological states
Lower 1/3	Absorption slightly less than middle 1/3, but can absorb what escapes middle 1/3 Vitamin B–12 absorption Reabsorption of bile salts	Increased resident flora almost 'colon-like' Deconjugation bile salts Initial metabolism of unabsorbed xenobiotics
Appendix or caecum	Limited function as a lymphoid organ	Possible extensive metabolism Post-absorptive fermentation
Large intestine	Active Na^+ absorption Absorption of H_2O, 0.5 l/day	Site of most active flora metabolism of xenobiotics Short-chain fatty acids promote mucosal growth

The luminal membranes of the enterocytes contain glycoprotein enzymes that are involved in digestion (disaccharidases, peptidases, etc.). The activities of these enzymes are a function of the position of the enterocytes on the villi; cells nearest the extrusion zones at the villus tips have higher activities than those at the crypts. The activities develop as the cells migrate from the crypts, where they are formed, to the villus tips, where extrusion takes place.

Secretion and reabsorption to form an entero–entero recirculation has been described recently (Schultz, 1984). In this process, substances secreted at the crypts or lower part of the villus are reabsorbed at the villus tips, and thus may form an entero–entero recirculation loop (see Fig. 3.1). This is similar to the familiar entero–hepatic recirculation of the bile acids and steroids (Fig. 3.2). In both of these loops, the circulating substances are conserved, lowering the metabolic work load of the host, and may serve the metabolic needs of the enteric bacteria, ensuring their survival. Thus, both entities, the host and its resident microbial flora, benefit.

D. The Fate of Luminal Nutrients

Diet, dysfunction, and disease, by altering appetite and food intake, influence the nutrient and bulk supply to the alimentary tract. Changes of motility, intestinal flora, bile and pancreatic secretions, enzymatic breakdown of nutrients, and the absorption of nutrient-hydrolysis products alter the production and loss of mucosal cells at the crypts and villus tip extrusion zones respectively. The absorbed nutrients affect (*i*) intestinal blood and lymph flows, (*ii*) the endocrine, paracrine and neural control of the alimentary tract by different local effects or through mediation via the hypothalmus, and (*iii*) the differentiation of enterocytes as they progress up the villi. Each of these phenomena, in turn, can decrease or increase enterocyte numbers and even their degree of maturation. The new mucosal cell population will have a changed absorptive–secretory capacity that may be measured and quantified on a per cell or on an organ basis. The focus here is on the absorption and secretion of ions and fluid by the small intestine, the net balance between these opposing forces leading to elimination by excretion.

Ingested food in man is primarily digested by acid hydrolysis or enzymatic cleavage by proteases, by lipases and by saccharidases found in the small intestine which is poorly populated by bacteria (Bentley *et al.*, 1972). In contrast in the ruminant, very dense microbial populations reside in the pre-gastric and post-gastric fermentation chambers and

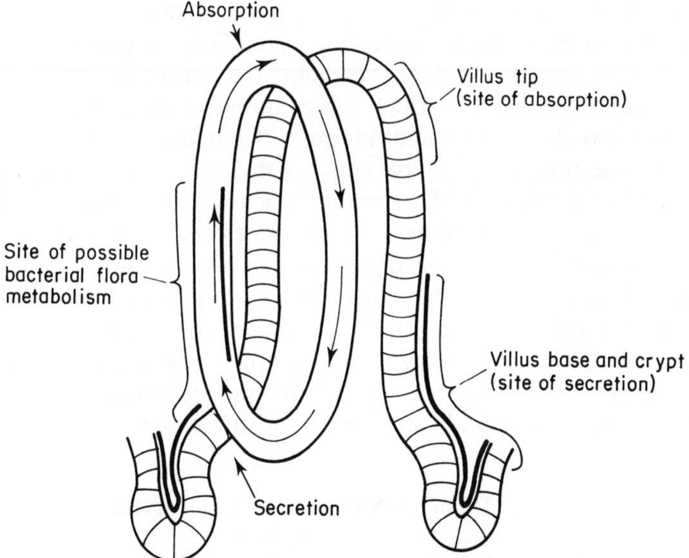

Fig 3.1 A diagram of entero–entero circulation.

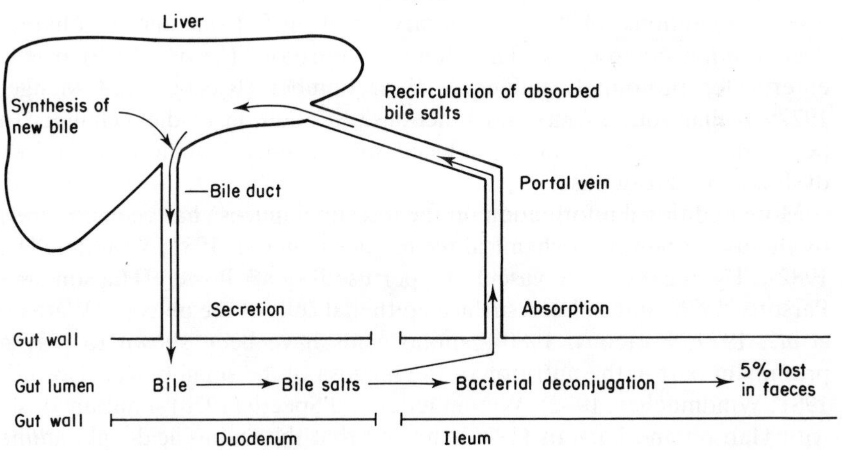

Fig 3.2 A diagram of entero–hepatic circulation.

organs in which bacteria, not endogenous host enzymes, degrade oligosaccharides, oligopeptides, and fibre. Grouping these two distinct fermentative organs together has helped to promote the study of the physiological mechanisms which are common to the rumen and colon in mammals (Wolin, 1981) and in man (Cummings, 1981). Differences between the rumen and colon exist in their epithelial linings (squamo-cuboidal in the rumen and columnar, mucus-producing in the colon) and in their bacterial populations (cellulose digesters and numerous protozoa in the rumen, hemi-cellulose digesters, and fewer protozoa in the colon). Despite these differences there are striking similarities: both organs absorb sodium at a high rate, secrete bicarbonate, and absorb the short-chain fatty acids (SCFA) produced by bacteria. This absorption of SCFA provides nutrients which can support the metabolic needs of the mucosal epithelial cells lining both the rumen and the colon.

E. Luminal Nutrition of Enterocytes

Enterocytes, the functional cells of the alimentary tract, are in a dynamic state, constantly being shed and renewed by mitosis; this concept of population dynamics has been reviewed by two recent symposia on intestinal adaptation (Robinson *et al.*, 1982; Polak *et al.*, 1982). The enterocytes, moreover, are unique in that they have two sources of nutrition. Not only do enterocytes, like other cells, obtain their nutriments from the interstitial fluid via the blood but they also, during digestion, receive a considerable supply from the normal food intake, the protein-aceous secretions of the alimentary tract and from the exfoliated, degenerating enterocytes. This 'luminal nutrition' (Levin, 1969) of the enterocytes profoundly influences their number (Riecken and Menge, 1977; Williamson, 1978a) and functions. In addition to diet, changes in population dynamics can be induced by the microbial flora and/or by dysfunction and disease.

More additional information on the intestinal mucosa has been obtained by the use of newer biochemical techniques (Evered, 1981; Windmueller, 1982). By means of a vascularly perfused small bowel (Hanson and Parsons, 1976) and isolated surface epithelial cells of the mucosa (Watford *et al.*, 1979; Porteous, 1980), amino acids have been shown to play a prominent part in the nutrition of the mucosa of the small bowel (Evered, 1981; Windmueller, 1982). Windmueller and Spaeth (1978) simultaneously with Hanson and Parsons (1978) showed that the amino acids, glutamine and aspartate, accounted for well over 70% of the CO_2 production of respiration and that during states of fasting these amino acids and ketone bodies were the preferred metabolic fuels for the small bowel mucosa. Oxidation of glucose and unesterified fatty acids constitute less than 10%

of the total oxidative fuels for the mucosa of fed animals. Further experiments revealed that in a contest between luminal and vascular metabolic substrates 45% of the total mucosal metabolism was derived from luminal nutrients such as glutamine, glutamate, and aspartate (Windmueller and Spaeth, 1980). In summary, the products of enzymatic digestion, in the main amino acids, support the metabolic welfare of the small intestinal mucosa, and half of the total support is derived from luminal contents.

In the fermentative organs, the products of bacterial fermentation nourish the colonic mucosa. Evidence to support this concept comes from experiments performed *in vitro* with mucosal sheets and colonocytes. Henning and Hird (1972) and McNeil *et al.* (1978) have shown that bacterial SCFA are absorbed in the colon along a concentration gradient from lumen to serosa without evidence of active transport. When these same bacterial SCFA are used in conjunction with those nutrients of value to the small intestinal mucosa, several points emerge. Amino acids, while of some importance in the proximal colon, become less important as a metabolic fuel in the distal colon (Roediger, 1980, 1982). In their place, SCFA ascend in utility and contribute mostly to the production of CO_2 by the mucosa. Disregarding regional differences along the length of the colon, epithelial cells prepared from the entire length of the colon reveal a preference of metabolic fuels in the following order: SCFA, ketone bodies, amino acids and glucose (Roediger, 1982). These conclusions are obtained from fed animals with luminal nutrients continually available. It appears that 70% of the energy supply is derived from bacterial fermentation products. Bacteria in the colon play a far greater role in nutrition of the mucosa from the lumen than do amino acids from the lumen in the small intestine. Thus, the dependence on luminal contents for nourishment of the mucosal epithelium is greatest in the distal gastro-intestinal tract.

The utility of bacterial SCFA for nutrition of the small intestine has been studied. SCFA do not stimulate oxygen consumption (Watford *et al.*, 1979; Porteous, 1980) of enterocytes as glutamine does, but SCFA are nevertheless oxidized. The extent to which bacterial SCFA can sustain the small intestinal mucosa metabolically has not yet been determined.

F. Physiological Effects of the Flora

1. *Morphology*

(a) The germ-free gut. The normal structure and morphology of the gastro-intestinal tract in germ-free animals are altered in ways that emphasize the importance of an animal's interaction with its indigenous

microbial flora in establishing its defences against microbial invasion while, at the same time, maintaining adequate host nutrition by normal alimentary tract function (Heneghan, 1965). In germ-free rodents the caecum is greatly enlarged and fails to develop its normal musculature and is filled with liquid contents (Gordon and Pesti, 1971); however, this does not happen in non-rodent species such as the germ-free chicken (Coates, 1973) and the germ-free dog (Heneghan *et al.*, 1971). The overall mass of the small intestine in each germ-free species, however, is decreased, and its surface area is smaller, whereas the villi of the small intestine are unusually uniform in shape and slender, with crypts, which are shorter and less populated with cells than in their respective conventional control animals (Gordon and Bruckner-Kardoss, 1961; Meslin *et al.*, 1973, 1974). The lamina propria is much thinner in germ-free animals, with a reduction in total cellularity (Abrams *et al*, 1963). The number of lymphocytes, plasma cells, and intraepithelial lymphocytes are all profoundly reduced (Crabbe *et al.*, 1970). The Peyer's patches of germ-free animals are smaller and do not show the development of germinal centres as do conventional animals (Crabbe *et al.*, 1970). The epithelial cell turnover rate in germ-free mice (Abrams *et al.*, 1963) and germ-free chickens (Rolls *et al.*, 1978) has been found to be approximately one-half that of their respective conventional controls. However, the villus/crypt cell ratio is always higher in germ-free mice, rats, chickens, pigs, and dogs than in their conventional counterparts, which indicates that less proliferating tissue is required to keep the germ-free mucosa intact (Heneghan, 1979). In general, manual stereological morphometric techniques have tended to confirm these morphological trends (Heneghan *et al.*, 1979).

(b) Bacteria and colonic mucosal cell growth. The size of the colon varies markedly in different species (Stevens, 1977). Carnivores have relatively small colons, while herbivores require large colons to ferment otherwise indigestible vegetable products. An important study from the Mayo Clinic (Stephen *et al.*, 1983) used ileal intubation and aspiration to measure the quantity of carbohydrate entering the colon of normal subjects after ingestion of meals containing 20 to 60 g of starch. From 5 to 10% of the ingested starch escaped small bowel absorption and ended up in the colon. Since subjects ingest several hundred grams of starch each day, large quantities of starch must reach the colon. These studies support the concept that large quantities of carbohydrate in the lumen support the turnover and growth of the colonic bacteria (Smith and Bryant, 1979).

The view has frequently been supported that bacteria stimulate cell growth in the colon to provide better protection against bacterial invasion. Whether bacteria through their physical presence or as a result of the fermentative products alone stimulate mucosal cell growth has recently become clear and should be discussed.

Control of mucosal growth and control of intestinal adaptation are mediated by various mechanisms, most of which have been reviewed recently (Williamson, 1978b; Johnson, 1979). Nutrition is one of these mechanisms. Over 27 years ago, Sander and colleagues (1959) showed that infusion of bacterial fatty acid in the rumen caused marked development of the ruminal mucosa while infusions of glucose and saline did not produce such an effect. These observations on mucosal growth have been confirmed in other ruminants such as sheep (Sakata and Tamate, 1978).

In the colon, cell renewal is markedly depressed by fasting (Hagemann and Stragand, 1977), elemental diets (Janne *et al.*, 1977), and interruption of the faecal stream either by colostomies (Terpstra *et al.*, 1981) or ligation (Stragand and Hagemann, 1977). The mechanisms involved are unclear but Stragand and Hagemann (1977) showed that physical exposure to luminal contents is needed to initiate colonic cell hyperplasia following induction of mucosal atrophy by deviation of the faecal stream. Many factors, for instance short-chain fatty acids, ammonia, and amines, are removed in a colon defunctioned by ligation or colostomy. Only fatty acids on their own have been tested for their effect on mucosal cell turnover. A mixture of bacterial fatty acids markedly stimulate the mitotic index in the defunctioned colon (Sakata *et al.*, 1980; Sakata and von Engelhardt, 1983), whereas control infusions with saline do not. While confirmation is needed the results indicate that the metabolic products of bacteria, rather than bacteria themselves, moderate cell proliferation. Hyperplasia of the colonic mucosa seen after surgical closure of colostomies (Terpstra *et al.*, 1981) is very likely related to the re-exposure to bacterial fatty acids. The hyperplasia of the colonic mucosal cells may possibly be linked to the pronounced effect n-butyrate has on nucleic acid metabolism in general (Kruh, 1982).

2. *Motility and Blood Flow*

In evaluating the influence of the microbial flora on total alimentary tract function, the effects of intestinal motility, peristalsis, and the rate of intestinal transit must be considered. Increased motor activity of alimentary tract smooth muscle usually represents a compromise between the host's requirements to mix the chyme as well as propel it posteriorly.

Colonic motility is designed to mix luminal contents with very slow forward propulsion to permit absorption of the bulk of the water and electrolytes entering the colon. In healthy persons, the colonic contents move toward the anus at a mean rate of only about 1 cm h^{-1} (Ritchie, 1968). A little studied, but possibly important, aspect of colonic motor activity is a functional 'sphincter' at the rectosigmoid area which slows forward progression of faecal matter. Decreased activity of this physiological valve may lead to diarrhoea, while hyperactivity could yield constipation.

The control of the colonic vasculature was reviewed by Anderson (1984). The colon does not autoregulate its blood flow as well as the remainder of the gut (Hanson and Johnson, 1967), i.e., no fall in colonic vascular resistance to maintain blood flow. As a result, when blood flow decrease, increased O_2 extraction tends to maintain O_2 uptake. Colonic blood flow responds to luminal contents, as exemplified by a marked increase in blood flow when free fatty acids are infused into the colonic lumen (Kvietys and Granger, 1981). Parasympathetic stimulation (non-vagal) enhances while sympathetic stimuli decrease colonic blood flow (Hullen, 1970). A variety of hormones influence colonic blood flow, for example vasoactive intestinal polypeptide (VIP) is a very potent mediator of colonic vasodilation (Eklund *et al.*, 1979).

Abrams and Bishop (1967) reported a slower intestinal transit in germ-free mice, and Gustafsson and Norman (1969) found a similar reduction in germ-free rats, although transit was modified by the composition of the diet. Using the non-absorbable marker, polyethylene glycol, Heneghan and Mittelbronn (1981) showed a somewhat slower intestinal transit in germ-free dogs and in intact germ-free rats. After caecectomy, however, intestinal transit was slightly faster in the germ-free rats than in caecectomized conventional rats. Since caecectomy also reduced the large variability in the timing of test meal appearance in the faeces, the enlarged caecum in germ-free rats represented a highly variable trap for a test meal, sometimes trapping large quantities and at other times small amounts. Proper interpretation of results based upon faecal appearance becomes very difficult, if not impossible.

3. *Secretion: Magnitude and Variety*

A variety of stimuli can convert the colon from an absorptive to a secretory organ, including bacterial toxins, bile acids, fatty acids, laxatives, and hormones, VIP and anti-diuretic hormone (ADH). Many of these stimuli increase the permeability of the colonic mucosa as well.

Cyclic AMP activity is thought to be important in colonic secretion. In the human colon, VIP is the most potent stimulator of cyclic AMP formation (Dupont *et al.*, 1980). Boige and co-workers (1984) carried out a number of studies indicating that α-adrenergic agents are potent inhibitors of VIP-induced cyclic AMP production. Thus, theoretically, these agents might be useful in the clinical management of various secretory diarrhoeal states.

Aldosterone enhances sodium transport out of the renal tubule and the colonic lumen. However, the kidney has several types of receptors for aldosterone, while the colon has just a single, high affinity receptor (Rafestin-Oblin *et al.*, 1984).

The net amount of fluid and ions absorbed relates to the amounts secreted by the small intestine. Such secretion is thought to arise mainly from the crypt regions and is influenced not only by nervous, paracrine, and hormonal control but also by luminal factors such as bacterial toxins and bile (Moon, 1980; Makhlouf, 1974). Alterations in any of these factors can lead to pathophysiological changes in the intestinal absorption and secretion of water and electrolytes. Ignored for many years, the secretory mechanisms of the intestine have become the subjects of intensive investigation (Field *et al.*, 1980).

4. *Absorption*

Absorption is influenced not only by gastric and intestinal motility but also by the functional state of the enterocytes and the ability of the blood and lymph to clear transferred substances from their contraluminal membrane. Gastric motility controls the amount of nutrients delivered to the small intestine for hydrolysis and absorption. Small intestinal motility affects the efficiency of absorption because it mixes and moves the luminal contents, preventing the development of localized high concentrations of hydrolysis products. The propulsive motility controls the residence or contact time that the mucosa has with the luminal contents and thereby can increase or reduce the ability of the intestine to absorb efficiently. The fibre content of the diet, acting as a bulking agent, plays a role in absorption because it can speed the passage of bowel contents and thus reduce absorption. The small intestine becomes less efficient as the fibre content of the diet increases (Southgate and Durnin, 1970).

Although colectomized humans may have normal longevity, the abnormal loss of water and electrolytes from an ileostomy could endanger life if dietary sodium were not plentiful (Clarke *et al.*, 1967). The normal colon has the ability to absorb about 5.0 l of isotonic sodium over a 24 hour period, while larger quantities entering the colon lead to diarrhoea (Debongnie and Phillips, 1978). Most fluid and electrolyte absorption from the colon depends on active sodium transport from the lumen against steep electrochemical gradients (Schultz *et al.*, 1977). This electrolyte transport seems to be dependent on the action of Na^+K^+-ATPase (Ferreira and Smith, 1968), which can be modified by mineralocorticoids that enhance sodium uptake (Levitan and Ingelfinger, 1965).

Potassium may be either absorbed or secreted by the colon, depending on the blood to lumen gradient (Salas-Coll *et al.*, 1976). The colon also rapidly absorbs free fatty acids produced during bacterial fermentation of carbohydrates (Ruppin *et al.*, 1980), thus conserving calories and reducing the osmotic load that would otherwise cause diarrhoea. In the absence of bacterial fermentation germ-free animals exhibit enlarged caeca filled with liquid contents plus very loose stools (Gustafsson and Norin, 1977). Also the colon appears to have smaller 'pores' than the small intestine and is thus less permeable to most non-electrolytes (Stevens, 1977). This may be important since a variety of bacterial toxins and xenobiotics normally reside in the colon.

(a) Absorption in germ-free intestine.   Absorptive capacity of the germ-free small intestine for *d*-xylose has been evaluated *in vitro* with isolated everted intestinal sacs and *in vivo* by intestinal perfusion and by disappearance of a test meal, by Heneghan (1963), who reported a twofold increase in *d*-xylose absorption in germ-free mice and rats. The rates of active sodium and glucose absorption were the same as in conventional animals. Scharrer and Riedel (1972) found no differences between germ-free and conventional rats in the uptake of oleic acid or of L-leucine from isolated small intestinal sacs (Riedel *et al.*, 1972). On the other hand, Tennant *et al.* (1971), who used a Cori experiment and determined absorption by the radioactivity remaining in each section of the alimentary tract after 6 hours, observed no differences in *d*-xylose or in oleic acid absorption between germ-free and conventional rats (Tennant *et al.*, 1968). The absorption of glucose (Coates *et al.*, 1981) and methionine (Yokota and Coates, 1982) were studied *in vivo* with both perfusion and loop techniques, and the absorption of each substance was similar in germ-free and conventional chicks, when calculated per unit length of intestine. Also, the methionine stayed in the gut wall of the germ-free birds much longer than in the conventional animals, even though the conventional intestinal wall is thicker (Yokota, 1981). However, free amino acid concentration in the caecum is 10 to 30 times higher in

germ-free than in conventional rats (Combe *et al.*, 1970). Combe *et al.* (1976) have published an excellent review of host/alimentary-tract-flora relationships in the digestion and absorption of fats, carbohydrates, proteins and minerals. Thus, while active transport seems unaffected by the presence or absence of a microbial flora, passive absorption tends to be increased in the germ-free state (Laroche *et al.*, 1964).

(b) Microbial overgrowth.   Abnormal small bowel function has been observed in a number of conditions characterized by excessive proliferation of luminal bacteria. Surgical blind-loops, strictures, enteroenterostomies, fistulas and diverticula involving the small intestine may all be associated with macrocytic anaemia and steatorrhoea. While it is generally agreed that bacteria contribute to the vitamin B-12 deficiency that causes the anaemia, the influence of folic acid deficiencies cannot be overlooked. However, the mechanisms by which the bacteria interfere with B-12 absorption are unclear. Gianella *et al.* (1972) have shown that bacteria can successfully compete with intrinsic factor for B-12 and that B-12 bound to bacteria can be removed by intrinsic factor. Arnold *et al.* (1974) and Evrard *et al.* (1965) have shown that germ-free rats with blind-loops do not exhibit steatorrhoea, but subsequent establishment of a 'normal' intestinal flora did result in 60–80% excretion of ingested fats. More recently, Heneghan and Mittelbronn (1981) demonstrated that vitamin B-12 absorption was similar in germ-free and conventional rats with or without caecectomy. However, vitamin B-12 absorption was increased in germ-free and monocontaminated dogs (60% absorption of test meal) compared with that in conventional animals (8% absorption of test meal). Further investigation is necessary to pinpoint the reasons for this species difference. Clearly, we have only begun to investigate the influence of the microbial flora on intestinal absorption.

(c) Sodium absorption in the colon.   Short-chain fatty acids (SCFA) stimulate sodium absorption in the colon of animals and man (Cummings, 1981; Roediger and Moore, 1981) by mechanisms which are dependent on mere diffusion of fatty acids through the mucosa along a concentration gradient. Oxidative respiration has been invoked as an explanation for stimulation of sodium absorption by SCFA in the colonic mucosa, but the proximal colon absorbs more sodium than the distal colon (Rechkemmer and von Engelhardt, 1983), when in fact bacterial fatty acids make a greater contribution to mucosal metabolism in the distal colon (Roediger, 1980). This suggests that mechanisms other than oxidative respiration, for example enzyme induction, may play a part in stimulation of sodium absorption. Irrespective of mechanisms, absence of bacterial

fatty acids leads to net luminal appearance of sodium (Roediger and Rae, 1982). Reintroduction of SCFA in the colon redresses the imbalance and restores the colonic mucosa to a resorptive state. Thus, fatty acids appear to have a trophic effect on the colonic mucosa not unlike in other fermentative organs, such as the rumen where withdrawal of SCFA severely restricts the functional capacity of the ruminal mucosa (Hecker, 1974). A trophic change due to SCFA may possibly explain the diarrhoea that occurs after closure of colostomy where the atrophied and defunctioned colon is incapable of absorbing a substantial water load (Tilson *et al.*, 1976). The above observations clearly point to a strong interdependence between luminal bacteria of the fermentative organs and their mucosal lining.

The action of SCFA on the colonic mucosa has been summarized in Table 3.2 and indicates the wide range of effects that these simple chemical substances can exert on the epithelium of the colon.

5. *Functional Relation Between Bacteria and Colonic Mucosa*

In order to maintain adequate production of SCFA for mucosal nutrition, the pH and pO_2, the degree of anaerobiosis, have to remain within narrow physiological ranges. Control of each is poorly understood but both conditions involve interaction between the colonic mucosa and bacterial population. Some interacting factors are listed in Table 3.3 and reviewed further.

(a) Maintenance of luminal pH. Luminal pH depends upon the production rate of SCFA by bacteria and the luminal appearance of bicarbonate which maintains the luminal pH at 7.4 with little variation (Wrong *et al.*, 1981). Bicarbonate is secreted at a high rate into the colon and controlled by carbonic anhydrase found in large quantities in the non-mucus surface epithelial cells of the colonic mucosa (Spicer *et al.*, 1982). Apart from maintaining luminal pH, bicarbonate also controls cellular pH through a process of bicarbonate exchange for luminal chloride anions and anions of bacterial fatty acids (butyrate and acetate). Lawson *et al.* (1983) have shown that luminal appearance of bicarbonate was raised when the rectal mucosa was exposed to sodium butyrate in dialysis bags. Bicarbonate appearance elevated the juxto-mucosal pH from 7.40 to 7.64, reflecting an interaction between bacterial metabolites and mucosa in health. In disease such as *E. coli* and colitis, exotoxins acting upon the colonic mucosa markedly stimulate bicarbonate secretion (Argenzio and Whipp, 1981). In this case, another bacterial product rather than the organism itself acts to induce metabolic changes in the colonic mucosa.

Table 3.2 *Known or suspected effects of bacterial fatty acids on the functions of the colonic epithelium*

Activity	Response	Source
Mitochondrial respiration	Endogenous respiration replaced by fatty acid oxidation	Roediger (1982)
Mitochondrial enzyme activity (HMG-CoA synthetase)	Likely stimulated	
DNA content	Likely stimulated	Terpstra *et al.* (1981)
Nucleic acid acylation	Enhanced	Kruh (1982)
Cell mitosis rate	Increased	Sakata *et al.* (1980, 1983)
Membrane enzyme activity (alkaline phosphatase)	Likely increased	
Microsomal enzyme activity	Likely increased	
Cytosol acylation	Unknown	

Table 3.3 *Interrelationships between the colonic mucosa and the colonic bacteria*

Mucosal metabolic products which benefit bacteria	Bacterial metabolic products which benefit mucosal cells
O_2	Short-chain fatty acids (SCFA): acetate, propionate, butyrate
Urea	NH_3
NO_3^-	NO_2^-
Lactate	Amines and other nitrogenous substances
K^+	
HCO_3^-	

(b) Regulation of anaerobiosis. The pO_2 on the luminal surface of the colonic mucosa ranges between 85 and 100 mm of mercury when measured by equilibration across dialysis membranes closely applied to the mucosa. The pO_2 in the centre of bacteria is less than 5 mm of mercury, and correspondingly the pCO_2 is much higher. Several poorly understood factors contribute to this extreme anaerobiosis. The mucosal interactions involved in this control are twofold: lactate production and availability of nitrate and nitrite.

Lactate produced in large quantities by the colonic mucosa (Roediger and Moore, 1981) diffuses into the lumen where it becomes available for metabolism by facultative anaerobes, especially to SCFA. It is possible that mucosally associated organisms are more likely to be lactate fermentors which assist in lactate removal and in turn production of fatty acids for mucosal nutrition. This metabolic shuttle aids in the maintenance of an anaerobic environment as some oxygen is removed in the process.

In aerobic respiration, hydrogen is passed via the cytochrome system to the terminal electron acceptor, which is oxygen. In anaerobic respiration bacteria use inorganic ions such as nitrate, nitrite, sulphate, and sulphite as an alternative to oxygen as a terminal electron acceptor. Micro-organisms which have the enzymes to reduce nitrate are mainly *Escherichia coli* and Pseudomonadaceae. The interdependence between nitrate, mucosa and bacteria is demonstrated by the fact that the colon extracts ingested nitrite. By using isotopically labelled nitrite, ingested or inhaled nitrite appears in the colonic lumen either as labelled ammonia or as labelled glutamate, no doubt due to nitrite which enters the colonic lumen directly from the circulation through the colonic mucosa (Witter *et al.*, 1979; Thayer *et al.*, 1982). Furthermore, large quantities of nitrite may enter the colon from the ileum. Measurements from ileostomies of ulcerative colitis patients indicate that levels of nitrite can be as high as 9.0 mM (Tannenbaum *et al.*, 1978), yet the appearance of nitrite in stool is very low. If nitrite is incubated in stool under anaerobic conditions almost all nitrite is reduced and appears as ammonia (Archer *et al.*, 1981). Thus, circulating and ingested nitrite contribute towards respiration of anaerobic bacteria thereby assisting in the maintenance of bacterial flora.

The action of nitrite anions traversing the colonic mucosa has not been studied before, but Roediger (1986) has recently shown that colonocytes are not endangered by nitrite (10 mM). Quite the opposite, nitrites up to 20 mM concentration stimulate oxidation of bacterial fatty acids, the major oxidative fuel for the colonic mucosa. Elsewhere such concentrations of nitrite are generally held to be detrimental to tissues. Other nitrogenous substances such as ammonia and methylamine, derived from nitrate and produced by bacteria, do not have a stimulatory effect on mucosal oxidation of fat. These observations suggest that anaerobic respiration of the colonic bacteria and aerobic respiration of the colonic mucosa are interrelated, and that nitrites may be mutually beneficial and not harmful, as previously believed.

(c) Dietary fibre. In the present world of nutrition (heavily populated by amateur, self-appointed experts), the marvellous effects of a high-fibre diet on a variety of diseases are considered to be a self-evident fact. In

reality, data from controlled studies to support the value of fibre are extremely scarce. The subject of fibre is further complicated by the heterogenicity of the raw material. Several well-performed studies on the influence of fibre on colonic function have been published recently (van Dokkum *et al.*, 1983; van Soest, 1984; Fleming *et al.*, 1983). These studies showed that ingestion of appreciable coarse fibre will increase the weight and frequency of stools. However, the physical and chemical form of the fibre is important. Finely ground fibre is much less effective than is the chemically identical, coarse fibre (van Dokkum *et al.*, 1983; van Soest, 1984). Fibres that are only minimally fermented (cellulose or corn bran) increase faecal weight to a greater extent than readily fermentable fibre (xylan and pectin). The latter are associated with high flatus output (Fleming *et al.*, 1983).

(d) Gas production.   Methane gas (CH_4) is an excretory product of man that is derived solely from the metabolism of a group of colonic organisms. There are wide individual variations in methane excretion, with some individuals consistently excreting large quantities of CH_4 (producers) and others excreting little or no CH_4 (non-producers) (Levitt and Ingelfinger, 1968). Spanish investigators studied the prevalence of CH_4 production in control subjects and patients with carcinoma of the colon (Pique *et al.*, 1984). The prevalence of CH_4 was much higher (91%) in patients with colon cancer than in controls (42%). Resection of the cancer reduced the prevalence of CH_4 production to 47%, while patients with unresectable tumours continued to have a high prevalence of CH_4 production. The authors postulate that the existence of the tumour may have influenced CH_4 production. CH_4 production also was investigated in patients with vascular disease (McKay *et al.*, 1983). Patients with aorto-iliac disease had a higher prevalence of CH_4 production (83%) than did control subjects or patients with femoro-popliteal disease (35%), and the authors conclude that gut ischaemia may enhance the proliferation of CH_4-producing bacteria, which are strict anaerobes.

(e) Colon cancer.   Two major hypotheses regarding the aetiology of colorectal cancer are that (*i*) long-chain fatty acids present in dietary fat, or endogenous bile acids, are converted to carcinogens or cocarcinogens by the action of gut bacteria (Hill, 1978); and (*ii*) a high-fibre diet dilutes and accelerates material through the gut, thereby reducing both the amount of time bowel flora have to produce carcinogens and the amount of time these carcinogens have to act on the bowel mucosa (Burkitt, 1971). The theory that a high-fibre diet is important in preventing cancers is based on somewhat inconsistent epidemiologic observations comparing

different countries and cultures. To look at this question more directly, a case-control study was done comparing bowel habits of people with colorectal cancer to their spouses and to hospitalized controls (Nakamura *et al.*, 1984). In a retrospective analysis comparing 100 persons in each group, no significant differences were found in the historical frequency of bowel movements, presence of constipation, or use of laxatives between cases and controls. The authors concluded that these data provide no support for the hypothesis that slow transit time increases the incidence of bowel cancer. This study does not, however, deal with the theory that the diluent effect of stool bulk may be an important protective factor, since the number of bowel movements does not necessarily reflect the bulk of stool passed.

Another case-control study performed in Greece studied the role of diet on the incidence of colorectal cancer in a population characterized by ethnic homogeneity, but substantial heterogeneity with respect to dietary habits (Manousos *et al.*, 1983). The series consisted of 100 patients with colorectal cancer and age- and sex-matched controls. Cancer patients reported significantly less frequent consumption of vegetables and, independently, more frequent consumption of meat, especially lamb and beef. Between the two extremes (high-vegetable, low-meat diet vs. high-meat, low-vegetable diet) a risk ratio of about eight appears to exist, which is of sufficient size and direction to explain a substantial part of the international variation in the incidence of colon cancer.

In a similar dietary study performed in 542 patients with colorectal cancer in Toronto, the major risk factor for colon cancer was saturated fat (Miller *et al.*, 1983). There was no demonstrated protective effect of dietary fibre. There was only a minor protective effect in females for cruciferous vegetables. For rectal cancer, a significant effect of saturated fat was only found for females in the highest consumption category. There was no protective effect for vegetable or dietary fibre.

The relationship between the intake of dietary fat and the subsequent development of colorectal cancer during a 15-year follow-up was investigated in 7074 men of Japanese ancestry living in Hawaii (Stemmermann *et al.*, 1984). Data on fat intake were obtained by 24-hour recall records at baseline examination. A significant negative association was found between colon cancer and the intake of saturated fat, whether assessed on the basis of grams per day or as a percentage of the caloric intake. The strongest negative relationship was found in cancer of the right colon.

Both epidemiologic and experimental evidence have implicated bile acids as an aetiological factor in the development and growth of colon cancer (Hill and Aries, 1971). High levels of dietary fat and high levels of faecal steroids, in particular bile acids, have been considered important, although the exact nature of this involvement was unclear (Reddy *et al.*, 1976).

6. *Alteration by Antibiotics*

Numerous human clinical situations have been observed where germ-free-like conditions exist or develop as the result of treatment of disease, as illustrated in the following examples. (1) Immune deficient human babies, brought up under germ-free conditions for protection from lethal infectious diseases, present some of the metabolic conditions found in germ-free rats (Kellogg, 1973). Several germ-free animal characteristics, such as absence of coprostanol formation (Gustafsson and Werner, 1968) are also encountered in children during the first year of life. (2) Endogenous trypsin and elastase showed sharply increased faecal levels in normal persons treated with antibiotics (Borgstrom *et al.*, 1977). When male conventional rats were fed by stomach tube for five days with either benzyl-penicillin, neomycin, erythromycin, ampicillin, tetracycline, oxy-tetracycline, kanamycin, or bacitracin-neomycin, symptoms characteristic of germ-free animals materialized. From the second or third day of treatment neither coprostanol nor stercobilin was produced, a germ-free animal pattern of the faecal mucins and bile acids was developed and the animals excreted active proteolytic enzymes (Gustafsson and Norin, 1977; Gustafsson *et al.*, 1977).

G. **Endocrine Function**

1. *Gut Hormones*

For many years, gut hormones meant gastrin, cholecystokinin, secretin and pancreozymin. Beginning in 1974 with the advent of radio-immuno-assay (RIA) technology, however, many gut peptides have been found in just about every tissue examined. The effects of gut peptides are potentiated by the so-called biogenic monoamines, which are synthesized from an amine precursor. Hence, the acronym APUD (amine precursor uptake and decarboxylation) has been given to these cells.

It is beyond the scope of this review to examine this rapidly expanding area of research; however, a summary of the presently known endocrine secretions of the various enterocytes is shown in Table 3.4. Thus, the influence of gut peptides on nutrient absorption and subsequent transport and metabolism is significant and the overlapping role of the intestinal

Table 3.4 *Enterocyte endocrine secretions*

Enterocyte Type	Location	Product	Major Action
A	Stomach	Pancreatic glucagon	Hepatic glycogenolysis
D	Pylorus, duodenum	Somatostatin	Local inhibition of endocrine cells
D_1	Stomach, intestines	Vasoactive intestinal peptide (VIP)	Ion/water secretion, gut motility
EC	Stomach, intestines, submucosal glands, appendix, etc.	Serotonin (5-HT), motilin, substance P	Gut motility
G	Pylorus, duodenum	Gastrin	Gastric acid secretion
I	Small intestine	Cholecystokinin	Pancreatic enzyme secretion, gallbladder emptying
K	Small intestine	Gastric inhibitory peptide (GIP)	Inhibition of gastric acid secretion
L	Small intestine, colon	Gut-type glucagon, pancreatic glucagon	Hepatic glycogenolysis
N	Small intestine	Neurotensin	
S	Small intestine	Secretin	Pancreatic and biliary ion/water secretion

microbial flora demands that the effects of gut peptides be established when postulating that the intestinal flora produces the observed effects. In the future, failure to establish the role of gut peptides will make interpretations concerning the effects of the microbial flora difficult if not impossible. Excellent reviews on gut peptides have been published by Creutzfeldt (1982) and Mutt (1982).

2. *Enterohepatic Circulation of Steroid Hormones*

The metabolism of the sex steroid hormones involves an enterohepatic circulation that is dependent upon biologically active excretion, bacterial deconjugation, and intestinal reabsorption similar to those of the bile acids. Approximately 60% of circulating oestrogens are conjugated in the form of glucuronides or sulphates and are excreted in the bile (Eriksson and Gustafsson, 1971). Deconjugation, the step prerequisite to mucosal cell reabsorption, is catalysed by the bacterial enzymes β-glucuronidase and sulphatase, and is nearly complete. Indeed, 97% of the oestrogens excreted in the faeces is in the deconjugated form, although virtually all of the oestrogens in the bile are conjugated.

Dietary fibre intake appears to have an effect on the intestinal metabolism of oestrogens. Faecal excretion of oestrogen was threefold higher among premenopausal vegetarian women than among omnivores (Goldin *et al.*, 1982). Urinary excretion of oestriol-3-glucuronide was also lower in vegetarians. These findings indicate a lesser enterohepatic circulation of oestrogens in vegetarian women, which may be related to reduced intestinal bacterial enzymatic activity in this population.

Another indication that the microflora is involved in oestrogen metabolism is the observation that oral antibiotics exert a profound effect on the enterohepatic circulation of oestrogen. Studies have shown that the urinary oestriol concentration is decreased following oral administration of ampicillin, penicillin, or neomycin (Aldercreutz *et al.*, 1975; Pulkkinen and Willman, 1971, 1973). The last antibiotic is of particular interest since it is poorly absorbed after oral administration, which indicates that the observed effect is due to changes in the population of the intestinal flora and not to any systemic properties of the drug.

Bacterial metabolism of the sex hormones includes oxidative and reductive reactions in addition to deconjugation (Eriksson and Gustafsson, 1971; Jarvenpaa *et al.*, 1980). The type of chemical reaction is dependent upon the degree of anaerobiosis in the medium and the concentration of bacteria (Lombardi *et al.*, 1978). When the bacterial concentration is high, simulating the colonic environment, the E_h is low. These conditions indicate anaerobiosis, and the predominant reactions are reductive. On the other hand, an oxygenated environment with a low concentration of micro-organisms mediates oxidative reactions.

These findings have important clinical significance. Failures of oral contraceptive pills have been associated with the concomitant use of oral antibiotics. Five pregnancies were reported among 88 women taking rifampin and oral contraceptives (Reimer, 1974). Other antibiotics that have been associated with birth-control failure include ampicillin, chloramphenicol and sulphamethoxypyridazine (Dossetar, 1975). These studies demonstrate the importance of the intestinal microflora in the metabolism of the sex steroid hormones.

H. The Role of Mucus

Mucus is the 'skin' of the alimentary tract and it serves as effectively as, and in a more versatile way than, the skin of the body. In 1856, Claud Bernard commented that mucus encloses the gastric juice like a vase as impermeable as if it were made of porcelain. Mucus does indeed form a coherent protective layer covering the living lining of the alimentary tract, and its integrity in health prevents both bacterial infection and biochemical damage. At the same time, it allows the regulated movement of simple molecules that will pass into the absorbing cells. Recently, a hydrogen ion concentration gradient across the mucus on human gastric mucosa has been demonstrated by using microelectrodes (Bahari et al., 1982); these data support the hypothesis that a 'mucus–bicarbonate' protective barrier exists. Also, comparisons between the glycoproteins isolated from normal and from malignant areas of the same surgical specimens showed that in the malignant tissue glycoproteins there was (1) a lower concentration of serine, (2) increased amounts of sialic acid and ester sulphate, and (3) a blood group antigenicity different from that of the hosts' red cells (Schrager and Oates, 1978).

For some time, elevated levels of mucus (Loesche, 1968), of amino acids that are typical of mucus (Combe and Pion, 1966) and of hexosamine have been found in the caecal contents of germ-free rats and mice, compared to their conventional counterparts. Lindstedt et al. (1965) demonstrated a fivefold increase in the concentration of hexosamine in the caecal contents of germ-free rats when compared to their conventional controls. Furthermore, this excess of mucus and related substances may contribute to the inhibition of water absorption and the increased liquid contents of the lower alimentary tract of gnotobiotic rodents (Csaky, 1968). On the other hand, Coates and Rolls (1981) found a fivefold increase in hexosamine concentrations in the caecal contents of germ-free chickens; this indicates a five times higher mucin concentration. Yet the chicks did not exhibit the caecal enlargement characteristic of germ-free rats. Thus, the accumulation of mucus itself does not produce caecal enlargement.

Since carbohydrate–protein macromolecules play an important role in the function of the mucociliary barrier system of the lungs, glycosaminoglycan (GAG) composition was studied in dog lungs (Radhakrishnamurthy *et al.*, 1983). Total GAG concentration was 47% higher, heparin sulphate and heparin concentrations were lower and the heparin sulphate fractions had lower total sulphate content in germ-free lungs than in the conventional. These data reemphasize the overall catabolic effect of the microbial flora on mucins.

The detailed pathways of glycolipid synthesis were studied by Umesaki *et al.* (1981a), who identified two major neutral glycolipids as glucosylceramide by column chromatography and asialo GM 1 by gas liquid chromatography. In a previous paper, Umesaki *et al.* (1981b) reported that the induction of a fucolipid in the microvillus membrane of the mouse intestinal mucosa by conventionalization was observed by monitoring the incorporation of radiolabelled fucose *in vivo*. These results suggest that conventionalization can induce the fucosyl asialo GM 1 in the microvillus membrane through the induction of a fucosyltransferase. Further studies in conventional mice are necessary to determine whether these changes are due to the action of the normal microbial flora or to the overall stress of conventionalization.

Physiologically significant micro-organisms present in the crypts of Lieberkuhn or in the mucus gel layer on the mucosa of the intestinal tract can be isolated by serial sectioning of the frozen intestinal wall (Gustaffson *et al.*, 1981). The sections with adherent bacteria were used to contaminate a series of small germ-free isolators, each harbouring 1 or 2 germ-free rats. Germ-free rats contaminated with a section of the caecal wall from a conventional rat, containing bacteria from the crypts of Lieberkuhn, demonstrated the formation of stercobilin from bilirubin and the degradation of intestinal mucin. One animal, monocontaminated with a *Peptostreptococcus* species, demonstrated a complete conventional animal mucin pattern in its intestinal contents.

I. Pancreatic Enzymes

The fate of the pancreatic endopeptidases, i.e., trypsin, chymotrypsin and elastase, after their activation and subsequent hydrolysis of ingested food proteins is poorly understood. These enzymes represent a major portion of the pancreatic enzymes, yet only trace amounts of them are normally eliminated in the faeces. Several possible metabolic pathways contributing to the disappearance of these enzymes during intestinal passage have been suggested, such as degradation by auto-digestion or binding to inhibitors produced by the intestinal mucosa.

The concentration of pancreatic trypsin in caecal contents was about the same in germ-free and conventional rats, but there was a striking difference in the faecal concentrations. In the germ-free rat the amount of active trypsin was the same as in the caecum, but in the conventional rat active trypsin could be demonstrated only in very low concentrations in faeces. These data have been confirmed with the use of very sensitive and specific immunochemical methods (Genell *et al.*, 1977) that showed that the faeces of germ-free rats had 50 times more pancreatic trypsin per gram than conventional rat faeces. Pancreatic elastase was found in large amounts in the small intestine of both germ-free and conventional rats. In the caecal contents and faeces of the conventional rat, no elastase could be demonstrated with either enzymatic or immunological methods; whereas, in the germ-free rat very large amounts, mainly inactive, were found. Pancreatic chymotrypsin could not be demonstrated in caecal contents, either in conventional or germ-free rats, but was easily found in the small intestine.

J. Practicality of Extrapolations to Man

The problem of extrapolating toxicological data from animals to man is very complex and still based on empirical approaches, but there are several components which have been summarized in a recent review by Garattini (1985): (*i*) different animal species dispose of chemicals in different ways; therefore doses of a chemical cannot be used as a basis for extrapolation. Modern toxicology tends, in fact, to utilize concentrations in blood and in target organs rather than doses; (*ii*) in several cases chemicals are transformed in the body and by the animal's microbial flora into other chemical species, metabolites. These metabolites are sometimes biologically active. Therefore, extrapolations do not necessarily reflect the concentrations of the administered compound but may relate to the concentration of the active metabolite(s); (*iii*) equal concentrations of a chemical (or of its active metabolite) do not mean equal biological activity in different animal species or in man. It is important to consider the sensitivity of the biological system on which a toxicological effect depends. This aspect can easily be measured in animals but only seldom in man; (*iv*) the toxic effects of a chemical are modulated by a number of factors which include age, sex, microbial flora, pathology, and previous and concomitant exposure to other chemicals. Analysis and control of all of these factors may be possible for acute exposure, but becomes almost impossible for chronic exposure. Much more research is needed to acquire and interpret all available data. Routine toxicology tests must be supplemented by a more scientific approach aiming at understanding the mechanisms of the toxic effect. Mathematical models are no substitute for poor information on the biological mechanisms of toxicity.

The physiological importance of the intestinal microflora in the human carcinogenic process is an area that still requires more basic research before any definite relationships are established. The large metabolic capacity of the flora in xenobiotic metabolism, together with the wealth of results obtained from experimental animals, make it extremely unlikely that the flora has no role to play. Goldman (1981) has published a review on the metabolism of xenobiotics by the intestinal flora and its role in cancer development. Furthermore, the metabolic events mediating the cancer-protecting effects of fibre in the diet are not known, even though these factors beneficially alter the metabolic activity and/or composition of the flora. Thus, by studying how these protective factors alter the metabolic activity, rather than the composition of the flora, by carrying out metabolic studies in germ-free and conventional animals, and by monitoring the mutagenicity of germ-free and conventional excreta, more light can be thrown on these beneficial phenomena.

Finally, the physiology of the germ-free animal represents the species conditions *per se*, without the interference of an entity — the flora — which is as large as one of the main organs of the body. To this must be added the fact that the flora is not well defined at the present, and that it might be influenced by changes in diet and life style. The wide use of antibiotics in combination with the fact that these might have a pertinent effect on the normal intestinal flora merits further caution. The influence of the flora in carcinogenesis and the metabolism of such compounds as bile acids, cholesterol, and steroid hormones also adds to the necessity of using germ-free animals as a tool to get to the baseline of these reactions and conditions.

K. Future Research

The most fruitful areas for future research, to establish the host–microbial relationships that are important in maintaining normal physiology and in understanding the pathophysiology of neoplastic disease and toxicology, should centre on the role of basic wide-ranging causative phenomena. These investigations should involve different species to assure the widest possible interpretations and applications of these findings. In this regard, more attention should be directed toward basic mechanisms of how the microbial flora produces its effects on the host and less attention towards which microbes do it. The same microbes may not produce the same effects in different species, but the basic mechanisms may be alike. Such a dilemma was seen in early research in strangulation obstruction and oral diseases in germ-free animals (Cohn *et al.*, 1967; Orland *et al.*, 1954); it was easy to design experiments that test the effects of different bacteria in gnotobiotes but difficult to establish critically the fundamental and universal pathophysiological mechanisms of neoplastic disease and toxicology.

Finally, Table 3.5 summarizes some of the areas that will be important as rapid advances are made in our knowledge of alimentary-tract/host-microflora function in health and disease.

1.   *Organ Xenografts in Nude Mice*

To improve the technique for transplantation of intestinal mucosal xenografts, both canine and human colonic mucosa was isolated by EDTA perfusion of the intact mesentery and by dissection from smooth muscle. The EDTA perfusion technique, which was a modification of methods of Hazel Cheng of the University of Toronto (Bjerknes and Cheng, 1981; Cheng *et al.*, 1984), produced remarkably pure and viable crypts (see Fig. 3.3). The mucosal tissue was rinsed in media with antibiotics, incubated *in vitro* for 1 hour or 24 hours at 37°C and transplanted into nude mice. Mucosal tissues isolated by dissection were placed subcutaneously (SubQ) with a covering membrane filter. EDTA isolated mucosal cells (EDTA) were placed at various sites or sealed inside membrane filter chambers. The dissected SubQ, the EDTA SubQ, and the intramuscular grafts had the greatest viability. Filter paper increased the vascularity around the grafts. Viable enterocytes were seen in grafts examined after 2–21 days growth *in vivo* and after 3–6 weeks with 11/14 or 78.6% of the transplanted grafts surviving. Figs. 3.4 and 3.5 show viable dog colonic mucosa, isolated by dissection, growing in nude mice and exhibiting grossly normal appearance at 1–2 weeks and 17 weeks after transplantation under a membrane filter (Harbin and Heneghan, 1985). Also, Fig. 3.6 shows viable human colonic mucosa, isolated by EDTA perfusion, growing in nude mice and exhibiting grossly normal

Table 3.5 *Summary of technologies that will influence toxicology research*

Technology	Application
Radioimmunoassay	Gut hormone quantitation in blood and tissues
Rheology of mucus	Study the 'protective' role of mucus in host and the 'nutritive' role of 'mucus' for gut microbes
Germ-free animals inoculated with human tissue both healthy and diseased	Use of the physiological characteristics of germ-free animals to study human diseases when microbes can't be cultured
Histochemistry with TEM and SEM	A better understanding of physiological processes at the molecular level
Microcomputers (a) Image analysis (b) Precise control of perfusion pumps	Data analysis and reporting (a) Three dimensional representation of alimentary tract morphology (b) Quantitative studies on luminal flow and intestinal absorption
Breath analysis	Application of this clincial technique in large experimental animals to study functional absorptive surfaces
Germ-free technology to protect immune-deficient animals from infectious disease	Long-term studies of human tissue and disease-causing organisms in an animal model that permits host-factor modulation

morphology at 12 weeks after transplantation intramuscularly (IM). Establishment of a baseline of successful growth of xenografted enterocytes will greatly increase the speed of the development of this technique.

When the growth and development of these xenografts has been standardized and 'baseline' studies completed it should be possible to carry out the following toxicological studies. Each nude mouse would receive transplants of colonic mucosa from four different species: rat, mouse, dog and human. Then the nude mice would be given certain toxic substances orally and their relative effects on the mucosa of four different

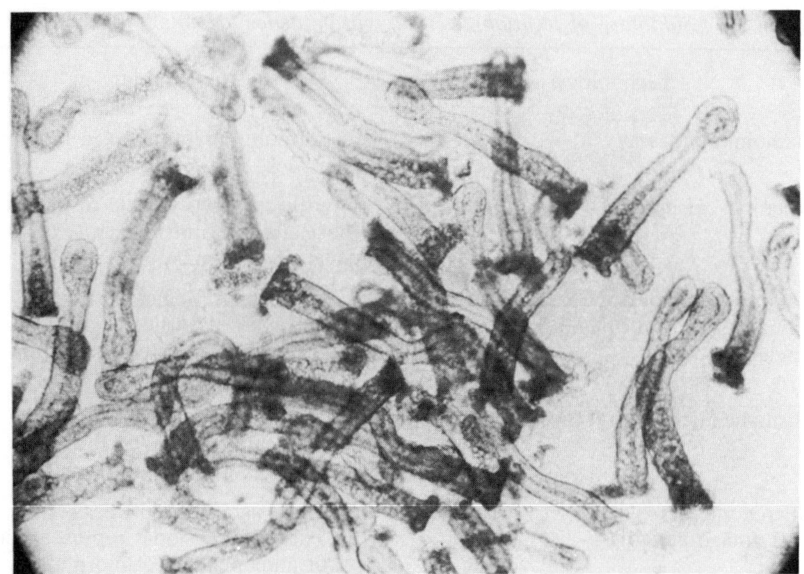

Fig 3.3 Normal control dog colon mucosa isolated by EDTA perfusion of mesenteric blood vessels. These pure colonic crypts are viable, 95% excluded Trypan Blue (100×).

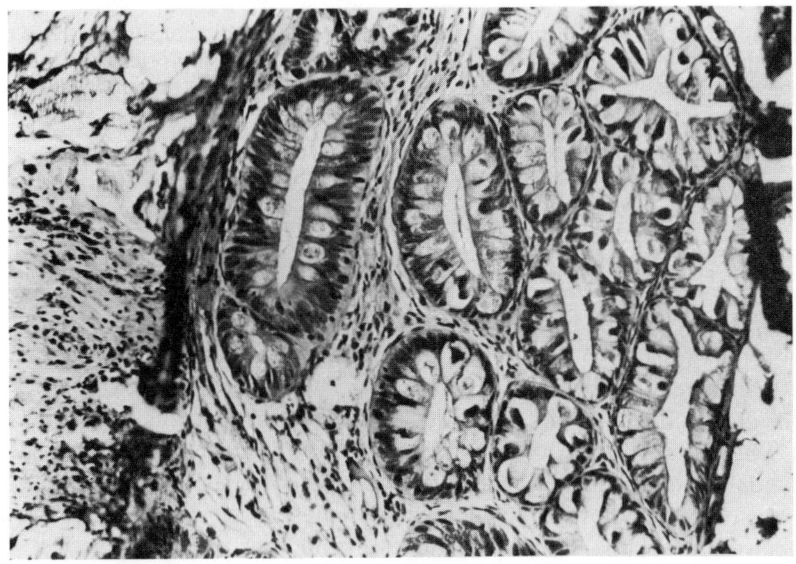

Fig 3.4 Dog colon mucosa isolated by dissection, 1–2 weeks after transplant SubQ with filter. Note the scattered pockets of viable crypts (300×).

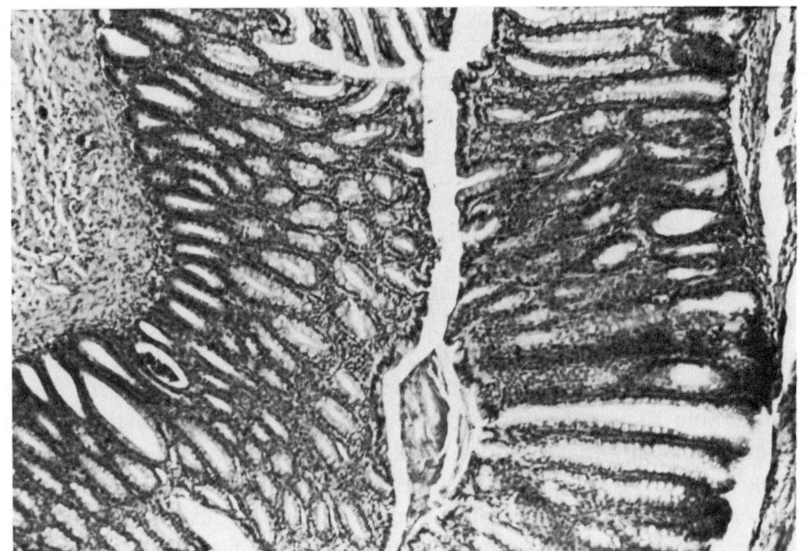

Fig 3.5 Dog colon mucosa isolated by dissection, 17 weeks after transplantation SubQ with filter. Complete regeneration of colonic crypts with a 'tree-like' shape of lumen in upper left corner (300×).

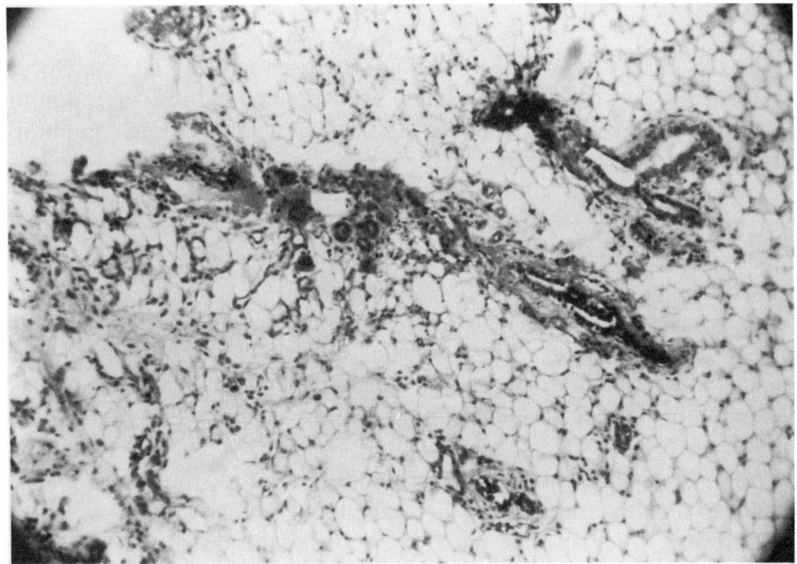

Fig 3.6 Human colon mucosa isolated by EDTA perfusion, 12 weeks after transplant IM. Note the numerous pockets of viable colonic crypts. In 6 week samples, similar regeneration was noted (50×).

species could be studied directly. Alternatively, the mucosal tissues would be exposed to varying concentrations of toxic substances before transplantation. This model system will help to bridge the gap between animal toxicology and the extrapolation to the human condition.

2. *Gnotobiotes Associated with a Human Flora*

A unique application of gnotobiotes was illustrated by the study of Phillips and Zierdt (1976), who showed that only in gnotobiotic guinea pigs inoculated with a human patient's flora were the parasites of *Blastocystis hominis* able to invade the intestinal mucosa and produce the disease. However, no pathology was observed in germ-free or monocontaminated guinea pigs. Even though one cannot expect all of the human microbes to become established in the gnotobiote, this study indicated that sufficient numbers can survive to produce a suitable model for human disease.

L. Summary and Conclusions

1. The descriptive phase of toxicology research is past. The rat, mouse, guinea pig and rabbit have been well defined. However, additional baseline studies are necessary in other species, so that more comparative investigations are possible.
2. The era of applied human toxicology and neoplastic disease research in experimental animals has begun. The many different species of animals available today have much to offer as models for the study of human toxicology and neoplastic disease.
3. Many new technologies, such as immunohistochemistry, radioimmunoassay, microcomputer-based image analysis, and radioactive-breath tests of intestinal absorption, have been developed for use in neoplastic research. These techniques should be applied to studies of toxicology and oncology.
4. Primarily experimental animals should be used to study basic mechanisms of health and disease in toxicology, not as screening tools to determine which specific bacteria produces the disease.
5. Experiments should be performed in as many different species of animals as possible to give the widest possible interpretation to the hypotheses being developed.

Acknowledgements

The investigations that formed the basis of this discussion were funded by the following grants: FR–00272 from the Animal Resources Branch, NIH, AM–18886 from the Digestive Diseases Branch, NIAMDD, NIH, 81–LMN/008–B31 from the Research and Development Program, Board of Regents, State of Louisiana, and PDT–223 from the American Cancer Society.

References

Abrams, G. D., Bauer, H. and Sprintz, H. (1963). Influence of the normal flora on mucosal morphology and cellular renewal in the ileum. *Lab. Invest.* **12**, 355–364.

Abrams, G. D. and Bishop, J. E. (1967). Effect of the normal microbial flora on gastrointestinal motility. *Proc. Soc. Exp. Biol. Med.* **126**, 301–304.

Adlercreutz, H., Martin, F., Tikkanen, M. J. and Pulkkinen, M. O. (1975). Effect of ampicillin administration on the excretion of twelve oestrogens in pregnancy urine. *Acta Endocrinol.* **80**, 551–557.

Anderson, P. O. (1984). Vascular control in the colon and rectum *Scand. J. Gastroenterol.* **19**, Suppl. 93, 65–78.

Archer, M. C., Saul, R. L., Lee, L. -J. and Bruce, W. R. (1981). Analysis of nitrate, nitrite and nitrosamines in human feces. *In "Gastrointestinal Cancer: Endogenous Factors"*, Banbury Report 7. pp. 321–327. Cold Spring Harbor Laboratory, Cold Spring Harbor, NY.

Argenzio, R. A. and Whipp, S. C. (1981). Effect of *Escherichia coli* heat-stable enterotoxin, cholera toxin and theophyllin on ion transport in porcine colon. *J. Physiol. (Lond.)* **320**, 469–487.

Arnold, G. A., Hines, D. P. and Nance, F. C. (1974). The blind-loop syndrome in germfree animals: Studies of B–12 absorption. *Gastroenterol.* **66**, A–7/661.

Bahari, H. M. M., Ross, I. N. and Turnberg, L. A. (1982). Demonstration of a pH gradient across the mucus layer on the surface of human gastric mucosa *in vitro. Gut* **23**, 513–516.

Bentley, D. W., Nichols, R. L., Condon, R. E. and Gorbach, S. L. (1972). The microflora of the human ileum and intra-abdominal colon: Results of direct needle aspiration at surgery and evaluation of the technique. *J. Lab. Clin. Med.* **79**, 421–429.

Bergstrand, O. and Holmstrom, B. (1978). Recent studies on transmissible agent in Crohn's disease. *Acta Chir. Scand.* [Suppl] **482**, 41–44.

Bjerknes, M. and Cheng, H. (1981). Methods for the isolation of intact epithelium from the mouse intestine. *Anat. Rec.* **199**, 565–574.

Boige, N., Munck, A. and Laburthe, M. (1984). Adrenergic versus VIPergic control of cyclic AMP in human colonic crypts. *Peptides* **5**, 379–383.

Borgstrom, A., Genell, S. and Ohlsson, K. (1977). Endogenous elevated fecal levels of pancreatic endopeptidases after antibiotic treatment. *Scand. J. Gastroenterol.* **12**, 525–529.

Bruckner, G. and Szabo, J. (1984). Nutrient absorption in gnotobiotic animals. *Adv. Nutr. Res.* **6**, 271–332.

Burkitt, D. P. (1971). Epidemiology of cancer of the colon and rectum. *Cancer*
   28, 3–13.
Cheng, H., Bjerknes, M. and Amar, J. (1984). Methods for the determination
   of epithelial cell kinetic parameters of human colonic epithelium isolated
   from surgical and biopsy specimens. *Gastroenterol.* **866**, 78–85.
Clarke, A. M. Chirnside, A., Hill, G. L., Pope, G. and Stewart, M. K. (1967).
   Chronic dehydration and sodium depletion in patients with established
   ileostomies. *Lancet* **2**, 740–743.
Coates, M. E. (1973). Gnotobiotic animals in nutrition research. *Proc. Nutr. Soc.*
   32, 53–58.
Coates, M. E., Cole, C. B., Fuller, R., Houghton, S. B. and Yokata, H. (1981).
   The gut microflora and the uptake of glucose from the small intestine of the
   chick. *Br. Poult. Sci.* **22**, 289–294.
Coates, M. E. and Gustafsson, B. E. (1984). "The Germ-free Animal in
   Research," Laboratory Animals Ltd., London, England, *Laboratory Animal
   Handbooks* **9**, 1–442.
Coates, M. E. and Rolls, B. A. (1981). Potato starch, gut flora and caecal size
   in the chick. *J. Sci. Food Agricult.* **32**, 481–484.
Cohn, I., Jr., Heneghan, J. B., Nance, F. C., Bornside, G. H., Cain, J. L., Yu,
   S.-K. and Labat, J. A. (1967). Germ-free surgical research: Current status.
   Ann. Surg. **166**, 518–529.
Combe, E., Demarne, Y., Gueguen, L., Ivorec-Szylit, O., Meslin, J. C. and
   Sacquet, E. (1976). Some aspects of the relationships between gastrointestinal
   flora and host nutrition. *World Rev. Nutr. Diet.* **24**, 1–57.
Combe, E. and Pion, R. (1966). Note sur la composition en acides amines du
   contenu de caecum de rats axeniques et de rats témoins. *Ann. Biol. Animale,
   Biochim. Biophys.* **6**, 255–259.
Combe, E., Pion, R. and Sacquet, E. (1970). Influence de la nature et du taux
   des proteines alimentaires sur la composition en acides amines du contenu
   du caecum axenique. *Ann. Biol. Animale, Biochim. Biophys.* **10**, 697–702.
Crabbe, P. A., Nash, D. R., Bazin, H., Eyssen, H. and Heremans, J. F. (1970).
   Immunohistochemical observations on lymphoid tissues from conventional
   and germfree mice. *Lab. Invest.* **22**, 448–457.
Creutzfeldt, W. (1982). Gastrointestinal peptides – role in pathophysiology and
   disease. *Scand. J. Gastroenterol.* [Suppl. 77] **17**, 7–20.
Csaky, T. Z. (1968). Intestinal water permeability regulation involving the
   microbial flora. *In* "The Germfree Animal in Research" (ed. M. E. Coates),
   pp. 151–159. Academic Press, London, U.K.
Cummings, J. H. (1981). Short chain fatty acids in the human colon. *Gut* **22**,
   763–779.
Debongnie, J. C. and Phillips, S. F. (1978). Capacity of the human colon to
   absorb fluid. *Gastroenterol.* **74**, 698–703.
Dossetar, J. (1975). Drug interaction with oral contraceptives. *Br. Med. J.* **4**,
   467–468.
Dupont, C., Laburthe, M., Broyart, J. P., Bataille, D. and Rosselin, G. (1980).
   Cyclic AMP production in isolated colonic epithelial crypts: A highly sensitive
   model for the evaluation of vasoactive intestinal peptide action in human
   intestine. *Eur. J. Clin. Invest.* **10**, 67–76.
Eklund, S., Jodal, M., Lundgren, O.I. and Sjoqvist, A. (1979). Effects of
   vasoactive intestinal polypeptide on blood flow, motility and fluid transport
   in the gastrointestinal tract of the cat. *Acta Physiol. Scand.* **105**, 461–468.

Eriksson, H. and Gustafsson, J. A. (1971). Excretion of steroid hormones in adults: Steroids in feces from adults. *Eur. J. Biochem.* **18**, 146–150.

Evered, D. F. (1981). Advances in amino acid metabolism in mammals. *Biochem. Soc. Trans.* **9**, 159–169.

Evrard, E., Sacquet, E., Raibaud, P., Charlier, H., Dickinson, A., Eyssen, H. and Hoet, P. P. (1965). Studies on conventional and gnotobiotic rats: Effect of intestinal bacteria on fecal lipids and fecal sterols. *In:* "Erahrungsforschung: Berichte und Mitteilungen" (eds K. Taufel and M. Ulmann), pp. 257. Academic Press of Berlin.

Ferreira, H. G. and Smith, M. W. (1968). Effect of a saline environment on sodium transport by the toad colon. *J. Physiol. (Lond.)* **198**, 329–343.

Field, M., Fordtran, J. S. and Schultz, S. G. (1980). "Secretory Diarrhea", pp. 1–227. Bethesda, MA, American Physiological Society.

Fleming, S. E., Marthinsen, D. and Kuhnlein, H. (1983). Colonic function and fermentation in men consuming high fiber diets. *J. Nutr.* **113**, 2535–2544.

Garattini, S. (1985). Toxic effects of chemicals: Difficulties in extrapolating data from animals to man. *Crit. Rev. Toxicol.* **16**(1), 1–29.

Genell, S., Gustafsson, B. E. and Ohlsson, K. (1977). Immunochemical quantitation of pancreatic endopeptidases in the intestinal contents of germfree and conventional rats. *Scand. J. Gastroenterol.* **12**, 811–820.

Gianella, R. A., Broitman, S. A. and Zamcheck, N. (1972). Competition between bacteria and intrinsic factor for vitamin B–12: Implications for vitamin B–12 malabsorption in intestinal bacterial overgrowth. *Gastroenterol.* **62**, 255–260.

Goldin, B. R., Aldercreutz, H., Gorbach, S. L., Warram, J. H., Dwyer, J. T., Swenson, L. and Woods, M. N. (1982). Estrogen excretion patterns and plasma levels in vegetarian and omnivorous women. *N. Eng. J. Med.* **307**, 1542–1547.

Goldman, P. (1981). The metabolism of xenobiotics by the intestinal flora. *In:* "Gastrointestinal Cancer: Endogenous Factors" Banbury Report 7, pp. 25–39. Cold Spring Harbor Laboratory, Cold Spring Harbor, New York.

Gorbach, S. L. (1975). Intestinal microflora in idiopathic inflammatory bowel disease. *In:* "Inflammatory Bowel Disease" (eds B. Kirsner and R. G. Shorter), p. 47–61. Lea and Febiger, Philadelphia.

Gordon, H. A. and Bruckner-Kardoss, E. (1961). Effect of normal microbial flora on intestinal surface area. *Am. J. Physiol.* **201**, 175–178.

Gordon, H. A. and Pesti, L. (1971). The gnotobiotic animal as a tool in the study of host microbial relationships. *Bacteriol. Rev.* **35**, 390–429.

Gustafsson, B. E. (1982). The physiological importance of the colonic microflora. *Scand. J. Gastroenterol.* [Suppl. 77] **17**, 117–131.

Gustafsson, B. E., Carlstedt-Duke, B. and Nord, C. -E. (1981). Mucosa related intestinal bacteria and host metabolism. *In:* "Recent Advances in Germfree Research" (eds S. Sasaki, A. Ozawa, and H. Hashimoto), pp. 249–254. Tokai University Press, Tokyo.

Gustafsson, B. E., Gustafsson, J. -A. and Carlstedt-Duke, B. (1977). Prolonged induction of germfree bile acid pattern in conventional rats by antibiotics. *Acta Med. Scand.* **201**, 155–160.

Gustafsson, B. E. and Maunsbach, A. B. (1971). Ultrastructure of the enlarged caecum in germfree rats. *Z. Zellforschung mikrosk. Anat.* **120**, 555–578.

Gustafsson, B. E. and Norin, K. E. (1977). Development of germfree animal characteristics in conventional rats on antibiotics. *Acta Path. Microbiol. Scand.* **85**, 1–8.

Gustafsson, B. E. and Norman, A. (1969). Influence of the diet on the turnover of bile acids in germfree and conventional rats. *Br. J. Nutr.* **23**, 429–442.

Gustafsson, J. -A. and Werner, B. (1968). Fetal sterols in infants bile acids and steroids 194. *Acta Physiol. Scand.* **73**, 305–310.

Hagemann, R. F. and Stragand, J. J. (1977). Fasting and refeeding: Cell kinetic response of the jejunum, ileum and colon. *Cell Tissue Kinet.* **10**, 3–9.

Hanson, K. M. and Johnson, P. C. (1967). Pressure-flow relationships in isolated dog colon. *Am. J. Physiol.* **212**, 574–578.

Hanson, P. J. and Parsons, D. S. (1976). The utilization of glucose and production of lactate by in vitro preparations of rat small intestine: Effects of vascular perfusion. *J. Physiol. (Lond.)* **255**, 775–795.

Hanson, P. J. and Parsons, D. S. (1978). Factors affecting the utilisation of ketone bodies and other substrates by rat jejunum: effects of fasting and of diabetes. *J. Physiol. (Lond.)* **278**, 55–67.

Harbin, S. and Heneghan, J. B. (1985). Growth of dog intestinal xenografts in nude mice. *In*: "Germfree Research: Microflora Control and its Application to the Biomedical Sciences" (ed. B. S. Wostmann). Alan R. Liss, New York. *Prog. Clin. Biol. Res.* **181**, 467–471.

Hecker, J. F. (1974). "Experimental Surgery on Small Ruminants", pp. 1–322. Butterworth, London, U.K.

Heneghan, J. B. (1963). Influence of microbial flora on xylose absorption in rats and mice. *Am. J. Physiol.* **205**, 417–420.

Heneghan, J. B. (1965). Imbalance of the normal microbial flora: The germfree alimentary tract. *Am. J. Digest. Dis.* **10**, 864–869.

Heneghan, J. B. (1973). Germfree research: A new approach in micro-ecology. *In*: "Germfree Research: Biological Effect of Gnotobiotic Environments" (ed. J. B. Heneghan), pp. 3–8. Academic Press, New York.

Heneghan, J. B. (1979). Enterocyte kinetics, mucosal surface area and mucus in gnotobiotes. *In*: "Clinical and Experimental Gnotobiotics" (eds. T. Fliedner, H. Heit, D. Niethammer and H. Pflieger), pp. 19–27. Gustav Fischer Verlag, Stuttgart.

Heneghan, J. B., Gordon, H. A. and Miniats, O. P. (1979). Intestinal mucosal surface area and goblet cells in germfree and conventional piglets. *In*: "Clinical and Experimental Gnotobiotics" (eds T. Fliedner, H. Heit, D. Niethammer and H. Pflieger), pp. 107–111. Gustav Fischer Verlag, Stuttgart.

Heneghan, J. B., Longoria, S. G. and Cohn, I., Jr. (1971). Gnotobiotic beagle dogs: maintenance, growth, and reproduction. *In*: "Defining the Laboratory Animal" (IVth Symposium, International Committee on Laboratory Animals), pp. 597–615. National Academy of Sciences, Washington, D.C.

Heneghan, J. B. and Mittelbronn, M. Y. (1981). Vitamin B–12 absorption in cecectomized gnotobiotic rats. *In*: "Proceedings of the 28th International Congress of Physiological Sciences Budapest, 1980" (eds T. Gati, L. G. Szollar and Gy. Ungvary). *Adv. Physiol. Sci. Nutr. Dig. Metab.* **12**, 453–457.

Henning, S. J. and Hird, F. J. R. (1972). Transport of acetate and butyrate in the hind-gut of rabbits. *Biochem. J.* **130**, 791–796.

Hill, M. J. (1978). Some leads to the etiology of cancer of the large bowel. *Surg. Annu.* **10**, 135–149.

Hill, M. J. and Aries, V. (1971). Faecal steroid composition and its relationship to cancer of the large bowel. *J. Path.* **104**, 129–139.

Hullen, L. (1970). Extrinsic nervous control of colonic motility and blood flow. *Acta Physiol. Scand.* **335**, 1–116.

Janne, P., Carpentier, Y. and Willems, G. (1977). Colonic mucosal atrophy induced by a liquid elemental diet in rats. *Am. J. Dig. Dis.* **22**, 808–812.

Jarvenpaa, P., Kosunen, T., Fotsis, T. and Aldercreutz, H. (1980). In vitro metabolism of estrogens by isolated intestinal micro-organisms and by human fecal microflora. *J. Steroid Biochem.* **13**, 345–349.

Johnson, L.R. (1979). Regulation of gastrointestinal mucosal growth. *World J. Surg.* **3**, 477–486.

Kellogg, T. F. (1973). Faecal bile acids and neutral sterols of gnotobiotic, antibiotic-fed normal, and normal human children. *In*: "Germfree Research: Biological Effect of Gnotobiotic Environments" (ed. J. B. Heneghan), pp. 79–81. Academic Press, New York.

Kruh, J. (1982). Effects of sodium butyrate, a new pharmacological agent, on cells in culture. *Mol. Cell Biochem.* **42**, 65–82.

Kvietys, P. R. and Granger, D. N. (1981). Effects of solute-coupled fluid absorption on blood flow and oxygen uptake in the dog colon. *Gastroenterol.* **81**, 450–457.

Laroche, M. J., Cottart, A., Sacquet, E. and Charlier, H. (1964). Absorption de quelques substances chimiques par le tracte gastrointestinal de rats aseptiques et classiques. *Ann. Pharm. Fr.* **22**, 333–339.

Lawson, M., Kwok, K., Kerr-Grant, A. and Roediger, W. E. W. (1983). A functional test to assess disease activity and severity in ulcerative colitis. *Gastroenterol.* **84**, 1226–1226.

Levin, R. J. (1969). The effects of hormones on the absorptive, metabolic and digestive functions of the small intestine. *J. Endocrinol.* **45**, 315–348.

Levitan, R. and Ingelfinger, F. J. (1965). Effect of d-aldosterone on salt and water absorption from the intact human colon. *J. Clin. Invest.* **44**, 801–808.

Levitt, M. D. and Ingelfinger, F. J. (1968). Hydrogen and methane production in man. *Ann. N.Y. Acad. Sci.* **150**, 75–81.

Lindstedt, G., Lindstedt, S. and Gustafsson, B. E. (1965). Mucus in intestinal contents of germfree rats. *J. Exp. Med.* **121**, 201–213.

Loesche, W. J. (1968). Protein and carbohydrate composition of cecal contents of gnotobiotic rats and mice. *Proc. Soc. Exp. Biol. Med.* **128**, 195–199.

Lombardi, P., Goldin, B. R., Boutin, E. and Gorbach, S. L. (1978). Metabolism of androgens and estrogens by human fecal microorganisms. *J. Steroid Biochem.* **9**, 795–801.

Manousos, O., Day, N. E., Trichopoulos, D., Gerovassilis, F., Tzonou, A. and Polychronopoulou, A. (1983). Diet and colorectal cancer: A case-control study in Greece. *Int. J. Cancer* **32**, 1–5.

McKay, L. F. Brydon, W. G., Eastwood, M. A. and Housley, E. (1983). The influence of peripheral vascular disease on methanogenesis in man. *Atherosclerosis* **47**, 77–81.

McNeil, N. I., Cummings, J. H. and James, W. P. T. (1978). Short chain fatty acid absorption by the human large intestine. *Gut* **19**, 819–822.

Makhlouf, G. M. (1974). The neuroendocrine design of the gut. *Gastroenterol.* **67**, 159–184.

Meslin, J. C., Sacquet, E. and Guenet, J. L. (1973). Action de la flora bacterienne sur la morphologie et al surface de la muqueuse de l'intestin grêle du rat. *Ann. Biol. Animale, Biochim. Biophys.* **11**, 334–335.

Meslin, J. C., Sacquet, E. and Raibaud, P. (1974). Action d'une flore microbienne qui ne déconjugue pas les sels biliaires sur la morphologie et la renouvellement cellulaire de la muqueuse de l'intestin grêle du rat. *Ann. Biol. Animale,*

Biochim. Biophys. **13**, 203–214.

Miller, A. B., Howe, G. R., Jain, M., Craib, K. J. P. and Harrison, L. (1983). Food items and food groups as risk factors in a case-control study of diet and colo-rectal cancer. *Int. J. Cancer* **32**, 155–161.

Moon, H. W. (1980). Luminal and mucosal factors of small intestine affecting pathogenic colonization. *In*: "Secretory Diarrhea" (eds M. Field, J. S. Fordtran, and S. G. Schultz), pp. 127–139. American Physiological Society, Bethesda, MA.

Mutt, V. (1982). Gastrointestinal hormones: A field of increasing complexity. *Scand. J. Gastroenterol.* [Suppl. 77] **17**, 133–152.

Nakamura, G. J., Schneiderman, L. J. and Klauber, M. R. (1984). Colorectal cancer and bowel habits. *Cancer* **54**, 1475–1477.

Orland, F. J., Blayney, J. R., Harrison, R. W., Reyniers, J. A., Trexler, P. C., Wagner, M., Gordon, H. A. and Luckey, T. D. (1954). Use of the germfree animal technique in the study of experimental caries. *J. Dent. Res.* **33**, 147–174.

Phillips, B. P. and Zierdt, C. H. (1976). *Blastocystic hominis*: pathogenic potential in human patients and gnotobiotes. *Exp. Parasitol.* **39**, 358–364.

Pique, J. M., Pallares, M., Cuso, E., Vilar-Bonet, J. and Gassull, M. A. (1984). Methane production and colon cancer. *Gastroenterol.* **87**, 601–605.

Polak, J. M., Bloom, S. R., Wright, N. A. and Daly, M. J. (1982). Adaptation pathophysiology of intestinal response to disease. *Scand. J. Gastroenterol.* **17**(74), 1–180.

Porteous, J. W. (1980). Glutamate, glutamine, aspartate, asparagine, glucose and ketone-body metabolism in chick intestinal brush-border cells. *Biochem. J.* **188**, 619–632.

Pulkkinen, M. O. and Willman, K. (1971). Maternal estrogen levels during penicillin treatment. *Br. Med. J.* **4**, 48–48.

Pulkkinen, M. O. and Willman, K. (1973). Reduction of maternal estrogen excretion by neomycin. *Am. J. Obstet. Gynecol.* **115**, 1153–1153.

Radhakrishnamurthy, B., Heneghan, J. B., Smart, F., Jeansonne, N. and Berenson, G. S. (1983). Glycosaminoglycan composition of germfree dog lungs. *Proc. Soc. Exp. Biol. Med.* **172**, 457–462.

Rafestin-Oblin, M. E., Lomes, M., Michel, J. B., Michaud, A. and Claire, M. (1984). Mineralocorticoid receptors in the epithelial cells of human colon and ileum. *J. Steroid Biochem.* **20**, 311–315.

Rechkemmer, G. and von Englehardt, W. (1983). Absorptive processes in different colonic segments of the guinea-pig and the effects of short chain fatty acids. *In*: "Colon and Nutrition" (eds H. Kasper and H. Goebell), p. 61. MTP Press Ltd, Lancaster, U.K.

Reddy, B. S., Narisawa, T., Weisburger, J. H. and Wynder, E. L. (1976). Promoting effect of sodium deoxycholate on colon adenocarcinoma in germfree rats. *J. Natl Cancer Inst.* **56**, 441–444.

Reimer, D. (1974). Rifampicin, "pill" do not go well together. *J. Am. Med. Assoc.* **227**, 608–608.

Riecken, E. O. and Menge, H. (1977). Nutritive effects of food constituents on the structure and function of the intestine. *Acta Hepatogastroenterogie* **24**, 389–399.

Riedel, G., Scharrer, E. and Losch, U. (1972). Resorptionstudien an keimfreien kuken: I. Amino-saurenresorption. *Zentralbl. Veterinarmed.* **A19**, 563–568.

Ritchie, J. A. (1968). Colonic motor activity and bowel function: I. Normal movement of contents. *Gut* **9**, 442–456.

Robinson, J. W. L., Dowling, R. H. and Riecken, E. O. (1982). "Mechanisms of Intestinal Adaptation", pp. 1–357. MTP Press Ltd, Lancaster, U.K.

Roediger, W. E. W. (1980). Role of anaerobic bacteria in the metabolic welfare of the colonic mucosa in man. *Gut* **21**, 793–798.

Roediger, W. E. W. (1982). Utilisation of nutrients by isolated epithelial cells of the rat colon. *Gastroenterol.* **83**, 424–429.

Roediger, W. E. W. (1986). Interrelationship between bacteria and mucosa of the gastrointestinal tract. *In*: "Microbial Metabolism in the Digestive Tract" (ed. M. J. Hill), pp. 201–209. CRC Press, Boca Raton, Fla.

Roediger, W. E. W. and Moore, A. (1981). Effect of short chain fatty acid on sodium absorption in isolated human colon perfused through the vascular bed. *Dig. Dis. Sci.* **26**, 100–106.

Roediger, W. E. W. and Rae, D. (1982). Trophic effect of short chain fatty acids on mucosal handling of ions by the defunctioned colon. *Br. J. Surg.* **69**, 23–25.

Rolls, B. A., Turvey, A. and Coates, M. E. (1978). The influence of the gut microflora and of dietary fibre on epithelial cell migration in the chick intestine. *Br. J. Nutr.* **39**, 91–98.

Ruppin, H., Bar-Meir, S., Soergel, K. H., Wood, C. M. and Schmitt, Jr., M. G. (1980). Absorption of short-chain fatty acids by the colon. *Gastroenterol.* **78**, 1500–1507.

Sakata, T., Hikosaka, K., Shiomura, Y. and Tamate, H. (1980). The stimulatory effect of butyrate on epithelial cell proliferation in the rumen of the sheep and its mediation by insulin: differences in vivo and in vitro studies. *In*: "Cell Proliferation in the Gastrointestinal Tract" (eds D. R. Appleton, J. P. Sunter, and A. J. Watson). Pitman, Tunbridge Wells, U.K.

Sakata, T. and Tamate, H. (1978). Rumen epithelial cell proliferation accelerated by rapid increase in intra-ruminal butyrate. *J. Dairy Sci.* **61**, 1109–1113.

Sakata, T. and von Englehardt, W. (1983). Stimulatory effect of short chain fatty acids on the epithelial cell proliferation in rat large intestine. *Comp. Biochem. Physiol.* **74A**, 459–462.

Salas-Coll, C. A., Kermode, J. C. and Edmonds, C. J. (1976). Potassium transport across the distal colon in man. *Clin. Sci. Molec. Med.* **51**, 287–296.

Sander, E. G., Warner, R. G., Harrison, H. N., and Loosli, J. K. (1959). The stimulatory effect of sodium butyrate and sodium propionate on the development of rumen mucosa in the young calf. *J. Dairy Sci.* **42**, 1600–1605.

Savage, D. C. (1977). Microbial ecology of the gastrointestinal tract. *Ann. Rev. Microbiol.* **31**, 107–133.

Savage, D. C. (1986). Gastrointestinal microflora in mammalian nutrition. *Ann. Rev. Nutr.* **6**, 155–178.

Scharrer, E. and Riedel, G. (1972). Resorptionsstudien bei keimfreien kuken: II. Die resorption von olsaure. *Z. Tierphysiol. Tierernaehrung Futtermittelkunde* **30**, 264–268.

Schrager, J. and Oates, M. D. G. (1978). Relation of human gastrointestinal mucus to disease states. *Br. Med. Bull.* **34**(1), 79–82.

Schultz, S. G., Frizzell, R. A. and Nellans, H. N. (1977). Active sodium transport and the electrophysiology of rabbit colon. *J. Membr. Biol.* **33**, 351–384.

Schultz, S. G. (1984). A cellular model for active sodium absorption by mammalian colon. *Ann. Rev. Physiol.* **46**, 435–451.

Smith, C. J. and Bryant, M. P. (1979). Introduction to metabolic activities of intestinal bacteria. *Am. J. Clin. Nutr.* **32**, 149–157.

Southgate, D. A. T. and Durnin, J. V. G. A. (1970). Calorie conversion factors: An experimental reassessment of the factors used in the calculation of the energy value of human diets. *Br. J. Nutr.* **24**, 517–535.

Spicer, S. S., Sens, M. A. and Tashian, R. E. (1982). Immunocytochemical demonstration of carbonic anhydrase in human epithelial cells. *J. Histochem. Cytochem.* **30**, 864–873.

Stemmermann, G. N., Nomura, A. M. Y. and Heilbrun, L. K. (1984). Dietary fat and the risk of colorectal cancer. *Cancer Res.* **44**, 4633–4637.

Stephen, A. M., Haddad, A. C. and Phillips, S.F. (1983). Passage of carbohydrate into the colon: Direct measurements in humans. *Gastroenterol.* **85**, 589–595.

Stevens, C. E. (1977). Comparative physiology of the digestive system. *In*: "Dukes' Physiology of Domestic Animals" (ed. M. J. Swenson), pp. 216–232. Cornell University Press, Ithaca, N.Y.

Stragand, J. J. and Hagemann, R. F. (1977). Effect of luminal contents on colonic cell replacement. *Am. J. Physiol.* **233**, E208–E211.

Tannenbaum, S. R., Fett, D., Young, V. R., Land, P. D. and Bruce, W. R. (1978). Nitrite and nitrate are formed by endogenous synthesis in the human intestine. *Science* **200**, 1487–1489.

Tennant, B., Reina-Guerra, M. and Harold, D. (1971). Influence of micro-organisms on intestinal absorption. *Ann. N.Y. Acad. Sci.* **176**, 262–272.

Tennant, B., Reina-Guerra, M., Harold, D. and Goldman, M. (1968). Influence of microorganisms on intestinal absorption: oleic acid ^{131}I and triolein ^{131}I absorption by germfree and conventional rats. *J. Nutr.* **97**, 65–69.

Terpstra, O. T., Dahl, E. P., Williamson, R. C. N., Ross, J. S. and Malt, R. A. (1981). Colostomy closure promotes cell proliferation and dimethylhydrazine-induced carcinogenesis in rat distal colon. *Gastroenterol.* **81**, 475–480.

Thayer, J. R., Chasko, J. H., Swartz, L. A. and Parks, N. J. (1982). Gut reactions of radioactive nitrite after intratracheal administration in mice. *Science* **217**, 151–153.

Tilson, M. D. Fellner, B. J. and Wright, H. K. (1976). A possible explanation for postoperative diarrhea after colostomy closure. *Am. J.Surg.* **131**, 94–97.

Umesaki, Y., Suzuki, A., Kasama, T., Tohyama, K., Mutai, M. and Yamakawa, T. (1981a). Presence of asialo GM 1 and glucosylceramide in the intestinal mucosa of mice and induction of fucoysl asiolo GM 1 by conventionalization of germ-free mice. *J. Biochem. (Tokyo)* **90**, 1731–1738.

Umesaki, Y., Tohyama, K. and Mutai, M. (1981b). Appearance of fucolipid after conventionalization of germfree mice. *J. Biochem. (Tokyo)* **90**, 559–561.

Van Dokkum, W., Pikaar, N. A. and Thissen, J. T. N. M. (1983). Physiological effects of fibre-rich types of bread. *Br. J. Nutr.* **50**, 61–74.

Van Soest, P. J. (1984). Some physical characteristics of dietary fibres and their influence on the microbial ecology of the human colon. *Proc. Nutr. Soc.* **43**, 25–33.

Watford, M., Lund, P. and Krebs, H. A. (1979). Isolation and metabolic characteristics of rat and chicken enterocytes. *Biochem. J.* **178**, 589–596.

Williamson, R. C. N. (1978a). Intestinal adaptation: Structural, functional and cytokinetic changes. *N. Eng. J. Med.* **298**, 1393–1402.

Williamson, R. C. N. (1978b). Intestinal adaptation: Mechanisms of control. *N. Eng. J. Med.* **298**, 1444–1450.

Windmueller, H. G. (1982). Glutamine utilization by the small intestine. *In*: "Advances in Enzymology", Vol. 53 (ed. A. Meisler), pp. 201–237. New York, John Wiley and Sons, New York.

Windmueller, H. G. and Spaeth, A. E. (1978). Identification of ketone bodies and glutamine as the major respiratory fuels *in vivo* for post absorptive rat small intestine. *J. Biol. Chem.* **253**, 69–76.

Windmueller, H. G. and Spaeth, A. E. (1980). Respiratory fuels and nitrogen metabolism *in vivo* in small intestine of fed rats. *J. Biol. Chem.* **255**, 107–112.

Witter, J. P., Gatley, S. J. and Balish, E. (1979). Distribution of nitrogen-13 from labelled nitrate (13NO-3) in humans and rats. *Science*, **204**, 411–413.

Wolin, M. J. (1981). Fermentation in the rumen and human large intestine. *Science* **213**, 1463–1468.

Wrong, O. M., Edmonds, C. J. and Chadwick, V. S. (1981). "The Large Intestine: Its Role in Mammalian Nutrition and Homeostasis", pp. 1–217. MTP Press Ltd, Lancaster, U.K.

Yokota, H. (1981). Intestinal absorption of nutrients in germfree chicken. *In*: "Recent Advances in Germfree Research" (ed. S. Sasaki, A. Ozawa and K. Hashimoto), pp. 343–346. Tokai University Press, Tokyo.

Yokota, H. and Coates, M. E. (1982). The uptake of nutrients from the small intestine of gnotobiotic and conventional chicks. *Br. J. Nutr.* **47**, 349–356.

4

Deconjugation of Biliary Metabolites by Microfloral β-glucuronidases, Sulphatases and Cysteine Conjugate β-lyases and their Subsequent Enterohepatic Circulation

G. L. LARSEN

A. Introduction

Bacteria resident in the gastro-intestinal (GI) tract of mammals have been shown to play a major role in the metabolism of xenobiotics, some of which are carcinogens and mutagens (Scheline, 1973; Goldman, 1978; Bakke *et al.*, 1981b). The capacity for such a contribution is not surprising when one considers that the GI flora represent over 400 different bacterial species, most of which are strict anaerobes; they number more cells than the whole of the host (Finegold *et al.*, 1975) and constitute a mass similar to other mammalian organs.

Most xenobiotics are nonpolar and therefore readily absorbed from the GI tract. On absorption from the GI tract, xenobiotics are transported by the portal blood initially to the liver for detoxication. The liver, to a large degree, governs what xenobiotic metabolites the flora will encounter and thus metabolize. In general, the liver tends to oxidize xenobiotics (i.e. cytochrome P450) and form xenobiotic glucuronic acid-, sulphate-, or glutathione-conjugates. Because of the high molecular weight and polar nature of these conjugates, they are extensively excreted in the bile and enter the small intestine where their absorption from the GI tract is highly variable. Some of these conjugates are absorbed throughout the GI tract while others are not. Conjugates that are not readily absorbed tend to move down the small intestinal tract to the caecum or large bowel where large populations of GI flora exist and where microfloral metabolism can take place.

A contrast exists in the microfloral and hepatic metabolism of xenobiotics. The GI flora tend to deconjugate and reduce the hepatic xenobiotic metabolites which results in the formation of lower molecular weight nonpolar molecules which are readily reabsorbed. β-Glucuronidase, sulphatase and more recently cysteine conjugate β-lyase (β-lyase, or C-S lyase) represent major classes of deconjugating enzymes of the microflora. Absorption of these nonpolar molecules and their transport by the portal blood to the liver for detoxication is termed enterohepatic circulation. Enterohepatic circulation is responsible for conservation and reutilization of endogenous substrates in the body, such as the bile acids and steroids. Many of the endogenous compounds that undergo enterohepatic circulation are excreted in the bile as glucuronide, sulphate and/or glutathione conjugates. Utilization of glutamic acid, sulphate, pyruvate and ammonia by the microflora for their metabolism and growth probably explains the presence of β-glucuronidase, sulphatase and β-lyase in the microflora. One important consequence of microbial deconjugation is that, while it conserves endogenous compounds in the body, it retards the elimination of xenobiotics from the body. Additionally, as will be discussed later, β-lyase cleavage results in the introduction of sulphur in the form of thiol into the xenobiotic molecule, changing its physical characteristics. This paper will discuss β-glucuronidase, sulphatase, and β-lyase deconjugation enzymes in the microflora which result in the formation of nonpolar metabolites which undergo enterohepatic circulation (see Table 4.1 and Fig. 4.1).

B.   β-glucuronidase

1.   *Activity and Distribution*

β-glucuronidase is present throughout the GI tract (Marsh *et al.*, 1953) and has been recognized as an important enzyme in the hydrolysis of xenobiotic glucuronides for some time. Glucuronides also represent the largest class of xenobiotic conjugates excreted in the bile (Table 4.1). The intestinal flora are considered to be the major source of β-glucuronidase (pH optimum 6.5) because hydrolysis of many xenobiotic glucuronides is dramatically reduced (>90%) in germ-free or antibiotic pretreated rats (Williams *et al.*, 1970; Grantham *et al.*, 1970). Antibiotics that reduce anaerobic bacteria also eliminate β-glucuronidase activity from rat caecal contents both *in vivo* and in cultures (Kent *et al.*, 1972).

High levels of β-glucuronidase are present in the lower bowel (caecum, large intestine) contents in most mammalian species, with very low levels of bacterial β-glucuronidase present in the small intestinal tract of man, rabbit, and guinea pig. The rat and mouse, with higher microbial

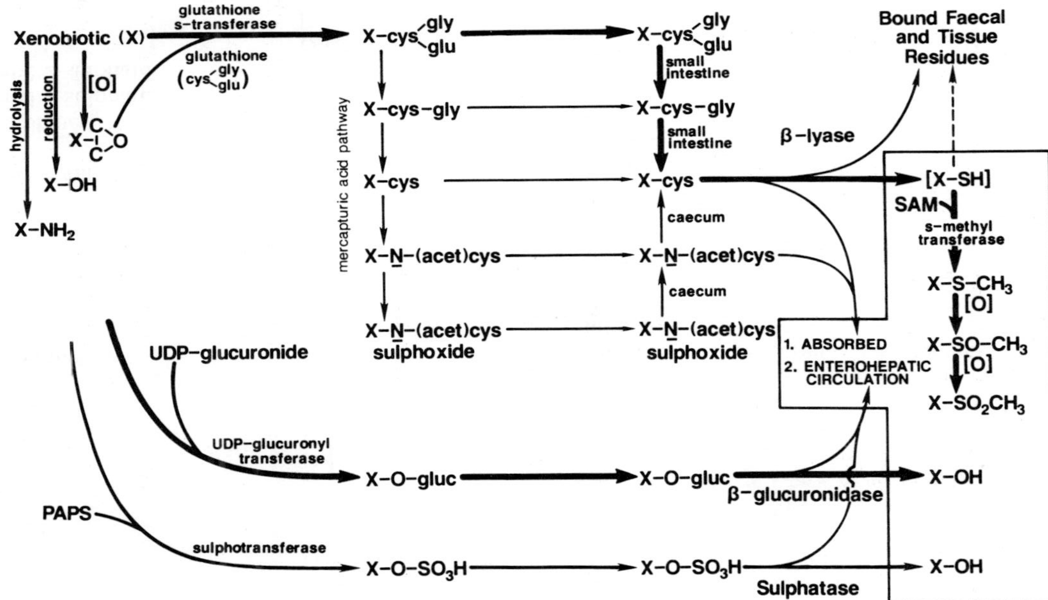

PHASE I (preconjugation) PHASE II (conjugation) TISSUE METABOLISM BILIARY SECRETION INTESTINAL METABOLISM BACTERIAL HYDROLYSIS (caecum and large intestine)

Fig 4.1 The metabolic pathway of biliary mercapturic-acid, glucuronide and sulphate ester conjugates of xenobiotics in the gastro-intestinal tract *in vivo*. The dashed line represents a suspected but unproven pathway. SAM is *S*-adenosylmethionine, PAPS is 3′-phosphoadenosine-5′phosphate.

Table 4.1 *Xenobiotic metabolites excreted in the bile undergoing enterohepatic circulation*

Xenobiotic	Compound[a] type	Animal[b] species	Biliary[c] conjugate hydrolysed	Reference
Phenol		R	gluc.	Layiwola *et al.* (1983)
Dichlorophen	D	R	gluc.	Dixon and Caldwell (1978)
Diethylstilboestrol	C	R	gluc.	Hanahan *et al.* (1953)
				Fischer *et al.* (1966)
				Clark *et al.* (1969)
Pregnanolone	D	R	gluc.	Long and Soyka (1975)
Chloramphenicol	D	R	gluc.	Glazko *et al.* (1949, 1952)
				Thompson *et al.* (1954)
Morphine	D	R	*O*-gluc.	Walsh and Levine (1975)
Vanillian, Isovanillin		R	gluc. sulphate	Strand and Scheline (1975)
1-α-Acetylmethadol	D	R	gluc.	Roerig *et al.* (1979)
Sulisatin	D	R	sulphate	Moreto *et al.* (1977)
Phenobarbital	D	R	gluc.	Klaassen (1971)
				Marselos *et al.* (1975)
Metronidazole	D	R	gluc.	LaRusso *et al.* (1978)
3,4,4′-Trichlorocarbanilide		M	*N*-gluc. *O*-sulphate	Hiles *et al.* (1978)
Biphenylyl 4-sulphate		R	gluc.	Hearse *et al.* (1969)
Cyclohexylphenyl 4-sulphate		R	gluc.	Hearse *et al.* (1969)
Cyclohexylphenyl 2-sulphate		R	gluc.	Hearse *et al.* (1969)
Prontosil	D	R	*N*-gluc.	Gingell *et al.* (1971)
Phenmetrazine	D	R	gluc.	Franklin *et al.* (1977)
Phenytoin	C	R	gluc.	El-Hawari and Plaa (1978)
3-Phenoxybenzoic acid	P	R	gluc.	Huckle *et al.* (1981)

Compound				
Warfarin	D	R	*O*-gluc. sulphate	Remmel *et al.* (1981)
Phenacetin	D	R	gluc.	Smith and Griffiths (1978)
Acetaminophen	D	M	glut.	Wong *et al.* (1981)
N,N-Di(2-chloroethyl)aniline	C	R	*O*-gluc.	Chipman *et al.* (1980)
Digitoxin		R		Volp and Lage (1978)
Mestranol	D	R	*O*-gluc.	Brewster *et al.* (1976) Löffler and Bolt (1980)
N-2-Fluorenylacetamide	C	R	*O*-gluc. sulphate	Grantham *et al.* (1970) Williams *et al.* (1970) King and Shayman (1974)
4-Acetylaminobiphenyl	C	R	*O*-gluc.	Wheeler *et al.* (1975)
Ethinyloestradiol	D	R,H	*O*-gluc. sulphate	Back *et al* (1978) Löffler and Bolt (1980) Maggs *et al.* (1983)
Phenylhydantoin	C	R	*O*-gluc.	El-Hawari and Plaa (1976)
Phenolphthalein	D	R	*O*-gluc.	Hirom *et al.* (1975)
Buprenorphine	D	R	gluc.	Brewster *et al.* (1981)
Carbenoxolone	D	R	*O*-gluc. sulphate	Iveson *et al.* (1971)
Methamphetamine	D	R	*O*-gluc.	Sakai *et al.* (1982)
4-Amino-2-(4-butanoyl-hexahydro-lH-1,4-diazepin-l-yl)-6,7-dimethoxyquinazoline HC1	D	R,Rb,H	*O*-gluc. *N*-gluc.	Yamato *et al.* (1982)
Lysergic acid	D	R	*O*-gluc.	Parker *et al.* (1980)
Diphenylacetic acid		R	aryl gluc.	Parker *et al.* (1980)
2-Nitrotoluene	C	R	*O*-gluc. glut.	Chism and Rickert (1985)
Carbofuran	P	R	gluc. sulphate	Marshall and Dorough (1979)
O-{3-[4-(2-Methoxyphenyl)-1-piperazinyl]-2-hydroxypropyl}-3-methoxybenzaldoxim dihydrochloride	D	R	*O*-gluc.	Illing and House (1981)

Cont'd

Table 4.1 *(Continued)*

Xenobiotic	Compound[a] type	Animal[b] species	Biliary[c] conjugate hydrolysed	Reference
4,4′-Dihydroxydiphenyl-(pyridyl-2)-methane	D	R	sulphate	Forth *et al.* (1972)
Valproic acid		R	acyl gluc.	Dickinson *et al* (1985)
Indomethacin	D	R,G,D,M	gluc.	Hucker *et al.* (1966)
2,4′,5-Trichlorobiphenyl		R	glut., merc., cys.-gluc., cys.-gly.	Bakke *et al.* (1982)
Bis-Methylthiotetrachloro-benzene	P	R	cysteine merc., cys.gly.	Bakke (1983)
3,5-Dibutyl-4-hydroxytoluene		R,M	gluc. merc.	Daniel *et al.* (1968)
Desacetylbisacodyl		R	gluc.	Vogt *et al.* (1965)
Glutethimide	D	D	gluc.	Keberle *et al.* (1962)
Nitropyrene	C	R	gluc. glut.	Morotomi *et al.* (1985) Medinsky *et al.* (1985)
Aflatoxin B$_1$	C	R	glut.	Degen and Neumann (1978) Wei *et al.* (1981)
Estrone	D	R	*O*-gluc. sulphate	Sim and Back (1985)
Estriol	D	R	gluc.	Tikkanen *et al.* (1973)
3-(4-Chlorophenyl)-thiazolo(3,2a)benzimidazole-2-acetic acid (Wy-18,251)	D	R	gluc.	Ruelius *et al.* (1985)

5H-Dibenzo(a,d)cyclohepten-5-ylidene (Wy-41,770)	D	R	gluc.	Ruelius *et al.* (1985)
3,3′-Dimethoxybenzidine	C	R	*N*-gluc.	Rodgers *et al.* (1983)
Diclofenac		R,D,M	ester gluc.	Stierlin and Faigle (1979)
Δ¹-tetrahydrocannabinol		R	gluc.	Widman *et al.* (1974)
Propachlor	P	R	ox-merc.	Larsen and Bakke (1981)
			glut.	Larsen and Bakke (1983)
			cyst.	
			gluc.	
2,6-Dinitrotoluene	C	R	gluc.	Long and Rickert (1982)
Oxyphenisatin	D	R	sulphate	Sund *et al.* (1979)
Safrole	C	R	glut.	Benedetti *et al.* (1977)
			gluc.	Fennel *et al.* (1984)
			merc.	
Benzidine	C	R	gluc.	Lynn *et al.* (1984)
			glut.	Frederick *et al.* (1985)
N-Hydroxy-*N*-2-fluorenylacetamide	C	R	gluc.	Weisburger *et al.* (1970)
Iopanoyl				
	D	D	gluc.	Goldberg *et al.* (1977)
				Thoeni *et al.* (1978)
Diflunisal	D	R	gluc.	Lin *et al.* (1985)
Benzo[a]pyrene	C	R	sulphate	Boroujerdi *et al.* (1981)
			gluc.	Chipman *et al.* (1981a,b)
Benzo[a]pyrene-4,5-epoxide	C	R	gluc.	Elmhirst *et al.* (1985)
			glut.	
Fenclofenac	D	B,M,R,GP,Rb	gluc.	Greenslade *et al.* (1980)
Naphthalene		R	glut.	Pue *et al.* (1982)
		R	gluc.	Bakke *et al.* (1983)
9-Hydroxy-9,10-dihydro-10-cysteinyl phenanthrene		R	merc.	Struble *et al.* (1986)
Naphthalene acetic acid	P	R	gluc.	Lethco and Brouwer (1966)
Pentachloromethylthiobenzene		R	merc.	Bakke *et al.* (1981a)

Cont'd

Table 4.1 (*continued*)

Xenobiotic	Compound[a] type	Animal[b] species	Biliary[c] conjugate hydrolysed	Reference
Carbaryl	P	R	gluc.	Struble *et al.* (1983a,b)
(Chloromethyl)thiazole	D	R	merc.	Bakke *et al.* (1981c)
			gluc. methylmercapto	Rafter and Bakke (1982)
Pentachloronitrobenzene	P	G,S	gluc. merc.	Aschbacher and Feil (1983)
Norethisterone	D	R	gluc.	Back *et al.* (1978, 1980)
Fluphenazine	D	D,M	gluc.	Dreyfuss *et al.* (1971)

[a] The compound types are P, pesticide; D, drug; C, carcinogen.
[b] The animal species are R, rat; M, monkey; H, human; Rb, rabbit, D, dog, G, goat; B, baboon, GP, guinea pig; and S, sheep.
[c] The biliary conjugates hydrolysed are gluc., glucuronide; glut., glutathione; ox-merc., *S*-oxide of the mercapturate; and merc., mercapturate.

populations in the small intestine, have higher levels of β-glucuronidase in these contents than man, rabbit and guinea pig (Hawksworth *et al.*, 1971). In the rat and mouse, therefore, xenobiotic glucuronides can undergo hydrolysis in the small intestine with subsequent enterohepatic circulation.

Mammalian β-glucuronidase (pH optimum 4.0–5.5) is present in small intestinal tissue and contents. Compared to rat caecal contents, the levels of β-glucuronidase in small intestinal contents, mucosa and wall were 3, 16 and 32%, respectively (Rod and Midtvedt, 1977). In the germ-free (GF) rat, levels of β-glucuronidase (pH optimum 4.5) exist in the contents of the small intestine and this activity decreases slightly from the small to the large intestine. In contrast, the conventional rat has β-glucuronidase activity in small intestinal contents similar to the GF rat, but this activity increases dramatically from the small intestine to the caecum (96.8% less). In addition, the pH optimum of the enzyme in the caecal contents is 6.5 in the conventional rat. The ratio of bacterial enzyme in the caecal contents to the mammalian enzyme in caecal mucosa at pH 6.5 is 24 : 1 (Rod and Midtvedt, 1977). Because the enzyme is found in lower quantity in the small intestine contents and limited hydrolysis of xenobiotic glucuronides occur in germ-free and antibiotic treated rats, the contribution of mammalian β-glucuronidase is considered to be low.

β-glucuronidase has been studied in *Escherichia coli* (Buehlar *et al.*, 1951). Mono-infection of germ-free rats with *E. coli* restored caecal β-glucuronidase to levels comparable to those found in the caecum of conventional rats while *Streptococcus pyrogenes* restored caecal β-glucuronidase to only 10% of that in conventional rats (Rod and Midtvedt, 1977). β-glucuronidase has been detected in strict-anaerobic strains of the intestinal bacteria of the genera *Peptostreptococcus*, *Corynebacterium*, *Propionibacterium*, *Bacteroides*, *Clostridium*, *Catenabacterium*, *Bifidobacterium*, *Streptococcus*, and *Lactobacillus* and the family of Enterobacteriaceae (Hawksworth *et al.*, 1971; Kent *et al.*, 1972). Recent *in vivo* studies with gnotobiotic rats have shown that β-glucuronidase was present in strains of the following intestinal bacteria: *Clostridium*, *Peptostreptococcus*, *Staphylococcus*, *Streptococcus*, *Escherichia*, and *Lactobacillus* (Gadelle *et al.*, 1985; Cole *et al.*, 1985). Two β-glucuronidases (β-gluc. I and β-gluc. II) have been isolated and characterized from the intestinal anaerobe *Clostridium perfringens*. β-gluc. I had a pH optimum of 7.2, pH stability below 7.0, and a molecular weight of 115 000. β-Gluc. II had a pH optimum of 6.0, pH stability at around 6.0, and a molecular weight of 195 000. The enzymes hydrolysed *p*-nitrophenylglucuronide, naphthol AS-B1 glucuronide and phenophthalein glucuronide (Sakaguchi and Murata, 1984). The specificity of the bacterial β-glucuronidase has not been extensively studied; however, it is clear from the diverse group of xenobiotics hydrolysed (Table 4.1) that the β-glucuronidases in the gut are not highly substrate specific. It would be of interest to determine if these β-glucuronidases can hydrolyse the C-glucuronide of Δ^6-tetrahydro-cannibinol which has been found in mouse liver (Levy *et al.*, 1978). Acyl glucuronides of valproic acids (glucuronidase-resistant glucuronides) are hydrolysed by esterases present throughout the GI tract, although these esterases were found to be most abundant in the caecum (Dickinson *et al.*, 1985).

Induction of β-glucuronidase was demonstrated with glucuronide conjugates and bile flow. Exclusion of bile dramatically lowers levels of β-glucuronidase in the rat caecum (Robertson *et al.*, 1982). Further, in a continuous-flow culture system of rat caecal bacteria, the bile acids chenodeoxycholic, cholic acid and substrate (p-nitrophenyl-β-D-glucuron-ide) increased β-glucuronidase levels (Mallett *et al.*, 1983). Matsushiro (1965) identified glucaro-1,4-lactone in human bile as the factor responsible for inhibition of bacterial β-glucuronidase by bile. Such an inhibitor in bile may help explain the low levels of β-glucuronidase activity in the small intestine.

2. *Toxic Consequences of Glucuronide Hydrolysis*

Notable examples of β-glucuronidase hydrolysis of toxic xenobiotic glucuronides in the GI tract are diethylstilboestrol (DES), benzo[a]pyrene, dinitropyrene (DNP) and chloroamphenicol (CP). DES was one of the first compounds demonstrated to undergo enterohepatic circulation. DES, a carcinogen, is excreted in the bile as a glucuronide conjugate which was hydrolysed in the GI tract (Fischer *et al.*, 1966). The β-glucuronidase activity was of bacterial origin because neomycin sulphate reduced the amount of DES-glucuronide hydrolysis 50-fold (Clark *et al.*, 1969).

Benzo[a]pyrene [b(a)p] is a ubiquitous environmental carcinogen. Renwick and Drasar (1976) found that biliary metabolites of b(a)p are hydrolysed to b(a)p diols and b(a)p by the intestinal bacteria. Regeneration of the original polyunsaturated hydrocarbon in the GI tract is important because b(a)p binds to DNA in colonic tissue [10-position of b(a)p and 2-amino groups of guanine] (Autrup *et al.*, 1978). Additionally, b(a)p is metabolized in the rat and excreted in the bile as the glucuronide (34–38% of the dose) and sulphate ester (9% of the dose, Boroujerdi *et al.*, 1981; Chipman *et al.*, 1981a,b). Kinoshita and Gelboin (1978) have shown that a DNA-bound derivative was produced by β-glucuronidase hydrolysis of b(a)p-3-glucuronide and this binding did not involve 3-hydroxy-b(a)p.

Such binding to genetic material of b(a)p during β-glucuronidase hydrolysis of b(a)p-glucuronide may initiate carcinogenesis, one of the three conditions conducive for the occurrence of chemical carcinogenesis (Farber, 1983). The other two conditions, proliferating cells and promotion of cancerous growth, also exist within the gut. Cell proliferation is a natural process in the gastro-intestinal tract because the mucosal cells are some of the fastest growing cells in the body: they are constantly dividing to replace cells sloughed off into the intestinal lumen. Tumours may be promoted in the gut by neutral steroids, bile acids and their bacterial metabolites (Narisawa *et al.*, 1974; Kelsey, 1983) or by b(a)p itself (Gelboin, 1980). Thus the conditions are present for b(a)p to cause cancer in the lower GI tract, which may explain the higher incidence of colon cancer in industrialized countries. Further, bile from rats or rabbits dosed with b(a)p is mutagenic to *Salmonella typhimurium* (Ames test) when β-glucuronidase is present (Connor *et al.*, 1979; Forti and Trieff, 1980; Chipman *et al.*, 1983; Kari *et al.*, 1984). Results reported by Ben-Itzhak *et al.* (1985) using a bioluminescence test (BLT) for genotoxic compounds verify these reports. Bile from b(a)p perfused rat liver showed no genotoxicity when β-glucuronidase and aryl sulphatase enzymes were not present in the BLT, however, with their presence, the genotoxicity levels increased 100-fold. Similar results have been reported for the carcinogen *N*-2-fluorenylacetamide (Grantham *et al.*, 1970; Williams *et al.*, 1970; King and Shayman, 1974).

Chloramphenicol was one of the earliest compounds reported to undergo enterohepatic circulation. Chloramphenicol is excreted in the bile of rats as a glucuronic acid conjugate. The glucuronide of chloramphenicol is hydrolysed by β-glucuronidase in the lower gut and the aglycone is subsequently reduced in the caecum to an aryl amine (Glazko *et al.*, 1949, 1952). This aryl amine is absorbed and subsequently undergoes enterohepatic circulation which causes a toxic effect on the thyroid gland (Thompson *et al.*, 1954). A similar mechanism is thought to occur in the metabolism of the carcinogen dinitrotoluene. 2,6-dinitrotoluene (2,6-DNT) is excreted as 2,6-dinitrobenzylalcohol glucuronide in perfused rat liver at a 3.6–8.6-fold higher level in male than female rats. A twofold greater level of covalent binding of 2,6-DNT to hepatic macromolecules in male versus female rat livers was observed (Long and Soyka, 1975). 2,4-dinitrotoluene-induced DNA repair requires the presence of the intestinal microflora (Mirsalis *et al.*, 1982), with a peak of DNA-repair activity 12 hours after dosing (Mirsalis and Butterworth, 1981). This lag period is consistent with excretion of 2,4-DNT conjugates in the bile, hydrolysis, reduction and enterohepatic circulation. Again, the protein binding and DNA damage caused by dinitrotoluene metabolites in the gut, which require the presence of intestinal flora, could initiate chemical carcinogenesis. Consistent with these observations is the tenfold increase in mutagenicity of the biliary metabolites of benzidine (an aromatic amine) in the Ames test when β-glucuronidase was present in the test (Lynn *et al.*, 1984).

C. Sulphate Esters

Less information is present in the literature on sulphatase hydrolysis of sulphate esters of xenobiotics. Endogenous sulphate esters are hydrolysed in the GI tract by sulphatases of bacterial origin (Eriksson, 1971; Eriksson and Gustafsson, 1970; Cowen *et al.*, 1975; Strand and Scheline, 1975; Sim and Back, 1985). Laxative sulphate esters [sulphate ester of 4,4′-dihydroxydiphenyl-(pyridyl-2)-methane (Forth *et al.*, 1972), sulisatin (Moreto *et al.*, 1977) and oxyphenisatin (Sund *et al.*, 1979)] are more effective, presumably because they are not effectively absorbed from the small intestine, and thus proceed to the large bowel where bacterial sulphatases hydrolyse the ester. Release of the laxative in the large bowel allows its pharmacological action to occur. Iodothyronine sulphate is hydrolysed in the intestinal tract of the rat by the anaerobic bacteria of the genera *Lactobacillus* and probably *Eubacterium* or *Lachrospira* (de Herder *et al.*, 1985). Aryl sulphatase has been detected in the strict anaerobes of the *Clostridium* genus (Huijghebaert *et al.*, 1982). The specificity of these bacterial sulphatases is broad, as indicated by the various sulphate esters that undergo hydrolysis in the GI tract (see Table 4.1). Some endogenous substrates, such as oestriol, are excreted as double conjugates (i.e. glucuronide and sulphate ester, oestriol-3-sulphate-16-glucuronate (Levitz and Katz, 1968). Deconjugation by β-glucuronidase in the small intestine results in a sulphate ester of lower molecular weight which may be absorbed intact with other sulphate esters excreted in the bile (Fries *et al.*, 1967; Denner *et al.*, 1969; Hearse *et al.*, 1969; Eriksson, 1971; Taylor *et al.*, 1978; Schwenk *et al.*, 1981). Oestrone sulphate is absorbed intact from the small intestine loops of rats (17% in 30 minutes (Schwenk *et al.*, 1981)) and is thought to undergo further metabolism, including hydrolysis in the liver.

Sulphate esters are excreted in the bile of rats treated with the carcinogens *N*-2-fluorenylacetamide and benzo(a)pyrene. These conjugates are hydrolysed in the lower GI tract and undergo enterohepatic circulation (Grantham *et al.*, 1970; Boroujerdi *et al.*, 1981). As described earlier, b(a)p is metabolized and excreted in rat bile as the b(a)p-sulphate (9% of dose). No mutagenicity was observed in the bile from rats treated with b(a)p and tested in the Ames test in the presence of aryl sulphatase, and this indicated that the sulphate ester does not contribute to mutagenicity of b(a)p on hydrolysis. With N-2-fluorenylacetamide, the mutagenicity of the sulphate ester is important because the N-sulphate ester of N-hydroxy-2-acetylaminofluorene (N-sulphoxy-2-aminofluorene) has been reported to be the ultimate carcinogenic metabolite in the livers of infant male mice (Lai *et al.*, 1985).

D. Cysteine Conjugate β-lyase

1. *Activity and Distribution*

Recently, a bacterial cysteine conjugate β-lyase has been shown to be a key enzyme in a pathway which results in the introduction of a thiol-, methylthio-, methylsulphinyl-, or methylsulphonyl- moiety into a xenobiotic. The sulphur in these groups originate from mammalian-xenobiotic mercapturic acid synthesis (mercapturic acid pathway, MAP) as shown in Fig. 4.1 (Larsen and Bakke, 1978, 1983; Bakke *et al.*, 1981b; Suzuki *et al.*, 1982; Tomisawa *et al.*, 1984; Larsen, 1985; Larsen and Stevens, 1985). Sulphur is introduced from glutathione at electrophilic centres in xenobiotics by glutathione-S-transferase. Xenobiotic glutathione conjugates are extensively excreted in the bile. The glutathione conjugates undergo degradation by γ-glutamyl transpeptidase and carboxypeptidase, which sequentially hydrolyse glutamic acid and glycine moieties, respectively, from the glutathione conjugates forming cysteine conjugates. γ-glutamyl transpeptidase is present in liver (Tanaka, 1974), bile (Rosalki, 1975) and jejunum microvilli (Kozak and Tate, 1982). A similar enzyme, γ-glutamyl cyclotransferase, is present in liver (Orlowski and Meister, 1973). Carboxypeptidase has been isolated and purified from pancreatic tissue (Marinkovic *et al.*, 1977) and has been detected in sheep small intestinal tissue (Ben-Ghedalia *et al.*, 1974). Similar glycine hydrolysing enzymes, aminopeptidase M and dipeptidase, are present in jejunum microvilli (Kozak and Tate, 1982). Because these mammalian enzymes are present in liver, bile, and upper small intestine, xenobiotic glutathione conjugates excreted from the liver with the bile are believed to undergo these reactions as they move through the small intestine. As a result, they reach the microflora as their respective cysteine conjugates. When propachlor was given as an oral dose to bile duct cannulated rats, the glutathione conjugate was the major metabolite excreted in the bile (Larsen and Bakke, 1981). The glutathione conjugate of propachlor is hydrolysed to the cysteine conjugate by the contents of the small intestine of pig or rat (Larsen and Bakke, 1983). Further, when propachlor was given as an oral dose, the cysteine, *N*-acetyl cysteine, and *S*-oxide of the *N*-acetyl cysteine conjugates were the only metabolites excreted with the faeces in germ-free rats (Bakke *et al.*, 1980).

The cysteine-, *N*-acetyl cysteine- and the *S*-oxide of the *N*-acetyl cysteine-conjugates of xenobiotics are also extensively excreted in the bile. The *S*-oxide of the *N*-acetyl cysteine conjugate of propachlor has been shown to undergo both reduction to a thio ether and *N*-deacetylation when incubated with pig caecal contents. The sequence of these reactions is not known. The *N*-acetyl cysteine conjugate of propachlor also undergoes *N*-deacetylation when incubated with pig caecal contents (Larsen and Bakke, 1983). In both cases, reduction and deacetylation in the caecum results in formation of the cysteine conjugate (Fig. 4.1).

Cysteine conjugates of xenobiotics present in the small intestinal tract from metabolism of MAP metabolites or biliary excretion can proceed by two routes. First, the cysteine conjugate may be absorbed intact and undergo enterohepatic circulation (Bakke *et al.*, 1981b). This occurs extensively in the metabolism of the cysteine conjugate of naphthalene (Bakke *et al.*, 1983). Secondly, the cysteine conjugate may pass on to areas in the GI tract that contain β-lyase activity where it is converted to its corresponding thiol. β-Lyases have been associated with intestinal bacteria (Saari and Schultze, 1965; Nishizuka, 1971; Bakke *et al.*, 1981b; Suzuki *et al.*, 1982). The caecum and large intestinal tract in the pig and rat contain extensive β-lyase activity of bacterial origin (Larsen and Bakke, 1983). Cysteine conjugate β-lyase has been isolated and characterized from the following bacteria: *Fusobacterium necrophorum* (Larsen *et al.*, 1983), *Fusobacterium varium* (Tomisawa *et al.*, 1984) and *Eubacterium limosum* (Larsen and Stevens, 1985). β-lyases isolated from *F. necrophorum*, *F. varium*, and *E. limosum* cleaved 2-*S*-cysteinyl-*N*-isopropyl-acetanilide (cysteine conjugate of propachlor), the cysteine conjugate of *p*-bromobenzene, and *S*-benzyl-L-cysteine, respectively, to their corresponding thiol, pyruvate and ammonia, in stoichiometric quantities characteristic of a β-lyase. These β-lyases also cleave a broad spectrum of *S*-alkyl- and *S*-aryl-L-cysteine conjugates. The β-lyase from *E. limosum* cleaved a number of other β-substituted alanines and naturally occurring compounds which can be considered derivatives of cysteine. One naturally occurring substrate, cystathione, was cleaved by the *E. limosum* β-lyase, indicating that it contains cystathionase activity (Larsen and Stevens, 1985). Although mammalian β-lyases are present, they do not metabolize the cysteine conjugate of propachlor or some *S*-alkyl- and *S*-aryl-L-cysteine conjugates (Stevens and Jakoby, 1983). Thus, the formation of a wide variety of novel thiol-containing metabolites probably depends on these bacterial β-lyases, in agreement with the *in vivo* work of Bakke *et al.* (1981b).

The β-lyases isolated from *E. limosum*, *F. necrophorum* and *F. varium* have different physical characteristics. For example, β-lyase from *F. necrophorum* and *F. varium* have molecular weights of 228 000 and 70 000, respectively, require pyridoxal 5-phosphate for stability and do not cleave cystathionine. β-Lyase from *E. limosum* is stable in the absence of pyridoxal 5-phosphate and is a dimeric protein composed of two subunits of about 38 000 molecular weight each. All three bacterial β-lyases have pH optimums of 7.8–8.0.

A general distribution of β-lyase activity in the intestinal bacteria was observed because 27 of 43 of the intestinal bacteria tested contained β-lyase activity (Larsen, 1985). Only in the genus *Fusobacterium* did all the species tested contain β-lyase activity. The β-lyases usually had higher specific activities for *S*-alkyl-linked cysteine conjugates. Notable exceptions were β-lyases isolated from *E. tenue* and *F. nucleatum*. The β-lyase isolated from *E. limosum* had at least 16-fold higher specific activity than β-lyase isolated from other gastro-intestinal bacteria. In addition, β-lyase was found in mixed populations of bacteria isolated from rat and chicken caeca (Table 4.2). β-lyase isolated from these sources catalysed the cleavage of *S*-aryl- and/or *S*-alkyl-L-cysteine conjugates of xenobiotics.

In the same study, β-lyases isolated from mammalian tissue cleaved only the *S*-aryl linked substrate [*S*-(2-benzathiazolyl)cysteine] and had lower specific activity levels (i.e. rat liver, 14-fold; rat intestinal mucosa, 60-fold) than the intestinal bacteria (Larsen, 1985).

Polynuclear aromatic hydrocarbons (PAH) are extensively oxidized to epoxides which subsequently are conjugated with glutathione and excreted in the bile as MAP metabolites. Studies by Bakke *et al.* (1983) and Struble *et al.* (1986) have shown that naphthalene and phenanthrene, respectively, follow this pathway. In addition to β-lyase formation of PAH thiols, two other processes occur which produce naphthols, naphthalene and phenanthrenols and phenanthrene. The first process, formation of phenols, is mediated by the intestinal flora and is dependent on their presence in the gut. The second process involves unstable MAP metabolites of naphthalene and phenanthrene which undergo a nonenzymatic decomposition. These two processes appear to occur with other MAP metabolites of PAH; the 4,5-oxide of b(a)p is excreted in the bile as a glutathione conjugate (Elmhirst *et al.*, 1985), and, as indicated earlier, Renwick and Drasar (1976) observed that b(a)p was formed when bile containing a b(a)p metabolite was incubated with intestinal microflora.

Aflatoxin B_1 (AFB_1) may also be metabolized by this pathway. The glutathione conjugate of AFB_1 has been found in rat bile (Degen and Neumann, 1978) and when rat-urinary AFB_1 conjugates were incubated

Table 4.2 *Distribution of cysteine conjugate β-lyase in homogenates of intestinal bacteria (from Larsen, 1985)*

Bacteria	Substrate (sp. activity, nmol/min per mg)	
	2-S-cysteinyl-N-isopropylacetanilide	S-(2-benzothiazolyl)cysteine
Bacteriodes		
bivius	—[b]	—
disiens	—	N.D.[b]
eggerthii	1.8	N.D.
fragilis	4.0	N.D.
furcosus	7.2	2.2
hypermegas	10.6	N.D.
multiacidus	—	—
uniformis	1.2	—
vulgatus	—	—
Bifidobacterium adolescentis	—	N.D.
Clostridium ramosum	7.2	N.D.
Coprococcus		
catus	—	—
comes	5.2	—
cutactus	3.3	N.D.
Escherichia coli		
(anaerobic)	—	—
(aerobic)	—	N.D.
Eubacterium		
aerofaciens	8.4	N.D.
biforme	—	N.D.
contortum	15.8	—
cylindroides	8.2	N.D.
dolicum	—	—
formicigenerans	—	—
hadrum	—	N.D.
limosum	256	69.4

Cont'd

with rat caecal microflora they appeared to be converted to metabolites believed to be AFB_1 and aflatoxin P_1 (Wei *et al.*, 1981).

2. Toxic Consequences of Bacterial β-lyase Activity

Thiols are generated by the microflora β-lyase cleavage of xenobiotic cysteine conjugates in the gut and are generally considered to be

Table 4.2 *(Continued)*

Bacteria	Substrate (sp. activity, nmol/min per mg)	
	2-*S*-cysteinyl-*N*-isopropylacetanilide	*S*-(2-benzothiazolyl)cysteine
ramulus	—	N.D.
siraeum	—	—
tenue	4.2	29.0
tortuosum	2.6	N.D.
ventriosum	2.0	N.D.
Fusobacterium		
naviforme	7.6	2.9
necrogenes	4.8	0.6
necrophorum	6.6	6.7
nucleatum	11.2	65.2
plauti	12.4	*N.D.*
varium	19.6	*N.D.*
Lactobacillus		
acidophilus	—	—
plantarium	—	N.D.
Megasphaera elsdenii	4.2	2.6
Peptostreptococcus productus	11.3	N.D.
Propionibacterium acnes	—	N.D.
Selenomonas ruminantium	—	—
Streptococcus faecalis		
(anaerobic)	11.3	1.1
(aerobic)	8.7	N.D.
Ruminococcus		
obeum	—	N.D.
torques	—	N.D.
Rat-caecal bacteria	24.7	0.8
Chicken-caecal bacteria	5.4	N.D.

[a] N.D., not determined.
[b] —, not detected.

toxic (Evans, 1967). The cysteine conjugates of hexachlorobutadiene, trichloroethylene and perchloroethylene were mutagenic in the Ames test when the rat kidney S9 fraction was present (Green and Odum, 1985). Because metabolic cofactors were not required, the activation was thought to be due to β-lyase. Rankin *et al.* (1986) reported that inhibition of β-lyase by (aminooxy)acetic acid reduced renal toxicity of *N*-(3,5-dichlorophenyl)succinimide. They suggest that the ultimate toxic metabolite is generated by action of β-lyase on a cysteine conjugate of

N-(3,5-dichlorophenyl)succinimide. Although mammalian β-lyase was used in these studies, the results suggest that mutagenic and toxic metabolites (thiols) are generated in the GI tract by bacterial β-lyase cleavage of xenobiotic cysteine conjugates. Other studies have shown catabolism of some MAP metabolites to be mutagenic, and nephrotoxic (Rannug *et al.*, 1978; Green *et al.*, 1983).

The thiols formed by β-lyase cleavage may proceed by two pathways. First, they can be absorbed by the intestinal mucosa where they are methylated or conjugated with glucuronic acid, or second, they can bind to macromolecules and form bound residues (Bakke *et al.*, 1980; Bakke, 1983). Methylation is thought to occur in the intestinal mucosa because no S-methyl transferase activity is present in the intestinal contents or in 43 individual intestinal bacteria tested (bacteria listed in Table 4.2), but was detected in the intestinal mucosa, liver and kidney (Weisiger *et al.*, 1980; Larsen, 1985). S-Glucuronides can undergo enterohepatic circulation during which the thiols are regenerated by the intestinal glucuronidases.

The methylthio (CH_3S-) containing metabolites can be oxidized in the liver or possibly in the intestinal mucosa to methylsulphinyl (CH_3SO-) and methylsulphonyl (CH_3SO_2-) containing metabolites. These metabolites represent only a transient detoxication, because they would be slightly more polar than the parent xenobiotic resulting in rapid absorption from the GI tract. They also would have new physical and chemical characteristics which not only add to the detoxication burden of the animal but also to subsequent compartments in the environment.

Furthermore, methylthio groups have recently been shown to undergo a glutathione-mediated turnover in two metabolites of hexachlorobenzene—pentachlorothioanisole and *bis*-methylthiotetrachlorobenzene (Bakke, 1983; Mulford *et al.*, 1986). These studies reported that in rats over 50% of the original methyl groups in pentachlorothioanisole were excreted as CO_2 and methane sulphinic acid and the process involved at least two passes in enterohepatic circulation. The data indicated that methylsulphonyl may be a good leaving group for reconjugation with glutathione and would continually generate new thiols in the GI tract on each pass of enterohepatic circulation. This turnover would prolong the residence time and increase the detoxication burden of these compounds in the body. Methylsulphonyl-containing metabolites of polychlorinated biphenyls have been shown to persist in lung tissue (Bakke *et al.*, 1982).

The β-lyase mediated formation of methylthio-containing xenobiotic metabolites, excreted in the urine and faeces, has been shown to function *in vivo* (Fig. 4.1). Bakke and Gustafsson (1984) have listed 32 xenobiotics of various structures which are metabolized to methylthio-containing metabolites, most of which are also metabolized by the MAP pathway. An alternative pathway for methylthio formation has been proposed from isolation of methylsulphides of 2-acetylacetaminofluorene isolated after alkaline hydrolysis of proteins from livers of rats dosed with 2-acetylaminofluorene (DeBaun *et al.*, 1970). Thus, isolation of methylthio-containing metabolites probably indicates that a xenobiotic is metabolized by the MAP pathway.

The other route thiols can take after β-lyase cleavage is formation of nonextractable faecal residues (Bakke *et al.*, 1980; Larsen and Bakke, 1983). This formation of nonextractable residues may result from the reaction of the xenobiotic thiols with endogenous thiols to form disulphides or from other known reactions thiols undergo which result in covalent bond formation. Chemical bonding of this type may cause binding of the xenobiotic to tissue macromolecules and consequently initiate chemical carcinogenesis.

E. Conclusions

Deconjugation of biliary metabolites by β-glucuronidase, sulphatase and β-lyase and their subsequent enterohepatic circulation has been discussed. A number of toxic or carcinogenic compounds, as well as numerous drugs, pesticides and endogenous compounds, are deconjugated by these enzymes. In general, these enzymes have been shown by *in vivo* and *in vitro* data to be primarily of microbial origin, to be present in the lower GI tract in relatively high levels, and hydrolyse or cleave a variety of xenobiotic conjugates (Table 4.1). In contrast, the levels of these enzymes in mammalian tissue or of mammalian origin in the GI tract appear to be low or nonexistent.

Regeneration of b(a)p, naphthalene and phenanthrene in the GI tract is significant because in the case of b(a)p a carcinogenic compound is formed in the GI tract and regenerated xenobiotics can be absorbed into the tissues where reactive intermediates can be formed. In addition, deconjugation of biliary metabolites by β-glucuronidase and β-lyase has been shown to produce mutagenic compounds in the Ames test.

The β-lyase pathway involves a number of enzymes of both bacterial and mammalian origin which may reverse the detoxication of the MAP. The glutathione degrading enzymes, γ-glutamyl transpeptidase and carboxypeptidase, are thought to be of mammalian origin, and inhibition of either of these enzymes would block β-lyase cleavage. The enteric β-lyase is considered to be the key enzyme in this pathway, because its action results in the introduction of sulphur in the form of a thiol-, methylthio-, methylsulphinyl- or methylsulphonyl- group into the xenobiotic, and MAP metabolites have been shown to produce metabolites which are of toxicological importance. This process may be regarded as a pathway involving metabolic activation by microfloral β-lyase. Methylation of thiol containing xenobiotics likely occurs in the intestinal mucosa with subsequent oxidation of these methylthio groups to methylsulphinyl and methylsulphonyl moieties probably occurring in the liver. β-glucuronidase, sulphatase, and β-lyase alter the chemical and physical properties of the xenobiotic conjugate however, because as thiols are chemically and biologically more reactive than alcohols, the β-lyase has the potential of producing a more reactive product in the GI tract. Further, the formation of this new xenobiotic increases the burden of detoxication on the animal.

A number of factors show that deconjugation of these xenobiotic conjugates and their subsequent enterohepatic circulation are relevant to humans. First, data on drug metabolism (Table 4.1) and endogenous compounds show that both biliary glucuronides and sulphate esters undergo hydrolysis and enterohepatic circulation in humans, as well as in other animal species. Second, the same bacteria containing these enzyme systems can be isolated from the GI tracts of humans and various other species of animals. Finally, β-lyase activity has been detected in mixed populations of bacteria isolated from the caeca of pig, rat (Larsen, 1985) and chicken (Bakke and Larsen, 1985) which would indicate the β-lyase would likely to be found in bacteria inhabiting the lower bowel of humans.

References

Aschbacher, P. W. and Feil, V. J. (1983). Metabolism of pentachloronitrobenzene by goats and sheep. *J. Agr. Food Chem.* **31**, 1150–1158.

Autrup, H., Harris, C. C., Trump, B. F. and Jeffrey, A. M. (1978). Metabolism of benzo(a)pyrene and identification of the major benzo(a)pyrene – DNA adducts in cultured human colon. *Cancer Res.* **38**, 3689–3696.

Back, D. J., Breckenridge, A. M., Challiner, M., Crawford, F. E., Orme, M. L. E., Rowe, P. H. and Smith, E. (1978). The effect of antibiotics on the enterohepatic circulation of ethinylestradiol and norethisterone in the rat. *J. Steroid Biochem.* **9**, 527–531.

Back, D. J., Breckenridge, A. M., Crawford, F. E., Cross, K. J., Orme, M. L. E., Percival, A. and Rowe, P. H. (1980). Reduction of the enterohepatic circulation of norethisterone by antibiotics in the rat: correlation with changes in the gut flora. *J. Steroid Biochem.* **13**, 95–100.

Bakke, J. E. (1983). Metabolism of Bis-methylthiotetrachlorobenzene in rats. *Chemosphere* **12**, 793–798.

Bakke, J. E., Aschbacher, P. W., Feil, V. J. and Gustafsson, B. E. (1981a). The metabolism of pentachloromethylthiobenzene in germ-free and conventional rats. *Xenobiotica* **11**, 173–178.

Bakke, J. E., Bergman, Å. L. and Larsen, G. L. (1982). Metabolism of 2,4′,5-trichlorobiphenyl by the mercapturic acid pathway. *Science* **217**, 645–647.

Bakke, J. E. and Gustafsson, J. -Å. (1984). Mercapturic acid pathway metabolites of xenobiotics: generation of potentially toxic metabolites during enterohepatic circulation. *TIPS* **5**, 517–521.

Bakke, J. E., Gustafsson, J. -Å. and Gustafsson, B. E. (1980). Metabolism of propachlor by the germfree rat. *Science* **210**, 433–435.

Bakke, J. E. and Larsen, G. L. (1985). Metabolism of 2-chloro-*N*-isopropylacetanilide in chickens. *Chemosphere* **14**, 1749–1754.

Bakke, J. E., Larsen, G. L., Aschbacher, P. W., Rafter, J. J., Gustafsson, J. -Å. and Gustafsson, B. E. (1981b). Role of gut microflora in metabolism of glutathione conjugates of xenobiotics. *In*: "Sulfur in Pesticide Action and Metabolism" (eds J. D. Rosen, P. S. Magee and J. E. Casida), pp. 165–178. American Chemical Society Symposium Series No. 158, Washington, DC.

Bakke, J. E., Rafter, J. J., Lindeskog, P., Feil, V. J., Gustafsson, J. -Å. and Gustafsson, B. E. (1981c). Metabolism of 2-acetamido-4-(chloromethyl)-thiazole in germfree and conventional rats. *Biochem. Pharmacol.* **30**, 1839–1844.

Bakke, J., Struble, C., Gustafsson, J. -Å. and Gustafsson, B. (1983). Enterohepatic circulation and catabolism of mercapturic acid pathway metabolites of naphthalene. *In*: "Extrahepatic Drug Metabolism and Chemical Carcinogenesis" (eds J. Rydström, J. Montelius and M. Bengtsson), pp. 257–266. Elsevier Science Publishers B.V., Amsterdam.

Benedetti, M. S., Malnöe, A. and Broillet, A. L. (1977). Absorption, metabolism and excretion of safrole in the rat and man. *Toxicology* **7**, 69–83.

Ben-Ghedalia, D., Tagari, H. and Bondi, A. (1974). Protein digestion in the intestine of sheep. *Br. J. Nutr.* **31**, 125–142.

Ben-Itzhak, J., Levi, Ben-Zion, Shor, R., Lanir, A., Bassan, H. M. and Witzur, S. (1985). The formation of genotoxic metabolites of benzo[a]pyrene by the isolated perfused rat liver, as detected by the bioluminescence test. *Mutation Res.* **147**, 107–112.

Boroujerdi, M., Kung, H., Wilson, A. G. E. and Anderson, M. W. (1981). Metabolism and DNA binding of benzo(a)pyrene *in vivo* in the rat. *Cancer Res.* **41**, 951–957.

Brewster, D., Humphrey, M. J. and McLeavy, M. A. (1981). Biliary excretion, metabolism and enterohepatic circulation of Buprenorphine. *Xenobiotica* **11**, 189–196.

Brewster, D., Jones, R. S. and Symons, A. M. (1976). Biliary excretion of Mestranol in the female rat: effect of neomycin pretreatment on enterohepatic recirculation. *Biochem. Soc. Trans.* **4**, 516–518.

Buehlar, H. J., Katzmann, P. A. and Doisy, E. A. (1951). Studies on β-glucuronidase from *E. Coli. Proc. Soc. Exp. Biol.* **76**, 672–676.

Chipman, J. K., Frost, G. S., Hirom, P. C. and Millburn, P. (1981a). Biliary excretion, systemic availability and reactivity of metabolites following intraportal infusion of [³H]benzo[a]pyrene in the rat. *Carcinogenesis* **2**, 741–745.

Chipman, J. K., Hirom, P. C., Frost, G. S. and Millburn, P. (1981b). The biliary excretion and enterohepatic circulation of benzo(a)pyrene and its metabolites in the rat. *Biochem. Pharmacol.* **30**, 937–944.

Chipman, J. K., Hirom, P. C. and Millburn, P. (1980). Biliary excretion and enterohepatic circulation of aniline mustard metabolites in the rat and the rabbit. *Biochem. Pharmacol.* **29**, 1299–1301.

Chipman, J. K., Millburn, P. and Brooks, T. M. (1983). Mutagenicity and *in vivo* disposition of biliary metabolites of benzo(a)pyrene. *Toxicol. Lett.* **17**, 233–240.

Chism, J. P. and Rickert, D. E. (1985). Isomer- and sex-specific bioactivation of mononitrotoluenes. Role of enterohepatic circulation. *Drug Metab. Dispos.* **13**, 651–657.

Clark, A. G., Fischer, L. J., Millburn, P., Smith, R. L. and Williams, R. T. (1969). The role of gut flora in the enterohepatic circulation of stilboestrol in the rat. *Biochem. J.* **112**, 17–18.

Cole, C. B., Fuller, R., Mallet, A. K. and Rowland, I. R. (1985). The influence of the host on expression of intestinal microbial enzyme activities involved in metabolism of foreign compounds. *J. Appl. Bact.* **59**, 549–553.

Connor, T. H., Forti, G., Sitra, P. and Legator, M. S. (1979). Bile as a source of mutagenic metabolites produced *in vivo* and detected by *Salmonella typhimurium. Environ. Mutagenesis* **1**, 269–276.

Cowen, A. E., Korman, M. G., Hofman, A. F. and Cass, O. W. (1975). Metabolism of lithocholate in healthy man. I. Biotransformation and biliary excretion of intravenously administered lithocholate, lithocholylglycine, and their sulfates. *Gastroenterol.* **69**, 59–66.

Daniel, J. W., Gage, J. C. and Jones, D.I. (1968). The metabolism of 3,5-Di-tert.-butyl-4-hydroxytoluene in the rat and in man. *Biochem. J.* **106**, 783–790.

DeBaun, J. R., Miller, E. C. and Miller, J. A. (1970). *N*-Hydroxy-2-acetylamino-fluorene sulfotransferase: Its probable role in carcinogenesis and in protein-(methyl-*S*-yl) binding in rat liver. *Cancer Res.* **30**, 577–595.

Degen, G. H. and Neumann, H. (1978). The major metabolite of Aflatoxin B$_1$ in the rat is a glutathione conjugate. *Chem. -Biol. Interact.* **22**, 239–255.

de Herder, W. W., Hazenberg, M. P., Otten, M. H., Pennock-Schröder, A. M. and Visser, T. J. (1985). Hydrolysis of iodothyronine sulfates by sulfatase activity of anaerobic bacteria from the rat intestinal tract. *FEMS Microbiol. Lett.* **27**, 79–83.

Denner, W. H. B., Olavesen, A. H., Powell, G. M. and Dodgson, K. S. (1969). The metabolism of potassium dodecyl [^{35}S]-sulfate in the rat. *Biochem. J.* **111**, 43–51.

Dickinson, R. G. Eadie, M. J. and Hooper, W. D. (1985). Glucuronidase-resistant glucuronides of valproic acid: consequences to enterohepatic recirculation of valproate in the rat. *Biochem. Pharmacol.* **34**, 407–408.

Dixon, P. A. F. and Caldwell, J. (1978). The fate of dichlorophen in the rat. *Eur. J. Drug Metab. Pharmacokin.* **3**, 95–98.

Dreyfuss, J., Ross, J. J. Jr. and Schreiber, E. C. (1971). Biological disposition and metabolic fate of fluphenazine-^{14}C in the dog and Rhesus monkey. *J. Pharmac. Sci.* **60**, 821–825.

El-Hawari, A. M. and Plaa, G. L. (1976). The role of the enterohepatic circulation in the disposition of diphenylhydantoin (DPH). *Proc. Can. Fed. Biol. Soc.* **19**, 45.

El-Hawari, A. M. and Plaa, G. L. (1978). Role of the enterohepatic circulation in the elimination of phenytoin in the rat. *Drug Metab.Dispos.* **6**, 59–69.

Elmhirst, T. R. D., Chipman, J. K., Ribeiro, O., Hirom, P. C. and Millburn, P. (1985). Metabolism and enterohepatic circulation of benzo(a)pyrene-4,5-epoxide in the rat. *Xenobiotica* **15**, 899–906.

Eriksson, H. (1971). Absorption and enterohepatic circulation of neutral steroids in the rat. *Eur. J. Biochem.* **19**, 416–423.

Eriksson, H. and Gustafsson, J. -Å. (1970). Steroids in germfree and conventional rats sulpho- and glucuronohydrolase activities of caecal contents from conventional rats. *Eur. J. Biochem.* **13**, 198–202.

Evans, C. L. (1967). The toxicity of hydrogen sulphide and other sulphides. *Q. J. Exp. Physiol.* **53**, 231–248.

Farber, E. (1983). Initiation of carcinogenesis with chemicals – A biological perspective. "Extrahepatic Drug Metabolism and Chemical Carcinogenesis", Abstract No. L2, 16, May 17–20. Stockholm.

Fennell, T. R., Miller, J. A. and Miller, E. C. (1984). Characterization of the biliary and urinary glutathione and acetylcysteine metabolites of the hepatic carcinogen hydroxysafrole and its 1'-Oxo metabolite in rats and mice. *Cancer Res.* **44**, 3231–3240.

Finegold, S. M., Flora, P. J., Atterbery, H. R. and Sutter, V. L. (1975). Fecal bacteriology of colonic polyp patients and control patients. *Cancer Res.* **35**, 3407–3417.

Fischer, L. J., Millburn, P., Smith, R. L. and Williams, R. T. (1966). The fate of ^{14}C-stilboestrol in the rat. *Biochem. J.* **100**, 69–72.

Forth, W., Nell, G., Rummel, W. and Andres, H. (1972). The hydragogue and laxative effect of the sulfuric acid ester and the free diphenol of 4,4'-dihydroxy-diphenyl-(pyridyl-2)-methane. *Naunyn-Schmiedeberg's Arch. Pharmacol.* **274**, 46–53.

Forti, G. C. and Trieff, N. H. (1980). Kinetics of uptake and biliary excretion of benzo(a)pyrene and mutagenic metabolites in isolated perfused rat liver, *Teratogen. Carcinogen. Mutagen.* **1**, 269–282.

Franklin, R. B., Dring, L. G. and Williams, R. T. (1977). The metabolism of phenmetrazine in man and laboratory animals. *Drug Metab. Dispos.* **5**, 223–233.

Frederick, C. B., Weis, C. C., Flammang, T. J., Martin, C. N. and Kadlubar, F. F. (1985). Hepatic N-oxidation, acetyl-transfer and DNA-binding of the acetylated metabolites of the carcinogen, benzidine. *Carcinogenesis* **6**, 959–965.

Fries, N., Knapstein, P., Wendlberger, F. and Oertel, G. W. (1967). Enterohepatischer Kresilauf Von C_{19}-Steroiden V: Resorption und reconjugation Von 7α-^{3}H-DHEA-^{35}S-Sulfat im Dünndarmdes menschen *in vivo*. *Acta Endocrinol.* **56**, 705–712.

Gadelle, D., Raibaud, P. and Sacquet, E. (1985). β-Glucuronidase activities of intestinal bacteria determined both *in vitro* and *in vivo* in gnotobiotic rats. *Appl. Environ. Microbiol.* **49**, 682–685.

Gelboin, H. V. (1980). Benzo[a]pyrene metabolism, activation and carcinogenesis: role and regulation of mixed-function oxidases and related enzymes. *Physiol. Reviews* **60**, 1107–1166.

Gingell, R., Bridges, J. W. and Williams, R. T. (1971). The role of the gut flora in the metabolism of prontosil and neoprontosil in the rat. *Xenobiotica* **1**, 143–156.

Glazko, A. J., Dill, W. A. and Wolf, L. M. (1952). Observations on the metabolic disposition of chloramphenicol (chloromycetin) in the rat. *J. Pharmacol. Exper. Therap.* **104**, 452.

Glazko, A. J., Wolf, L. M., Dill, W. A. and Bratton, A. C. Jr. (1949). Biochemical studies on chloramphenicol (chloromycetin). II. Tissue distribution and excretion studies. *J. Pharmacol. Exper. Therap.* **96**, 445–449.

Goldberg, H. I., Lin, S. K., Thoeni, R., Moss, A. A. and Brito, A. (1977). Recirculation of iopanoic acid after conjugation in the liver. *Invest. Radiol.* **12**, 537–541.

Goldman, P. (1978). Biochemical pharmacology of the intestinal flora. *Ann. Rev. Pharmacol. Toxicol.* **18**, 523–539.

Grantham, P. H., Horton, R. E., Weisburger, E. K. and Weisburger, J. H. (1970). Metabolism of the carcinogen N-2-fluorenylacetamide in germ-free and conventional rats. *Biochem. Pharmacol.* **19**, 163–171.

Green, T., Nash, J. A., Odum, J. and Howard, E.G. (1983). The renal metabolism of a glutathione conjugate of the carcinogen hexachloro-1,3-butadiene: evidence for the formation of a mutagenic metabolite in the rat kidney. "Extrahepatic Drug Metabolism and Chemical Carcinogenesis Meeting," Abstract No. B.23, 126, May 17–20. Stockholm.

Green, T. and Odum, J. (1985). Structure/activity studies of the nephrotoxic and mutagenic action of cysteine conjugate of chloro- and fluoroalkenes. *Chem-Biol. Interact.* **54**, 15–31.

Greenslade, D., Havler, M. E., Humphrey, M. J., Jordan, B. J. and Rance, M. J. (1980). Species differences in the metabolism and excretion of fenclofenac. *Xenobiotica* **10**, 753–760.

Hanahan, D. J., Daskalakis, E. G., Edwards, T. and Dauben Jr., H. P. (1953). The metabolic pattern of C^{14}-diethylstilbestrol. *Endocrinology* **53**, 163–170.

Hawksworth, G., Drasar, B. S. and Hill, M. J. (1971). Intestinal bacteria and the hydrolysis of glycosidic bonds. *J. Med. Microbiol.* **4**, 451–459.

Hearse, D. J., Powell, G. M., Olavesen, A. H. and Dodgson, K. S. (1969). The influence of some physico-chemical factors on the biliary excretion of a series of structurally related aryl sulphate esters. *Biochem. Pharmacol.* **18**, 181–195.

Hiles, R. A., Caudill, D., Birch, C. G. and Eichhold, T. (1978). The metabolism and disposition of 3,4,4'-trichlorocarbanilide in the intact and bile duct-cannulated adult and in the newborn Rhesus monkey (M. mulatta). *Toxicol. appl. Pharmacol.* **46**, 593–608.

Hirom, P. C., Millburn, P. and Parker, R. J. (1975). The enterohepatic circulation of ³H-phenolphthalein in the rat. *Br. J. Pharmacol.* **56**, 355–356.

Hucker, H. B., Zacchei, A. G., Cox, S. V., Brodie, D. A. and Cantwell, N. H. R. (1966). Studies on the absorption, distribution and excretion of indomethacin in various species. *J. Pharmacol. Exp. Therap.* **153**, 237–249.

Huckle, K. R., Chipman, J. K., Hutson, D. H. and Millburn, P. (1981). Metabolism of 3-phenoxybenzoic acid and the enterohepatorenal disposition of its metabolites in the rat. *Drug Metab. Dispos.* **9**, 360–368.

Huijghebaert, S. M., Mertens, J. A. and Eissen, H. J. (1982). Isolation of a bile salt sulfatase-producing *Clostridium* strain from rat intestinal microflora. *Appl. Environ. Microbiol.* **43**, 185–192.

Illing, H. P. A. and House, E. S. A. (1981). Enterohepatic circulation in rat and dog of ¹⁴C-O-[3-(4-<2-methoxyphenyl>-1-piperazinyl)-2-hydroxypropyl]-3-methoxy-benzaldoxim dihydrochloride and its demethylated metabolite. *Eur. J. Drug Metab. Pharmacokin.* **6**, 303–312.

Iveson, P., Lindup, W. E., Parke, D. V. and Williams, R. T. (1971). The metabolism of carbenoxolone in the rat. *Xenobiotica* **1**, 79–95.

Kari, F. W., Kauffman, F. C. and Thurman, R. G. (1984). Characterization of mutagenic glucuronide formation from benzo(a)pyrene in the nonrecirculating perfused rat liver. *Cancer. Res.* **44**, 5073–5078.

Keberle, H., Hoffmann, K. and Bernhard, K. (1962). The metabolism of glutethimide (doriden). *Experientia* **15**, 105–111.

Kelsey, M. I. (1983). *In vitro* effect of bile acids. *In*: "Experimental Colon Carcinogenesis" (eds M. Autrup and G. M. Williams), p. 241. CRC Press, Boca Raton, FL.

Kent, T. H., Fischer, L. J. and Marr, R. (1972). Glucuronidase activity in intestinal contents of rat and man and relationship to bacterial flora (36510). *Proc. Soc. Exp. Biol. Med.* **140**, 590–594.

King, C. M. and Shayman, M. A. (1974). Reaction *in vivo* of N-hydroxy-2-fluorenylacetamide (N-hydroxy-FAA) with RNA and DNA of gastrointestinal tract and liver of the rat. *Proc. Am. Assoc. Canc. Res.* **15**, 42.

Kinoshita, N. and Gelboin, H. V. (1978). β-Glucuronidase catalyzed hydrolysis of benzo(a)pyrene-3-glucuronide and binding to DNA. *Science* **199**, 307–309.

Klaassen, C. D. (1971). Biliary excretion of barbiturates. *Br. J. Pharmac.* **43**, 161–166.

Kozak, E. M. and Tate, S. S. (1982). Glutathione-degrading enzymes of microvillus membranes. *J. Biol. Chem.* **257**, 6322–6327.

Lai, C. C., Miller, J. A., Miller, E. C. and Liem, A. (1985). *N*-Sulfoöxy-2-aminofluorene is the major ultimate electrophilic and carcinogenic metabolite of *N*-hydroxy-2-acetylaminofluorene in the livers of male C57BL/6J × C3H/HeJF$_1$ (B6C3F$_1$) mice. *Carcinogenesis* **6**, 1037–1045.

Larsen, G. L. (1985). Distribution of cysteine conjugate β-lyase in gastrointestinal bacteria and in the environment. *Xenobiotica* **15**, 199–209.

Larsen, G. L. and Bakke, J. E. (1978). Studies on the origin of the methylsulfonyl-containing metabolites from propachlor. *J. Environ. Sci. Health B* **5**, 495–504.

Larsen, G. L. and Bakke, J. E. (1981). Enterohepatic circulation in formation of propachlor (2-chloro-*N*-isopropylacetanilide) metabolites in the rat. *Xenobiotica* **11**, 473–480.

Larsen, G. L. and Bakke, J. E. (1983). Metabolism of mercapturic acid-pathway metabolites of 2-chloro-*N*-isopropylacetanilide (propachlor) by gastrointestinal bacterial. *Xenobiotica* **13**, 115–126.

Larsen, G. L., Larson, J. D. and Gustaffson, J. -Å. (1983). Cysteine conjugate β-lyase in the gastrointestinal bacterium *Fusobacterium necrophorum*. *Xenobiotica* **13**, 689–700.

Larsen, G. L. and Stevens, J. L. (1985). Cysteine conjugate β-lyase in the gastrointestinal bacterium *Eubacterium limosum*. *Mol. Pharmacol.* **29**, 97–103.

La Russo, N. F., Lindmark, D. G. and Müller, M. (1978). Biliary and renal excretion, hepatic metabolism, and hepatic subcellular distribution of metronidazole in the rat. *Biochem. Pharmacol.* **27**, 2247–2254.

Layiwola, P. J., Linnecar, D. F. C. and Knights, B. (1983). Hydrolysis of the biliary glucuronic acid conjugate of phenol by the intestinal mucus/flora of goldfish (*Carassius auratus*). *Xenobiotica* **13**, 27–29.

Lethco, E. J. and Brouwer, E. A. (1966). The metabolism of naphthaleneacetic acid-l-C^{14} in rats. *J. Agr. Food Chem.* **14**, 532–535.

Levitz, M. and Katz, J. (1968). Enterohepatic metabolism of estriol-3-sulfate-16-glucosiduronate in women. *J. Clin. Endocrinol. Metab.* **28**, 862–868.

Levy, S., Yagen, B. and Mechoulam, R. (1978). Identification of a C-glucuronide of Δ^6-tetrahydrocannabiol as a mouse liver conjugate *in vivo*. *Science* **23**, 1391–1392.

Lin, J. H., Yeh, K. C. and Duggan, D.E. (1985). Effect of enterohepatic circulation on the pharmacokinetics of diflunisal in rats. *Drug Metab. Dispos.* **13**, 321–326.

Löffler, V. S. and Bolt, H. M. (1980). Unterschungen zum enterohepatischen kreislauf von östradiol und Äthinylöstradiolbei der Ratte. *Arzneim.-Forsch.* **30**, 810–813.

Long, R. J. and Soyka, L. F. (1975). Biliary excretion and enterohepatic circulation of pregnanolone in the rat. *Biochem. Pharmacol.* **24**, 1067–1072.

Long, R. M. and Rickert, D. E. (1982). Metabolism and excretion of 2,6-dinitro[^{14}C]toluene *in vivo* and in isolated perfused rat livers. *Drug Metab. Dispos.* **10**, 455–458.

Lynn, R. K., Garvie-Gould, C. T., Milam, F., Scott, K. F., Eastman, C. L., Ilias, A. M. and Rodgers, R. M. (1984). Disposition of the aromatic amine, benzidine, in the rat: characterization of mutagenic urinary and biliary metabolites. *Toxicol. Appl. Pharmacol.* **72**, 1–14.

Maggs, J. L., Grabowski, P. S. and Park, B. K. (1983). The enterohepatic circulation of the metabolites of 17α-ethynyl [^{3}H]estradiol in the rat. *Xenobiotica* **13**, 619–626.

Mallett, A. K., Bearne, C. A. and Rowland, I. R. (1983). Metabolic activity and enzyme induction in rat fecal microflora maintained in continuous culture. *Appl. Environ. Microbiol.* **46**, 591–595.

Marinkovic, D. V., Marinkovic, J. N., Erdös, E. G. and Robinson, C. J. G. (1977). Purification of carboxypeptidase β from human pancreas. *Biochem. J.* **163**, 253–260.

Marselos, M., Dutton, G. and Hänninen, O. (1975). Evidence that D-glucaro-1,4-lactone shortens the pharmacological action of drugs being disposed via the bile as glucuronides. *Biochem. Pharmacol.* **24**, 1855–1858.

Marsh, C. A., Alexander, F. and Levvy, G. A. (1953). Glucuronide decomposition in the digestive tract. *Nature* **170**, 163.

Marshall, T. C. and Dorough, H. W. (1979). Biliary excretion of carbamate insecticides in the rat. *Pestic. Biochem. Physiol.* **11**, 56–63.

Matsushiro, T. (1965). Identification of glucaro-1,4-lactone in bile as a factor responsible for inhibitory effect of bile on bacterial β-glucuronidase. *Tohoku, J. exp. Med.* **85**, 330–339.

Medinsky, M. A., Shelton, H., Bond, J. A. and McClellan, R. O. (1985). Biliary excretion and enterohepatic circulation of l-nitropyrene metabolites in Fischer-344 rats. *Biochem. Pharmacol.* **34**, 2325–2330.

Mirsalis, J. C. and Butterworth, B. E. (1981). Induction of DNA repair in hepatocytes from rats treated *in vivo* with dinitrotoluene. *Environ. Mutagen* **3**, 316.

Mirsalis, J. C., Hamm, T. E. Jr., Sherrill, J. M. and Butterworth, B.E. (1982). Role of gut flora in the genotoxicity of dinitrotoluene. *Nature* **295**, 322–323.

Moreto, M., Goñalons, E., Mylonakis, N., Giraldez, A. and Torralba, A. (1977). Enterohepatic circulation of sodium sulisatin and its effects on glucose absorption in the rat. *J. Pharm. Pharmac.* **29**, 446–448.

Morotomi, M., Nanno, M., Watanabe, T., Sakurai, T. and Mutai, M. (1985). Mutagenic activation of biliary metabolites of l-nitropyrene by intestinal microflora. *Mutation Res.* **149**, 171–178.

Mulford, D. J., Bakke, J. E., Feil, V. J. and Bergman. Ă. (1986). Methylthioturnover in the metabolism of chlorinated thioanisoles by rats. 191st ACS National Meeting, New York City, NY Abst. No. 37, "Agrochemicals".

Narisawa, T., Magadia, N. E., Weisburger, J. M. and Wynder, E. L. (1974). Promoting effect of bile acids on colon carcinogenesis after intrarectal instillation of N-methyl-N^1-nitro-N-nitrosoguanidine in rats. *J. Natl. Cancer Inst.* **53**, 1093–1097.

Nishizuka, Y. (1971). *S*-Alkyl-*L*-cysteine lyase (*pseudomonas*). *In*: "Methods in Enzymology" (eds S. P. Colowick and N. D. Kaplan), Vol XVIIB, pp. 470–474. Academic Press.

Orlowski, M. and Meister, A. (1973). γ-Glutamyl cyclotransferase distribution, isozymic forms, and specificity. *J. Biol. Chem.* **248**, 2836–2844.

Parker, R. J., Hirom, P. C. and Millburn, P. (1980). Enterohepatic recycling of phenolphthalein, morphine, lysergic acid diethylamide (LSD) and diphenyl acetic acid in the rat. Hydrolysis of glucuronic acid conjugates in the gut lumen. *Xenobiotica* **10**, 689–703.

Pue, M. A., Frost, G. S. and Hirom, P. C. (1982). The enterohepatic circulation of a glutathione conjugate of naphthalene in the rat. *Biochem. Soc. Trans.* **10**, 112 (Abstract).

Rafter, J. J. and Bakke, J. E. (1982). Biliary metabolites of the anti-inflammatory drug 2-acetamido-4-(chloromethyl)thiazole. *Drug. Metab. Dispos.* **10**, 654–656.

Rankin, G. O., Teets, V. and Yang, D. (1986). Effect of cysteine conjugate β-lyase inhibition on N-(3,5-dichlorophenyl)succinimide-induced nephrotoxicity in the fischer 344 rat. *Fed. Am. Soc. Exp. Biol.* **45**, 571.

Rannug, U., Sundvall, A. and Ramel, C. (1978). The mutagenic effect of 1,2-dichloroethane on *Salmonella Typhimurium* I. Activation through conjugation with glutathione *in vitro*. *Chem. Biol. Interact.* **20**, 1–16.

Remmel, R. P., Pohl, L. R. and Elmer, G. W. (1981). Influence of the intestinal microflora on the elimination of warfarin in the rat. *Drug Metab. Dispos.* **9**, 410–414.

Renwick, A. G. and Drasar, B. S. (1976). Environmental carcinogens and large bowel cancer. *Nature* **263**, 234–235.

Robertson, A. M., Lee, S. P., Lindop, R., Stanley, R. A., Thomsen, L. and Tasman-Jones, C. (1982). Biliary control of β-glucuronidase activity in the luminal contents of the rat ileum, cecum, and rectum. *Cancer Res.* **42**, 5165–5166.

Rod, T. O. and Midtvedt, T. (1977). Origin of intestinal β-glucuronidase in germfree, mono-contaminated and conventional rats. *Acta path. microbiol. scand. B* **85**, 271–276.

Rodgers, R. M., Garvie-Gould, C., Scott, K. F., Milam, D. F. and Lynn, R. K. (1983). Metabolism, distribution, and excretion of the carcinogenic aromatic amine, 3,3′-dimethoxybenzidine in the rat. Formation of mutagenic urinary and biliary metabolites. *Drug. Metab. Dispos.* **11**, 293–300.

Roerig, D. L., Hasegawa, A. T. and Wang, R. I. H. (1979). Role of enterohepatic circulation in the analgesic action of l-α-acetylmethadol in the rat. *Drug Metab. Dispos.* **7**, 306–309.

Rosalki, S. B. (1975). Gamma-glutamyl transpeptidase. *Ad. Clin. Chem.* **17**, 53–107.

Ruelius, H. W., Young, E. M., Kirkman, S. K., Schillings, R. T., Sisenwine, S. F. and Janssen, F. W. (1985). Biological fate of acyl glucuronides in the rat. The role of rearrangement, intestinal enzymes and reabsorption. *Biochem. Pharmacol.* **34**, 451–452.

Saari, J. C. and Schultze, M. D. (1965). Cleavage of S-(1,2-dichlorovinyl)-L-cysteine by *Escherichia coli* B[1]. *Arch. Biochem. Biophys.* **109**, 595–602.

Sakaguchi, Y. and Murata, K. (1984). β-Glucuronidases of *Clostridium perfringens. Zentralbl Bakeriol. Microbiol. Hygser. A.* **257**, 308–316.

Sakai, T., Niwaguchi, T. and Murata, T. (1982). Distribution and excretion of methamphetamine and its metabolites in rats. I. Time-course of concentrations in blood and bile after oral administration. *Xenobiotica* **12**, 233–239.

Scheline, R. R. (1973). Metabolism of foreign compounds by gastrointestinal microorganisms. *Pharmacol. Rev.* **25**, 451–532.

Schwenk, M., Frank, B., Bolt, H. M. and Winne, D. (1981). Intestinal first-pass effects of estrone sulfate and estrone in the rat. *Arzneim-Forsch./Drug Res.* **31**, 1254–1257.

Sim, S. M. and Back, D. J. (1985). Intestinal absorption of oestrone, oestrone glucuronide and oestrone sulphate in the rat in situ – I. Importance of hydrolytic enzymes on conjugate absorption. *J. Steroid Biochem.* **22**, 781–788.

Smith, G. E. and Griffiths, L. A. (1978). Metabolism of a biliary metabolite of Phenacetin and other acetanilides of the intestinal microflora. *Experimentia* **15**, 418–419.

Stevens, J. and Jakoby, W. B. (1983). Cysteine conjugate β-lyase. *Molec. Pharmacol.* **23**, 761–765.

Stierlin, H. and Faigle, J. W. (1979). Biotransformation of diclofenac sodium (voltaren) in animals and in man. II. Quantitative determination of the unchanged drug and principal phenolic metabolites, in urine and bile. *Xenobiotica* **9**, 611–621.

Strand, L. P. and Scheline, R. R. (1975). The metabolism of vanillin and isovanillin in the rat. *Xenobiotica* **5**, 49–63.

Struble, C. B., Feil, V. J., Pekas, J. C. and Gerst, J. W. (1983a). Biliary secretion of ^{14}C and identification of 5,6-dihydro-5,6-dihydroxycarbaryl glucuronide as a biliary metabolite of [14C] carbaryl in the rat. *Pestic. Biochem. Physiol.* **19**, 85–94.

Struble, C. B., Larsen, G. L., Feil, V. J. and Bakke, J. E. (1986). Metabolism of 9-hydroxy-9,10-dihydro-10-cysteinylphenanthrene in rats. *In*: "Polynuclear Aromatic Hydrocarbons: Chemistry, Characterization and Carcinogenesis"; Proceedings of the 9th International Symposium on Polynuclear Aromatic Hydrocarbons. 893–900. Battelle Press, Columbus, OH.

Struble, C. B., Pekas, J. C. and Gerst, J. W. (1983b). Enterohepatic circulation and biliary secretion of 5,6-dihydro-5,6-dihydroxy[14C]carbaryl glucuronide in the rat. *Pestic. Biochem. Physiol.* **19**, 95–103.

Sund, R. B., Hol, L. and Strobraten, A. (1979). Studies in the rat on the absorption, biliary excretion, laxative action and interference with intestinal transport of some oxyphenisatin derivatives. *Acta Pharmacol. Toxicol.* **44**, 251–259.

Suzuki, S., Tomisawa, H., Ichihara, S., Fukazawa, H. and Tateishi, M. (1982). A C-S bond cleavage enzyme of cysteine conjugates in intestinal microorganisms. *Biochem. Pharmacol.* **31**, 2137–2140.

Tanaka, M. (1974). A histochemical study on the activity of gamma-glutamyl transpeptidase in liver disease. *Acta. Path. Jap.* **24**, 651–665.

Taylor, A. J., Powell, G. M., Howes, D., Black, J. G. and Olavesen, A. H. (1978). Metabolism of the surfactants sodium undecyltriethoxy sulfate and sodium dodecyltriethoxy sulfate in the rat. *Biochem. J.* **174**, 405–412.

Thoeni, R. F., Goldberg, H. I., Moss, A. A., Lin, S. K. and Brito, A. C. (1978). Observation on the metabolism of iopanoyl (telepaque) glucuronide in dogs treated with antibiotics. *Investigative Rad.* **13**, 241–246.

Thompson, R. Q., Sturtevant, M., Bird, O. D. and Glazko, A. J. (1954). The effect of metabolites of chloramphenicol (chloromycetin) on the thyroid of the rat. *Endocrinology* **55**, 665–681.

Tikkanen, M. J., Pulkkinen, M. O. and Adlercreutz, H. (1973). Effect of ampicillin treatment on the urinary excretion of estriol conjugates in pregnancy. *J. Steroid Biochem.* **4**, 439–440.

Tomisawa, H., Suzuki, S., Ichihara, S., Fukazawa, H. and Tateishi, M. (1984). Purification and characterization of C-S lyase from *Fusobacterium varium*. *J. Biol. Chem.* **259**, 2588–2593.

Vogt, W., Schmidt, G. and Dakhil, T. (1965). Die bedeutung der Glucuronidebildung und-spaltung für das Schicksal von dihydroxy-diphenyl-pyridyl-methan. *Arch. exp. Path. u. Pharmak.* **250**, 488–495.

Volp, R. F. and Lage, G. L. (1978). The fate of a major biliary metabolite of digitoxin in the rat intestine. *Drug Metab. Dispos.* **6**, 418–424.

Walsh, C. T. and Levine, R. R. (1975). Studies of the enterohepatic circulation of morphine in the rat. *J. Pharmacol. Exp. Ther.* **195**, 303–309.

Wei, C., Macy, J. M. and Hsieh, O.P.H. (1981). Biotransformation of Aflatoxin B_1 and its conjugated metabolites by rat gastrointestinal microfloras. *Appl. Environ. Microbiol.* **41**, 549–551.

Weisiger, R. A., Pinkus, L. M. and Jakoby, W. B. (1980). Thiol *S*-methyltransferase: suggested role in detoxication of intestinal hydrogen sulfide. *Biochem. Pharmacol.* **29**, 2885–2887.

Weisburger, J. H., Grantham, P. H., Horton, R. E. and Weisburger, E. K. (1970). Metabolism of the carcinogen N-hydroxy-N-2-fluorenyl-acetamide in germ-free rats. *Biochem. Pharmacol.* **19**, 151–162.

Wheeler, L. A., Soderberg, F. B. and Goldman, P. (1975). The reduction of N-hydroxy-4-acetylaminobiphenyl by the intestinal microflora in the rat. *Cancer Res.* **35**, 2962–2968.

Widman, M., Nordqvist, M., Agurell, S., Lindgren, J. and Sandberg, F. (1974). Biliary excretion of Δ^1-tetrahydrocannabinol and its metabolites in the rat. *Biochem. Pharmacol.* **23**, 1163–1172.

Williams, J. R., Grantham, P. H., Marsh, H. H., Weisburger, J. H. and Weisburger, E. K. (1970). Participation of liver fractions and of intestinal bacteria in the metabolism of *N*-hydroxy-*N*-2-fluorenylacetamide in the rat. *Biochem. Pharmacol.* **19**, 173–188.

Wong, L. T., Whitehouse, L. W., Solomonraj, G. and Paul, C. J. (1981). Pathways of disposition of acetaminophen conjugates in the mouse. *Toxicol. Lett.* **9**, 145–151.

Yamato, C., Takahashi, T., Kinoshita, K. and Fujita, T. (1982). The metabolic fate of 4-amino-2-(4-butanoylhexahydro-1H-1,4-diazepin-1-yl)-6,7′-dimethoxyquinazoline HC1. *Xenobiotica* **12**, 549–559.

5

Hydrolysis of Glycosides and Esters

JOSEPH P. BROWN

A. Introduction

During the past two decades an increasing appreciation has developed for the role of the intestinal microflora in the metabolic transformation of both exogenous and endogenous substances (Williams, 1972; Drasar and Hill, 1974; Scheline, 1973; Goldman, 1978). The intestinal flora in man has been compared to the liver both in size and diversity of its metabolic transformations. The microbial metabolism of substances in the bowel is largely dissimulative and may either complement or counteract hepatic metabolism. In the latter case microbial deconjugation of biliary metabolites (e.g. glucuronides, sulphates and amides) may result in their enterohepatic circulation and delayed excretion. The toxicological consequences of gut microflora metabolism have been reviewed recently (Rowland, 1981; Simon and Gorbach, 1984).

In this chapter I will focus on the role of the intestinal microflora in hydrolysing glycosides and esters and the toxicological implications of such transformations. In general the role of gut flora in carbohydrate catabolism has not been studied in great detail. Studies with germ-free and conventional rats suggest that intestinal glucosidase and disaccharidases are partially inactivated by intestinal microflora. Alternatively the degradation of gastro-intestinal mucins and blood group substances seems almost entirely due to the action of extracellular bacterial enzymes (Hoskins and Boulding, 1981).

Numerous plant glycosides present in man's diet (e.g. the flavonoids, cyanogenic glycosides, amygdalin, cycasin, esculin etc.) are hyrolysed by the intestinal flora releasing various aglycones. The latter may exert important physiological or toxic effects.

While several groups of bacteria (viz., *E. coli*, enterococci, lactobacilli, clostridia, bacteroides and bifidobacteria) possess β-glucosidase activity, the dominant position of lactobacilli, bacteroides and bifidobacteria among the intestinal flora indicates their major role in the intestinal hydrolysis of dietary β-glycosides (Hawksworth *et al.*, 1971).

ROLE OF THE GUT FLORA IN TOXICITY AND CANCER
ISBN 0-12-599920-8

B. Glycosides

1. *Intestinal Microbial Glycosidases*

(a) Mucin degradation. Hoskins and Boulding (1981) have studied glycosidase activities related to mucin degradation in anaerobic cultures derived from human faeces. Intracellular and extracellular activities of four glycosidases were measured with chromogenic p-nitrophenyl glycosides and validated with the release of the corresponding sugars from mucin glycoproteins (Table 5.1). Intracellular β-D-galactosidase, β-N-acetyl-glucosaminidase and sialidase were present in bacteria at all levels of inocula ($\geq 10^{-11}$g). Alternatively extracellular activities were consistently present at levels above 10^{-8}g. Microbial α-L-fucosidase activity was intracellular in all cultures examined. The authors suggest that the degradation of mucin is due to the extracellular glycosidase activities of a relatively minor subpopulation of the intestinal microflora. While the identities of the species involved are unknown, two species, *Ruminococcus torques* and *Bifidobacterium bifidum* are known to ferment porcine gastric mucin and could be present at appropriate concentrations in the lower human bowel.

(b) Laminarin degradation. Salyers *et al.* (1977) have examined the microbial degradation of laminarin, a well characterized β(1→3)-glucan similar to those found in plant and fungal cell walls. Laminarinase [β(1→3) glucanohydrolase, E.C. 3.2.1.6] can possess up to three types of activity: (*i*) β-glucosidase (EC 3.2.1.21) which hydrolyses low molecular weight glucose-containing substrates such as di- and trisaccharides and p-nitrophenyl-β-D-glucosides; (*ii*) exoglucanase that releases single glucose units from the non-reducing end of laminarin; and (*iii*) endoglucanase that releases dimer, trimer or higher β(1→3) oligomers of glucose from laminarin (Chesters and Bull, 1963). In the three species of *Bacteroides* studied, laminarinase activity was induced by laminarin and was predominantly intracellular. β-glucosidase activity was found in all three species and was induced by glucose containing disaccharides as well as by laminarin. The β-glucosidases of the three *Bacteroides* species differed in activity level, induction pattern and sensitivity to inhibition by D-glucono-1,5-lactone. These results contrast with those observed for other micro-organisms where β-D-(1→3) glucanase systems were extracellular and constitutive (Chesters and Bull, 1963). While the species studied represent significant components of the human faecal flora ranging from a low of 1.9% for *B. distasonis* to 8.9% for *B. thetaiotaomicron* (Finegold *et al.*, 1974; Moore and Holdeman, 1974; Holdeman *et al.*, 1976) it is still

somewhat uncertain how significant a role the intracellular laminarinase plays *in vivo* in the degradation of extracellular plant polysaccharides. However the β-D-glucosidase activity of these species is likely to be significant in the hydrolysis of lower molecular weight xenobiotic glycosides in the lower bowel.

Reddy *et al.* (1984) studied the intracellular glycosidases of *Bacteroides ovatus* from the human colon and found that crude hemicellulose, a heteroxylan, induced *in vitro* the formation largely of β-1,4-xylosidase but that significant levels of β-1,4-glucosidase, α-1,4- and α-1,6-gluco-sidases were also found.

2.   *Cycasin and Related Azoxyglycosides*

Studies of the mode of toxic action of cycasin represent an important historical precedent in the subject matter of this chapter. There are, approximately 100 species of cycad plants in nine genera, i.e. *Bowenia, Ceratozamia, Cycas, Dioon, Encephalartos, Microcycas, Macrozamia, Stangeria* and *Zamia*. These species are indigenous to the tropics or subtropics. The major acutely toxic effects resulting from ingestion of the plants are gastro-intestinal and neurologic. Probably the method of preparation of cycads for food use removes the toxic material (Farnsworth *et al.*, 1976) since few toxic effects have been noted in man.

Identification of toxic principles in cycads began in 1941 with the isolation of macrozamin (methyl-ONN-azoxy)methyl-β-D-primveroside from the Australian cycad *Macrozamia spiralis* (Cooper, 1941). Over the next three decades other glycosides of methylazoxymethanol were isolated from cycads and identified, notably: Cycasin, (methyl-ONN-azoxy)methyl-β-D-glucopyranoside (Fig. 5.1); Neocycasin A, (methyl-ONN-azoxy)-methyl-β-laminaribiopyranoside; Neocycasin B, (methyl-ONN-azoxy)-methyl-β-gentiobiopyranoside; Neocycasin C, (methyl-ONN-azoxy)-methyl-β-laminaritetrapyranoside; and Neocycasin E, (methyl-ONN-azoxy)methyl-β-cellobiopyranoside. The first observation bearing on the potential oncogenicity of the azoxyglycosides was that of Laqueur *et al.* (1963) with nuts of *Cycas circinalis* fed to laboratory animals. Subsequent studies showed that seedmeal and husk were also oncogenic in rats and guinea pigs, inducing tumours in liver and/or kidney (Farnesworth *et al.*, 1976). Laqueur *et al.* (1963) proposed that the oncogenic principle was a metabolite of cycasin, namely the aglycone, methylazoxymethanol. This conclusion was based on the fact that the carcinogenicity of cycasin, while readily observed in conventional rats, was lacking in the germ-free rat, even when excessive amounts were fed for periods over two years. Cycasin

Table 5.1 *Glycoside degrading and related activities of mammalian intestinal microflora*

Activity	Substrate	Source	Comment/Product(s)	Reference
β-D-galactosidase	*p*-nitrophenyl glycoside	Human faecal culture	Validation with asialo-α_1-acid glycoprotein	Hoskins and Boulding (1981)
β-*N*-acetylglucosaminidase	"	"	Validation with asialoagalacto-α_1-acid glycoprotein	"
α-L-fucosidase	"	"		"
Sialidase	Serum orosomucoid	"	*N*-acetylneuramimic acid release	"
Laminarinase (exo+endo)	Laminarin	*Bacteroides* spp.	Reducing sugar release	Salyers *et al.* (1977)
β-D-glucosidase	*p*-nitrophenyl glycoside	"	"	"
β-D-xylosidase	"	"	"	Reddy *et al.* (1984)
α-D-glucosidase	"	"	"	"
Dianthrone reductase	Sennoside A	*Clostridium sphenoides*	8-glucosyl rhein anthrone	Kobashi *et al.* (1980)
β-D-glucosidase	8-glucosylrhein anthrone	"	Rhein anthrone, rhein, sennidin	"
α-L-rhamnosidase	Rutin, quercitrin	*Streptococcus faecium* VGH-1, and *Streptococcus* sp. FRP-17	Quercetin and quercetin-3-*O*-β-D-glucoside	Macdonald *et al.* (1984)
β-D-glucosidase	Quercetin 3-*O*-D-glucoside		Quercetin	

β-D-glucosidase	Rutin	*Butyrivibrio fibrisolvens* D1, *Selenommas iruminantium* GA192)	Quercetin	Cheng *et al.* (1969, 1971)
C-ring fission	Rutin	*Peptostreptococcus* sp.	Phenolic acids, etc.	"
	Rutin	*Butyrivibrio* sp. C₃	Phenolic acids, etc.	"
	Quercitrin	"	"	"
	Naringin	"	"	"
β-glycosidase	Hesperidin	"	Hesperetin	"
C-ring fission	Hesperetin	Rat caecal flora	Phenolic acids, etc.	Honohan *et al.* (1976)
β-glycosidase	Apiin	"	Apigenin	Griffiths and Smith (1972a,b)
C-ring fission	Apigenin	"	Phenolic acids	
β-glycosidase and	Myricitrin	"	Phenolic acids	"
C-ring fission	Myricetin	"	Phenolic acids	
β-glucosidase	Stevioside	"	Steviol	Wingard *et al.* (1980)
	Rebaudioside A	"	Steviol	
β-glucosidase	3-phenoxybenzyl glucoside	"	3-phenoxybenzyl alcohol	Mikami *et al.* (1984, 1985)
	3-phenoxybenzyl gentiobioside	"	"	
	3-phenoxybenzyl gentiotrioside	"	"	
	3-phenoxybenzyl glucopyranose	"	3-phenoxybenzoic acid	"
β-glucosidase	Miserotoxin	Sheep and cattle rumin flora	3-nitropropanol	Muir *et al.* (1984)
β-glucosidase	3-hydroxycarbofuran glucoside	Rat caecal flora	3-hydroxycarbofuran	Marshall and Dorough, (1984)

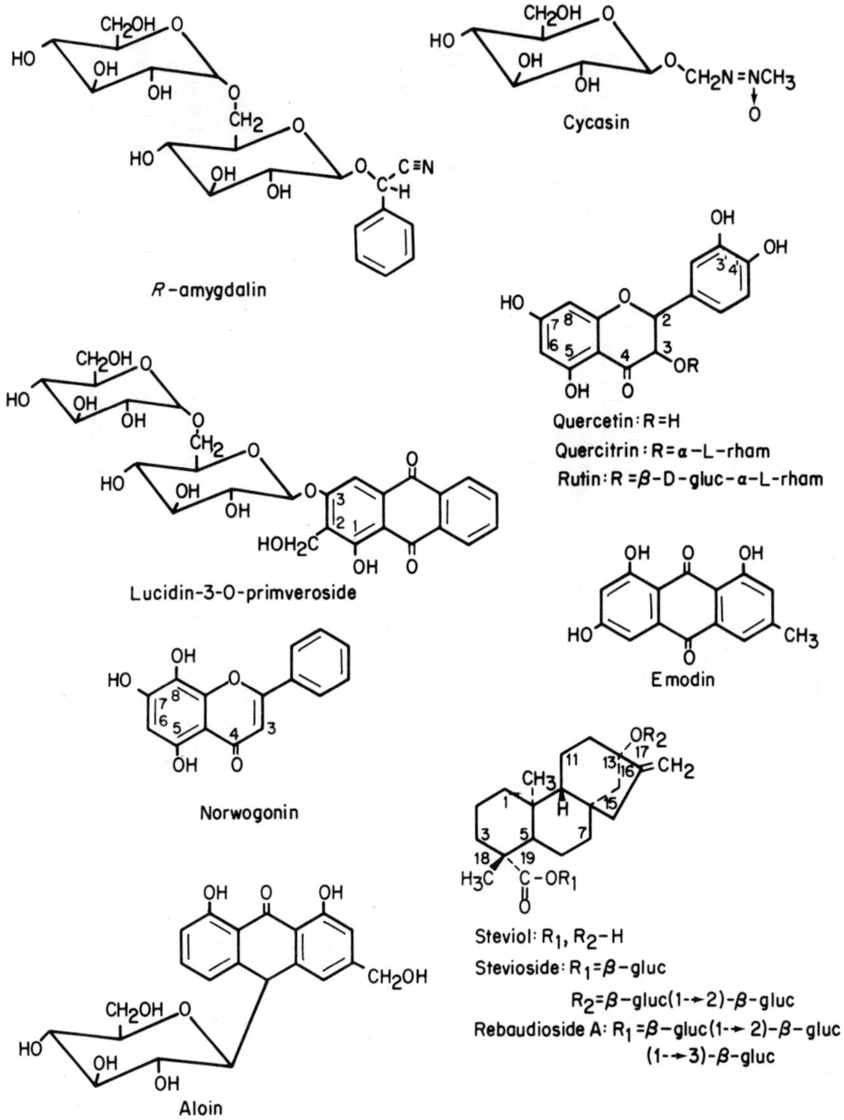

R-amygdalin

Cycasin

Quercetin: R=H
Quercitrin: R=α-L-rham
Rutin: R =β-D-gluc-α-L-rham

Lucidin-3-O-primveroside

Emodin

Norwogonin

Steviol: R$_1$, R$_2$-H
Stevioside: R$_1$=β-gluc
R$_2$=β-gluc(1→2)-β-gluc
Rebaudioside A: R$_1$ =β-gluc(1→ 2)-β-gluc
(1→3)-β-gluc

Aloin

Fig 5.1 Structures of some glycosides.

was found to be nearly quantitatively excreted by germ-free rats (Spatz
et al., 1966) and to be non-toxic when administered parenterally
(Kobayashi and Matsumoto, 1964). Furthermore germ-free rats monoassociated with salicin-fermenting lactobacilli metabolized cycasin, whereas

similar animals associated with non-salicin-fermenting lactobacilli were incapable of cycasin hydrolysis (Spatz *et al.*, 1967). Thus all available evidence supports the idea that intestinal microbial β-glycosidase activities are solely responsible for the hydrolysis of cycasin and presumably related azoxyglycosides.

While cycasin was non-oncogenic in germ-free rats, the aglycone methylazoxymethanol (MAM) and the synthetic methylazoxymethanol acetate (MAM Ac) were highly tumorigenic in these animals. Tumour formation in the lower intestine, liver and kidneys was independent of route of dose administration in germ-free rats. Curiously the tumour incidence in the intestinal tract of conventional rats treated with MAM and was about twice as high as that seen in germ-free animals. This effect has not been fully explained but could result either from physiological and morphological differences between the germ-free and conventional tracts, or perhaps from a microbial role in potentiating or promoting initial mucosal injury caused by exposure to the aglycone (Laqueur *et al.*, 1967).

The fate of the aglycone following hydrolytic release from the glycoside is not certain. Methyl azoxymethanol may spontaneously decompose to reactive methylcarbonium ions in a manner similar to that proposed for activated dimethylnitrosamine. Alternatively enzymatic pyridine nucleotide-dependent oxidation of MAM to a reactive aldehyde form may also be of toxicological significance (Feinberg and Zedeck, 1980). The possibility that another degradation intermediate diazomethane could be involved has also been suggested.

In addition to oncogenicity MAM has demonstrated teratogenicity and a wide range of genotoxic effects. The latter have been reviewed recently by Morgan and Hoffmann (1983). While cycasin is non-mutagenic in the *Salmonella* microsome assay, MAM and enzymatically hydrolysed cycasin (Table 5.2) are directly mutagenic, causing base pair substitutions in strain TA1535 and related strains (Matsushima *et al.*, 1979; Tamura *et al.*, 1980). Other genotoxic effects noted with MAM acetate include: DNA damage in repair assays in *Escherichia coli* and *Bacillus subtilis*; mutation, inter- and intragenic recombination in *Saccharomyces cerevisiae*: sex-linked recessive lethal mutations in *Drosophila melanogaster*; mutations, chromosome aberrations and sister chromatid exchanges in Chinese hamster cells *in vitro*; unscheduled DNA synthesis in HeLa cells, rat hepatocyte cultures, and human skin cultures *in vitro*; and DNA strand breakage in rat liver and other tissues following parenteral administration. A test for morphological sperm abnormalities following parenteral administration of MAM Ac to mice was negative.

Table 5.2 *Plant glycosides hydrolysed by intestinal microflora to mutagens*

Class	Glycoside	Treatment	Aglycone	Gene mutation in *Salmonella*	Reference
Azoxy					
	Cycasin	F	Methylazoxymethanol (MAM)	+	Taumura *et al.* (1980)
	Neocycasin A	F		+	"
	MAM glucosiduronic acid	F		−	"
	Macrozamin	F		−	"
Cyanogenic					
	Amygdalin	[a]	Mandelonitrile	+	Fenselau *et al.* (1977)
Anthraquinone					
	Lucidin 3-*O*-primveroside	C	Lucidin	+	Brown (1980)
	Chrysazin glucoside	C	Chrysazin	+	Brown and Dietrich (1979a)
	Quinizarin glucoside	C	Quinizarin	+	"
	Franguloside	F, C/M	Emodin	+	Tamura *et al.* (1980)
	Alizarin-2-*O*-glucoside	C	Alizarin	+	
	Emodin-1-(8)-*O* glucoside	C	Emodin	+	Brown and Dietrich (1979a)
	Aloin	C/M	Aloe emodin anthrone	−[b]	"

	Compound	Enzyme	Aglycone	Mutagenic	Reference
	Carminic acid	C/M	3,5,6,8-OH, 1-CH$_3$, 2-CO$_2$H AQ	−[b]	"
Flavonol					
	Quercitrin	F, C/M	Quercetin	+	Brown and Dietrich (1979b), Tamura *et al.* (1980)
	Rutin	F, C/M	Quercetin	+	
	Robinin	F, C/M	Kaempferol	+	"
	Isoquercitrin	H	Quercetin	+	Nagao *et al.* (1981)
	Hyperin	H	Quercetin	+	"
	Astragazin	H	Kaempferol	+	"
	Kaempferitrin	H	Kaempferol	+	"
	Tiliroside	H	Kaempferol	+	"
Diterpenoids					
	Stevioside	C	Steviol	+[c]	Wingard *et al.* (1980)
	Rebaudioside A	C	Steviol	+[c]	Pezzuto *et al.* (1985)
Miscellaneous					
	8-hydroxyquinoline glucoside	F/M	8-hydroxyquinoline	+	Tamura *et al.* (1980)

Symbols: F, fecalase; C, cecalase; M, microsomal S9; H, hesperidinase/naringinase

Notes: [a] Aglycone mutagenic but glycoside not tested

[b] No evidence of hydrolysis of C-C bond

[c] Mutagenicity and microbial hydrolysis were done separately.

In addition to indicating a mechanism of oncogenicity, though the molecular details are uncertain, this body of genetic toxicity data may indicate a potential for heritable mutations in man or domestic animals ingesting cycads.

3.   *Cyanogenic Glycosides*

Many plants contain cyanogenic glycosides such as amygdalin (Fig. 5.1) and prunasin, notably certain members of the Rosaceae (e.g. wild cherries, *Prunus* spp.). Exposure to dietary cyanide from ingestion of these plants can result in acute poisoning or chronic neurological disease in domestic animals and in man. For example cassava roots, which are an important staple crop in many tropical countries, contain cyanogenic glycosides which are usually removed by food preparation (soaking, roasting or sun drying) prior to consumption. When the roots are eaten without preparation, which can result from food shortage during a drought, the dietary cyanide intake can be high. Cyanide detoxification is accomplished by enzymatic conversion to thiocyanate, which depends on the availability of sulphur-containing amino acids. Thus deficiency of these amino acids can exacerbate the effects of dietary cyanide exposure resulting in nutritional neuropathies, e.g. spastic paraparesis (Cliff *et al.*, 1985).

The expectation that the intestinal metabolism of cyanogenic glycosides would be similar to that of the azoxyglycosides discussed above is complicated by the finding of neutral $\beta(1{\rightarrow}6)$ and $\beta(1{\rightarrow}1)$ glucosidases in human and animal tissues. Newmark *et al.* (1981) studied the ability of various tissues to hydrolyse the sugar residues from amygdalin (D-mandelonitrile-β-D-gentiobiopyranoside); prunasin (D-mandelonitrile-β-D-glucopyranoside), glucocerebroside and 4-methylumbrelliferyl-β-D-glucopyranoside. Enzymes that catalysed the cleavage of glucose from amygdalin and prunasin were present in the small intestine and intestinal contents and kidneys of germ-free rats. Data obtained with human surgical specimens confirm the localization of these glycosidases in the small intestine. The hydrolysis of gentiobiose was not detected in specimens hydrolysing cyanogenic glucosides, indicating a specificity for aryl and or alkyl glucosides. The biological roles of these mammalian β-glucosidases and their natural substrates are unknown. While it is likely that lower bowel microbial β-glycosidases act on glycosides reaching that point of the intestinal tract, the relative contributions of microbial and host enzymes in the intestinal hydrolysis of cyanogenic glycosides are unknown.

In addition to the metabolic release of cyanide, the aglycone of amygdalin and prunasin, mandelonitrile, has demonstrated mutagenic activity for *Salmonella typhimurium* strains TA98 and TA100 which was enhanced by exogenous microsomal enzymes of rat liver induced by Aroclor. The β-glucoside of mandelonitrile showed mutagenicity only in the presence of Aroclor-induced microsomal fraction. Amygdalin was also found to be mutagenic in host-mediated assays with the same tester strains (Fenselau *et al.*, 1977).

4. *Quinones*

(a) Benzoquinones and naphthoquinones. Certain hydroxybenzoquinones are widely distributed in plants (Myrsinaceae) and have been used for medicinal purposes because of their antihelminthic and purgative properties (Thomson, 1971). Substituted 1,4-naphthoquinones occur in nature as various pigments and K vitamins. Some of these compounds such as lawsone (2-hydroxynaphthoquinone) are used as dye stuffs while others such as juglone (5-hydroxynaphthoquinone), 7-methyljuglone and plumbagin (2-methyl-5-hydroxynaphthoquinone) are used in fold medicines (Thomson, 1971).

Although these quinones have not yet been described as occurring in glycoside form, their phenolic nature and potential genetic toxicity bear mentioning if only to complement the more extensive discussion of the natural anthraquinones below. Tikkanen *et al.* (1983b) studied the mutagenicities of approximately 30 natural and synthetic benzo- and naphthoquinones. None of the 13 benzoquinones tested was mutagenic in *Salmonella typhimurium* strains TA98, TA100 and TA2637, six of the naphthoquinones tested were mutagenic for TA2637 with exogenous activation including plumbagin, juglone and 7-methyljuglone. All the mutagenic napthoquinones contained one or two hydroxyl groups and/or methyl groups.

(b) 9,10-anthraquinones. Derivatives of 9,10-dioxoanthracene, the 9,10-anthraquinones (AQs), represent the largest group of naturally occurring quinones. The majority of these compounds isolated from higher plants and fungi are phenolic (Mathis, 1966). Naturally occurring and synthetic AQs have been used as colorants in foods, drugs, cosmetics, hair dyes and textiles. Certain plant AQ glycosides, particularly those from *Cassia*, *Rhamnus* and *Rheum* spp., traditionally have found use in purgative preparations (Van Os, 1976a).

The hydroxy anthraquinones are mainly distributed among the higher plants and fungi. Aside from rhubarb (*Rheum palmatum*) and possibly *Cassia*, none of the plants would normally be considered edible. As noted above, mixtures of AQs, in plant-derived medicinal preparations have long been employed as laxatives, e.g. sennae folium and sennae fructus (*Cassia augustifolia*), aloe (*Aloe ferox*), frangulae cortex (*Rhamnus frangula*), cascara sagrada (*R. purshiana*) and rhamicatharticae fructus *(R. cathartica)*. The active ingredients in these preparations, such as chrysophanol (1,8-dihydroxy-3-methyl-AQ), aloe-emodin (1,8-dihydroxy-3-hydroxymethyl-AQ), emodin (1,6,8-trihydroxy-3-methyl-AQ; Fig. 5.1) and physcion (1,8-dihydroxy-3-methyl-6-methoxy-AQ), are present as free aglycones, anthrones (9,10-dihydro-AQs), homodianthrones, hetero-dianthrones and also as a variety of *O*- and *C*-glycosides of the oxidized (quinone) forms, or of the reduced monosomers and dimers (Van Os, 1976). The most commonly found sugars are glucose or rhamnose at C-8 or occasionally C-1 in the form of *O*-glycosides. *O*-rhamnose at C-6 and *O*-glucose at C-8 may be found in the same molecule. To date *C*-glycosides have only been observed at the C-10 position.

Data on the metabolic fate of AQs and their glycoside comes mainly from studies on those compounds used therapeutically, such as the natural and synthetic cathartic AQs (Fairbairn, 1976). The mode of action of cathartic AQ glycosides is unknown, although they may act by inhibiting colonic membrane Na^+-K^+ ATPase and causing net movement of H_2O and Na^+ into the intestinal lumen.

If aglycones reach the small intestine, either because they are ingested as such, or are released by acid hydrolysis in the gastric juice, there is a strong possibility that they will be absorbed in a manner similar to other lipophilic substances. The aqueous solubility of the 1,8-dihydroxy-AQs and anthrones is rather low at pH 7.4 (<0.8 mg l^{-1}), whereas carboxylated 1,8-dihydroxy-AQs and anthrones such as rhein (1,8-dihydroxy-3-carboxylate-AQ) are much more water soluble (*c.* 0.5 g l^{-1}) and would be less well absorbed (Breimer and Baars, 1976; Van Os, 1976b). These absorbed phenolic aglycones are glucuronated in the liver, partly excreted in the urine and partly returned to the intestine via the bile. As water soluble glucuronides they eventually reach the colon, where intestinal bacterial action can again release the aglycone. A study of intestinal absorption in rats showed that only 30–40% of an oral dose of 1,8-dihydroxy-AQ (chrysazin, danthron) could be recovered in urine and faeces.

The AQ glycosides, being polar, hydrophilic and of higher molecular weight, are poorly absorbed in the small intestine, and pass directly to the large bowel where bacterial enzymes can release the aglycones.

Kobashi *et al.* (1980) have studied the degradation of sennosides A and B, the isomeric (10–10′) homodianthrone derivatives of rhein 8-*O*-glucoside isolated from the purgatives rhei rhizonia and sennae folium, by human faecal micro-organisms. Three types of activity were observed, namely glucoside hydrolysis, dianthrone reduction and dianthrone isomerization. *Clostridium sphenoides* metabolized sennoside A (10–10′ trans) largely to the aglycone sennidin but via 8-glucosylrhein anthrone and rhein anthrone (i.e. reductive dimer cleavage, glucoside hydrolysis and oxidative dimerization). *Clostridium butyricum* and *Bifidobacterium adolescentis* also possessed β-glucosidase activity and were capable of producing sennidin. A second group of organisms lacked glycosidase activity but could cleave and isomerize the dianthrone glucosides. *Eubacterium rectale*, *E. linosum*, *E. lentum*, *Peptostreptococcus intermedius*, *Clostridium perfringens* and *Lactobacillus brevis* were observed to produce unidentified glycosides, but not sennoside B. Several other faecal organisms investigated had no ability to metabolize sennoside A: *Bacteroides thetaiotaomicron*, *B. vulgatus*, *Bif. longum*, *Bif. bifidum*, *Streptococcus faecalis*, *Peptostreptococcus anaerobus*, *Veillonella alcalescens*, *Proteus mirabilis* and *Escherichia coli*. The fate of monoanthrone glycosides may resemble that of the AQ aglycones rather than AQ glycosides, since the emetic property of these agents is thought to be related to early absorption in the stomach or duodenum (Van Os, 1976b). The subsequent metabolism of AQ aglycones released in the colon is unclear. Bacterial reduction of 1,8-dihydroxy-AQ (danthron) to the anthrone (anthralin) has been demonstrated (Schmid, 1952), leading to the hypothesis that the active cathartic principles may not be the AQs but rather free anthrones and their tautomeric anthranols. It is clear that the glycosides themselves have no cathartic action either when administered parenterally or when introduced directly into the empty colon. It seems likely that whatever form is cathartically active, it does not need to be absorbed by the colonic mucosa in order to exert its action, although some absorption no doubt takes place.

Blair *et al.* (1977) reported foetal exposure to the drug danthron. Out of 160 maternity cases surveyed, 24 had taken an AQ type laxative at some stage during pregnancy. Administration of the drug at the time of induction of labour resulted in absorption from the maternal intestine, placental transport and excretion by foetal kidneys into the liquor. In mothers and babies the drug appeared as the glucuronide.

In addition to the cathartic effects noted above, other undesirable effects have been noted. Chrysazin (1,8-dihydroxyanthraquinone) was observed to induce intestinal tumours in rats (Mori *et al.* 1985). Emodin (4,5,7-trihydroxy-2-methylanthraquinone) has been shown to be a diarrhoeagenic toxicant in Dekalb cockerels with a mean lethal oral dose of 3.7 mg kg^{-1} body weight (Wells *et al.*, 1975). Luteoskyrin, a *bis*-polyhydroxy anthraquinone derivative, induced hepatotoxicity and hepatocarcinogenicity in mice (Uraguchi *et al.*, 1972).

The genetic effects of anthraquinones have been reviewed by Brown (1980). The results of testing some 80 phenolic AQs and related compounds in the *Salmonella*/microsome assay have been reported by Brown and Brown (1976), Brown and Dietrich (1979a) and Tikkanen *et al.* (1983a). A high percentage of the hydroxy AQs exhibited mutagenicity for strains sensitive to frame shifting mutagens, particularly TA1537 but also in some cases for TA1538 and TA98. Activity with strain TA100 was seen in a few cases. Of particular note were aloe-emodin, anthragallol (1,2,3-trihydroxy-AQ), purpurin (1,2,4-trihydroxy-AQ), emodin, rhein, alizarin (1,2-dihydroxy-AQ), physcion, chrysophanol (1,8-dihydroxy-2-methyl-AQ), anthralin and chrysazin. Only a few compounds exhibited significant exogenous metabolic activation (e.g. lucidin 2-ethyl ether) or showed an obligatory requirement for microsomal activation (e.g. chrysophanol). All of these possessed alkyl or *O*-alkyl function groups. The most mutagenic member of the phenolic AQs tested was lucidin (1,3,-dihydroxy-2-hydroxymethyl-AQ). This compound was recently identified as the mutagenic principle in *Rubia tinctorum* L. (madder) root (Yasui and Takeda, 1983).

Anthraquinone glycosides were in general non-mutagenic in the *Salmonella* assay. The *O*-β-D-glucosides of three AQs which were directly mutagenic for *Salmonella* TA1537 were non-mutagenic without activation but exhibited low activity with the Aroclor induced S9 microsomal fraction, namely, chrysazin monoglucoside, quinizarin monoglucoside and franguloside. Alizarin 2-*O*-β-glucoside, emodin-1(8)-*O*-β-D-glucoside, and lucidin 3-*O*-β-D-primveroside (Fig. 5.1) were non-mutagenic, as were the glucoside tetraacetates of alizarin, chrysazin and quinizarin. When these compounds were treated with enzymic extracts of rat intestinal bacteria, all the glycosides including the tetraactates were mutagenic owing to the release of the aglycones. In addition to the *O*-glycosides, two AQ *C*-glucosides, namely aloin (10-glucopyranosyl (1,8-dihydroxy,3-(hydroxy-methyl)-9(10H)-anthracenone)) and carminic acid (7-α-D-glucopyranosyl-9,10-dihydro-3,5,6,8-tetrahydroxy-1-methyl-9,10-dioxo-2-anthracene carboxylic acid) were tested with the same procedures and found non-mutagenic. This finding is consistent with the known chemical stability of the *C*-glucoside link (Fairbairn, 1962; Van Os, 1976a).

The non-mutagenicity of AQ glycosides should be interpreted with caution with respect to the *Salmonella*/microsome assay since it may result from the poor permeability of these organisms for these highly polar molecules. The anthracycline and anthracyclinone antibiotics are known to require their amino sugar substituents to bind effectively to DNA (Berg and Eckhardt, 1970).

In addition to inducing gene mutations in bacteria certain phenolic AQs and anthrones have also demonstrated activity in bacterial DNA repair assays, cytogenetic effects in plant root tip preparations and binding to mammalian DNA *in vitro* (Brown, 1980).

The mode of action of those hydroxy AQs, which are directly mutagenic in *Salmonella* and show few obvious structural correlations with mutagenic potency, is unknown. However it seems likely that a non-specific free radical mechanism may be involved (Nagata *et al.*, 1968). Alkyl substituted phenolic AQs which often show a significant or absolute requirement for exogenous metabolic activation may operate through the same ultimate free radical mechanism or via distinct reactive species. Masuda and Ueno (1984) observed that the metabolic activation of emodin to a direct acting mutagen for *Salmonella* was accomplished through selective ring hydroxylation (i.e. 2-hydroxyemodin). The mutagenic product has the same 1,2,3-trihydroxy substitution pattern as anthragallol, a potent direct acting mutagen, and so the same mechanism may be operative. Chesis *et al.* (1984) have proposed that one-electron reduction of quinones mediated by NADPH–cytochrome P-450 reductase results in metabolites mutagenic for *Salmonella*, whereas 2-electron reduction yields non-mutagens.

The naturally occurring or synthetic hydroxyanthraquinones, whether ingested as food constituents, food contaminants, or as drugs or medicinal preparations, can demonstrate all of the complex interactions between intestinal microflora and host metabolism: microbial hydrolysis of glycosides and glucuronides; microbial and host metabolism of aglycones; enterohepatic circulation of aglycones and metabolites; toxic and physio-logical effects of the aglycones on the host. We will see this pattern become even more complex in the discussion of the flavonoids below.

5.   Flavonoids

(a) Chemistry and occurrence. The basic structural feature of the flavonoid compounds is the 2-phenylbenzo[α]pyrane or flavane nucleus comprising 2 benzene rings, A and B, linked through a heterocyclic pyrane C ring (Fig. 5.1). The importance of these compounds as potential environmental mutagens and carcinogens stems from their widespread occurrence in human foods and their use in more purified forms as drugs and food supplements. The flavonoids are one of the more numerous groups of natural products. About 2000 individual members of the class have been described and as a group the flavonoids are universally distributed among vascular plants. For quercetin, the most common flavonol, over 70 glycosidic combinations have been fully characterized

and many more partly analysed. Nearly as many glycosides have been described for the other two common flavonols, kaempferol and myricetin. Adding the known glycosides of the rarer flavonols and flavones brings the total number of separate compounds to about 400. The most common glycosides of quercetin occurring in food plants are the 3-*O*-galactoside (hyperin), 3-*O*-glucoside (isoquercitin), 3-*O*-glucuronide (quercituron), 3-*O*-rhamnoside (quercitin), 3-*O*-rhamnoside-galactoside (bioquercitin), 3-*O*-rutinoside (rutin), 7-*O*-glucoside (quercimeritrin), and 4'-*O*-glucoside (dipiraeoside) (Kuhnau, 1976). For kaempferol the analogous galactoside (trifolin), glucoside (astragalin), rhamnoside (afzelin) and rutinoside (nicotiflorin) are also common.

(b) Biological effects.   Claims have long been made for vitamin-like activity for certain groups of food flavonoids, however no conclusive data have been obtained demonstrating their dietary necessity. The antioxidant property of the flavonoids is due to their phenolic nature, the antioxidant effect increasing with the degree of hydroxylation of the A and B rings. Antimicrobial activity of flavonoids for a variety of bacteria (staphylococci, *Escherichia coli*, salmonellae), viruses and fungi seems pronounced in the methylated, lipophilic flavones such as nobiletin, tangeretin and sinensetin. Similarly certain methylated flavones and flavonols have exhibited cytotoxic effects on human carcinoma cells. The chief therapeutic claims for flavonoids involve a number of physiological and biochemical effects, including smooth muscle relaxation, anti-inflammation, diuretic effects and decrease in capillary fragility in vascular disorders (McClure, 1975). The mechanisms of these effects are largely unknown, although enzyme inhibition and copper chelation have been suggested as likely causes.

(c) Metabolic fate.   The fate of orally ingested food flavonoids in mammals is similar in its initial stages to that of other plant glycosides. The flavonoid glycosides, being hydrophobic and of higher molecular weight than aglycones, are poorly absorbed in the small intestine. Since they are largely β-glucosides they are poorly hydrolysed by mammalian intestinal digestive enzymes and pass largely unaltered to the lower bowel.

The importance of the gut microflora in the metabolism of these compounds was first suggested by Booth and Williams (1963). They observed the hydrolysis of rutin (quercetin-3-*O*-β-rutinoside) to 3-hydroxyphenylpropionic acid by faecal and caecal extracts from rats. In an earlier study (Booth *et al.*, 1958) it was found that hesperidin (2*S*-hesperetin-7-*O*-β-rutinoside) was similarly degraded when administered orally to rats, being excreted in urine as the aglycone hesperetin, its glucuronide and at least 7 ring fission products including

3,4-dihydroxyphenylpropionic acid, 3-methoxy-4-hydroxyphenylpropionic acid, 3-hydroxycinnamic acid, 3-hydroxyphenylpropionic acid, 3-hydroxyhippuric acid, 3-hydroxybenzoic acid and 3-methoxy-4-hydroxybenzoic acid.

Griffiths and Smith (1972a,b) studied the metabolic fate of a wide variety of flavonoids: (*i*) a group of polyphenolic compounds, many with 3',4',5'-trihydroxylation of the B ring as in myricetin (3,5,7,3',4',5'-hexahydroxyflavone), and (*ii*) a group of compounds related in structure to apigenin (4',5,7-trihydroxyflavone). In the case of the polyhydroxy compounds, those with free 5,7,4'-hydroxyl groups were susceptible to ring fission after oral administration to rats. Similar products were formed from compounds with 3',4',5'-hydroxylation during anaerobic incubation with rat intestinal microflora *in vitro*. The importance of the microflora *in vivo* was indicated by the suppression of the products 3,5-dihydroxy-phenylacetic and 3-hydroxyphenylacetic acid following oral administration of the antibiotic neomycin. For the group of flavonoids related to apigenin the presence of free 5-,7- and 4'-hydroxyl groups was also essential for ring fission.

A later study of the metabolic fate of hesperetin [3-^{14}C] has demonstrated the cooperative nature of microbial and mammalian catabolism of flavonoids (Honohan *et al.*, 1976). The primary product of hesperetin-[3-^{14}C] found in the urine of rats following oral administration and after anaerobic incubation with rat caecal contents was 3-hydroxy-4-methoxyphenylpropionic acid. The labelled flavanone was completely degraded to phenylpropionic acids, benzoic acids, their conjugated derivatives, and CO_2; the latter accounted for 40% of the dose. However, very little $^{14}CO_2$ was produced when hesperetin-[3-^{14}C] was incubated with rat caecal flora. These data suggest that the catabolism of the propyl chain of the B ring metabolites is mediated by mammalian and not bacterial enzymes. This conclusion is in agreement with the earlier findings of Griffiths and Smith (1972a) that 4-hydroxybenzoic acid could not be formed by gut microbial action *in vitro*.

Intraperitoneal injection of hesperetin-[3-^{14}C] to a bile duct cannulated rat resulted in biliary excretion of the entire dose, showing that the animal is unable to effect ring fission. The specific microflora components responsible for the intestinal degradation of various dietary flavonoids has not been studied extensively. Cheng *et al.* (1969, 1971) isolated a number of strains of *Butyrivibrio* spp. from the bovine rumen capable of degrading rutin anaerobically. Also they observed that *Butyrivibrio fibrisolvens* D1 and *Selenomonas ruminantium* GA192 hydrolysed the glycosidic bond of rutin and further dissimilated the sugar without affecting ring fission and yielding the insoluble aglycone. Alternatively

Peptostreptococcus sp. B178 degraded rutin and *Butyrivibrio* sp. C_3 degraded rutin, quercetin and naringin, all to water soluble products, indicating ring fission. The latter organism fermented the sugar moiety of hesperidin, but did not cleave the heterocyclic ring. Also it could not catabolize quercetin or taxifolin, suggesting a role for the glycoside bond in enzyme induction, specificity, or perhaps membrane transport of glycosides subject to ring fission. In addition to the strains above some 40 additional organisms were tested for ability to degrade rutin and all proved negative, including: *Bacteroides* spp.; *Borrelia* sp.; *Eubacterium* spp.; *Lachnospira multiparus; Lactobacillus* spp.; *Peptostreptococcus* spp.; *Ruminococcus* spp.; *Succinomonas amylolytica*; and *Succinovibrio* spp.

Recently Macdonald *et al.* (1983, 1984) have investigated the hydrolysis of rutin and quercitrin by bacteria derived from human saliva and faeces. Cell-free extracts of human saliva cultures hydrolysed rutin but not quercitrin, whereas similar extracts of faecal bacteria hydrolysed both glycosides. The bulk of the activity in both preparations was found to be inducible. With faecal preparations both rutin and quercitrin induced respective hydrolytic activity, whereas in salivary preparations only rutin hydrolysis was induced by rutin. A faecal isolate *Streptococcus* sp. strain FRP-17, and strain VGH-1 of *Streptococcus faecium* hydrolysed rutin to quercetin and were also active on *O*-nitrophenyl-β-D-glucoside. Several closely related species lacked β-glucosidase, namely: *S. faecalis*; *S. bovis*; *S. pneumoniae*; *S. sanguis* (I and II); and *S. pyogenes* (groups A, B and C). Furthermore it was observed that the hydrolysis of rutin by these organisms led to the intermediate, quercetin-3-*O*-D-glucopyranoside indicating the presence of α-rhaminosidase activity as well as β-glucosidase. In a separate study (Mader and Macdonald, 1985) it was observed that various bile acids (chenodeoxycholic acid, deoxycholic acid and cholic acid) enhance the ability of rutin and quercetin hydrolysing organisms to successfully compete with other microbial populations. Since bile acids have been linked to bowel cancer both epidemiologically and in animal models the authors suggest a possible connection with flavonol exposure in the bowel.

Gugler *et al.* (1975) have examined the pharmacokinetics of quercetin in six human subjects after single intravenous (100 mg) and oral (4 g) doses. A sensitive fluorometric method, allowing detection of 0.1 μg ml^{-1} of quercetin in biological fluids, was used. The plasma data were analysed according to a 2-compartment open model with half-lives of 8.8 $\pm$ 1.2 minutes (0–40 minutes) α-phase and 2.4 $\pm$ 0.2 hours (40–540 minutes) β-phase. Protein binding was estimated to exceed 98%. The apparent volume of distribution was only 0.34 $\pm$ 0.03 l kg^{-1}, and 7.4% $\pm$ 1.2% of the i.v. dose was excreted in the urine as a conjugate while 0.65% of the dose was excreted unchanged. The total body plasma clearance of quercetin in normal subjects averaged 571 ml min^{-1} and renal clearance was 4.6 ml min^{-1}. Oral administration of 4 g quercetin to 4 subjects (50–65 mg kg^{-1}) resulted in no measurable plasma concentration (<0.1 g ml^{-1}). No quercetin conjugates were detected in the urine of any subject at any time after dosing. Analysis of faeces for quercetin up to 72 hours following oral administration showed recovery of 53 ± 5% of the dose. Only traces of quercetin were recovered from the faeces after 72 hours. The authors concluded that less than 1% of the unaltered quercetin is absorbed from the gastro-intestinal tract and ascribe the remainder of the dose to microbial degradation in the lower bowel. A recent study by Brown and Griffiths (1983) with bile duct cannulated rats revealed that after a high oral dose of 50 mg of the glycoside rutin, both isorhamnetin (3'-methoxyquercetin) and quercetin were detected in bile as conjugates together with an unidentified aglycone. Oral administration of quercetin resulted in quercetin and isorhamnetin conjugates in the bile. In an earlier comparison study 50 mg doses of naringin, naringenin, hesperidin and hesperetin resulted in 48 hour biliary excretion of 11.4, 7.5, 1.9 and 3.2% of the respective doses, primarily as glucuronide conjugates (Hackett *et al.*, 1979).

In another study (Ueno *et al.*, 1983) [^{14}C]quercetin labelled in the C-4 position or carbonyl of the C ring was orally administered to bile duct cannulated rats. Approximately 20% of the dose was absorbed from the digestive tract, more than 30% was recovered as $^{14}CO_2$ and about 30% was excreted unchanged in the faeces. Urinary and biliary excretion values were 9 and 12% of dose respectively, again indicating the potential importance of enterohepatic circulation in the metabolic fate of dietary flavonoids. Biliary metabolites included the glucuronide and sulphate conjugates of [^{14}C]quercetin, 3'-*O*-methyl[^{14}C]quercetin and 4'-*O*-methyl[^{14}C]quercetin.

Petrakis *et al.* (1959) have carried out the most complete study of tissue distribution of radioactivity following oral administration of a single 5 mg randomly ^{14}C-labelled dose of quercetin. In a rat sacrificed 12 hours after dosing only about 80% of the administered radioactivity was recovered, and over half or 44% was found in the intestinal contents, mostly the lower bowel. Of the absorbed radioactivity, the most was found in the lungs (12% of dose) and large intestinal wall (3% of dose). Much smaller amounts were found in the blood, kidneys, and gastric walls (<1% of dose total). Respired CO_2 accounted for 15% of the dose and urinary excretion was 4%. No ^{14}C label was detected in liver, spleen, heart or brain. No radioactive quercetin was found in the urine.

In summary, there is little evidence at present that after ingestion of food flavonoids, free aglycones persist in the general or enteohepatic circulations. While this conclusion is reassuring it should be pointed out that no adequate metabolism studies have been conducted with [^{14}C] labelled glycosides and even studies with the free aglycone quercetin have not involved identification of metabolite residues in such critical organs as the stomach and large intestine. Also the studies cited showed a rather poor recovery of ^{14}C activity.

(d) Toxicity and oncogenicity. The food flavonoids are virtually non-toxic with respect to acute exposures but relatively few in depth toxicity studies have been reported. Ambrose *et al.* (1952) reported low toxicity of quercetin to rats and rabbits for study durations up to 410 days at up to 1% in the diet. This study employed far too few animals and was of insufficient duration to detect a weakly oncogenic effect, however. Conflicting oncogenicity studies were published in 1980 and 1981. Saito *et al.* (1980) found no significant difference in tumour incidences in ddY mice fed a 2% quercetin diet and a control diet. Pamukcu *et al.* (1980) fed rats a basic diet supplemented with 0.1% quercetin for 58 weeks. They observed multiple ileal intestinal neoplasms including adenoma (4), fibroadenoma (7), and adenocarcinoma (9, 3 with mesenteric metastases). Also found were 5 bladder tumours, papillary or senile transitional cell carcinomas. Hirono *et al.* (1981) and Morino *et al.* (1982) found no evidence for oncogenicity of quercetin or rutin in ACI rats or golden hamsters. In the latter study the compounds were administered at up to 10% in the diet and some groups were also treated with croton oil, a tumour promoter. Similarly Stoewsand *et al.* (1984) found quercetin at 0.1% and 0.2% in the diet non-carcinogenic in Fischer rats.

The effect of quercetin on the two-stage carcinogenesis of the rat urinary bladder was evaluated by Hirose *et al.* (1983). No tumours or hyperplasia were observed in animals given 5% quercetin as initiator in the diet for 4 weeks followed by 0.001% *N*-butyl-*N*-(4-hydroxybutyl)-nitrosamine (BHBN) for 29 weeks. Furthermore administration of 5.0% quercetin diet in 25 weeks after initiation with 0.01% BHBN for 4 weeks did not promote bladder carcinogenesis. No lesions were detected in rats fed 5.0% quercetin diet only. Kato *et al.* (1985) found quercetin lacked initiating activity for rat liver with phenobarbital and partial hepatectomy as promoters or promoting activity (Kato *et al.*, 1984) with methylazoxy-methanol acetate as initiator. Quercetin has also been observed to exhibit antagonistic effects to a tumour virus (Luczak and Wleklik, 1985) and promoters (Nishino *et al.*, 1984a,b,c).

While the balance of these results could indicate that quercetin is a non-oncogen or at most a very weak one, the discrepancy of the Pamukcu *et al.* (1980) study is disturbing and cannot easily be accounted for by strain, dietary or environmental conditions. One difference noted by Morino *et al.* (1982) was the presence in their quercetin of 5,7,3′-trihydroxy-4′-methoxy flavone (diosmetin) as an impurity. As the authors note diosmetin would need to be a potent inhibitor of carcinogenesis to explain the discrepancy. Alternatively Stavric (1984) has reviewed the published quercetin oncogenicity data and recent unpublished data by the same Pamukcu group showing that both quercetin and rutin induced liver tumours in SD and Fischer rats. He concluded that differences in strain of test animal and basal diets could partially explain the variations in oncogenicity observed.

(e) Genetic toxicity. The genetic effects of various flavonoid compounds have been surveyed by a number of authors, notably Sugimura *et al.* (1977), MacGregor and Jurd (1978), Brown and Dietrich (1979b), Brown (1980), Nagao *et al.* (1981), and Elliger *et al.* (1984). Early studies on flavonoid mutagencity in *Salmonella* indicated that the most important structural feature required for activity in strains TA98, TA1537 and TA100 was the presence of a C3-OH, which is basic to the flavonol structure. The C5-OH also seemed significant. Flavonols lacking free hydroxyl groups on the B ring (e.g. galangin) or having only one OH group (e.g. kaempferol) showed an absolute requirement for microsomal activation in order to exhibit mutagenicity in the *Salmonella* tester strains. In contrast quercetin with 3′,4′ hydroxylation of the B ring was shown to be subject to activation by soluble (S100) constitutive enzymes. More recently Nagao *et al.* (1981) and Elliger *et al.* (1984) have detected significant mutagenic activity for a number of flavones without 3-OH substitution, notably wogonin (5,7-dihydroxy-8-methoxyflavone), norwogonin (5,7,8-trihydroxyflavone; Fig. 5.1) and isowogonin (5,8-dihydroxyflavone). Activity with these compounds was seen largely with strain TA100. These authors observed that norwogonin was also subject to activation by constitutive soluble enzymes from the rat liver, but that in distinction with flavonol activation mentioned above, NADP appeared to be an important cofactor and B ring oxidation was apparently not involved. While a quinone methide has been proposed as the mutagenic product of flavonol activation it would appear that flavones have a distinct mechanism of action.

As noted above flavonoids, including mutagenic flavones and flavonols, occur in nature largely as glycosides. Glycosides of mutagenic flavonols are non-mutagenic in the *Salmonella* assay unless treated with appropriate glycosidases. Brown and Dietrich (1979a,b) observed mutagenicity of rutin (quercetin-3-*O*-gluc-rham) and robinin (kaempferol-3-*O*-gal-rham-

7-O-rham) only after treatment with mixed glycosidases from rat caecal bacteria or *Helix pomatia*. Nagao *et al.* (1981) similarly observed mutagenic activity for isoquercitrin (quercetin-3-O-gluc), hyperin (quercetin-3-O-gal), astragalin (kaempferol-3-O-gluc), kaempferitrin (kaempferol-3-O-rham-7-O-rham) and tiliroside (kaempferol-3-O-(6-coumaroyl)gluc) only after treatment with hesperidinase from *Aspergillis niger*.

Genetic effects of flavonoids in other test systems are somewhat limited. Quercetin, the most mutagenic and widespread flavonol studied in *Salmonella* assays, also exhibited mutagenic activity in *E. coli* (Hardigree and Epler, 1978), L5178Y mouse lymphoma cells *in vitro* (Meltz and MacGregor, 1981), V79 Chinese hamster cells (Maruta *et al.*, 1979), chromosomal aberrations in Chinese hamster ovary cells *in vitro* (Carver *et al.*, 1983), cell transformation in hamster embryo cells (Umezawa *et al.*, 1977), and sex-linked recessive lethals in *Drosophila melanogaster* (Watson, 1982).

Alternatively, the non-mutagenicity of quercetin has also been observed in both *in vitro* and *in vivo* tests, notably in the mouse micronucleus test and a *Salmonella* TA98 host mediated assay in the mouse (Aeschbacher *et al.*, 1982).

(f) Dietary exposure.   Flavonol glycosides, particularly glycosides of the flavonols quercetin and kaempferol, are found in the edible portions of the majority of food plants, e.g. citrus and other fruits and berries; leafy vegetables; roots, tubers and bulbs; herbs and spices; legumes; cereal grains; tea and cocoa. Tea, coffe, cocoa, fruit jams, red wine, beer and vinegar account for about 25% of flavonol intake. The estimated daily intake of all flavonols in the average American diet is about 1 g. About 170 mg are accounted by 4-oxoflavonols (i.e. flavones, flavanones, chalcones, etc.). The majority of this quantity is probably composed of flavones (apigenin glycosides and luteolin glycosides) and flavonols (kaempferol glycosides and quercetin glycosides) (Kuhnau, 1976; Herrmann, 1976). The intake of promutagenic flavonol glycosides has been estimated to be about 50 mg (quercetin equivalents) per day (Brown, 1980).

Mutagenic activity for *Salmonella* in a number of food extracts has been attributed to flavonols or other flavones, notably in: Sumac spice (Seino *et al.*, 1978); Japanese pickles (Takahashi *et al.*, 1979); teas (Nagao *et al.*, 1979; Uyeta *et al.*, 1981); wine (Tamura *et al.*, 1980); and citrus fruit juices (Mazaki *et al.*, 1982).

(g) Conclusions.   The toxicological significance of dietary exposure to food flavonols and flavones has been a subject of scientific debate (Aeschbacher, 1982; Knudsen, 1982; Sugimura, 1982). Of concern are

the demonstrated widespread occurrence in common foodstuffs, the microbial release of mutagenic aglycones in the intestinal tract, the broad variety of genetic toxicities in various *in vitro* systems and the conflicting, albeit largely negative, oncogenicity and related data in experimental animals. Mitigating factors such as microbial C ring fission in the gut, rapid excretion of absorbed aglycone with low tissue residues, lack of mutagenicity in whole animal tests and potential anti-carcinogenic effects (Nagase *et al.*, 1964; Wattenberg and Leong, 1970) may ultimately be shown to reduce the risk from exposure to these agents to negligible levels. For the present however it would seem prudent not to ingest excess quantities of flavonols or their glycosides, such as rutin, in the form of so-called vitamin supplements.

6.   Diterpenoids — ent-kaurene Glycosides

Because of the sweetness of its leaves, the Paraguayan shrub *Stevia rebaudiana* Bertoni has been the subject of scientific interest for several decades. Extracts of the plant and stevioside (19-*O*-β-glucopyranosyl-13-*O*-[β-glucopyranosyl (1→2)]-β-glucopyranosyl-13-hydroxykaur-16-en-19-oic acid), its major sweet constituent, are available in Japan as commercial sweeteners for a variety of foods, soft drinks and confectionery.

Stevioside (Fig. 5.1) is one of eight sweet *ent*-kaurene glycosides in *S. rebaudiana*, the others being steviolbioside, rebaudiosides A-E (Fig. 5.1) and dulcoside A. Wingard *et al.* (1980) have studied the fate of stevioside, rebaudioside A and steviol-17-[^{14}C] in the intestinal tract of the rat. They observed that stevioside and rebaudioside A were completely hydrolysed to steviol (Fig. 5.1) by anaerobic whole-cell suspensions of rat caecal bacteria *in vitro*. Furthermore it was demonstrated that steviol-17-[^{14}C] was virtually completely absorbed by the intestinal tract after oral or intracaecal administration. The radioactivity was largely excreted in the bile, indicating a potential for enterohepatic circulation of the steviol aglycone. Very little ^{14}CO$_2$ (0.02% of dose) was observed, demonstrating the stability of the exocyclic methylene label. The authors predicted similar metabolic fate in man for the *ent*-kaurene glycosides.

Pezzuto *et al.* (1985) have evaluated the mutagenicity of steviol and a variety of steviol glycosides in *Salmonella typhimurium* TM 677 with and without activation by exogenous post mitrochrondial liver fraction (S9) from Aroclor 1254 induced rats. They found six glycosides to be non-mutagenic, namely stevioside, steviolbioside, dulcoside A and rebaudiosides A, B and C. On the other hand steviol showed substantial mutagenic activity which appeared to be dependent on inducible (Aroclor 1254 or phenobarbital) cytochrome P450 mediated metabolism. Isosteviol (13-

methyl-16-oxo derivative), a known decomposition product of stevioside, had no mutagenic activity. Furthermore, the synthetic 16-methyl derivatives (α and β isomers), *ent*-kaurenoic acid and steviol 16,17-epoxide were also non-mutagenic. Genetic toxicity data for steviol in other systems are not yet available thus it is premature to judge the significance of these findings. However they seem to fit the pattern established with other groups of plant glycosides.

7. Steroid Glycoside Prodrugs

As noted in several examples presented above, colon-specific delivery of bioactive compounds is known to occur naturally in man through the liberation of aglycones from poorly absorbed plant glycosides following ingestion. Release of aglycones is mediated by glycosidases produced by various colonic bacteria. In addition, the azo-reductase activity of the intestinal bacteria has been used to deliver therapeutic agents to the lower bowel; sulphasalazine (Goldman, 1978) and a polymer-based prodrug system (Brown *et al.*, 1983) both deliver, after reduction of their azo bonds, 5-aminosalicylate to the colon. Only recently have prodrug glycosides been prepared and evaluated for their ability to exploit intestinal microbial glycosidases to effect such site-specific action (Friend and Chang, 1984, 1985).

The 21-yl-β-D-glucosides and galactosides of dexamethazone, prednisolone, hydrocortisone, and fluorocortisone and the 21-yl-β-D-cellobiosides of prednisolone were prepared and subjected to hydrolysis by contents of rat stomach, proximal small intestine, distal small intestine and caecum. All of the glycosides were slowly hydrolysed by stomach and proximal intestinal contents, more rapidly by distal contents and most rapidly by caecal contents. The findings varied substantially, hydrolytic susceptibility decreasing in the following order with distal intestinal contents: prednisolon-21-yl-β-D-galactoside, prednisolon-21-yl-β-D-glucoside, prednisolon-21-yl-β-D-cellobioside, dexamethason-21-yl-β-D-galactoside, dexamethason-21-yl-β-D-glucoside. Hydrolysis rate of the cellobioside was half that of the glucoside and one quarter that of galactoside.

Hydrolysis of all the prodrugs in caecal contents was rapid (109–665 nmol $min^{-1}g^{-1}$ wet weight) with the exceptions of hydrocortison-21-yl-β-D-glucoside and fluorocortison-21-yl-β-D-glucoside (30–40 nmol $min^{-1}g^{-1}$). These activities were generally comparable with the following *p*-nitrophenyl glycoside controls: glucoside (454 nmol $min^{-1}g^{-1}$); galactoside (1620 nmol $min^{-1}g^{-1}$); and cellobioside (96 nmol $min^{-1}g^{-1}$). Friend and Chang (1984) observed a good correlation between intestinal absorption of the prodrug glycosides and the apparent 1-octanol: 0.01M phosphate buffer partition coefficients. They predict that disaccharide or oligosaccharide carriers might be preferable or even necessary for lower bowel delivery of larger, more lipophilic, drug molecules. It is still unknown whether such steroid prodrugs demonstrate efficacious anti-inflammatory activity in the lower bowel in animal model systems or in man.

8. Miscellaneous Glycosides

(a) Phenoxybenzyl alcohol. 3-phenoxybenzyl alcohol (PB alc) and 3-phenoxybenzoic acid (PB acid) are common major metabolites in plants of the photostable pyrethoid insecticides (e.g. cypermethrin, deltamethrin, fenvalerate) and could appear in certain food plants as residues. The alcohol and acid occur in plants mainly as glycoside conjugates. Mikami *et al.* (1984) showed that PB acid is converted in various plants into conjugates by esterification with glucose, malonyl glucose, disaccharides (gentiobiose, cellobiose, glucosylxylose) and two types of triglucose. Mikami *et al.* (1985) have compared the metabolism in rats of PB alc and its mono-, di- and triglucoside conjugates and the monoglucoside of PB acid.

Upon single oral administration to rats, 1-(3-phenoxybenzyl)-β-D-glucopyranoside, 1-(3-phenoxybenzyl)-β-D-gentiobioside and 1-(3-phenoxybenzyl)-β-D-gentiotrioside or 1-(3-phenoxybenzoyl)-β-D-glucopy-ranose were rapidly hydrolysed and extensively eliminated in the urine, mostly as the sulphate conjugate of 3-(4-hydroxyphenoxy)benzoic acid. Faecal elimination was relatively minor whereas biliary excretion was about 42% of the ^{14}C radiolabelled doses; the glucuronides of PB alc, PB acid, and 3-(4-hydroxyphenoxy)benzoic acid were major metabolites. The biliary glucuronides were hydrolysed in the small intestine to aglycones, which were re-absorbed and metabolized to the sulphate conjugate of 3(-4-hydroxyphenoxy)benzoic acid. The mono-, di- and triglucosides of PB acid were absorbed mainly as PB acid and to lesser degrees as the intact glycosides.

The various glycosides and glucosides were assessed for degradation by rat caecal contents *in vitro*. The glucosides were more readily degraded than the glucuronides. Hydrolysis of the gentiotrioside and gentiobioside occurred by sequential removal of the terminal sugar. The authors concluded that the gut microflora were largely responsible for cleavage of the glucosides of PB alc and PB acid, although the small intestinal mucosa exhibited a somewhat higher hydrolytic activity *in vitro* (7 to 43 nmol min^{-1}g^{-1} tissue). The glucose ester of PB acid was considered to be more readily hydrolysed in rats than the glucosyl ether because of a lower recovery in urine and faeces of germ-free rats, although this compound was not assessed for degradation by the rat caecal bacteria.

(b) Hydroxycarbofuran. The description of the metabolic fate of 3-phenoxybenzyl alcohol above is typical of most pesticides which undergo extensive conjugative metabolism in both plant and animal systems. Usually such conjugates are considered much less toxicologically significant than the parent materials or non-conjugated intermediary metabolites. Exceptions to this usual pattern might be exemplified by carbofuran (2,3-dihydro-2, 2-dimethyl-7-benzofuranyl-*N*-methylcarbamate). This insecticide is partially oxidized to 3-hydroxycarbofuran (3-OH-C) in plants and animals, and both the parent and metabolite have similar toxicities. In animals 3-OH-C is further degraded and effectively excreted. On the other hand, many plants form the 3-*O*-glucoside of hydroxycarbofuran (3-OH-C-gluc) as a major residue. Marshall and Dorough (1984) have studied the metabolic fate of orally administered [^{14}C-ring] hydroxycarbofuran 3-*O*-glucoside and its aglycone in the rat. They observed that the glucoside, unlike the aglycone, was poorly absorbed. At 3 hours, 55.7% of the dose was in the caecum, 40% of this as the unaltered glucoside and 9% as the 3-OH benzofuran-7-glucuronide. Only 1% of the glucoside dose was found in the colon, indicating effective microbial hydrolysis of the 3-*O*-glucoside. Intracaecal administration of hydroxycarbofuran 3-*O*-glucoside resulted in rapid glycoside hydrolysis. Slower hydrolysis was also observed in the duodenum and ileum, and the authors conclude that little if any intact glucoside is absorbed from the gastro-intestinal tract. The importance of biliary excretion was shown in bile duct cannulated rats where after 6 hours 6% of a glucoside dose had been excreted in bile, compared to 23% of the 3-OH-C dose. Thus ingestion of glucosides of 3-OH-C is unlikely to result in less exposure to the toxic aglycone.

(c) Nitropropanol. Miserotoxin (3-nitro-1-propyl-β-D-glucopyranoside) is synthesized by *Astragalus* spp. (Leguminosae) and is toxic to livestock. In cattle and sheep the glucoside is readily hydrolysed after ingestion by ruminal microorganisms releasing the aglycone, 3-nitropropanol (NPOH). Miserotoxin is much less toxic to rats due to a lower level of microbial hydrolysis in the intestinal tract. Recent evidence suggests that nitropropanol is metabolized in mammals to nitropropionic acid (NPA) (Muir *et al.*, 1984). The latter compound is also a toxic constituent of certain legume forages, although NPA and NPOH do not occur together. Monogastric animals are more susceptible to NPA than ruminants which can apparently rapidly detoxify NPA. NPA may exert its toxic action through inhibition of mitochondrial respiratory enzymes.

C. Esters

1. *Esterification of Bile Acids and Sterols*

(a) Methyl deoxycholate. Edenharder and Hammann (1985) screened 2476 isolates of predominant human intestinal bacteria freshly isolated from the faeces of 51 subjects for their cholate transforming capacities. While 74 isolates dehydroxylated cholate at C7, resulting in the formation of deoxycholate, 28 isolates formed multiple products including the ketonic bile acids 3α, 12α-dihydroxy-7-keto and 3-keto, 7α, 12α-dihydroxy-5-β-cholanic acids, as well as the previously unidentified deoxycholic acid C-24 methyl ester. The latter metabolite was produced anaerobically by strains of most saccharolytic *Bacteroides* spp. (e.g. *B. distasonis*, *B. eggerthii*, *B. fragilis*, *B. incommunis*, *B. thetaiotaomicron*, *B. uniformis*, *B. variabilis* and *B. vulgatus*). It was also detected with a few strains of *Eubacterium* and *Lactobacillus* species. The authors suggest esterification via transfer of a C_1-unit, since no exogenous methanol was necessary. The frequency of bacterial methyl deoxycholate formation from cholate was comparable with that of 7α dehydroxylation, i.e. 3–4% of total isolates. Curiously both abilities were lost after serial subculturing as pure cultures. In mixed faecal cultures bile acid esterification seemed much less frequent than 7α dehydroxylation. While the function of esterification is uncertain, such esters are less soluble and exhibit less antibacterial activity. Thus esterification could serve as a detoxification mechanism for the bacteria. Other potentially toxic properties of the methyl ester have not yet been investigated.

(b) Ethyl lithocholate. Lithocholic acid (3α-hydroxy-5β-cholan-24-oic acid) is an important bile acid formed in the faeces of animals and humans fed high beef-fat diets, and is associated with higher incidences of large bowel cancer. The metabolism of [^{14}COOH]-lithocholic acid by rat intestinal flora was studied by Kelsey and Sexton (1976). The authors used mixed faecal cultures derived from animals fed a conventional or high-meat diet for 6 months. Aliquots of a 7 hour anaerobic culture were incubated with [^{14}C]-lithocholate. Cultures from the high meat diet converted lithocholate to isolithocholate (3β-hydroxy-5β-cholan-24-oic acid, 14%), ethyl lithocholate (ethyl-3α-hydroxy-5β-cholan-24-oate, 10%) and ethyl isolithocholate (4%). The corresponding figures for the conventional diet cultures were 12%, 7% and 5% respectively. It was observed that anaerobic conditions were necessary for esterification and that ethyl lithocholate could be produced by certain faecal micro-organisms including two strains of *Bacteroides* sp., *Citrobacter* sp. and *Peptococcus*

                    J. P. BROWN

productus I. The toxicological properties of these ethyl esters have not
been adequately investigated, although they have not yet been detected
in human faeces (Macdonald *et al.*, 1983).

(c) 3-hydroxyl esterification.   A novel bile and sterol conjugation mechanism has been reported by Quistad *et al.* (1982) and Miyamoto *et al.* (1986)
for acid metabolites of the pyrethroid insecticides fluvalinate and
fenvalerate respectively. Conjugates of 2-chloro-4-trifluromethylanilino-
3-methylbutanoic acid with the 3-OH of cholic, taurochenodeoxycholic
and taurocholic acids were observed to be significant secondary metabolites
formed in faeces of the cow, chicken and rat at 5–12% of the administered
oral doses of [^{14}CF$_3$]-fluvalinate. Similarly, esters of 4-chlorophenyl-
isovaleric acid (CPIA) and the 3-OH of cholesterol have been observed
in mice and rats fed fenvalerate.

The site of formation of the bile acid esters is unknown, but is thought
to be enteric and possibly mediated by intestinal microflora. The
cholesterol ester is formed from only one of the four optical isomers of
fenvalerate, namely [$2R,\alpha S$], and is thought to arise via liver microsomal
transesterification, although other tissues demonstrated esterifying activity,
notably brain, kidney and spleen in rodents, dog and Rhesus monkey.
The CPIA-cholesterol ester is believed to be the cause of granulomatous
changes observed in liver, spleen and/or lymph nodes of animals fed
fenvalerate.

Since the pyrethoid insecticides are relatively poorly absorbed from the
gastro-intestinal tract, the role of the microflora in their transformations
may be more significant than is currently recognized and should be
investigated further.

2.   *Ester Hydrolysis*

While the hydrolysis of xenobiotic esters is usually thought to be
mediated by mammalian intestinal or hepatic carboxylesterases capable of
hydrolysing carboxyl esters, thiol esters and aromatic amides (Inoue *et
al.*, 1979), the intestinal microflora can play a subsidiary role in ester
hydrolysis.

Scheline (1968) found that mixed rat caecal bacteria hydrolysed methyl
gallate to gallic acid, pyrogallol and resorcinol.

Yano and Takahashi (1981) evaluated the ability of *Escherichia coli* R-
12 KL98 to hydrolyse a series of *trans*-cinnamyl esters. *Trans*-cinnamyl
acetate is found in cassia oil from *Cinnamomum sieboldii* (Lauraceae)
which has been used as a food flavouring. The one to six carbon aliphatic

esters were tested and only the *trans*-cinnamyl formate was significantly hydrolysed (20%).

Di-(2-ethylhexyl)phthalate (DEHP) is a widely used plasticizer and is recognized as an environmental contaminant. Since it is used in the manufacture of polyvinylchloride, human exposure via such items as blood bags and food wrappers is likely. While the acute toxicity of DEHP is relatively low, chronic toxicity includes testicular atrophy and hepatocarcinogenicity in rodents (Gray *et al.*, 1982; Northrup *et al.*, 1982). DEHP and numerous related compounds have been found non-mutagenic for *Salmonella* (Zeiger *et al.*, 1985). Rowland (1974) and Rowland *et al.* (1977) studied the enteric metabolism of a series of phthalic acid diesters in the rat. The rates of hydrolysis *in vitro* of dimethyl-, di ethyl-, di-n- butyl-, dicyclohexyl-, di-n-octyl and di-(2-ethylhexyl)phthalate were highest with small intestinal contents and much lower with stomach or caecal contents. Dimethyl-, diethyl- and di-n-butyl phthalates were more rapidly hydrolysed probably solely by mammalian enzymes, either of pancreatic or mucosal origin. With DEHP it has been shown that the metabolism by intestinal contents *in vitro* can be reduced, but not eliminated, by incorporation of antibiotics (Rowland, 1974). Thus intestinal bacterial enzymes may play a role in the hydrolysis of DEHP and probably dioctyl- and dicyclohexyl phthalates, at least in the rat. In all cases, the product of hydrolysis was the mono ester. Since mono-(2-ethylhexyl)phthalate (MEHP) was shown to induce testicular atrophy and peroxisome proliferation in the liver, hydrolysis of phthalate diesters does not result in significant detoxification, but rather appears to promote intestinal absorption. After a single oral dose of DEHP (2.8 g kg^{-1}) plasma concentrations of 9 mg l^{-1} DEHP and 63 mg l^{-1} MEHP were reached in 3 hours (Teirlynck and Belpaire, 1985). An absorption threshold has been reported at a dose of about 0.5 mg kg^{-1} DEHP below which no DEHP reaches the liver. When [7-^{14}C] DEHP was administered to rats, 19% of the dose was excreted in the urine within 72 hours, the remainder being excreted in the faeces (98.3% total recovery). Multiple dosing with DEHP (2.8 g kg^{-1} per day for 7 days) resulted in no accumulation of DEHP or MEHP in plasma.

References

Aeschbacher, H. -U. (1982). The significance of mutagens in food. *Prog. Clin. Biol. Res.* **109**, 349–362.

Aeschbacher, H. -U., Meier, H. and Ruch, E. (1982). Nonmutagenicity *in vivo* of the food flavonol quercetin. *Nutr. Cancer* **4**, 90–98.

Ambrose, A. M., Robbins, D. J. and de Eds, F. (1952). Comparative toxicities of quercetin and quercitrin. *J. Am. Pharm. Assoc. Sci. Ed.* **41**, 119–122.

Berg, H. and Eckhardt, K. (1970). Zur Interaktion von Anthracyclinen und Anthracyclinonen mit DNS. *Z. Naturf.* **25B**, 362–367.

Blair, A. W., Burdon, M., Powell, J., Gerrard, M. and Smith, R. (1977). Fetal exposure to 1,8-dihydroxyanthraquinone. *Biol. Neonate* **31**, 289–293.

Booth, A. N. and Williams, R. T. (1963). Dehydroxylation of catechol acids by intestinal contents. *Biochem. J.* **88**, 66–67P.

Booth, A. N., Jones, F. T. and De Eds, F. (1958). Metabolic fate of hesperidin, Epio-Dictyol, Homoeriodictyol, and Diosmin, *J. Biol. Chem.* **230**, 661–668.

Breimer, D. D. and Baars, A. J. (1976). Pharmacokinetics and metabolism of anthraquinone laxatives. *Pharmacol.* **14**, Suppl. 1, 30–47.

Brown, J. P. (1977). Role of gut bacterial flora in nutrition and health: A review of recent advances in bacteriological techniques, metabolism and factors affecting flora composition. *CRC Crit. Rev. Food Sci. Nutr.* **8**, 229–336.

Brown, J. P. (1980). A review of the genetic effects of naturally occurring flavonoids, anthraquinones and related compounds. *Mutat. Res.* **75**, 243–277.

Brown, J. P. and Brown, R. J. (1976). Mutagenesis by 9,10-anthraquinone derivatives and related compounds in *Salmonella typhimurium. Mutat. Res.* **40**, 203–224.

Brown, J. P. and Dietrich, P. S. (1979a). Mutagenicity of anthraquinone and benzanthrone derivatives in the Salmonella/microsome test: Activation of anthraquinone glycosides by enzymic extracts of rat cecal bacteria. *Mutat. Res.* **66**, 9–24.

Brown, J. P. and Dietrich, P. S. (1979b). Mutagenicity of plant flavonols in the Salmonella/mammalian microsome test: Activation of flavonol glycosides by mixed glycosidases from rat cecal bacteria and other sources. *Mutat. Res.* **66**, 223–240.

Brown, J. P., McGarraugh, G. V., Parkinson, T. M., Wingard, R. E. and Onderdonk, A. B. (1983). A polymeric drug for treatment of inflammatory bowel disease. *J. Med. Chem.* **26**, 1300–1307.

Brown, S. and Griffiths, L. A. (1983). New metabolites of the naturally occurring mutagen, quercetin, the pro-mutagen, rutin and of taxifolin. *Experientia* **39**, 198–200.

Carver, J. H., Carrano, A. V. and MacGregor, J. T. (1983). Genetic effects of the flavonols quercetin, kaempferol, and galangin on Chinese hamster ovary cells *in vitro*. Mutat. Res. **113**, 45–60.

Cheng, K. J., Jones, G. A., Simpson, F. J. and Bryant, M. P. (1969). Isolation and identification of rumen bacteria capable of anaerobic rutin degradation. *Can. J. Microbiol.* **15**, 1365–1371.

Cheng, K. J., Krishnamurty, H. G., Jones, G. A. and Simpson, F. J. (1971). Isolation and identification of products, produced by the anaerobic degradation of naringen by *Butyrivibrio* sp. *Can. J. Microbiol.* **17**, 129–131.

Chesis, P. L., Levin, D. E., Smith, M. T., Ernster, L. and Ames, B. N. (1984). Mutagenicity of quinones: Pathways of metabolic activation and detoxification. *Proc. Natl Acad. Sci. USA* **81**, 1696–1700.

Chesters, C. G. C. and Bull, A. T. (1963). The enzymic degradation of laminarin. *Biochem. J.* **86**, 28–46.

Cliff, J., Lundqvist, P., Martensson, J., Rosling, H. and Sorbo, B. (1985). Association of high cyanide and low sulphur intake in cassava-induced spastic paraparesis. *Lancet* **ii**, 1211–1213.

Cooper, J. M. (1941). Isolation of a toxic principle from the seeds of *Macrozamia spiralis. J. Proc. R. Soc. N.S. Wales* **74**, 450–545.

Crayford, J. V. and Hutson, D. H. (1980). The metabolism of 3-phenoxybenzoic acid and its glucoside conjugate in rats. *Xenobiotica* **10**, 355–364.

Drasar, B. S. and Hill, M. J. (1974). "Human Intestinal Flora". Academic Press, San Franciso.

Edenharder, R. and Hammann, R. (1985). Deoxycholic acid methyl ester – a novel bacterial metabolite of cholic acid. *System. appl. Microbiol.* **6**, 18–22.

Elliger, C. A., Henika, P. R. and MacGregor, J. T. (1984). Mutagenicity of flavones, chromones and acetophenones in *Salmonella typhimurium*. New structure-activity relationships. *Mutat. Res.* **135**, 77–86.

Fairbairn, J. W. (1964). The analysis and standardization of anthraquinone drugs. *Planta Med.* **12**, 260–264.

Fairbairn, J. W. (1976). The Lugano Symposium Proceedings. *Pharmacology* **4**, Suppl. 1.

Farnsworth, N. R., Bingel, A. S., Fong, H. H. S., Saleh, A. A., Christenson, G. M. and Stauffer, S. M. (1976). Oncogenic and tumor-promoting spermatophytes and pteridophytes and their active principles. *Cancer Treat. Rep.* **60**, 1171–1214.

Feinberg, A. and Zedeck, M. S. (1980). Production of a highly reactive alkylating agent from the organospecific carcinogen methyl azoxymethanol by alcohol dehydrogenase. *Cancer Res.* **40**, 4446–4450.

Fenselau, C., Pallante, S., Batzinger, R. P., Benson, W. R., Barron, R. P., Sheinin, E. B. and Maienthal, M. (1977). Mandelonitrile–glucuronide: Synthesis and characterization. *Science* **198**, 625–626.

Finegold, S. M., Attebery, H. R. and Sutter, V. L. (1974). Effect of diet on human fecal flora: comparison of Japanese and American diets. *Amer. J. Clin. Nutr.* **27**, 1456–1469.

Friend, D. R. and Chang, G. W. (1984). A colon-specific drug-delivery system based on drug glycosides and the glycosidases of colonic bacteria. *J. Med. Chem.* **27**, 261–266.

Friend, D. R. and Chang, G. W. (1985). Drug glycosides: potential prodrugs for colon-specific drug delivery. *J. Med. Chem.* **28**, 51–57.

Goldman, P. (1978). Biochemical pharmacology of the intestinal flora. *Am. Rev. Pharmacol. Toxicol.* **18**, 523–39.

Gray, T. J. B., Rowland, I. R., Foster, P. M. D. and Gangolli, S. D. (1982). Species differences in the testicular toxicity of phthalate esters. *Toxicol. Lett.* **11**, 141–147.

Griffiths, L. A. and Smith, G. E. (1972a). Metabolism of apigenin and related compounds in the rat: metabolite formation *in vivo* and by the intestinal microflora *in vitro*. *Biochem. J.* **128**, 901–911.

Griffiths, L. A. and Smith, G. E. (1972b). Metabolism of myricetin and related compounds in the rat: metabolite formation *in vivo* and by the intestinal microflora *in vitro*. *Biochem. J.* **130**, 141–151.

Gugler, R., Leschik, M. and Dengler, H. J. (1975). Disposition of quercetin in man after single oral and intravenous doses. *Eur. J. Clin. Pharmacol.* **9**, 229–234.

Hackett, A. M., Marsh, I., Barrow, A. and Griffiths, L. A. (1979). The biliary excretion of flavonones in the rat. *Xenobiotica* **9**, 491–502.

Hardigree, A. A. and Epler, J. L. (1978). Comparative mutagenesis of plant flavonoids in microbial systems. *Mutat. Res.* **88**, 231–239.

Hawksworth, G., Drasar, B. S. and Hill, M. J. (1971). Intestinal bacteria and the hydrolysis of glycosidic bonds. *J. Med. Microbiol.* **4**, 451–459.

Herrmann, K. (1976). Flavonols and flavones in food plants: a review. *J. Food Technol.* **11**, 433–448.

Hirono, I., Ueno, I., Hosaka, S., Takanashi, H., Matsushima, T., Sugimura, T. and Natori, S. (1981). Carcinogenicity examination of quercetin and rutin in ACI rats. *Cancer Lett.* **13**, 16–21.

Hirose, M., Fukushima, S., Sakata, T., Inui, M. and Ito, N. (1983). Effect of Quercetin on two-stage carcinogenesis of the rat urinary bladder. *Cancer Letters*, **21**, 23–27.

Holdeman, L. V., Good, I. J. and Moore, W. E. C. (1976). Human fecal flora: Variation in bacterial composition within individuals and a possible effect of emotional stress. *Appl. Environ. Microbiol.* **31**, 359–375.

Honohan, T., Hale, R. L., Brown, J. P. and Wingard, R. E. (1976). Synthesis and metabolic fate of hesperetin-3-^{14}C. *J. Agric. Food Chem.* **24**, 906–911.

Hoskins, L. C. and Boulding, E. T. (1981). Mucin degradation in human colon ecosystems. *J. Clin. Invest.* **67**, 163–172.

Inoue, M., Morikawa, M., Tsuboi, M. and Sugiura, M. (1979). Species difference and characterization of intestinal esterase on the hydrolysing activity of ester-type drugs. *Jap. J. Pharmacol.* **29**, 9–16.

Kato, K., Mori, H., Fujii, M., Bunai, Y., Nishikawa, A., Shima, H., Takahashi, M., Kawai, T. and Hirono, I. (1984). Lack of promotive effect of quercetin on methylazoxymethanol acetate carcinogenesis in rats. *J. Toxicol. Sci.* **9**, 319–325.

Kato, K., Mori, H., Fujii, M., Bunai, Y., Nishikawa, A., Shima, H., Takahashi, M. and Hirono, I. (1985). Absence of initiating activity by quercetin in the rat liver. *Ecotoxicol. Environ. Saf.* **10**, 63–69.

Kelsey, M. I. and Sexton, S. A. (1976). The biosynthesis of ethyl esters of lithocholic acid and isolithocholic acid by rat intestinal microflora. *J. Steroid Biochem.* **7**, 641–647.

Knudsen, I. (1982). Natural, processed, and artificial mutagens in foods — significance and consequences. *Prog. Clin. Biol. Res.* **109**, 305–326.

Kobashi, K., Nishimura, T., Kusaka, M., Hattori, M. and Namba, T. (1980). Metabolism of sennosides by human intestinal bacteria. *Planta Med.* **40**, 225–236.

Kobayashi, A. and Matsumoto, H. (1964). Studies on methylazoxymethanol, the aglycone of cycasin (toxic constituent of *Cycas circinalis* nuts): isolation, biological chemical properties. *Arch. Biochem. Biophys.* **110**, 373–380.

Kuhnau, J. (1976). The flavonoids, a class of semi-essential food components: Their role in human nutrition. *World Rev. Nutr. Diet.* **24**, 117–191.

Laqueur, G. L., Michelson, O., Whiting, M. G. and Kurland, L. T. (1963). Carcinogenic properties of nuts from *Cycas circinalis* L. indigenous to Guam. *J. Natl Cancer Inst.* **31**, 919–951.

Laqueur, G. L., McDaniel, E. G. and Matsumoto, H. (1967). Tumor reduction in germfree rats with methylazoxymethanol (MAM) and synthetic MAM acetate. *J. Natl Cancer Inst.* **39**, 355–371.

Luczak, M. and Wleklik, M. (1985). Rozwoj i regres ja guzow indukowanych przez wirus M-MSV u myszy pod wplywem podawania rutyny i kwercetyny. *Med. Dosw. Mikrobiol.* **37**, 196–201.

Macdonald, I. A., Bussard, R. G., Hutchinson, D. M. and Holdeman, L. V.

(1984). Rutin-induced β-glucosidase activity in *Streptococcus faecium* VGH-1 and *Streptococcus* strain FRP-17 isolated from human feces: Formation of the mutagen, quercetin, from rutin. *Appl. Environ. Microbiol.* **47**, 350–355.

Macdonald, I. A., Bokkenheuser, V. D., Winter, J., McLernon, A. M. and Mosbach, E. H. (1983). Degradation of steroids in the human gut. *J. Lipid Res.* **24**, 675–700.

Macdonald, I. A., Mader, J. A. and Bussard, R. G. (1983). The role of rutin and quercitrin in stimulating flavonol glycosidase activity by cultured cell-free microbial preparation of human feces and saliva. *Mutat. Res.* **122**, 95–102.

MacGregor, J. T. and Jurd, L. (1978). Mutagenicity of plant flavonoids: structural requirements for mutagenic activity in *Salmonella typhimurium. Mutat. Res.* **54**, 297–309.

Mader, J. A. and Macdonald, I. A. (1985). Effect of bile acids on formation of the mutagen quercetin, from two flavonol glycoside precursors by human gut bacterial preparations. *Mutat. Res.* **155**, 99–104.

Marshall, T. C. and Dorough, H. W. (1984). Comparative disposition of 3-hydroxy carbofuran glucoside and its aglycone in rats. *J. Agric. Food Chem.* **32**, 882–886.

Maruta, A., Enaka, K. and Umeda, M. (1979). Mutagenicity of quercetin and kaempferol on cultured mammalian cells. *Gann* **70**, 273–276.

Masuda, T. and Ueno, Y. (1984). Microsomal transformation of emodin into a direct mutagen. *Mutat. Res.* **125**, 135–144.

Mathis, C. (1966). *In*: "Comparative Phytochemistry" (ed. T. Swain), pp. 245–270. Academic Press, New York.

Matsushima, T., Matsumoto, H., Shirai, A., Sawamura, M. and Sugimura, T. (1979). Mutagenicity of the naturally occurring carcinogen cycasin and synthetic methylazoxymethanol conjugates in *Salmonella typhimurium. Cancer Res.* **39**, 3780–3782.

Mazaki, M., Ishii, T. and Uyeta, M. (1982). Mutagenicity of hydrolysates of citrus fruit juices. *Mutat. Res.* **101**, 283–291.

McClure, J. W. (1975). *In*: "The Flavonoids" (eds J. B. Harborne, T. J. Mabry and H. Mabry), p. 970. Academic Press, New York.

Meltz, M. L. and MacGregor, J. T. (1981). Activity of the plant flavonol quercetin in the mouse lymphoma L5178Y TK +/− mutation, DNA single-strand break, and Balb/c3T3 chemical transformation assays. *Mutat. Res.* **88**, 317–324.

Mikami, N., Wakabayashi, N., Yamada, H. and Miyamoto, J. (1984). New conjugated metabolites of 3-phenoxybenzoic acid in plants. *Pestic. Sci.* **15**, 531–542.

Mikami, N., Yoshimura, J., Kaneko, H., Yamada, H. and Miyamoto, J. (1985). Metabolism in rats of 3-phenoxybenzyl alcohol and 3-phenoxybenzoic acid glucoside conjugates formed in plants. *Pestic. Sci.* **15**, 33–45.

Miyamoto, J., Kaneko, H. and Okuno, Y. (1986). *In*: "Xenobiotic Conjugation Chemistry" (eds G. D. Paulson, J. Caldwell, D. H. Hutson, and J. J. Menn), Vol. 229, pp. 268–281. ACS Symposium Series, American Chemical Society, Washington, D.C.

Moore, W. E. C. and Holdeman, L. V. (1974). Human fecal flora: the normal flora of 20 Japanese-Hawaiians. *Appl. Environ. Microbiol.* **27**, 961–979.

Morgan, R. W. and Hoffmann, G. R. (1983). Cycasin and its mutagenic metabolites. *Mutat. Res.* **114**, 19–58.

Mori, H., Sugie, S., Niwa, K., Takahashi, M. and Kawai, K. (1985). Induction of intestinal tumors in rats by chrysazin. *Brit. J. Cancer* **52**, 781–783.

Morino, K., Matsukura, N., Kawachi, T., Ohgaki, H., Sugimura, T. and Hirono, I. (1982). Carcinogenicity test of quercetin and rutin in golden hamsters by oral administration. *Carcinogenesis* **3**, 93–97.

Muir, A. D., Majak, W., Pass, M. A. and Yost, G. S. (1984). Conversion of 3-nitropropanol (miserotoxin aglycone) to 3-nitropropionic acid in cattle and sheep. *Toxicol. Lett.* **20**, 137–141.

Nagao, M., Takahashi, Y., Yamanaka, H. and Sugimura, T. (1979). Mutagens in tea and coffee. *Mutat. Res.* **68**, 101–106.

Nagao, M., Morita, N., Yahagi, T., Shimizo, M., Kuroyanagi, M., Fukuoka, M., Yoshihira, K., Natori, S., Fujino, T. and Sugimura, T. (1981). Mutagenicities of 61 flavonoids and 11 related compounds. *Environ. Mutagen.* **3**, 401–419.

Nagase, S., Fujimaki, C. and Isaka, H. (1964). Effect of administration of quercetin on the production of experimental liver cancers in rats fed 4-dimethylaminoazobenzene. *Proc. Jpn Cancer Assoc.* pp. 26–27.

Nagata, C., Inomata, M., Kodama, M. and Tagashira, Y. (1968). Electron spin resonance study on the interaction between the chemical carcinogens and tissue components, III. Determination of the structure of the radical produced either by stirring 3,4-benzopyrene with albumin or incubating it with liver homogenates. *Gann* **159**, 289–298.

Newmark, J., Brady, R. O., Grimley, P. M., Gal, A. E., Waller, S. G. and Thistlethwaite, J. R. (1981). Amygdalin (Laetrile) and prunasin β-glucosidases: Distribution in germ-free rat and in human tumor tissue. *Proc. Natl Acad. Sci. U.S.A.* **78**, 6513–6516.

Nishino, H., Iwashima, A., Fujiki, H. and Sugimura, T. (1984a). Inhibition by quercetin of the promoting effect of teleocidin on skin papilloma formation in mice initiated with 7,2-dimethylbenz[a]anthracene. *Gann* **75**, 113–116.

Nishino, H., Nishino, A., Iwashima, A., Tanaka, K. and Matsuura, T. (1984b). Quercetin inhibits the action of 12-*O*-tetradecaoylphorbol-13-acetate, a tumor promotor. Oncology **41**, 120–123.

Nishino, H., Naito, E., Iwashima, A., Tanaka, K., Matsuura, T., Fujiki, H. and Sugimura, T. (1984c). Interaction between quercetin and Ca2+–calmodulin complex: possible mechanism for anti-tumor-promoting action of the flavonoid. *Gann* **75**, 311–316.

Northrup, S., Martis, L., Ulbricht, R., Garber, J., Miripol, J. and Schmitz, T. (1982). Comment on the carcinogenic potential of di(2-ethylhexyl) phthalate. *J. Toxicol. Environ. Health* **10**, 493–518.

Pamukcu, A. M., Yalciner, S., Hatcher, J. F. and Bryan, G. T. (1980). Quercetin, a rat intestinal and bladder carcinogen present in bracken fern (*Pteridium aquilinum*). *Cancer Res.* **40**, 3468–3472.

Petrakis, P. L., Kallianos, A. G., Wender, S. H. and Shetlar, M. R. (1959). Metabolic studies of quercetin labelled with C^{14}. *Arch. Biochem. Biophys.* **85**, 264–271.

Pezzuto, J. M., Compadre, C. M., Swanson, S. M., Dhammika Nanayakkara, N. P. and Kinghorn, A. D. (1985). Metabolically activated steviol, the aglycone of stevioside is mutagenic. *Proc. Natl Acad. Sci. U.S.A.* **82**, 2478–2482.

Quistad, G. B., Staiger, L. E. and Schooley, D. A. (1982). Xenobiotic conjugation: a novel role for bile acids. *Nature* **296**, 462–464.

Reddy, N.R., Palmer, J. K., Pierson, M. D. and Bothast, R. J., (1984). Intracellular glycosidases of human colon *Bacteroides ovatus* B4–11. *Appl. Environ. Microbiol.* **48**, 890–892.

Rowland, I. R. (1974). Metabolism of di-(2-ethylhexyl) phthalate by the contents of the alimentary tract of the rat. *Food Cosmet. Toxicol.* **12**, 293–302.

Rowland, I. (1981). The influence of the gut microflora on food toxicity. *Proc. Nutr. Soc.* **40**, 67–74.

Rowland, I. R., Cottrell, R. C. and Phillips, J. C. (1977). Hydrolysis of phthalate esters by the gastro-intestinal contents of the rat. *Food. Cosmet. Toxicol.* **15**, 17–21.

Salyers, A. A., Palmer, J. K. and Wilkins, T. D. (1977). Laminarinase (β-glucanase) activity in *Bacteroides* from the human colon. *Appl. Environ. Microbiol.* **33**, 1118–1124.

Saito, D., Shirai, A., Matsushima, T., Sugimura, T. and Hirono, I. (1980). Test of carcinogeneity of quercetin, a widely distributed mutagen in food. *Teratogen. Carcinogen. Mutagen.* **1**, 213–221.

Scheline, R. R. (1968). The metabolism of drugs and other compounds by the intestinal bacteria. *Acta Pharmacol. Toxicol.* **26**, 332–342.

Scheline, R. R. (1973). Metabolism of foreign compounds by gastrointestinal microorganisms. *Pharmacol. Rev.* **25**, 451–523.

Schmid, W. (1952). Zum Wirkungsmechanismus diatetischer und medikamentoser Darnmittel. *Arzneim. Forsch.* **2**, 6–20.

Seino, Y., Nagao, M., Yahagi, T., Sugimura, T., Yasuda, T. and Nishimura, S. (1978). Identification of a mutagenic substance in a spice, sumac, as quercetin. *Mutat. Res.* **58**, 225–229.

Simon, G. L. and Gorbach, S. L. (1984). Intestinal flora in health and disease. *Gastroenterol.* **86**, 174–193.

Spatz, M., McDaniel, E. G. and Laqueur, G. L. (1966). Cycasin excretion in conventional and germfree rats. *Proc. Soc. Exp. Biol. Med.* **121**, 417–422.

Spatz, M., Smith, D. W. E., McDaniel, E. G. and Laqueur, G. L. (1967). The role of intestinal microorganisms in determining cycasin toxicity. *Proc. Soc. Exp. Biol. Med.* **124**, 691–697.

Stavric, B. (1984). Mutagenic food flavonoids. *Fed. Proc.* **43**, 2454–2458.

Stoewsand, G. S., Anderson, J. L., Boyd, J. N., Hrazdina, G., Babish, J. G., Walsh, K. M. and Losco, P. (1984). Quercetin — a mutagen, not a carcinogen, in Fischer rats. *J. Toxicol. Environ. Health* **14**, 105–114.

Sugimura, T., Nagao, M., Yahagi, T., Seino, Y., Shirai, A., Sawamura, M., Natori, S., Yoshihira, K., Fukuoka, M. and Kuroyanagi, M. (1977). Mutagenicity of flavone derivatives. *Proc. Jpn Acad.* **53B**, 194–197.

Sugimura, T. (1982). Mutagens, carcinogens and tumor promoters in our daily food. *Cancer* **49**, 1970–1982.

Takahashi, Y., Nagao, M., Fujino, T., Yamaizumi, Z. and Sugimura, T. (1979). Mutagens in Japanese pickle identified as flavonoids. *Mutat. Res.* **68**, 117–123.

Tamura, G., Gold, C., Ferro-Luzzi, A. and Ames, B. N. (1980). Fecalase: a model for activation of dietary glycosides to mutagens by intestinal flora. *Proc. Natl Acad. Sci. U.S.A.* **77**, 4961–4965.

Teirlynck and Belpaire (1985). Disposition of orally administered di-(z-ethylhexyl)phthalate and mono-(2-ethylhexyl)phthalate in the waf. *Arch. Toxicol*

57, 226–230.

Thomson, R. H. (1971). "Naturally Occurring Quinones". Academic Press, London.

Tikkanen, L., Matsushima, T. and Naturi, S. (1983a). Mutagenicity of anthraquinones in the Salmonella preincubation test. *Mutat. Res.* **116**, 297–304.

Tikkanen, L., Matsushima, T., Natori, S. and Yoshihira, K. (1983b). Mutagenicity of natural naphthoquinones and benzoquinones in the *Salmonella* microsome test. *Mutat. Res.* **124**, 20–34.

Ueno, I., Nakano, N. and Hirono, I. (1983). Metabolic fate of [^{14}C] quercetin in the ACI rat. *Japan. J. Exp. Med.* **53**, 41–50.

Umezawa, K., Matsushima, T., Sugimura, T., Hirakawa, T., Tanaka, M., Katoh, Y. and Takayama, S. (1977). *In vitro* transformation of hamster embryo cells by quercetin. *Toxicol. Lett.* **1**, 175–178.

Uraguchi, K., Saito, M., Noguchi, Y., Takahashi, K., Enomoto, M. and Tatsuno, T. (1972). Chronic toxicity and carcinogenicity in mice of the purified mycotoxins, luteoskyrin and cyclochlorotine. *Food Cosmet. Toxicol.* **3**, 193–207.

Uyeta, M., Taue, S. and Mazaki, M. (1981). Mutagenicity of hydrolysates of tea infusions. *Mutat. Res.* **88**, 233–240.

Van Os, F. H. L. (1976a). Anthraquinone derivatives in vegetable laxatives. *Pharmacol.* **14**, Suppl. 1, 7–17.

Van Os, F. H. L. (1976b). Some aspects of the pharmacology of anthraquinone drugs. *Pharmacol.* **14**, Suppl. 1, 18–29.

Watson, W. A. F. (1982). The mutagenic activity of quercetin and kaempferol in *Drosophila melanogaster. Mutat. Res.* **103**, 145–147.

Wattenberg,, L. W. and Leong, J. L. (1970). Inhibition of the carcinogenic action of benzo(a)pyrene by flavones. *Cancer Res.* **30**, 1922–1925.

Wells, J. M., Cole, R. J. and Kirksey, J. W. (1975). Emodin, a toxic metabolite of *Aspergillus wentii* isolated from weevil-damaged chestnuts. *Appl. Microbiol.* **30**, 26–28.

Williams, R. T. (1972). Toxicologic implications of biotransformation by intestinal microflora. *Toxicol. appl. Pharmacol.* **23**, 769–781.

Wingard, R. E., Brown, J. P., Enderlin, F. E., Dale, J. A., Hale, R. L. and Seitz, C. T. (1980). Intestinal degradation and absorption of the glycosidic sweeteners stevioside and rebaudioside A. *Experientia* **36**, 519–520.

Yano, K. and Takahashi, Y. (1981). Hydrolysis of trans-cinnamyl esters by the entero bacterial cells (*Escherichia coli*). *Lab. Pract.* **30**, 468.

Yasui, Y. and Takeda, N. (1983). Identification of a mutagenic substance, in *Rubia tinctorum* L. (madder) root, as lucidin. *Mutat. Res.* **121**, 185–190.

Zeiger, E., Haworth, S., Mortelmans, K. and Speck, W. (1985). Mutagenicity testing of di(2-ethylhexyl)phthalate and related chemicals in *Salmonella. Environ. Mutagen.* **7**, 213–232.

6

Metabolism of Nitro Compounds

DOUGLAS E. RICKERT

A. Introduction

Nitroaromatic compounds comprise an important class of chemicals which includes antibiotic, antiparasitic and radiosensitizing drugs, and environmental contaminants resulting from the combustion of fossil fuels and explosives. They are intermediates in the manufacture of several thousand consumer products, accounting for nearly 10% of the sales of the chemical industry (Hartter, 1984). The nitro group on nitroaromatic compounds can be reduced by mammalian or bacterial enzymes. For compounds whose first metabolic products are easily reoxidized by molecular oxygen (e.g. a nitroanion radical (Mason and Holtzman, 1975)), the aerobic environment found in mammalian tissues will mitigate against formation of isolatable metabolites. Reduced metabolites formed from such compounds are more likely to arise from metabolism by obligate anaerobic bacteria in the oxygen-poor environment of the distal small intestine, caecum and large intestine. Chemicals can encounter the obligate anaerobes of the intestine in three ways: (*i*) they may be poorly absorbed after ingestion and remain in the intestine long enough to be swept to the distal small intestine and caecum by peristalsis; (*ii*) they (or their metabolites) may partition across the intestinal wall from the blood; (*iii*) they (or their metabolites) may be excreted in the bile. Of the compounds to be discussed below, the nitrobenzenes probably encounter the anaerobic bacteria of the intestine after partitioning from the blood. The nitrotoluenes and nitropyrenes are excreted in the bile of rats and arrive in the lower small intestine and caecum as metabolites. In all cases biotransformation by the intestinal microflora apparently accounts for quantitatively and biologically significant metabolites.

ROLE OF THE GUT FLORA IN TOXICITY AND CANCER
ISBN 0-12-599920-8

B. Nitrobenzenes

Reduction of nitrobenzenes by intestinal microorganisms was noted in early work by Bray and his co-workers (1953). The 2,3,5,6- and 2,3,4,5-tetrachloroaniline excreted by rabbits after oral doses of 2,3,5,6- or 2,3,4,5-tetrachloronitrobenzene, respectively, could be formed in incubations of intestinal contents with the tetrachloronitrobenzenes. Nitrobenzene, 2- and 4-nitrotoluene, and several other nitroaromatic compounds were also reduced in incubations with rabbit intestinal contents. It was unclear from this work whether reduction by mammalian or microbial enzymes was more important to the disposition of nitrobenzenes *in vivo*.

Since the reduction of nitrobenzene to nitrosobenzene and phenylhydroxylamine had been shown to be important in the methaemoglobinaemia produced by nitrobenzene administration (Kiese, 1974), Reddy *et al.* (1976) reasoned that if reduction of nitrobenzene by intestinal microflora was more important than reduction by mammalian enzymes, germ-free rats should be resistant to nitrobenzene-induced methaemoglobinaemia. They gave conventional, germ-free or antibiotic treated Sprague–Dawley rats nitrobenzene (200 mg kg^{-1} p.o.) and measured methaemoglobin levels in the blood over a period of 7 hours. Methaemoglobin levels in conventional rats reached 30–40% during the first 2 hours after nitrobenzene administration; no measurable methaemoglobin was formed in germ-free or antibiotic treated rats. When nitrobenzene reduction was measured (as aniline formed) in homogenates from various tissues, the liver, kidney and gut wall of germ-free and conventional rats were similar, but nitrobenzene reduction by gut contents from germ-free rats was less than 2% of that observed in conventional rats. These data indicated that the gut microflora were necessary for the production of methaemoglobinaemia in rats, and suggested that the majority of nitrobenzene reduction in intact rats occurred in the gut microflora.

Levin and Dent (1982) compared the *in vitro* reduction of nitrobenzene by hepatic microsomes and caecal contents of Fischer-344 rats. Metabolism of nitrobenzene to isolatable products by rat hepatic microsomes under aerobic conditions was slow (<22 pmol metabolized/min/mg protein). Nitrobenzene was readily reduced by incubations containing caecal contents under anaerobic conditions. Concentrations of the presumed methaemoglobinogenic metabolites, nitrosobenzene and phenylhydroxylamine, peaked after 60 minutes of incubation, while the concentration of aniline continued to increase throughout the entire 180 minute incubation, eventually accounting for nearly all of the nitrobenzene metabolized. Nitrobenzene was reduced to aniline by hepatic microsomes under anaerobic conditions but at less than 1% the rate of reduction by rat caecal contents (4.4. nmol min^{-1}g^{-1} liver *vs.* 668 nmol min^{-1}g^{-1} caecal contents). Since the liver and caecal contents are of approximately equal weight, these data support the hypothesis that most of the *in vivo* reduction of nitrobenzene in rats is due to metabolism by intestinal microflora.

The major identified urinary metabolites of nitrobenzene in Fischer-344 rats are 3- and 4-nitrophenol, which apparently arise from ring hydroxylation of nitrobenzene, and 4-hydroxyacetanilide, which is formed through an aniline intermediate (Levin and Dent, 1982; Rickert *et al.*, 1983a). Antibiotic treated and control animals excreted a similar percentage of a nitrobenzene dose as the two oxidized metabolites, 3- and 4-nitrophenol, but excretion of the reduced metabolite, 4-hydroxyacetanilide, accounted for only 0.9% of the dose in antibiotic treated animals compared to 16.2% of the dose in control animals (Levin and Dent, 1982). Thus, it is clear that the intestinal microflora are major determinants in the metabolism and acute toxicity of nitrobenzene.

C. Nitrotoluenes

The nitrotoluenes are important intermediates in the manufacture of dyes and plastics. 2-nitrotoluene is genotoxic, and a mixture of dinitrotoluene isomers as well as purified 2,6-dinitrotoluene is hepatocarcinogenic in rats (Doolittle *et al.*, 1983; Rickert *et al.*, 1984). The metabolism of various nitrotoluenes by rat, mouse or human intestinal contents has been studied, as the covalent binding and genotoxicity of these compounds is dependent upon intestinal microflora. Hepatic unscheduled DNA synthesis, a measure of DNA repair, was increased in conventional rats, but not in germ-free rats, treated with either 2,6-dinitrotoluene (Mirsalis *et al.*, 1982) or 2-nitrotoluene (Doolittle *et al.*, 1983). Conventional Fischer-344 rats given a dose of radiolabelled 2,4-dinitrotoluene excreted four major metabolites. Two of the metabolites, 2,4-dinitrobenzoic acid and 2,4-dinitrobenzyl glucuronide, resulted from benzyl carbon oxidation or benzyl carbon oxidation followed by glucuronidation, respectively. The other two metabolites, 4-*N*-acetyl-2-nitrobenzoic acid and 2-amino-4-nitrobenzoic acid, had undergone nitro group reduction as well as benzyl carbon oxidation (Rickert *et al.*, 1981). Whereas conventional rats excreted approximately 16% of a dose of 2,4-dinitrotoluene as the latter two metabolites, germ-free rats excreted only about 2% of the dose as those metabolites. This suggests that the most important site for reduction of 2,4-dinitrotoluene is in the intestinal microflora.

Caecal contents of male Swiss–Webster mice, male and female Fischer-344 rats, human ileal contents from a patient with an ileostomy, and human faecal samples reduced 2,4-dinitrotoluene under anaerobic conditions to 2-nitroso-4-nitrotoluene, 4-nitroso-2-nitrotoluene, 4-amino-2-nitrotoluene and 2-amino-4-nitrotoluene (Guest *et al.*, 1982). Prolonged incubation yielded 2,4-diaminotoluene, but intermediate hydroxylamino-nitro-, aminonitroso- or hydroxylaminonitrosotoluenes could not be isolated. It is possible that those compounds are sufficiently reactive to covalently bind to macromolecules of the microflora. This is supported by the fact that only 42–90% of the added 2,4-dinitrotoluene could be recovered from the incubation mixtures, and that when 2-amino-4-nitrotoluene or 4-amino-2-nitrotoluene were incubated with rat caecal contents, only about 30% of the added substrate was recovered as either parent compound or 2,4-diaminotoluene. In an *in vivo* study approximately 10% of a dose of 2,4-dinitrotoluene was covalently bound to caecal contents 8 hours after administration of 35 mg kg^{-1} (Rickert *et al.*, 1983b).

Caecal contents from Fischer-344 rats reduced the nitro group at the 4 position of 2,4-dinitrotoluene more rapidly than that at the 2 position (Guest *et al.*, 1982). Consequently, 4-amino-2-nitrotoluene concentrations in incubations of 2,4-dinitrotoluene with caecal contents were three to five times higher than were 2-amino-4-nitrotoluene concentrations. 2-amino-4-nitrotoluene was converted to 2,4-diaminotoluene more rapidly than 4-amino-2-nitrotoluene. It would be interesting to compare the relative rates of reduction of isomeric nitrotoluenes across microbial species to determine whether all have similar substrate specificities.

One can calculate from *in vitro* experiments that the caecal contents of Fischer-344 rats contain 10 to 20 times the reducing capacity of the liver, even if comparisons are made under conditions of reduced oxygen (Guest *et al.*, 1982). This suggests that, like nitrobenzene, the nitrotoluenes are primarily reduced by intestinal microorganisms. It should be noted, however, that the toxicity of 2-nitrotoluene and 2,6-dinitrotoluene derives not from reduction of the parent compound but from a product of (di)nitrobenzyl alcohol reduction. 2-nitrotoluene and 2,6-dinitrotoluene are rapidly absorbed from the small intestine, oxidized at the benzyl carbon and conjugated to yield 2-nitrobenzyl glucuronide and 2,6-dinitrobenzyl glucuronide which are extensively excreted in the bile. Intestinal microflora hydrolyse the glucuronide and reduce a nitro group to yield 2-aminobenzyl alcohol and 2-amino-6-nitrobenzyl alcohol which are reabsorbed. Further sulphotransferase-dependent metabolism results in electrophilic products which covalently bind to DNA (Rickert *et al.* 1984; Rickert, 1986). Detailed *in vitro* studies of the microbial metabolism of 2-nitrobenzyl alcohol and 2,6-dinitrobenzyl alcohol have not been reported, but there is little reason to believe that their metabolism would differ markedly from that of 2,4-dinitrotoluene.

D. Nitropyrenes

The nitropyrenes are environmental contaminants which are products of combustion and are found in urban air particulates and diesel exhaust (Wang *et al.*, 1980; Pedersen and Siak, 1981). They are very potent mutagens in the Ames *Salmonella* test, and their mutagenicity appears to be dependent upon reduction (Mermelstein *et al.*, 1981; Messier *et al.*, 1981; Howard *et al.*, 1983a). When intestinal microfloras from rats were incubated with radiolabelled 1-nitropyrene (3.7 mM), the parent compound rapidly disappeared and three metabolites were found (Howard *et al.*, 1983b). 1-aminopyrene accounted for over 85% of the ethyl acetate extractable radioactivity, with the other two metabolites accounting for 12–13%. Of the individual obligate anaerobes tested, *Bacteroides thetaiotaomicron*, *Clostridium perfringens*, *Peptococcus anaerobius*, *Clostridium* sp. and *Peptostreptococcus productus* converted over 95% of the added 1-nitropyrene (3.7 mM) to 1-aminopyrene during a 6 hour incubation. *Bifidobacterium infantis* and *Citrobacter* sp. converted about 70% of the added 1-nitropyrene in the same time. *Lactobacillus acidophilus* incubated under anaerobic conditions and *Escherichia coli* and three strains of *Salmonella typhimurium* incubated under either aerobic or anaerobic conditions reduced only 10–20% of the added 1-nitropyrene to 1-aminopyrene. Thus, a number of bacteria are capable of effecting 1-nitropyrene reduction, but the rates vary widely. Human intestinal microflora in semicontinuous culture reduced 1-nitropyrene to 1-aminopyrene, but they also produced *N*-formyl-1-aminopyrene (Manning *et al.*, 1986). The latter metabolite has not been reported to occur in other systems. It seems unlikely that human microflora, but not rodent microflora, are capable of forming *N*-formyl-1-aminopyrene. A more plausible explanation is that sufficiently long incubation times were used in the semicontinuous culture system (>24 hours; Manning *et al.*, 1986) to allow concentrations of the metabolite to accumulate to measurable levels.

Reduction of 1-nitropyrene by intestinal microflora is clearly important *in vivo*. El-Bayoumy *et al.* (1983) found 1-aminopyrene in the faeces of conventional but not germ-free Fischer-344 rats. In a more extensive study, 4,5-dihydro-4,5-dihydroxy-1-nitropyrene, 1-nitro-3-hydroxypyrene, 1-nitro-6-hydroxypyrene, 1-nitro-8-hydroxypyrene, 1-aminopyrene, 1-amino-6-hydroxypyrene and 1-amino-8-hydroxypyrene (or their glucuronide conjugates) were identified in urine and faeces of conventional Fischer-344 rats given an oral dose of 1-nitropyrene (El-Bayoumy *et al.*, 1984). The same metabolites were found in urine and faeces of germ-free rats, except those which had undergone nitroreduction. Although

1-acetylaminopyrene was identified as a metabolite of 1-nitropyrene in the bile of isolated perfused liver preparations and *in vivo* (Bond *et al.*, 1984; Medinsky *et al.*, 1985), and 1-acetylaminopyrene and 1-aminopyrene were identified in isolated perfused lung preparations (Bond and Mauderly, 1984), the rates of conversion were slow, and liver and lung probably do not contribute greatly to the reduction of 1-nitropyrene *in vivo*. It is not clear what metabolites are toxic to mammalian systems. The hydroxylated metabolites probably arise from epoxides; similar metabolites are responsible for the toxicities associated with polycyclic aromatic hydrocarbons. The mutagenicity for *Salmonella typhimurium* is probably due to reduced products, but whether those formed from 1-nitropyrene by intestinal microflora are responsible for any mammalian toxicity remains to be demonstrated.

The dinitropyrenes are even more potent mutagens in the Ames *Salmonella typhimurium* test than 1-nitropyrene (Mermelstein *et al.*, 1981), and while no studies specifically examining the metabolism of these compounds by intestinal microflora have appeared, they are readily reduced by *Salmonella typhimurium* (Bryant, *et al.*, 1984). 1,6-dinitro-pyrene does not require intestinal microflora to yield a genotoxic response in rat liver. While it induced unscheduled DNA repair in primary cultures of rat or human hepatocytes, it produced no unscheduled DNA repair in hepatocytes isolated from rats treated *in vivo* (Butterworth *et al.*, 1983). These data suggest that either the dinitropyrenes are reduced by mammalian enzymes or that their activation to genotoxic metabolites requires oxidation.

References

Bond, J. A. and Mauderly, J. L. (1984). Metabolism and macromolecular covalent binding of [^{14}C]-1-nitropyrene in isolated perfused and ventilated rat lungs. *Cancer Res.* **44**, 3924–3929.

Bond, J. A., Medinsky, M. A. and Dutcher, J. S. (1984). Metabolism and biliary excretion of [^{14}C]-1-nitropyrene in rats and isolated perfused livers. *Toxicol. appl. Pharmacol.* **75**, 531–538.

Bray, H. G., Hybs, Z., James, S. P. and Thorpe, W. V. (1953). The metabolism of 2:3:5:6- and 2:3:4:5-tetrachloronitrobenzenes in the rabbit and the reduction of aromatic nitro compounds in the intestine. *Biochem. J.* **53**, 266–273.

Bryant, D. W., McCalla, D. R., Lultschik, P., Quilliam, M. A. and McCarry, B. E. (1984). Metabolism of 1,8-dinitropyrene by Salmonella typhimurium. *Chem.-Biol. Interact.* **49**, 351–368.

Butterworth, B. E., Earle, L. L., Strom, S., Jirtle, R. and Michalopoulos, G. (1983). Induction of DNA repair in human and rat hepatocytes by 1,6-dinitropyrene. *Mutat. Res.* **122**, 73–80.

Doolittle, D. J., Sherrill, J. M. and Butterworth, B. E. (1983). Influence of intestinal bacteria, sex of the animal, and position of the nitro group on the hepatic genotoxicity of nitrotoluene isomers *in vivo*. *Cancer Res.* **43**, 2836–2842.

El-Bayoumy, K., Sharma, C., Louis, Y. M. Reddy, B. and Hecht, S. S. (1983). The role of intestinal microflora in the metabolic reduction of 1-nitropyrene to 1-aminopyrene in conventional and germfree rats and in humans. *Cancer Lett.* **19**, 311–316.

El-Bayoumy, K., Reddy, B. and Hecht, S. S. (1984). Identification of ring oxidized metabolites of 1-nitropyrene in the faeces and urine of germfree F344 rats. *Carcinogenesis* **5**, 1371–1373.

Guest, D., Schnell, S. R., Rickert, D. E. and Dent, J. G. (1982). Metabolism of 2,4-dinitrotoluene by intestinal microorganisms from rat, mouse, and man. *Toxicol. appl. Pharmacol.* **64**, 160–168.

Hartter, D. R. (1984). The use and importance of nitroaromatic chemicals in the chemical industry. *In*: "Toxicity of Nitroaromatic Compounds" (ed. D. E. Rickert), pp. 1–13. Hemisphere Publishing Co., Washington, D.C.

Howard, P. C., Heflich, R. H., Evans, F. E. and Beland, F. A. (1983a). DNA adducts formed in vitro and in Salmonella typhimurium upon metabolic reduction of the environmental mutagen 1-nitropyrene. *Cancer Res.* **43**, 2052–2058.

Howard, P. C., Beland, F. A. and Cerniglia, C. E. (1983b). Reduction of the carcinogen 1-nitropyrene to 1-aminopyrene by rat intestinal bacteria. *Carcinogenesis* **4**, 985–990.

Kiese, M. (1974). "Methemoglobinemia: A comprehensive treatise", p. 128. CRC Press, Inc., Cleveland.

Levin, A. A. and Dent, J. G. (1982). Comparison of the metabolism of nitrobenzene by hepatic microsomes and cecal microflora from Fischer-344 rats *in vitro* and the relative importance of each *in vivo*. *Drug. Metab. Dispos.* **10**, 450–454.

Manning, B. W., Cerniglia, C. E. and Federle, T. W. (1986). Biotransformation of 1-nitropyrene to 1-aminopyrene and N-formyl-1-aminopyrene by the human intestinal microbiota. *J. Toxicol. Environ. Health* **18**, 339–346.

Mason, R. P. and Holtzman, J. L. (1975). Mechanism of microsomal and mitrochondrial nitroreductase. Electron spin resonance evidence for nitroaromatic free radical intermediates. *Biochemistry* **14**, 1626–1632.

Medinsky, M. A., Shelton, H., Bond, J. A. and McClellan, R. O. (1985). Biliary excretion and enterohepatic circulation of 1-nitropyrene metabolites in Fischer-344 rats. *Biochem. Pharmacol.* **34**, 2325–2330.

Mermelstein, R., Kiriazides, D. K., Butler, M., McCoy, E. C. and Rosenkranz, H. S. (1981). The extraordinary mutagenicity of nitropyrenes in bacteria. *Mutat. Res.* **89**, 187–196.

Messier, F., Lu, C., Andrews, P., McCarry, B. E., Quilliam, M. A. and McCalla, D. R. (1981). Metabolism of 1-nitropyrene and formation of DNA adducts in Salmonella typhimurium. *Carcinogenesis* **2**, 1007–1011.

Mirsalis, J. C., Hamm, T. E., Jr., Sherrill, J. M. and Butterworth, B. E. (1982). Role of gut flora in genotoxicity of dinitrotoluene. *Nature (Lond.)* **295**, 322–323.

Pedersen, T. C. and Siak, J. -S. (1981). The role of nitroaromatic compounds in the direct-acting mutagenicity of diesel particle extracts. *J. appl. Toxicol.* **1**, 54–60.

Reddy, B. G., Pohl, L. R. and Krishna, G. (1976). The requirement of the gut flora in nitrobenzene-induced methemoglobinemia in rats. *Biochem. Pharmacol.* **25**, 1119–1122.

Rickert, D. E., Bond, J. A., Long, R. M. and Chism, J. P. (1983a). Metabolism and excretion of nitrobenzene by rats and mice. *Toxicol. appl. Pharmacol.* **67**, 206–214.

Rickert, D. E., Schnell, S. R. and Long, R. M. (1983b). Hepatic macromolecular covalent binding and intestinal disposition of [14C]dinitrotoluenes. *J. Toxicol. Environ. Health* **11**, 555–567.

Rickert, D. E., Long, R. M., Krakowka, S. and Dent, J. G. (1981). Metabolism and excretion of 2,4-[14C]dinitrotoluene in conventional and axenic Fischer-344 rats. *Toxicol. appl. Pharmacol.* **59**, 574–579.

Rickert, D. E., Butterworth, B. E. and Popp, J. A. (1984). Dinitrotoluenes: Acute toxicity, metabolism and oncogenicity. *CRC Crit. Rev. Toxicol.* **13**, 217–234.

Rickert, D. E. (1987). Metabolism of nitroaromatic compounds. *Drug. Metab. Rev.* 18, 23–53.

Wang, C. Y., Lee, M. -S., King, C. M. and Warner, P. O. (1980). Evidence for nitroaromatics as direct-acting mutagens of airborne particulates. *Chemosphere* **9**, 83–87.

7

Nitrate, Nitrite and *N*-Nitroso Compounds
The Role of the Gut Microflora

A. K. MALLETT

A. Introduction

Nitrate is a widely distributed environmental contaminant which has come under increasing scrutiny in recent years due to the toxic effects of its reduction product, nitrite. The bacterial population colonizing the mammalian intestinal tract is capable of performing this transformation with the potential subsequent induction of methaemoglobinaemia or the formation of genotoxic *N*-nitroso compounds.

The involvement of the gastro-intestinal microflora in the toxicity and metabolism of nitrate within the body is described in the following sections.

B. Sources of Ingested Nitrate

Nitrate is the predominant form of nitrogen oxides present in the diet of man and laboratory animals, and is present in substantial quantities in most sources of water and in plants (WHO, 1978; 1984). Nitrites are also widely distributed, but generally occur at much lower levels than nitrates (WHO, 1978; 1984). Nitrate enters the environment as a consequence of the oxidation of organic nitrogen by soil bacteria (Payne, 1973) or the leaching of natural mineral deposits or fertilizers from the soil (Ryden *et al.*, 1984; White, 1984). Water-borne sources of nitrate become increasingly important as contamination of the water table increases, and may supply 70–80% of the total nitrate intake (Chilvers *et al.*, 1984). On a global basis, the highest *per capita* intake of total nitrate is found in the USA and UK (Hartman, 1982), with a typical value of 1–1.5 mmol/day.

ROLE OF THE GUT FLORA IN TOXICITY AND CANCER
ISBN 0-12-599920-8

C. Endogenous Formation of Nitrate *in vivo*

In addition to exposure from preformed nitrate from the above sources, experimental studies in man and laboratory animals have suggested a number of biological pathways resulting in the *de novo* formation of nitrate and nitrite by microbial or mammalian metabolic processes. Initial evidence of endogenous nitrate synthesis came from observations that urinary nitrate excretion exceeded nitrate intake in humans consuming a low-nitrate diet (Mitchell *et al.*, 1916; Tannenbaum *et al.*, 1978; Kurzer and Calloway, 1981), but was subject to criticisms on methodological grounds. The major contention revolves around the problems of achieving constant, reproducible baseline measurements during nitrate balance studies of this kind (Hartman, 1982). Urinary nitrate estimations are suggested to be subject to appreciable quenching, possibly leading to an under-estimation of output (Hartman, 1982), whilst dietary analyses may be incapable of completely accounting for all of the nitrate present in the rations (Bartholomew and Hill, 1984). Nitrate excretion exhibits marked daily fluctuations (Tannenbaum *et al.*, 1978; Green *et al.*, 1981) suggesting a complex pharmacodynamic system requiring equilibration periods in excess of those presently used (Hartman, 1982; Bartholomew and Hill, 1984). Finally an excess of urinary nitrate is only apparent in the rat (Green *et al.*, 1981) or ferret (Dull and Hotchkiss, 1984a) when the intake of oral nitrate is at a low level, suggesting that endogenous nitrate synthesis is responsive to exogenous nitrate exposure. A recent nitrate balance study in humans employing HPLC detection of nitrate demonstrated a consistent excess of urinary nitrate over ingested nitrate/nitrite averaging 0.87 mmol/day (Lee *et al.*, 1986). The conclusions drawn from the majority of nitrate balance studies would, however, appear to be equivocal on the occurrence of endogenous nitrate synthesis.

More conclusive evidence for nitrate formation *in vivo* has come from experimental studies concerned with the metabolic fate of inorganic nitrogen within the body, and has been aided by the use of $[^{15}N]$-labelled precursors. Bacterial enzymes were initially implicated in a scheme of heterotrophic nitrification, since gut micro-organisms isolated from the rat, guinea pig and man could oxidize acetohydroxamate and hydroxylamine to nitrate when cultured aerobically *in vitro* (Ralt *et al.*, 1981). Such bacterial pathways were proposed as responsible for the nitrate/nitrite detected in human intestinal contents (Tannenbaum *et al.*, 1978), although other studies have returned much lower values and questioned the occurrence of this reaction (Saul *et al.*, 1981). Bacterial nitrification is an aerobic process, dependent upon free oxygen (Payne, 1973), and would be hindered by the highly anaerobic conditions present in the large intestine

(Moore and Holdeman, 1974; Moore *et al.*, 1978). The intestinal microflora readily assimilates inorganic nitrogen into bacterial cell mass (Forsythe and Parker, 1985; Takahashi and Kametaka, 1986), suggesting the availability of free ammonia to fuel this process would be limiting. The low redox potential and reducing conditions found in the hindgut (Schröder and Johansson, 1973) would thus more likely favour reduction and denitrification of nitrate (Saul *et al.*, 1981), and Witter *et al.* (1982) found no oxidation of ammonium sulphate, hydroxylamine or acetohydroxamate to nitrate under anaerobic conditions *in vitro*.

Balance studies comparing germ-free and conventional flora rats showed no differences in the apparent excess of urinary nitrate over nitrate intake (Green *et al.*, 1981; Witter *et al.*, 1982), suggesting, despite any shortcomings of the methodology (*vide supra*), that the gut microflora was not involved in endogenous nitrate synthesis. A search for potential substrates for conversion to nitrate, by mammalian processes, revealed that conventional flora rats given [^{15}N]-ammonium salts excreted [^{15}N]-nitrate in the urine, demonstrating that ammonia was a precursor of endogenously synthesized nitrate (Table 7.1). The conversion of ammonia to nitrate was however very low, but increased dramatically following activation of the reticuloendothelial system with *Escherichia coli* endotoxin, with a smaller increase in response to inflammatory reactions provoked by carrageenan, carbon tetrachloride or turpentine (Wagner *et al.*, 1983a; Saul and Archer, 1984). Stuehr and Marletta (1985) compared nitrate synthesis in strains of mice possessing specific genetic lymphoreticular defects. C3H/HeJ mice, which are hyporesponsive to *E. coli* endotoxin, showed no stimulation of nitrate synthesis following immune challenge, whereas endotoxin-responsive C3H/He mice excreted elevated levels of urinary nitrate. Related studies *in vitro* demonstrated that thioglycolate-elicited peritoneal macrophages from C3H/He, but not C3H/HeJ, mice generated nitrate and nitrite when cultured with endotoxin (Stuehr and Marletta, 1985). Such activated macrophages have also recently been shown to produce *N*-nitroso compounds *in vitro* (Miwa *et al.*, 1987), suggesting that immune cells may be involved in the conversion of nitrate/nitrite to toxic products. Nitrate synthesis may also occur in man during inflammatory illness, since an increase in urinary nitrate is seen in infants (Hegesh and Shiloah, 1982) and adults (Wagner and Tannenbaum, 1982) suffering from diarrhoea.

Studies into the biochemical mechanism of nitrate formation *via* ammonia have shown that liver slices exhibit increased nitrate production after exposure to paraquat or 2,4-dinitrophenol (Dull and Hotchkiss, 1984b), two potent uncouplers of cellular electron transport systems. These observations, together with the demonstration that xanthine/

Table 7.1 *Incorporation of [^{15}N]ammonium into urinary [^{15}N]nitrate* in vivo

Species	Treatment	Percent conversion to [^{15}N]nitrate	Reference
Rat	[^{15}N]-ammonium acetate [^{15}N]-ammonium acetate plus *E. coli* endotoxin	0.003 0.055	Wagner *et al.* (1983a)
Rat	[^{15}N]-ammonium chloride [^{15}N]-hydroxylamine	0.008 4.7	Saul and Archer (1984)
Ferret	[^{15}N]-ammonium sulphate	0.010	Dull and Hotchkiss (1984a)

xanthine oxidase co-oxidizes ammonia to nitrate *in vitro* (Dull and Hotchkiss, 1984b; Nagano and Fridovich, 1985), supports the proposals (Wagner *et al.*, 1983a; Saul and Archer, 1984) that active oxygen species (i.e. superoxide, hydroxyl radical) are needed for nitrate formation. However Wagner *et al.* (1985b) reported that nitrate synthesis *in vivo* was not directly proportional to the dose of ammonia administered, and not regulated directly through changes in plasma ammonia concentration (Wagner *et al.*, 1985b). Nitrate synthesis *in vivo* may therefore be regulated by the availability of oxidizing species generated by the reticuloendothelial system rather than the availability of nitrogen-containing precursors.

Atmospheric nitrogen oxides may also be oxidized to nitrate *in vivo*, since rats exposed to 8.8 p.p.m. NO_2 excrete increased levels of urinary nitrate for three days after treatment (Saul and Archer, 1983). Yoshida *et al.* (1983) found that approximately 55% of inhaled [^{15}N]-NO appeared in the urine of the rat over 48 hours, and was identified as being in the form of nitrate and urea. On the basis of these findings it was estimated that a man breathing air containing 0.1 p.p.m. NO_2 might be absorbing as much as 3.6 mg nitrite per day (Saul and Archer, 1983).

Through these mechanisms endogenous synthesis may generate an amount of nitrate each day equal to that ingested in the diet (Saul and Archer, 1983; 1984) with attendant toxicological risks for the host.

D. Fate of Nitrate in the Body

In most mammals, nitrate is absorbed from the proximal small intestine and enters the total body water to be subsequently excreted in the urine (see Fig. 7.1). The pharmacokinetic factors governing the distribution of nitrate within the body have been extensively reviewed (Hartman, 1982) and will not be considered in detail, although it should be noted that important differences are found in the excretion of nitrate by man and laboratory animals. Thus about 60–70% of an oral dose of nitrate is excreted in urine by man in the first 24 hours (Wagner *et al.*, 1983b; Bartholomew and Hill, 1984) while in the rat this value is attained after 72 hours (Wang *et al.*, 1981), with only minor excretion *via* the faeces for both species.

Oral nitrate also exhibits salivary–intestinal recirculation in man (Hartman, 1982) and the dog (Fritsch and de Saint Blanquat, 1985), and is secreted into the distal sections of the alimentary tract in the rat (Witter *et al.*, 1979), potentially influencing its metabolism and toxicity. The concentration and distribution of nitrate in the various regions of the rat intestinal tract may be altered by pre-exposure to nitrate, since Lin and Lai (1982) found detectable residues in the stomach, small intestine and large intestine of rats fed a diet containing 0.5% nitrate. A portion of an oral [^{15}N]-nitrate challenge may be retained in the body, with the bacterial

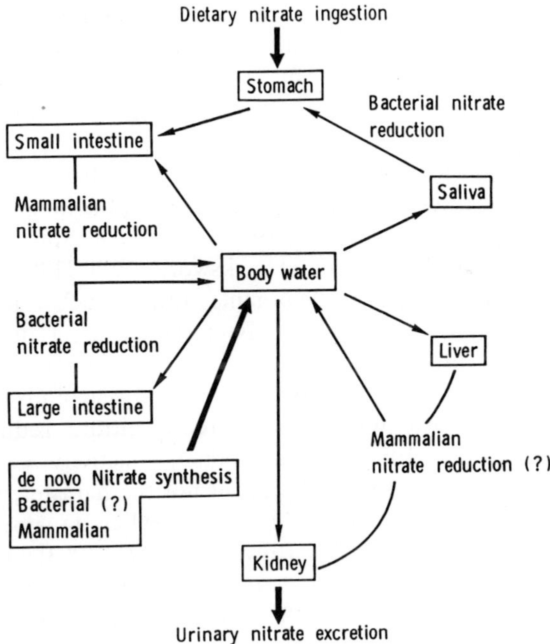

Fig 7.1 Nitrate disposition *in vivo*. The emboldened arrows indicate the major points at which nitrate is postulated to enter or leave the body.

population of the large intestine playing a major role in this process (Schultz *et al.*, 1985). An increase in urinary nitrate excretion following oral nitrate challenge is reported in the ferret after bacterial decontamination of the gut by treatment with neomycin sulphate and mycostatin (Dull and Hotchkiss, 1984a), and the recovery of oral nitrate in the urine is greater for germ-free rats than for their conventional flora counterparts (Witter *et al.*, 1982; Schultz *et al.*, 1985). The gut flora would thus appear to be an important determinant of nitrate disposition.

Bacterial metabolism of nitrate is a reductive step, and is associated with two molybdoproteins that differ in their ancilliary cofactors and electron donors according to bacterial type, cellular location and metabolic function (Payne, 1973). In some cases, this reduction is assimilatory and results in the incorporation of nitrate nitrogen into microbial amino acids, a reaction catalysed by a number of facultative or obligate anaerobic bacteria (Payne, 1973). The activity of this nitrate reductase is induced by the presence of reduced nitrogenous compounds in the environment, but is only expressed by a limited number of organisms when grown on a minimal medium (Payne, 1973). Other bacteria reduce far more nitrate under anaerobic conditions than is needed for synthetic reactions; under these conditions, dissimilatory nitrate reduction is coupled to phosphorylation (Ota, 1982), with increased ATP production during fermentation (Hasan and Hall, 1975). However, both assimilatory and dissimilatory nitrate reduction result in production of nitrite which may be available to interact with mammalian tissues.

Nitrate reduction has been detected in the microbial population of the rat small and large intestine (Mallett *et al.*, 1983a), the human achlorhydric stomach (Green and Tannenbaum, 1982), the saliva (Spiegelhalder *et al.*, 1976) and the infected bladder (Hawksworth and Hill, 1971). Faecal micro-organisms may also degrade organic nitrates, such as pentaerythritol tetranitrate (King and Fung, 1984). Bacterial nitrate reduction may be induced in the rat intestinal and stomach flora by diets containing nitrate (Lin and Lai, 1982). Colonisation of the rat gastrointestinal tract by certain lactobacilli also appears to increase nitrate reduction in gut contents (Lin and Lai, 1982). Nitrate reductase activity is also increased in the rat or mouse caecal microflora, but not the hamster, following the administration of diets containing high-methoxyl content pectin (Wise *et al.*, 1982; Mallett *et al.*, 1983a; Rowland *et al.*, 1983). However, the most active site for the bacterial reduction of nitrate in man is the oral microflora (Spiegelhalder *et al.*, 1976; Walters and Smith, 1981) which reduces nitrate recirculated in the saliva. Indeed, approximately one quarter of ingested nitrate is recirculated in saliva and roughly 20% of this is reduced to nitrite by microbial activities in the oral cavity (Spiegelhalder *et al.*, 1976).

Nitrate is also metabolized by certain ill-defined mammalian pathways detected in the tissues of germ-free animals. Schultz *et al.* (1985) reported the recovery of [^{15}N]-ammonia and urea in the urine of germ-free rats, which accounted for up to 5% of the administered [^{15}N]-nitrate, indicating mammalian nitrate reduction. Cytosolic liver enzymes such as xanthine oxidase (Fridovich and Handler, 1962) or aldehyde oxidase (Rajagopalan *et al.*, 1962) use nitrate as an alternative terminal electron acceptor, and may contribute to the activity reported for liver, kidney, spleen and intestine (Schultz *et al.*, 1985). Ward *et al.* (1985, 1986) demonstrated the presence of a heat-labile, nitrate-reducing activity located in the gut mucosa of the germ-free rat. This activity was approximately ten times greater in the small intestinal mucosa than in the stomach (Ward *et al.*, 1986). The reduction of organic nitrates has been described for kidney and liver homogenates (Maier *et al.*, 1980) and is catalysed by glutathione : polyolnitrate oxidoreductase (Needleman, 1975). Despite the undoubted ability of mammalian enzymes to reduce nitrate, the importance of such pathways is likely to be minor in comparison to the highly efficient bacterial reduction present along the alimentary tract.

E. Toxic Consequences of Nitrate Reduction

The microbial reduction of nitrate may be associated with certain toxicological events for the host animal arising from the chemical reactivity of the resulting nitrite.

1. *Methaemoglobinaemia*

Nitrite and oxyhaemoglobin in blood undergo a chemical co-oxidation to yield nitrate and methaemoglobin (Kosaka *et al.*, 1979) at levels which exceed the capacity of host enzymes to restore the function of the respiratory pigment. The nitrate regenerated in this manner may then undergo bacterial reduction and further compromise the host. Methaemoglobinaemia is clinically important since the modified respiratory pigment cannot transport oxygen to the tissues (de Bruin, 1976). The nitrite produced by the nitrate-reducing bacteria of the oral cavity or the achlorhydric stomach is potentially available to interact in this manner.

Infants from areas where the drinking water is rich in nitrate are particularly at risk since they drink more than adults on a body weight basis, have a less efficient methaemoglobin reductase system and possess a stomach microflora rich in nitrate reducing bacteria (Green and Tannenbaum, 1982). Blood methaemoglobin is also significantly increased in residents from non-industrial regions in comparison with values of industrial populations (3.9% and 1.3% of haemoglobin as methaemoglobin, respectively) and mirrors the higher nitrate content of the drinking water found in the rural community (Woebkenberg *et al.*, 1981). Nitrate reduction in rodents may also induce methaemoglobinaemia, and Wise *et al.* (1982) reported nitrate-induced methaemoglobinaemia in rats exhibiting increased gut microbial nitrate reductase activity. Generally, however, methaemoglobin values are small in man, compatible with a generally low daily intake of nitrate/nitrite (Hartman, 1982).

2. *N-nitroso compounds*

(a) Factors influencing in vivo *formation.* Nitrate, following microbial reduction to nitrite, occurs as nitrous acid (the protonated form of nitrite) at low pH, and induces genotoxic changes in mammalian and microbial systems (reviewed by Hartman (1982) and Green and Tannenbaum (1982)). Several feeding studies have suggested that nitrite is not a strong carcinogen (Green and Tannenbaum, 1982), although it may induce lymphomas in rats (Newberne, 1979). Nitrite can, however, combine with certain amino groups and yield carcinogenic or mutagenic *N*-nitroso compounds (Bartsch and Montesano, 1984). Factors influencing the formation of *N*-nitroso compounds (i.e. nitrosamines, nitrosamides) have been extensively reviewed (Challis *et al.*, 1980; Singer, 1980; Archer, 1984; Reed and Walters, 1985) and will not be considered in detail here. Nitrosation occurs via an acid catalysed mechanism, where nitrite exists as the nitrosonium ion (NO^+), nitrous acidium ion (H_2ONO^+) or nitrous anhydride (N_2O_2), with the rate of reaction dependent upon the availability of these nitrogen species (Archer, 1984). Various chemicals, including thiocyanate and ascorbate, are reported to catalyse or inhibit this process (Archer, 1984).

In addition to producing the nitrite necessary for nitrosation to occur, bacteria may play a further role and promote nitrosation by certain non-enzymic mechanisms. Early studies of microbial nitrosation of amines employed prolonged incubation periods in complex media (Hashimoto *et al.*, 1975; Coloe and Hayward, 1976) which could result in a decrease in pH of the incubation, resulting in acid catalysed nitrosation. Indeed,

Archer *et al.* (1975) proposed a non-enzymic mechanism for bacterial nitrosation involving hydrophobic interaction of secondary amines and cellular components at low pH, although Tannenbaum *et al.* (1977) considered that micellar catalysis by microbial components was also possible in a non-acidic environment.

Recent studies using pure cultures of bacteria *in vitro* have shown that microbial enzymes are directly involved in catalysing the formation of *N*-nitroso compounds. Resting cells of *Escherichia coli* nitrosate a variety of secondary amines at neutral pH (Suzuki and Mitsuoka, 1984; Calmels *et al.*, 1985; Leach *et al.*, 1985). Other intestinal bacteria were able to perform this function (Suzuki and Mitsuoka, 1984; Calmels *et al.*, 1985) but were in general oxygen-tolerant types (i.e. facultative anaerobes) which make a relatively minor contribution to the gut ecosystem (Moore *et al.*, 1978). Of thirty-two obligate anaerobic species tested for nitrosating ability only one (*Peptococcus asaccharolyticus*) was positive (Suzuki and Mitsuoka, 1984). However, certain denitrifying bacteria (e.g. *Pseudomonas aeruginosa*) exhibit an increase in nitrosating ability after anaerobic pre-culture in the presence of nitrate or nitrite, with yields 10 to 100 times greater than *E. coli* isolates grown under similar conditions (Leach *et al.*, 1987; Calmels *et al.*, 1987a).

Studies on mechanisms of bacterial nitrosation have revealed that the system responsible is sensitive to heat denaturation or other cellular disruption, and displays Michaelis–Menten kinetics, suggesting an enzymic process (Calmels *et al.*, 1985; Leach *et al.*, 1985). Calmels *et al.* (1987b) demonstrated a loss of nitrosating activity in *E. coli* mutants lacking nitrate reductase/formate hydrogenlyase activity, and inhibition when cysteine or sodium tungstate were present in the culture medium. The ability of *E. coli* to nitrosate is not, however, linked to nitrite reductase activity (Calmels *et al.*, 1987a). Other studies have suggested that the responsible enzyme is located in the inner membrane of the cell, possibly associated with membrane-bound respiratory proteins (O'Donnell *et al.*, 1987). These data suggest that a molybendum-containing nitrate reductase may be involved in the catalysis of nitrosation by *E. coli*.

The kinetics of bacterial nitrosation therefore differ markedly from those for acid-catalysed nitrosation, and may be of clinical significance in the endogenous formation of *N*-nitroso compounds within the body, but may be antagonized by competing bacterial pathways capable of degrading certain nitrosamines (Rowland and Grasso, 1975a, 1975b; Kawabata and Miyakoshi, 1976). Once formed, *N*-nitroso compounds interact with biological material or enter reactions with other chemical groups (Singer *et al.*, 1980; Challis, 1985). Present evidence indicates the involvement of micro-organisms in the nitrate-dependent induction of gastric and bladder tumours associated with *N*-nitroso compound formation, but is comparatively weak for the generation of nitrosation products in the hindgut.

(b) Endogenous nitrosation of amino acids.   One of the principal methods used to monitor nitrosation reactions *in vivo* follows the urinary excretion of certain *N*-nitrosoamino acids, such as nitrosoproline (Ohshima *et al.*, 1982; Wagner *et al.*, 1982) and nitrosothioproline (Tsuda *et al.*, 1983; Ohshima *et al.*, 1984). The stability of these compounds (Daily *et al.*, 1975; Chu and Magee, 1981) and their apparent lack of genotoxicity (Daily *et al.*, 1975; Fidder *et al.*, 1984) makes them suitable for studies on the mechanism of nitrosation in man. For example, L-nitrosoproline exhibits chemical constants comparable to some other amines known to yield carcinogenic nitroso derivatives (Mirvish, 1975), and has been used as the basis of a model for predicting the formation of carcinogenic nitrosamines *in vivo* (Ohshima *et al.*, 1983).

Nitrosoproline formation varies with the intake of nitrate/nitrite or proline (Wagner *et al.*, 1982; Ohshima *et al.*, 1982, 1983), with a presumed role of the oral microflora in the reduction of nitrate to nitrite. Wagner *et al.* (1985a) have shown that orally administered [^{15}N]-nitrate was incorporated into urinary nitrosoproline by six subjects consuming a low nitrate diet, although the contribution from [^{15}N]-nitrosamino acid varied between 13–52% of the total ([^{14}N] plus [^{15}N]) nitrosoproline present in the urine. Pre-existing nitrate/nitrite already present in the body (either dietary or formed from endogenous synthesis) would account for the source of the remaining nitroso-nitrogen, and could explain the observation that the nitrosation of proline by the rat (Mallett *et al.*, 1985) and ferret (Dull *et al.*, 1986) proceeds equally in the presence or absence of oral nitrate administration. Irrespective of its source, however, nitrate should require reduction to nitrite prior to entering into nitrosation reactions. Nevertheless, antibiotic-treated (Mallett *et al.*, 1984) or germ-free rats (Mallett *et al.*, 1985; Ward *et al.*, 1986) excrete readily quantifiable amounts of nitrosoproline (Table 7.2), possibly indicating the involvement of mammalian nitrate reductase pathways or pre-existing nitrite in this process.

In addition to the nitrosation of simple amino acid precursors, nitrosation reactions may occur using the N-atoms present in peptides and proteins, although this reaction has yet to be demonstrated to occur *in vivo*. The chemical synthesis of certain *N*-nitroso peptides has, however, been reported (Challis *et al.*, 1984; Kubacka and Scanlan, 1984). The fate of these compounds in the body is presently unknown, although some are stable enough to suggest possible absorption through the stomach or

Table 7.2 *Urinary excretion of nitrosoproline by germ-free, antibiotic-treated and conventional microflora rats given nitrate and proline*

Treatment	Strain	NPRO excretion (%)[a]			Reference
		CV	AB	GF	
1.25 g $NaNO_3$/kg bwt 250 mg L-PRO/kg bwt 40 μCi L-[U-^{14}C] PRO/kg bwt	Sprague-Dawley	100 100	100 78	– –	Mallett *et al.* (1984)
1.25 g $NaNO_3$/kg bwt 250 mg L-PRO/kg bwt 40 μCi L-[U-^{14}C] PRO/kg bwt	Fischer F344	100	–	134	Mallett *et al.* (1985)
2% $NaNO_3$ (water) 1% L-PRO (diet)	Wistar	100 100	– –	4 54	Ward *et al.* (1986)
1% $NaNO_3$ (water) 0.5% L-PRO (diet)	Wistar	100	–	55	Ward *et al.* (1986)

Abbreviations used: NPRO, nitrosoproline; L-PRO, L-proline; $NaNO_3$, sodium nitrate; bwt, bodyweight; CV, conventional microflora; AB, antibiotic-treated; GF, germ-free; –, not done.
[a] NPRO excretion as a percentage of excretion in CV rats.

duodenum (Challis *et al.*, 1984) with the potential for genotoxicity in other tissues.

(c) Sites of nitrosamine formation in vivo. Nitrosamine formation in the stomach can be catalysed by secreted gastric acid using nitrite produced by the nitrate-reducing activities of the oral microflora (Spiegelhalder *et al.*, 1976). Nitrosation may also occur under the very different physicochemical conditions present in individuals with gastric achlorhydria due to, for example, pernicious anaemia or partial gastrectomy. Pernicious anaemia is caused by the lack of an endogenously produced intrinsic factor necessary for the uptake of vitamin B12, and is invariably accompanied by failure to secrete gastric acid. Partial gastrectomy, and more recently selective vagotomy, are surgical treatments for peptic ulcer with an associated loss of acid secreting ability by the gastric mucosa. One consequence of an increased stomach pH (Reed *et al.*, 1985) is the continuous bacterial colonization of the lumenal contents by micro-organisms exhibiting nitrate-reducing properties (Bartholomew *et al.*, 1980; Bockler *et al.*, 1983; Reed *et al.*, 1985). Both pernicious anaemia (Blackburn *et al.*, 1968) and partial gastrectomy (Dahm *et al.*, 1979) are associated with an increased risk of gastric neoplasia, and *N*-nitroso compounds are thought to be involved in the pathogenesis of these changes (Ruddell *et al.*, 1978; Schlag *et al.*, 1980; Reed *et al.*, 1985). Caygill *et al.* (1985) have postulated that an increase in nitrosamine formation in the achlorhydric patient may also be linked to an increased risk of cancers at other sites in the body, following absorption of nitroso compounds from the stomach. The occurrence of *N*-nitroso compounds in normal gastric contents has been reported by several authors (Mysliwy *et al.*, 1974; Mueller *et al.*, 1983), and is increased in the rat following colonization of the stomach by nitrate reductase positive strains of bacteria (Hashimoto *et al.*, 1976). *N*-nitroso compounds detected in human blood are probably derived from gastric sources (Fine *et al.*, 1977; Kowalski *et al.*, 1980).

The generation of *N*-nitroso compounds *in vivo* may explain the increased incidence of gastric cancer in areas where drinking water contains high concentrations of nitrate (Hill *et al.*, 1973; Tannenbaum *et al.*, 1979), although some recent studies in the UK have produced conflicting findings with a negative association between nitrate intake and cancer incidence (Beresford, 1985; Forman *et al.*, 1985). It has been suggested, however, that such data sl.ould be interpreted with caution given that methodological, social and other confounding factors may have unduly influenced the outcome of these latter studies (Pocock, 1985). Epidemiological investigations suggest an additional association with a high intake of 'starchy' food (Wynder *et al.*, 1963; Modan *et al.*, 1974).

The provision of extra carbohydrate to the oral or stomach microflora may increase bacterial metabolism or numbers, with a concomitant increase in the ability of the bacteria to reduce nitrate to nitrite. A similar effect has been reported with pectin (a fermentable carbohydrate) on the caecal microflora (Wise *et al.*, 1982), with an associated increase in the nitrate-dependent production of nitrosamines *in vitro* (Mallett *et al.*, 1983b).

N-nitroso compounds are also formed in saliva under *in vitro* incubation conditions (Tannenbaum *et al.*, 1977; Hart and Walters, 1983), yet the amount is unlikely to be as great as that detected in the stomach due to the unfavourable pH and shorter residence time. Nonetheless, Hart and Walters (1983) found compounds corresponding to nitrosamines and nitrosamides in saliva, while studies by Ellen *et al.* (1982) showed the presence of dimethylnitrosamine in human saliva, although the absolute amount was independent of the nitrate intake.

The infected urinary bladder presents an ideal site for nitrosation since the numbers of bacteria, supply of nitrate and amine and residence time are optimal, and *N*-nitroso compounds have been detected at this site (Radomski *et al.*, 1978; Brooks *et al.*, 1978). The organisms encountered in single or mixed population bladder infections are similar to those encountered in the hindgut, yet the greatest degree of nitrosation is associated with the facultatively anaerobic bacterium *E. coli*; this organism also exhibits an active nitrate reductase pathway (Hawksworth and Hill, 1971). It should be noted, however, that nitrosation reactions probably do not occur in the uninfected bladder, so the presence of *N*-nitroso compounds in urine samples may reflect glomerular filtration of products formed at other sites in the body. A certain degree of care is therefore required before assigning an origin to any *N*-nitroso compounds found in urine.

The generation of *N*-nitroso compounds in the lower regions of the gut was suggested by reports of nitrosamines in human faeces (Wang *et al.*, 1978; Varghese *et al.*, 1978). The production of these materials may result from bacterial action using nitrite (produced from nitrate by the oral or hindgut microflora) and certain amines present in the diet or produced by bacterial catabolism of peptides (Drasar and Hill, 1974). Hashimoto *et al.* (1976) reported the appearance of dimethylnitrosamine in small intestine and caecal contents of rats pretreated with five bacterial strains shown to produce nitrosamines *in vitro*, and then fed diets containing dimethylamine and nitrate. The continuous exposure of the gut to such compounds could initiate neoplastic changes in the bowel. However, the amount of nitroso compounds detected in faecal samples is very low, and subject to problems arising from artefact formation and contamination (Archer *et al.*, 1981). In addition, other workers have failed to detect nitrosamines in faeces (Archer *et al.*, 1981; Eisenbrand *et al.*, 1981; Lee *et al.*, 1981). Faeces also contain very low levels of nitrate and nitrite (Archer *et al.*, 1981; Saul *et al.*, 1981) suggesting limited availability of nitrosating equivalents in the hindgut, although isotope studies have demonstrated the appearance of orally administered nitrate/nitrite in the large intestine of the rat (Witter *et al.*, 1979). Thus a role for *N*-nitroso compounds in carcinogenesis of the large bowel remains unsubstantiated.

While the extent of nitrosation by the hindgut microflora *in vivo* is open to question, several studies have demonstrated the practicality of this reaction using *in vitro* techniques. ^{14}C-dimethylamine and nitrite yield dimethylnitrosamine when incubated anaerobically with rat intestinal contents at pH 7.0, and nitrosamine formation is markedly decreased by antibiotic treatment or heat denaturation of the gut contents (Klubes *et al.*, 1972), suggesting a role for the gut microflora. Nitrosamines were also detected when human faeces were incubated anaerobically with nitrosamine precursors (dimethylamine/dipropylamine/morpholine and nitrite) (Lee *et al.*, 1981) although, paradoxically, the extent of nitrosation increased when faeces were autoclaved. Hill and Hawksworth (1971) assessed the nitrosation potential of 107 strains of faecal bacteria (aerobes and anaerobes) from five genera, and reported the nitrate-dependent formation of diphenylnitrosamine in a proportion of all organisms at a pH apparently near neutrality; the possession of nitrate reductase activity was a prerequisite for this reaction.

F. Conclusions

Current evidence indicates a role for the bacterial population of the gut in determining the disposition of nitrate/nitrite within the body, and should be considered along with the other nitrogen-utilizing activities of the flora reported in this volume (Chapter 10). Bacterial reduction of nitrate to nitrite is associated with certain toxicological events, perhaps the most important of which is the formation of genotoxic *N*-nitroso compounds. Traditionally, orally ingested, dietary nitrate has been viewed as the major source of substrate for these reactions, although current evidence strongly suggests that the *de novo* production of nitrate/nitrite within the body to be of equal concern. Regardless of its origins, however, bacterial reduction must be viewed as a reaction of paramount importance when considering the pharmacology and toxicology of nitrate *in vivo*.

Acknowledgment

The author is grateful for support from the UK Ministry of Agriculture, Fisheries and Food.

References

Archer, M. C. (1984). Catalysis and inhibition of N-nitrosation reactions. *In*: "N-Nitroso Compounds: Occurrence, Biological Effects and Relevance to Human Cancer". (eds I. K. O'Neil, R. C. von Borstel, C. T. Miller, J. Long and H. Bartsch), pp. 263–274. International Agency for Research on Cancer, Lyon.

Archer, M. C., Yang, H. S. and Okun, J. D. (1975). Acceleration of nitrosamine formation at pH 3.5 by microorganisms. *In*: "Environmental Aspects of N-Nitroso Compounds" (eds E. A. Walker, M. Castegnara, L. Griciute and R. E. Lyle), pp. 239–246. International Agency for Research on Cancer, Lyon.

Archer, M. C., Saul, R. L., Lee, L. -J. and Bruce, W. R. (1981). Analysis of nitrate, nitrite and nitrosamines in human feces. *In*: "Banbury Report 7 — Gastrointestinal Cancer: Endogenous Factors" (eds W. R., Bruce, P. Correa, M. Lipkin, S. R. Tannenbaum and T. D. Wilkins), pp. 321–330. Cold Spring Harbor Laboratory, New York.

Bartholomew, B. A., Hill, M. J., Hudson, M. J., Ruddell, W. S. J. and Walters, C. L. (1980). "Gastric Bacteria, Nitrate, Nitrite and Nitrosamines in Patients with Pernicious Anaemia and in Patients Treated with Cimetidine" (eds E. A. Walker, L. Griciute M. Castegnara, M. Börzsönyil and W. Davis), pp. 595–608. International Agency for Research on Cancer, Lyon.

Bartholomew, B. and Hill, M. J. (1984). The pharmacology of dietary nitrate and the origin of urinary nitrate. *Fd Chem. Toxicol.* **22**, 789–795.

Bartsch, H. and Montesano, R. (1984). Relevance of nitrosamines to human cancer. *Carcinogenesis* **5**, 1381–1393.

Beresford, S. A. A. (1985). Is nitrate in drinking water associated with the risk of cancer in the urban UK? *Int. J. Epidemiol.* **14**, 57–63.

Blackburn, E. K., Callender, S. T., Dacie, J. V., Doll, R., Girdwood, R. H., Mollin, D. L., Saracci, R., Stafford, J., Thompson, R. B. Varadi, S. and Wetherly-Mein, G. (1968). Possible association between pernicious anaemia and leukemia: a prospective study of 1,625 patients with a note on the very high incidence of gastric cancer. *Int. J. Cancer* **3**, 163–170.

Bockler, R., Meyer, H. and Schlag, P. (1983). An experimental study of bacterial colonisation, nitrite and nitrosamine production in the operated stomach. *J. Cancer Res. Clin. Oncol.* **105**, 62–66.

Brooks, J. B., Cherry, W. B., Thacker, L. and Alley, C. C. (1978). Analysis by gas chromatography of amines and nitrosamines produced *in vivo* and *in vitro* by *Proteus mirabilis*. *J. Infect. Dis.* **126**, 143–153.

Calmels, S., Ohshima, H., Vincent, P. Gounot, A. M. and Bartsch, H. (1985). Screening of microorganisms for nitrosation catalysis at pH 7 and kinetic studies on nitrosamine formation from secondary amines by *E. coli* strains. *Carcinogenesis* **6**, 911–915.

Calmels, S., Ohshima, H. and Bartsch, H. (1987a). Nitrosamine formation by denitrifying and non-denitrifying bacteria: implication of nitrite- and nitrate-reductase in nitrosation catalysis. *J. Gen. Microbiol.* (submitted).

Calmels, S., Ohshima, H., Rosenkranz, H., McCoy, E. and Bartsch, H. (1987b). Biochemical studies on the catalysis of nitrosation by bacteria. *Carcinogenesis* **8**, 1085–1088.

Caygill, C., Hill, M. J., Craven, J., Hall, R. and Miller, C. (1985). Relevance of gastric achlorhydria to human carcinogenesis. *In*: "N-Nitroso Compounds:

Occurrence, Biological Effects and Relevance to Human Cancer" (eds I. K. O'Neill, R. C. von Borstel, C. T. Miller, J. Long and H. Bartsch), pp. 895–900. International Agency for Research on Cancer, Lyon.

Challis, B. C. (1985). Nutrition and nitrosamine formation. *Proc. Nutr. Soc.* **44**, 95–100.

Challis, B. C., Outram, J. R. and Shuker, D. E. G. (1980). New pathways for the rapid formation of N-nitrosamines under neutral and alkaline conditions. *In*: "N-Nitroso Compounds: Analysis Formation and Occurrence" (eds E. A. Walker, L., Gricuite, M. Castegnara and W. Davis), pp. 43–58. International Agency for Research on Cancer, Lyon.

Challis, B. C., Milligan, J. R. and Mitchell, R. C. (1984). Synthesis and stability of N-nitrosodipeptides. *J. Chem. Soc. Chem. Commun.* 1050–1051.

Chilvers, C., Inskip, H., Caygill, C., Bartholomew, B., Fraser, P. and Hill, M. (1984). A survey of dietary nitrate in well-water users. *Int. J. Epidem.* **13**, 324–331.

Chu, C. and Magee, P. N. (1981). Metabolic fate of nitrosoproline in the rat. *Cancer Res.* **41**, 5072–5076.

Coloe, P. J. and Hayward, N. J. (1976). The importance of prolonged incubation for the synthesis of dimethylnitrosamine by enterobacteria. *J. Med. Microbiol.* **9**, 211–223.

Dahm, D., Eichfass, H. P. and Koch, W. (1979). Gastric cancer in stump after Bilroth II resection: the influence of gastroenteric anastomosis. *Front. gastrointest. Res.* **5**, 164–169.

Daily, R. E., Braunberg, R. C. and Blaschka, A. M. (1975). The absorption, distribution and excretion of [^{14}C] nitrosoproline by rats. *Toxicology* **3**, 23–28.

de Bruin, A. (1976). "Biochemical Toxicology of Environmental Agents". Elsevier, Amsterdam.

Drasar, B. S. and Hill, M. J. (1974). "Human Intestinal Flora". Academic Press, London.

Dull, B. J. and Hotchkiss, J. H. (1984a). Nitrate balance and biosynthesis in the ferret. *Toxicol. Lett.* **23**, 79–89.

Dull, B. J. and Hotchkiss, J. H. (1984b). Activated oxygen and mammalian nitrate biosynthesis. *Carcinogenesis* **5**, 1161–1164.

Dull, B. J., Hotchkiss, J. H. and Vecchio, A. J. (1986). Basal N-nitrosoproline formation and excretion in the ferret. *Fd Chem. Toxicol.* **24**, 843–845.

Eisenbrand, G., Spiegelhalder, B. and Preussman, R. (1981). Analysis of human biological specimens for nitrosamine content. *In*: "Banbury Report 7 — Gastrointestinal Cancer: Endogenous Factors" (eds W. R. Bruce, P. Correa, M. Lipkin, S. R. Tannenbaum and T. D. Wilkins), pp. 275–283. Cold Spring Harbor Laboratory, New York.

Ellen, G., Schuller, P. L., Bruijns, E., Foreling, P. G. A. M. and Baadenhuijsen, H. (1982). Volatile N-nitrosoamines nitrate and nitrite in saliva of healthy volunteers after administration of large amounts of nitrate. *In*: "N-Nitroso Compounds: Occurrence and Biological Effects" (eds H. Bartsch, I. K. O'Neill, M. Castegnara, M. Okada and W. Davis), pp. 365–378. International Agency for Research on Cancer, Lyon.

Fidder, W., Miller, A. J., Pensabene, J. W. and Doerr, R. C. (1984). Investigation of the mutagenicity of N-nitrothiazondine using the Ames *Salmonella* test. *In*: "N-Nitroso Compounds: Occurrence, Biological Effects and Relevance to Human Cancer" (eds I. K. O'Neill, R. C. von Borstell, C. T. Miller, J.

Long and H. Bartsch), pp. 95–100. International Agency for Research on Cancer, Lyon.

Fine, D. H., Ross, P., Rounbehler, D. P., Silvergleid, A. and Song, L. (1977). Formation *in vivo* of volatile N-nitrosamines in man after ingestion of cooked bacon and spinach. *Nature* **265**, 753–755.

Forman, D., Al-Dabbagh, S. and Doll, R. (1985). Nitrates, nitrites and gastric cancer in Great Britain. *Nature* **313**, 620–625.

Forsythe, S. J. and Parker, D. S. (1985). Nitrogen metabolism by the microbial flora of the rabbit caecum. *J. appl. Bacteriol.* **58**, 363–369.

Fridovich, I. and Handler, P. (1962). Xanthine oxidase V. Differential inhibition of the reduction of various electron acceptors. *J. Biol. Chem.* **237**, 916–921.

Fritsch, P. and de Saint Blanquat, G. (1985). Excretion of nitrates and nitrites in saliva and bile in the dog. *Fd Chem. Toxicol.* **23**, 655–659.

Green, L. C., Tannenbaum, S. R. and Goldman, P. (1981). Nitrate synthesis and reduction in germfree and conventional rat. *Science* **212**, 56–58.

Green, L. C. and Tannenbaum, S. R. (1982). Nitrate, nitrite and N-nitrosocompounds: Biochemistry metabolism toxicity and carcinogenicity. *In*: "Human Nutrition" (eds A. Neuberger and T. H. Jukes), pp. 87–140, MTP Press, Lancaster.

Hart, R. J. and Walters, C. L. (1983). The formation of nitrite and N-nitroso compounds in salivas *in vitro* and *in vivo*. *Fd Chem. Toxicol.* **21**, 749–753.

Hartman, P. E. (1982). Nitrates and nitrites: ingestion, pharmacodynamics and toxicology. *In*: "Chemical Mutagens — Principles and Methods for their Detection" (eds F. J. de Serres and A. Hollaender) Vol. 7, pp. 211–294. Plenum Press, New York.

Hasan, S. M. and Hall, J. B. (1975). The physiological function of nitrate reduction in *Clostridium perfringens*. *J. Gen. Microbiol.* **87**, 120–128.

Hashimoto, S., Kawai, Y. and Mutai, M. (1975). *In vitro* N-nitrosodimethylamine formation by some bacteria. *Infec. Immun.* **11**, 1405–1406.

Hashimoto, S., Yokokura, T., Kawai, Y. and Mutai, M. (1976). Dimethylnitrosamine formation in the gastro-intestinal tract of rats. *Fd Cosmet. Toxicol.* **14**, 553–556.

Hawksworth, G. M. and Hill, M. J. (1971). Bacteria and the *N*-nitrosation of secondary amines. *Br. J. Cancer* **25**, 520–527.

Hegesh, E. and Shiloah, J. (1982). Blood nitrates and infantile methaemoglobinemia. *Clin. Chem. Acta.* **125**, 107–115.

Hill, M. J. and Hawksworth, G. (1971). Bacterial production of nitrosamines *in vitro* and *in vivo*. *In*: "N-Nitroso Compounds — Analysis and Formation" (eds P. Bogorski, R. Preussman, E. A. Walker and W. Davis), pp. 116–121. International Agency for Research on Cancer, Lyon.

Hill, M. J., Hawksworth, G. M. and Tattershall, G. (1973). Bacteria, nitrosamines and cancer of the stomach. *Br. J. Cancer* **28**, 562–567.

Kawabata, T. and Miyakoshi, S. (1976). Microbial formation of nitrospyrolidine from nitrosoproline. *In*: "Environmental N-Nitroso Compounds — Analysis and Formation" (eds E. A.Walker, P. Bogorski and L. Gricuite), pp. 261–266. International Agency for Research on Cancer, Lyon.

King, S.-Y. P. and Fung, H.-L. (1984). Rapid microbial degradation of organic nitrates in rat excreta: re-examination of the urinary and fecal metabolite profiles of pentaerythritol tetranitrate in the rat. *Drug. Metab. Disp.* **12**, 353–357.

Klubes, P., Cerna, I., Rabinowitz, A. D. and Jondorf, W. R. (1972). Factors affecting dimethylnitrosamine formation from simple precursors by rat intestinal bacteria. *Fd Cosmet. Toxicol.* **10**, 757–767.

Kosaka, H., Imaizumi, K., Imai, K. and Tyuma, I. (1979). Stoichiometry of the reaction of oxyhemoglobin with nitrite. *Biochim. Biophys. Acta* **581**, 184–190.

Kowalski, B., Miller, C. T. and Sen, N. P. (1980). Studies on the *in vivo* formation of nitrosamines in humans after ingestion of various meals. *In*: "N-Nitroso Compounds: Analysis, Formation and Occurrence" (eds E. A. Walker, L. Gricuite, M. Castegnara and M. Börzsönyi), pp. 467–477. International Agency for Research on Cancer, Lyon.

Kubacka, W. and Scanlan, R. A. (1984). Kinetics of nitrosation of four dipeptides N terminal in proline. *J. Agric. Fd Chem.* **32**, 404–406.

Kurzer, M. S. and Calloway, D. H. (1981). Nitrate and nitrogen balances in men. *Am. J. Clin. Nutr.* **34**, 1305–1313.

Leach, S. A., Challis, B., Cook, A. R., Hill, M. J. and Thompson, M. H. (1985). Bacterial catalysis of the N-nitrosation of secondary amines. *Biochem. Soc. Transact.* **13**, 380–381.

Leach, S. A., Cook, A. R., Challis, B. C., Hill, M. J. and Thompson, M. H. (1987). Bacterially mediated *N*-nitrosation reactions and endogenous formation of *N*-nitroso compounds. *In*: "The Relevance of *N*-nitroso Compounds to Human Cancer: Exposure and Mechanisms" (eds H. Bartsch, I. O'Neill, and R. Schulte-Herman.), pp. 396–403. International Agency for Research on Cancer, Lyon.

Lee, K., Greger, J. L., Consaul, J. R., Graham, M. S. and Chinn, B. L. (1986). Nitrate, nitrite balance and *de novo* synthesis of nitrate in humans consuming cured meats. *Am. J. Clin. Nutr.* **44**, 188–194.

Lee, L., Archer, M. C. and Bruce, W. R. (1981). Absence of volatile nitrosamines in feces. *Cancer Res.* **41**, 3992–3994.

Lin, J. -K. and Lai, C. -C. (1982). Effects of lactobacillus, antacids and antibiotics on the levels of nitrite in the gastrointestinal tracts of rats fed sodium nitrate. *Fd Chem. Toxicol.* **20**, 197–204.

Maier, G.A., Arena, C. and Fung, H. -L. (1980). Relationship between *in vivo* nitroglycerin metabolism and *in vitro* organic nitrate reductase activity in rats. *Biochem. Pharmacol.* **29**, 646–648.

Mallett, A. K., Rowland, I. R. and Wise, A. (1983a). Interaction between pectin and rat hindgut microflora. *Appl Environ. Microbiol.* **45**, 116–121.

Mallett, A. K., Rowland, I. R. and Wise, A. (1983b). Diet-related production of mutagens by the rat gut flora. *Toxicologist* **2**, abstr. 287.

Mallett, A. K., Rowland, I. R., Cottrell, R. C. and Gangolli, S. D. (1984). Nitrosproline formation in control and antibiotic-treated rats given nitrate and proline. *Cancer Lett.* **25**, 231–235.

Mallett, A. K., Rowland, I. R., Walters, D. G., Gangolli, S. D., Cottrell, R. C. and Massey, R. C. (1985). The role of oral nitrate in the nitrosation of [^{14}C] proline by conventional microflora and germ-free rats. *Carcinogenesis* **6**, 1585–1588.

Mirvish, S. S. (1975). Formation of N-nitroso compounds: chemistry, kinetics and *in vivo* occurrence. *Toxicol. appl. Pharmacol.* **31**, 325–351.

Mitchell, H. H., Shonle, H. A. and Grindley, H. S. (1916). The origin of the nitrates in urine. *J. Biol. Chem.* **24**, 461–490.

Miwa, M., Stuehr, D. J., Marletta, M. A. and Wishnok, J. S. (1987).

N-nitrosamine formation by macrophages. *In*: "The Relevance of *N*-nitroso Compounds to Human Cancer: Exposure and Mechanisms" (eds H. Bartsch, I. O'Neill. and R. Schulte-Herman), pp. 340–344. International Agency for Research on Cancer, Lyon.

Modan, B., Lubin, F., Barell, V., Greenberg, R. A., Modan, M. and Graham, S. (1974). The role of starches in the etiology of gastric cancer. *Cancer* **40**, 1887–1891.

Moore, W. E. C. and Holdeman, L. V. (1974). Special problems associated with the isolation and identification of intestinal bacteria in fecal flora studies. *Am. J. Clin. Nutr.* **27**, 1450–1455.

Moore, W. E. C., Cato, P. and Holdeman, L. V. (1978). Some current concepts in intestinal bacteriology. *Am. J. Clin. Nutr.* **31**, 533–539.

Mueller, R. L., Hasgel, H. -J., Greim, G., Ruppin, H. and Domschke, W. (1983). The endogenous synthesis of cancerogenic N-nitroso-compounds: bacterial flora and nitrite formation in the healthy human stomach. *Zbl. Bakt. Hyg.* **B178**, 297–315.

Mysliwy, T. S., Wick, E. L., Archer, M. C., Shank, R. C. and Newberne, P. M. (1974). Formation of N-nitrosopyrrolidine in a dog's stomach. *Br. J. Cancer* **30**, 279–283.

Nagano, T. and Fridovich, I. (1985). The co-oxidation of ammonia to nitrite during the aerobic xanthine oxidase reaction. *Arch. Biochem. Biophys.* **241**, 596–601.

Needleman, P. (1975). "Organic Nitrates", Springer, New York.

Newberne, P. M. (1979). Nitrite promotes lymphoma incidence in rats. *Science* **204**, 1079–1082.

O'Donnell, C. M., Edwards, C., Corcoran, G. D., Wave, J. and Edwards, P. R. (1987). *In vitro* production of nitrosamines by bacteria isolated from the operated stomach. *In:* "The relevance of *N*-nitroso Compounds to Human Cancer: Exposure and Mechanisms" (eds H. Bartsch, I. O'Neill and R. Schulte-Herman), pp. 400–403. International Agency for Research on Cancer, Lyon.

Ohshima, H., Bereziat, J. -C. and Bartsch, H. (1982). Monitoring N-nitrosamino acids excreted in the urine and faeces of rats as an index of endogenous nitrosation. *Carcinogenesis* **3**, 115–120.

Ohshima, H., Mahon, G. A. T., Wahrendorf, J. and Bartsch, H. (1983). Dose response study of N-nitrosoproline formation in rats and a deduced kinetic model for predicting carcinogenic effects caused by endogenous nitrosation. *Cancer Res.* **43**, 3653–3657.

Ohshima, H., O'Neill, I. K., Friesen, M., Pignatelli, B. and Bartsch, H. (1984). Presence in human urine of new sulphur-containing N-nitrosamino acids: N-nitrosotriazolidine 4-carboxylic acid and N-nitroso-2-methylthiazolidine 4-carboxylic acid. *In*: "N-Nitroso Compounds: Occurrence, Biological Effects and Relevance to Human Cancer" (eds I. K. O'Neill, R.C. von Borstel, C. T. Miller, J. Long and H. Bartsch), pp. 77–85. International Agency for Research on Cancer, Lyon.

Ota, A. (1982). Phosphorylation coupled to nitrate respiration. *Int. J. Biochem.* **14**, 341–346.

Payne, W. J. (1973). Reduction of nitrogenous oxides by microorganisms. *Bacterial Rev.* **37**, 409–452.

Pocock, S. J. (1985). Nitrates and gastric cancer. *Human Toxicol.* **4**, 471–474.

Radomski, J. L., Greenwald, D., Hearn, W. L., Block, N. L. and Woods, F. M. (1978). Nitrosamine formation in bladder infections and its role in the etiology of bladder cancer. *J. Urol.* **120**, 48–50.

Rajagopalan, K. V., Fridovich, I. and Hander, P. (1962). Hepatic aldehyde oxidase. I. Purification and properties. *J. Biol. Chem.* **237**, 922–928.

Ralt, D., Gomez, R. F. and Tannenbaum, S. R. (1981). Conversion of acetohydroxamate and hydroxylamine to nitrite by intestinal microorganisms. *Eur. J. appl. Microbial. Biotechnol.* **12**, 226–230.

Reed, P. I. and Walters, C. L. (1985). The relationship between food, nitrosamines and gastric cancer. *In*: "Food and the Gut" (eds J. O. Hunter and V. Alun Jones), pp. 135–149. Baillière Tindall, Eastbourne.

Reed, P. I., Summers, K., Smith, P. L. R., Walters, C. L., Bartholomew, B. A., Hill, M. J., Venitt, S., House, F. R., Hornig, D. H. and Bonjour, J. -P. (1985). Effect of gastric surgery for benign peptic ulcer and ascorbic acid therapy on concentrations of nitrite and N-nitroso compounds in gastric juice. *In*: "N-Nitroso Compounds: Occurrence, Biological Effects and Relevance to Human Cancer" (eds I. K. O'Neill, R. C. von Borstel, C. T. Miller, J. Long and H. Bartsch), pp. 975–979. International Agency for Research on Cancer, Lyon.

Rowland, I. R. and Grasso, P. (1975a). The bacterial degradation of nitrosamines. *Biochem. Soc. Transact.* **3**, 185–188.

Rowland, I. R. and Grasso, P. (1975b). Degradation of N-nitrosamines by intestinal bacteria. *Appl. Microbiol.* **29**, 7–12.

Rowland, I. R., Mallett, A. K. and Wise, A. (1983). A comparison of the activity of five microbiol enzymes in cecal content from rats, mice and hamsters and response to dietary pectin. *Toxicol. appl. Pharmacol.* **69**, 143–148.

Ruddell, W. S. J., Bone, E. S., Hill, M.J. and Walters, C. L. (1978). Pathogenesis of gastric cancer in pernicious anemia. *Lancet* **1**, 521–523.

Ryden, J. C., Ball, P. R. and Garwood, E. A. (1984). *Nature* 311, 50–53.

Saul, R. L., Kabir, S. H., Cohen, Z., Bruce, W. R. and Archer, M. C. (1981). Reevaluation of nitrate and nitrite levels in the human intestine. *Cancer Res.* **41**, 2280–2283.

Saul, R. L. and Archer, M. C. (1983). Nitrate formation in rats exposed to nitrogen dioxide. *Toxicol. appl. Pharmacol.* **67**, 284–291.

Saul, R. L. and Archer, M. C. (1984). Oxidation of ammonia and hydroxylamine to nitrate in the rat and *in vitro*. *Carcinogenesis* **5**, 77–81.

Schröder, H. and Johansson, A. K. (1973). Redox potential in caecal contents of the rat and azo reduction of salicyl-azo-sulphapyridine. *Xenobiotica* **3**, 233–246.

Schlag, P., Bockler, R., Ulrich, H., Peter, M., Merkle, P. and Herfarth, C. H. (1980). Are nitrite and N-nitroso compounds in gastric juice risk factors for carcinoma in the operated stomach. *Lancet* **1**, 727–729.

Schultz, D. S., Deen, W. M., Karel, S. F., Wagner, D. A. and Tannenbaum, S. R. (1985). Pharmacokinetics of nitrate in humans: role of gastrointestinal absorption and metabolism. *Carcinogenesis* **6**, 847–852.

Singer, S. S. (1980). Transnitrosation by nitrosamines and nitrosoureas. *In*: "N-Nitroso Compounds: Analysis, Formation and Occurrence" (eds E. A. Walker, L. Cricuite, M. Castegnaro, M. Börzsönyil and W. Davis), pp. 111–118. International Agency for Research on Cancer, Lyon.

Singer, S. S., Singer, G. M. and Cole, B. B. (1980). Alicyclic nitrosamines and nitrosamides as transnitrosating agents. *J. Org. Chem.* **45**, 4931–4935.

Spiegelhalder, B., Eisenbrand, G. and Preussman, R. (1976). Influence of dietary nitrate on nitrite content of human saliva: possible relevance to *in vivo* formation of N-nitroso compounds. *Fd Cosmet. Toxicol.* **14**, 545–548.

Stuehr, D. J. and Marletta, M. A. (1985). Mammalian nitrate biosynthesis: Mouse macrophages produce nitrite and nitrate in response to *Escherichia coli* lipopolysaccharide. *Proc. Natl Acad. Sci. USA* **82**, 7738–7742.

Suzuki, K. and Mitsuoka, T. (1984). N-Nitrosamine formation by intestinal bacteria. *In*: "N-Nitroso Compounds: Occurrence, Biological Effects and Relevance to Human Cancer" (eds I. K. O'Neill, R. C. von Borstel, C. T. Miller, J. Long and H. Bartsch), pp. 275–281. International Agency for Research on Cancer, Lyon.

Takahashi, M. and Kametaka, M. (1986). The fate of urea-N by the anaerobic culture of cecal microbes of rats. *Agric. Biol. Chem.* **80**, 773–775.

Tannenbaum, S. R., Archer, M. Correa, P., Cuello, C. and Haenszel, W. (1977). Nitrate and the etiology of gastric cancer. *In*: "Origins of Human Cancer" (eds H. H. Hyatt, J. D. Watson and J. A. Winstern), pp. 1609–1625, Cold Spring Harbor Laboratory, New York.

Tannenbaum, S. R., Fett, D., Young, V. R., Land, P. D. and Bruce, W. R. (1978). Nitrite and nitrate are formed by endogenous synthesis in the human intestine. *Science* **200**, 1487–1489.

Tannenbaum, S. R., Moran, D., Rand, W., Cuello, C. and Correa, P. (1979). Gastric cancer in Colombia. IV. Nitrite and other ions in gastric contents from a high risk region. *J. Natl Cancer Inst.* **62**, 9–12.

Tsuda, M., Hirayama, T. and Sugimura, T. (1983). Presence of N-nitroso-L-thioproline and N-nitroso-L-methylthioprolines in human urine as major N-nitroso compounds. *Gann* **74**, 331–333.

Varghese, A. J., Land, P. C., Furrer, R. and Bruce, W. R. (1978). Non-volatile N-nitroso compounds in human feces. *In*: "Environmental Aspects of N-nitroso compounds" (eds E. A. Walker, M. Castegnara, L. Gricuite, R. E. Lyle and W. Davis), pp. 257–264. International Agency for Research on Cancer, Lyon.

Wagner, D. A. and Tannenbaum, S. R. (1982). Enhancement of nitrate biosynthesis by *Escherichia coli* lipolysaccharide. *In*: "Banbury Report 12 — Nitrosamines and Human Cancer" (ed. P. N. Magee), pp. 437–443. Cold Spring Harbor Laboratory, New York.

Wagner, D. A., Shuker, D. E. G., Hasic, G. and Tannenbaum, S. R. (1982). Endogenous nitrosoproline synthesis in humans. *In*: "Banbury Report 12 — Nitrosamines and Human Cancer" (ed. P. N. Magee), pp. 319–333. Cold Spring Harbor Laboratory, New York.

Wagner, D. A., Young, V. R. and Tannenbaum, S. R. (1983a). Mammalian nitrate biosynthesis: Incorporation of $^{15}NH_3$ into nitrate is enhanced by endotoxin treatment. *Proc. Natl Acad. Sci.* **80**, 4518–4521.

Wagner, D. A., Schultz, D. S., Deen, W. M., Young, V. R. and Tannenbaum, S. R. (1983b). Metabolic fate of an oral dose of [^{15}N]-labelled nitrate in humans: effect of diet supplementation with ascorbic acid. *Cancer Res.* **43**, 1921–1925.

Wagner, D. A., Shuker, D. E. G., Bilmazes, C., Obiedzyinski, M., Young, V. R. and Tannenbaum, S.R. (1985a). Modulation of endogenous synthesis of N-nitrosamino acids in humans. *In*: "N-Nitroso Compounds: Occurrence, Biological Effects and Relevance to Human Cancer" (eds I. K. O'Neill, R. C. von Borstel, C. T. Miller, J. Long and H. Bartsch), pp. 223–230.

International Agency for Research on Cancer, Lyon.

Wagner, D. A., Moldawer, L. L., Pomposelli, J. J., Tannenbaum, S. R. and Young, V. R. (1985b). Nitrate biosynthesis in the rat: Precursor-product relationships with respect to ammonia. *Biochem J.* **232**, 547–551.

Walters, C. L. and Smith, P. L. R. (1981). The effect of water-bourne nitrate on salivary nitrite. *Fd Cosmet. Toxicol.* **19**, 297–302.

Wang, C. F., Cassens, R. G. and Hoekstra, W. G. (1981). Fate of ingested ^{15}N-labelled nitrate and nitrite in the rat. *J. Fd Sci.* **46**, 745–748.

Wang, T., Kakizoe, T., Dion, P., Furrer, R., Varghese, A. J. and Bruce, W. R. (1978). Volatile nitrosamines in normal human faeces. *Nature*, **276**, 280–281.

Ward, F. W., Coates, M. E. and Walker, R. (1985). Nitrate reduction in germfree rats. *In*: "Germfree Research: Microflora Control and its Application to the Biomedical Sciences" (eds B. S. Wostman, J. R. Pleasants, B. A. Teah, M. Pollard and M. Wagner), pp. 123–125. Alan R. Liss Inc., New York.

Ward, F. W., Coates, M. E. and Walker, R. (1986). Nitrate reduction, gastrointestinal pH and N-nitrosation in gnotobiotic and conventional rats. *Fd Chem. Toxicol.* **24** 17–22.

White, R. E. (1984). Nitrate leaching from grassland. *Nature* **311**, 10.

WHO, (1978). "Nitrates, Nitrites and *N*-Nitroso Compounds (Environmental Health Criteria 5)". World Health Organisation, Geneva.

WHO (1984). Nitrate and nitrite. *In*: "Guidelines for Drinking-Water Quality volume 2. Health Criteria and Other Supporting Information", pp. 128–134. World Health Organisation, Geneva.

Wise, A., Mallett, A. K. and Rowland, I. R. (1982). Dietary fibre, bacterial metabolism and toxicity of nitrate in the rat. *Xenobiotica* **12**, 111–118.

Witter, J. P., Balish, E. and Gatley, S. J. (1979). Distribution of nitrogen-13 from labelled nitrate ([13]NO_3^-) and nitrite ([13]NO_2^-) in germfree (GF) and conventional flora (CV) rats. *Appl. Environ. Microbiol.* **38**, 870–874.

Witter, J. P., Salish, E. and Gatley, S. J. (1982). Origin of excess urinary nitrate in the rat. *Cancer Res.* **42**, 3654–3658.

Woebkenberg, N. R., Mostardi, R. A., Ely, D. L. and Worstell, D. (1981). *Envir. Res.* **26**, 347–351.

Wynder, E. L., Knet, J., Dungal, N. and Segi, M. (1963). An epidemiological investigation of gastric cancer. *Cancer* **16**, 1461–1469.

Yoshida, K., Kasama, K., Kitabatake, M. and Imai, M. (1983). Biotransformation of nitric oxide, nitrite and nitrate. *Int. Arch. Occup. Environ. Hlth.* **52**, 103–115.

8

Intense Sweeteners and the Gut Microflora

A. G. RENWICK

A. Introduction

The intense sweeteners which are currently available widely throughout the world may be divided into two groups — organic acids and peptides (Renwick, 1986). The latter, aspartame and thaumatin, are digested in the upper intestine and thus have little potential for interaction with the gut microflora. The organic acids, saccharin, cyclamate and acesulfame-K, are incompletely absorbed from the gut and thus an interaction is possible, either by the sweetener altering the microbial flora, or the bacteria metabolizing the sweetener. These three sweeteners are considered in chronological order of their discovery, followed by stevioside which is an intensely sweet glycoside currently available in only a few countries, including Japan (Fig. 8.1).

B. Saccharin

The establishment of an acceptable daily intake (ADI) for the human ingestion of food components such as intense sweeteners is based on high dose animal toxicity studies. In such studies dietary levels of the sweetener may be as high as 10% w/w. Such intakes can produce profound perturbations of homeostatic mechanisms, including the metabolic activity of the intestinal microflora. Such an effect has been reported in rats fed saccharin containing diets and is associated with alterations in carbohydrate and protein digestion and in microbial catabolism. The relationship of the reported metabolic changes to the increase in bladder tumours found in rats fed similar high dietary levels is unclear. Saccharin is not a typical electrophilic carcinogen since it is an anion which is not metabolized *in vivo* (see Renwick (1985) for a review) and does not bind to DNA of the target organ (Lutz and Schlatter, 1977). Thus tumour development is probably by some indirect mechanism which is secondary to the

ROLE OF THE GUT FLORA IN TOXICITY AND CANCER
ISBN 0-12-599920-8

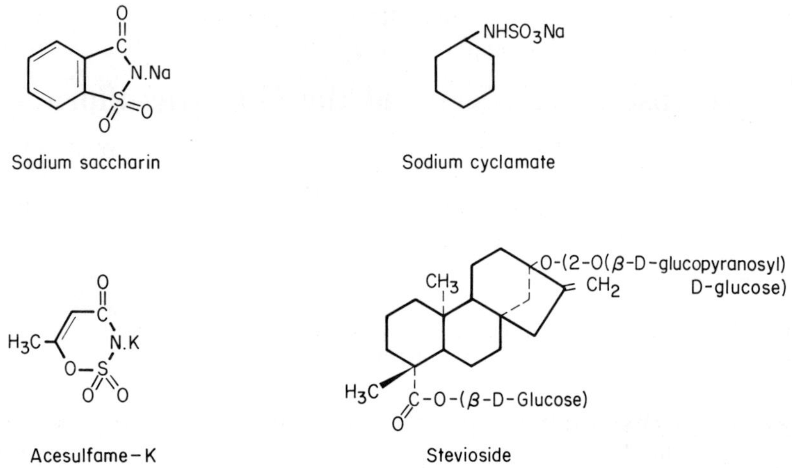

Sodium saccharin

Sodium cyclamate

Acesulfame–K

Stevioside

Fig 8.1   The intense sweeteners discussed in this chapter.

biochemical and physiological changes produced in rats at high dietary levels. The resultant profound differences between test animals and controls renders the interpretation of the toxicity findings and their extrapolation to man complex and contentious.

Saccharin has been used as an intense sweetener for most of this century (Arnold *et al.*, 1983) with almost continuous debate concerning its safety. The debate has intensified in recent years since a number of high dose feeding studies have reported an increased incidence of bladder tumours in treated male rats. The experimental conditions necessary for this effect to be demonstrated include high dietary levels of sodium saccharin (equal or greater than 3% w/w), and neonatal administration. A significant increase in tumour incidence has been found consistently only in studies in which saccharin was given throughout a two-generation protocol or when the dams and pups were given saccharin-containing diets from birth (Arnold *et al.*, 1980; Schoenig *et al.*, 1985; Taylor *et al.*, 1980).

Most single generation studies have not shown an increased incidence of bladder tumours in saccharin-fed animals (see Oser (1985) for a review). Exceptions to this are a study in the ACI strain of rat which also showed a high incidence of infection by the bladder parasite *Trichosomoides crassicauda* (Fukushima *et al.*, 1983a), and the F_0 (parental) generation of the study by Arnold *et al.* (1980). This latter study is of interest since the F_0 animals were only 32 days old when started on saccharin diet, which is younger than in other single generation studies. Thus it appears that the period of lactation and weaning may be critical for the development of bladder tumours in male rats fed very high dietary levels of saccharin. This period covers both the maturation of the target organ, the bladder, which occurs during the first 28 days of life (Ayres *et al.*, 1985) and also the development of the adult gut flora at weaning. This temporal relationship suggests that the marked changes in the gut flora of the rat described below may be linked to bladder tumour development in this species.

1. *Evidence of alterations in the organisms present in the gut lumen*

Although the addition of sodium saccharin to the medium inhibited the *in vitro* growth of intestinal bacteria (Anderson and Kirkland, 1980; Naim *et al.*, 1985), *in vivo* administration at up to 7.5% in the diet did not produce a marked reduction in the total aerobes or anaerobes present in the caecum (Anderson and Kirkland, 1980; Mallett *et al.*, 1985a) or faeces (Sims and Renwick, 1983). Anderson and Kirkland (1980) reported the deletion of an unidentified caecal organism in rats fed 7.5% sodium saccharin for 10 days, but Sims and Renwick (1983) found significant increases in the numbers of both aerobes and anaerobes in the faeces of rats fed 7.5% sodium saccharin for 2 months, with no obvious change in the composition of the bacteria present. An increase in total caecal bacteria was found by Mallett *et al.* (1985a) in rats fed 5% sodium saccharin for 20 weeks, but this was due to caecal enlargement rather than an increased concentration. Although saccharin administration does not apparently alter the composition of the intestinal flora markedly, it produces a number of differences in the metabolic capacity of the caecal organisms. These changes accompany a profound dose-dependent enlargement of the caecum (Lawson and Hertzog, 1981; Anderson, 1983, 1985; Sims and Renwick, 1983).

2. *Changes in carbohydrate metabolism*

Addition of high concentrations of saccharin *in vitro* inhibits a wide range of hydrolytic enzymes, including porcine amylase (Anderson, 1985), rat small intestinal amylase (Naim *et al.*, 1985), sucrase and isomaltase (Anderson, 1985) and the production of glucose on incubation of rat small intestinal contents with laboratory rat food (Anderson, 1985). Although the concentrations of saccharin necessary were very high (up to 100 mg ml^{-1}), they were compatible with the dietary levels fed to animals. Rat caecal β-glucuronidase, but not β-glucosidase, was inhibited both *in vivo* and *in vitro* by saccharin (Mallett *et al.*, 1985a).

An *in vivo* consequence of this inhibitory activity was the accumulation in the faeces of a polysaccharide, which would produce an osmotic effect and lead to caecal enlargement (Anderson, 1983, 1985). This polysaccharide probably arose from incomplete digestion of a dietary component rather than synthesis by a faecal organism (Anderson, 1983, 1985). Accumulation of reducing sugars in the caecum was reported by Naim *et al.* (1985), who suggested that it may arise from saccharin inhibition of bacterial growth and utilization of carbohydrate. Saccharin at concentrations of approximately 2% inhibits *in vitro* the glycolytic enzymes of *Streptococcus mutans* (Linke and Kohn, 1984) and the anaerobic fermentation of glucose by rat intestinal bacteria (Pfeffer *et al.*, 1985). Saccharin caused a decrease in caecal volatile fatty acids, especially butyrate, and an increase in lactate, both *in vivo* and on *in vitro* incubation (Anderson, 1985).

In a recent publication Anderson *et al.* (1987) showed that replacement of dietary starch by glucose did not influence the extent of caecal enlargement produced by 5% sodium saccharin. This indicates that dietary polysaccharide is not essential for caecal enlargement, and also that saccharin may affect the absorption of glucose and its utilization by the gut flora (see above). However, the importance of dietary carbohydrates in caecal enlargement was questioned by the finding that significant caecal enlargement still occurred even if the dietary carbohydrate was replaced by fat (Anderson *et al.*, 1987). The authors drew particular attention to the fact that the addition of 5% saccharin to a high fat – low carbohydrate diet did not cause the normally observed increase in urine volume or decrease in urine osmolality. Since these are factors which have been shown to correlate with the development of bladder tumours within a group of F_1 male rats fed 7.5% saccharin in normal diet (Schoenig *et al.*, 1985), Anderson *et al.* concluded that altered intestinal carbohydrate metabolism plays a key role in tumour development. However interpretation of this study is complicated by the fact that the dietary perturbation produced by the substitution of 65% starch by 28.9% lard plus 41% cellulose also resulted in a number of other changes. The animals given 5% saccharin in high fat diet showed the lowest body weight gain and the highest water consumption. The high water intake, but low urine volume suggests that there was significantly greater loss of water by other routes such as the faeces. Also the animals fed high fat diet excreted only 31% of the saccharin intake in the urine, compared with 83% in the starch groups indicating impaired absorption of saccharin. The

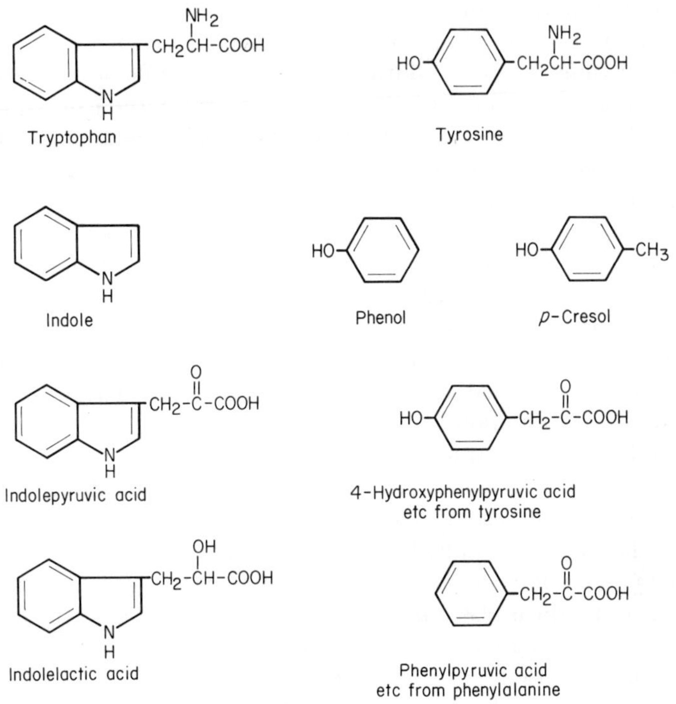

Tryptophan

Tyrosine

Indole

Phenol

p-Cresol

Indolepyruvic acid

4-Hydroxyphenylpyruvic acid
etc from tyrosine

Indolelactic acid

Phenylpyruvic acid
etc from phenylalanine

Fig 8.2 The aromatic amino acids and their metabolites discussed in this chapter.

abnormal fluid balance and saccharin absorption in the high fat/saccharin group demonstrate the presence of other major variables that would not be present in the F_1 animals fed 7.5% saccharin in the IRDC study (Schoenig *et al.*, 1985). Comparison of the changes found by Anderson *et al.* (1987) using high fat diet with the correlations of Schoenig *et al.* (1985) using normal diet is therefore of questionable validity. Conclusions based on such a comparison, for example that bladder tumorigenesis may be causally related to altered carbohydrate metabolism in the gut (but not to sodium excretion or microbial protein catabolism which showed the usual sodium saccharin induced increases, albeit reduced, in the presence of the high fat saccharin diet) must be regarded as premature.

3. *Changes in Protein Metabolism*

The initial observation suggesting that saccharin could interfere with protein digestion (Carlson *et al.*, 1923) has been confirmed recently by studies on the *in vitro* inhibition of urease and proteases such as pepsin and papain (Lok *et al.*, 1982). The *in vivo* significance of this was shown by Sims and Renwick (1983) during studies on the influence of saturation of renal tubular secretion of anions due to saccharin (Sweatman and Renwick, 1980) on the elimination of tryptophan metabolites. Dietary saccharin produced a dose dependent increase in the daily elimination of indican, which is formed from the microbial metabolism of tryptophan to indole (Fig. 8.2) followed by hydroxylation and conjugation with sulphate. The enzyme tryptophanase which converts tryptophan to indole is present largely in the caecum and colon of normal rats. Administration of high saccharin diets did not cause either a redistribution or increase in the enzyme activity, but rather a transient loss of activity followed by a return to near normal amounts after two weeks. The cause of the increased indole formation and indican excretion was accumulation in the caecum of both the substrate tryptophan (about 40-fold at 7.5% saccharin diet) and protein (ninefold at 7.5% saccharin) (Sims and Renwick, 1983). These changes were accompanied by a three- to fourfold increase in the weight of the caecal contents. Evidence for an altered pattern of microbial tryptophan metabolites was provided by a massive increase in indolelactic acid (Fig. 8.2), which was almost undetectable in animals fed saccharin-free diet, and increased up to 60-fold at 7.5% saccharin in the diet. Further evidence of inhibition of proteolysis was shown by *in vitro* studies on pepsin, suggesting that impaired digestion of protein was the principal source of the changes. This conclusion seems to be at variance with the data of Naim *et al.* (1982, 1985) who reported higher levels of proteolytic activity in the large intestines and caecum of rats fed a diet containing 2.5% saccharin. This higher activity was also found when saccharin was added *in vitro* to prolonged incubations of trypsin and chymotrysin. The authors (Naim *et al.*, 1985) concluded that the increased activity *in vivo* was not due to stimulated enzyme output from the pancreas, but rather that the inhibition of proteolytic activity would increase the survival of active enzymes in the lower portions of the intestine.

These observations concerning saccharin and protein digestion are of particular interest since various studies have indicated a link between experimental bladder cancer and protein, tryptophan and other amino acids.

(i) The incidence of spontaneous bladder tumours in rats can be increased markedly by feeding a high protein diet (Ross and Bras, 1973).

(ii) The protease inhibitor leupeptin acts as a promoter of bladder cancer in rats (Kakizoe *et al.*, 1977).

(iii) High dietary levels of leucine, isoleucine (Nishio *et al.*, 1986) and tryptophan (Radomski *et al.*, 1977; Cohen *et al.*, 1979; Fukushima *et al.*, 1983b) are promoters of bladder cancer in rats.

(iv) A sevenfold increase in dietary tryptophan caused a focal hyperplasia of the bladder epithelium in dogs (Radomski *et al.*, 1971).

(v) Microbial metabolites of aromatic amino acids may act as co-carcinogens or promoters of cancer development. Indole is a more potent co-carcinogen for the urinary bladder than the parent amino acid tryptophan (Dunning and Curtis, 1958; Oyasu *et al.*, 1972), while indoleacetic acid is a weak co-carcinogen (Dunning and Curtis, 1958). Simple phenols, such as cresol, which are microbial metabolites of tyrosine (Fig. 8.2), are cancer promoters using a mouse skin model (Boutwell and Bosch, 1959; Wynder and Hoffman, 1968).

The various changes in protein and tryptophan metabolism were found when saccharin was given during a two-generation protocol (Sims and Renwick, 1985). During lactation, saccharin increased the concentrations of indican in maternal plasma and milk and in the stomach contents of suckling pups. The urinary excretion of indican was increased in the F_1 animals fed 7.5% saccharin diet and the maximum amount (expressed as mg/kg/day) occurred soon after weaning. Analysis of urines collected between 13 and 24 months from the IRDC cancer bioassay on saccharin confirmed that increased formation of indole and excretion of indican was a consistent and permanent change (Lawrie *et al.*, 1985). The toxicological significance of indican with respect to saccharin effects thus appears to be high, but various factors suggest that it may be more important as an indicator of other changes, rather than a directly significant metabolite. For example, substitution of dietary starch by fat and cellulose reduced the extent of saccharin induced caecal enlargement to about 40% of that in rats fed a starch based diet (Anderson *et al.*, 1987). The saccharin induced increase in indican excretion was about 38% of that in rats fed a starch based diet. This close correlation suggests that the accumulation of protein may be the major cause of both caecal enlargement and indican excretion.

Evidence that indican may not be of direct importance in the development of bladder tumours comes from the IRDC two-generation study which contained two additional groups of rats fed 5% saccharin diet; one group received saccharin only during gestation and then returned to normal diet, and the other group had normal diet during gestation and started saccharin diet at birth via the dam (F_0 group). No bladder tumours were found in the former group but the incidence in the F_0 group was similar to those given 5% saccharin in a full two-generation protocol.

The studies on indican excretion by Sims and Renwick (1985) included a group transferred to 7.5% saccharin from birth. The excretion of indican in this group was not identical to that in the F_1 group since transient loss of tryptophanase occurred in the dam during lactation. Thus these pups did not acquire a 'saccharin adapted' gut flora and the excretion of indican did not reach that of the F_1 group until 11 weeks of age. Interestingly, the concentrations of indolelactic acid were greatly elevated in maternal plasma, and in the plasma and caecal contents of both F_1 and F_0 groups of saccharin treated pups from three weeks of age onwards. Unfortunately the potency of this metabolite as a promoter of bladder cancer has never been studied.

Saccharin diets also caused an increased total microbial metabolism of tyrosine associated with an altered pattern of metabolites (Lawrie *et al.*, 1985). Daily excretion of *p*-cresol was increased both on short term feeding and in the 13–24 month urines from the IRDC study, whilst phenol excretion was almost totally abolished. The increase in *p*-cresol excretion was related linearly to the dose over the range 0–5% sodium saccharin after 20 weeks on saccharin diets, with a 30–40-fold increase in daily *p*-cresol, compared with only 2–3-fold increase in indican, at the 5% dietary level (Lawrie and Renwick, 1987). At earlier time points (6 and 10 weeks) animals fed high dietary saccharin concentrations (5 and 7.5%) showed wide inter-individual variability with some animals excreting little *p*-cresol. In consequence the dose–effect relationship was almost bell-shaped (Fig. 8.3). The slow adaptation of *p*-cresol excretion at high dietary levels is consistent with an initial suppression of bacterial metabolism, similar to that seen in tryptophanase (Sims and Renwick, 1983). However, the excretion of indican was directly proportional to dietary level, even at 6 weeks (Fig. 8.4). The excretion of phenol at 6 weeks was unaffected at dietary levels of 1% sodium saccharin or less, but was strongly suppressed at 2% or more. Some recovery of phenol excretion occurred by 20 weeks continuous administration at higher dietary levels, suggesting slow adaptation of the gut microflora (Lawrie and Renwick, 1987). Initially when animals were given 7.5% saccharin diet there was a transient decrease in all three metabolites (indican, *p*-cresol and phenol), but by 20 days on diet only phenol excretion remained suppressed.

4. *Changes in Saccharin Metabolism*

Despite incomplete absorption from the gut such that it provides a potential substrate for microbial enzymes, radiolabelled saccharin was not

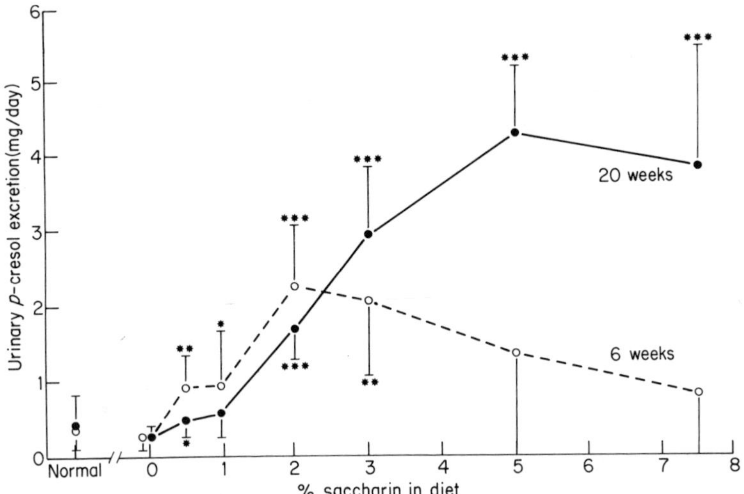

Fig 8.3 The urinary excretion of *p*-cresol in rats fed diets containing 0–7.5% sodium saccharin *ad libitum* (from Lawrie and Renwick (1987)).
*p<0.05, **p<0.01, ***p<0.001 compared with 0% group by Students' *t*-test for unpaired data.

metabolized either when given as a single dose (Ball *et al.*, 1977) or when given to F_1 male rats maintained on a 5% saccharin diet *ad libitum* (Sweatman and Renwick, 1979). In addition *in vitro* incubation with faeces from normal rats and rats maintained on saccharin diet did not result in any biotransformation of saccharin. The faeces of animals maintained on cyclamate diet, and which were shown to hydrolyse cyclamate to cyclohexylamine *in vitro* (see below), were also unable to metabolize the saccharin molecule (Ball *et al.*, 1977).

5.   Conclusions

High dietary levels of saccharin cause caecal enlargement in rats, which is associated with accumulation of carbohydrates and protein. When rats are first given saccharin diet there is a transient decrease in tryptophanase activity and the excretion of indican, *p*-cresol and phenol. Following a period of acclimatization to the diet, which may need many weeks to stabilize, the amounts of bacterial metabolites in both the urine and caecal contents indicate an altered pattern of metabolic reactions. The excretion of indican and *p*-cresol is increased while phenol is suppressed. The caecal contents contain increased amounts of lactic and indolelactic acids, but less propionic, butyric and indolepropionic acids, and tyramine.

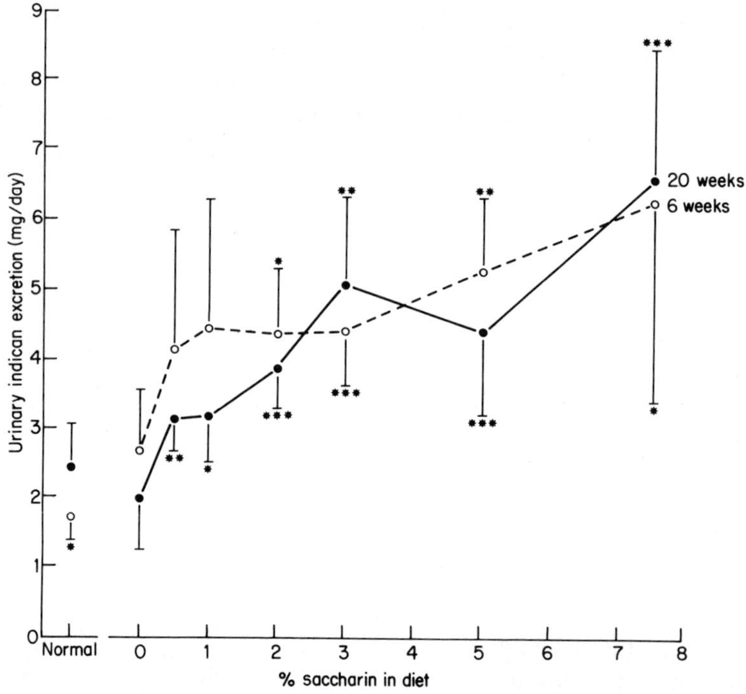

Fig 8.4 The urinary excretion of indican in rats fed diets containing 0–7.5% sodium saccharin *ad libitum* (from Lawrie and Renwick (1987)).
*P<0.05, **P<0.01, ***P<0.001 compared to 0% groups by Students' *t*-test for unpaired data.

Of these changes indolelactic acid is probably the most interesting since this increases in saccharin-fed animals from almost undetectable levels to become a major caecal tryptophan metabolite, and also it is increased in lactating females and neonatal F_0 and F_1 animals (Sims and Renwick, 1985). The relationships between the dietary concentration of saccharin and concentrations of indolelactic acid and tryptamine in the caecum and of phenol in the urine show a large change at approximately 2–3% dietary levels (Sims and Renwick, 1983; Lawrie and Renwick, 1987). This level corresponds to that necessary to demonstrate an increase in tumour incidence in F_1 male rats (Schoenig *et al.*, 1985). Although this could be a coincidence, the many biochemical differences between control and treated animals complicate the interpretation of the toxicity data. The relevance of phenomena seen at such high dietary levels to human risk evaluation is questioned by the report that significant changes in the elimination of microbial metabolites were not found in human volunteers given daily doses of saccharin (1 g) for 4 weeks (Roberts and Renwick, 1985; Lawrie and Renwick, 1987). This would be consistent with the recent review of the extensive published epidemiological evidence which concluded that there was no overall association between human bladder cancer and the consumption of intense sweeteners (Morgan and Wong, 1985).

C. Cyclamate

Cyclamate was banned in the UK and USA in 1969 following reports of an increased incidence of bladder tumours in rats fed a mixture of cyclamate, saccharin and cyclohexylamine, which is the microbial metabolite of cyclamate (Price *et al.*, 1970). The decision that cyclamate was responsible was based partly on the finding of a single bladder tumour in a group of rats given cyclohexylamine alone, and the fact that seven out of eight animals in the high dose cyclamate study converted cyclamate to cyclohexylamine. The latter observation however needs to be put into the context that 55 out of the 60 animals in the high group were converters (Price *et al.*, 1970). In addition bladder tumours were found in three out of 23 rats given cyclamate as part of a metabolism study (Friedman *et al.*, 1972). Re-examination of the histology data in the study of Price *et al.* (1970) revealed that there were 12 tumours, 9 in males and 3 in females, and there was no apparent association between tumour development and cyclohexylamine exposure (Bopp *et al.*, 1986). Subsequent attempts to replicate this observation using cyclamate alone, a cyclamate : saccharin mixture or cyclohexylamine have proved unsuccessful. Reviews of these data by a number of national and international bodies (e.g. the National Cancer Institute and the National Academy of Sciences – National Research Council in the USA; the Joint Expert Committee on Food Additives (JECFA) of the WHO) have concluded that neither cyclamate nor cyclohexylamine has been shown to be carcinogenic (Bopp *et al.*, 1986). Cyclamate continues to be available for human use in over 40 countries around the world, including Germany, Switzerland and Australia. Since cyclamate is not carcinogenic, its level of use is set by the toxicological profile of both cyclamate and its major metabolite cyclohexylamine. Cyclohexylamine is more toxic than cyclamate and therefore this sweetener represents a rare example where the level of use is set by the possible formation and toxicity of its metabolite (JECFA, 1977). Since the metabolite is formed by the gastro-intestinal flora, this sweetener is an excellent example of the importance of the gut bacteria in the toxicological assessment of an a nutrient.

1. *The Induction of Cyclamate Metabolism*

Early studies on the fate of radiolabelled cyclamate reported that it was eliminated in the urine and faeces unchanged (Taylor *et al.*, 1951; Miller *et al.*, 1966). However in 1966 Kojima and Ichibagase detected cyclohexylamine as a minor urinary metabolite in cyclamate treated dogs and humans. Cyclohexylamine was subsequently detected as a urinary metabolite of ^{14}C-cyclamate in rats, rabbits, guinea pigs and man, providing the individuals had received cyclamate chronically prior to the radiolabelled dose (Renwick and Williams, 1972b).

The induction of cyclamate metabolism is highly variable, both between species and between different individuals. Soon after the initial report of cyclamate metabolism a number of groups either set up metabolism studies in rats or incorporated metabolism studies into chronic toxicity investigations. Not all investigators could obtain converter rats in their colonies (Collings, 1971) whilst others found wide inter-individual variability (Oser *et al.*, 1968; Sonders *et al.*, 1969; Renwick and Williams, 1972b; Renwick, 1976, 1986; Bickel *et al.*, 1974) with some individuals metabolizing up to 45% of a test dose. Introduction of converter rats into a colony gave rapid transfer of cyclamate metabolizing ability (Collings, 1971). Individual animals which had developed metabolizing ability showed wide temporal fluctuations on repeated study (Oser *et al.*, 1968; Renwick, 1986) despite being maintained on the same cyclamate diet under apparently identical conditions.

Cyclamate metabolism has been reported in man following a single dose of cyclamate, but this has generally been at a low level, with most of the cyclohexylamine excreted in the second to fourth day after dosing (Asahina *et al.*, 1971; Renwick and Williams, 1972b). The daily excretion of cyclohexylamine increases during chronic administration to human volunteers with a plateau being reached after about 5–10 days (see Renwick (1983) for a review). During repeated dosing the percentage of the daily dose metabolized in different individuals ranges from undetectable to 60% with a highly skewed distribution (Fig. 8.5). During chronic regular cyclamate dosing there are wide daily fluctuations of ± 50% or more around the mean steady state excretion for that particular individual (Davis *et al.*, 1969; Collings, 1971; Litchfield and Swan, 1971; Renwick and Williams, 1972b). Part of this fluctuation is probably due to variable accumulation of cyclamate in the distal bowel, providing a variable amount of substrate available for metabolism, since the excretion of cyclohexylamine correlated with the extent of constipation (Davis *et al.*, 1969).

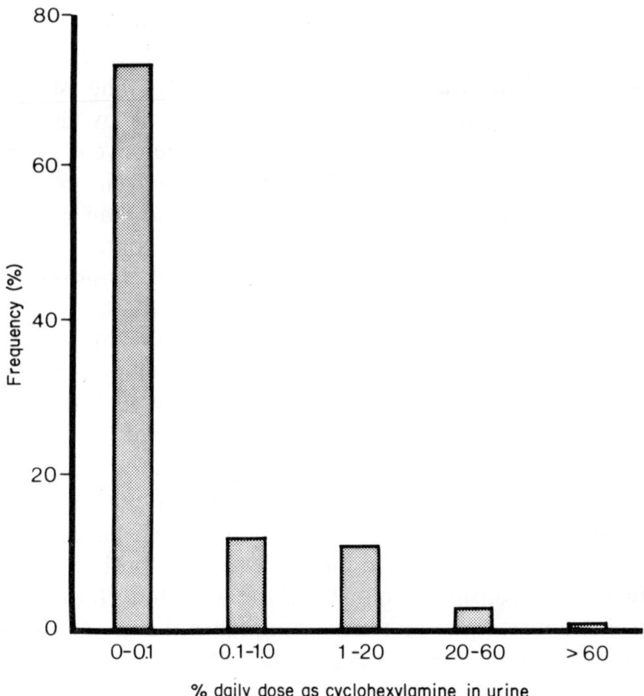

Fig 8.5 The distribution of cyclamate metabolizing ability in the human population during chronic intake (from Renwick (1983)).

2. The Site of Cyclamate Metabolism

Evidence implicating the gut flora as the site of cyclamate metabolism in rats was published soon after the initial report of cyclohexylamine excretion by Kojima and Ichibagase (1966). Renwick and Williams (1969) reported the conversion of cyclamate to cyclohexylamine *in vitro* by the lower gut contents but not the tissues of cyclamate pretreated rats. No conversion occurred in the presence of gut contents from untreated rats. In addition, they showed that orally administered cyclamate was converted to cyclohexylamine (38% of dose) but only 0.9% was metabolized following intraperitoneal dosing to pretreated rats. Almost simultaneously Sonders *et al.* (1969) reported a 47-fold difference in the extent of metabolism of oral and intravenous cyclamate and that neomycin treatment abolished the excretion of cyclohexylamine in a cyclamate receiving 'converter' rat.

Subsequent publications confirmed and extended these observations. The importance of the oral route of administration was confirmed in pigs (Collings, 1971) and rats (Bickel *et al.*, 1974). The suppression of cyclohexylamine excretion in converting individuals by the co-administration of antibiotics was shown in rats using neomycin or gentamicin (Bickel *et al.*, 1974), in guinea pigs using streptomycin (Asahina *et al.*, 1972b), in pigs using neomycin (Collings, 1971) and man using ampicillin (Collings, 1971). *In vitro* metabolism by intestinal contents and/or faeces was demonstrated for rats (Dalderup *et al.*, 1970; Drasar *et al.*, 1972; Bickel *et al.*, 1974; Tesoriero and Roxon, 1975; Mallett *et al.*, 1985b), guinea pigs (Asahina *et al.*, 1972b; Drasar *et al.*, 1972), rabbits (Drasar *et al.*, 1972), dogs (Goldberg *et al.*, 1969), pigs (Collings, 1971) and man (Drasar *et al.*, 1972). Conversely incubation of tissues from known cyclamate pretreated converting rats (Prosky and O'Dell, 1971; Drasar *et al.*, 1972), guinea pigs (Asahina *et al.*, 1972b; Drasar *et al.*, 1972) or rabbits (Drasar *et al.*, 1972) has been reported not to result in the formation of cyclohexylamine. Other findings which have supported the conclusion that the gut flora are the principal and probably the sole site of cyclamate metabolism in animals and man include (*i*) the transfer of activity from converting to non-converting rats either by natural or forced coprophagy (Collings, 1971; Bickel *et al.*, 1974), (*ii*) the rapid loss of acquired cyclamate metabolizing ability on cessation of chronic cyclamate ingestion in both rats (Renwick and Williams, 1972b; Bickel *et al.*, 1974) and man (Renwick and Williams, 1972b), (*iii*) the rapid and extensive absorption and excretion of cyclohexylamine following intracaecal or intracolonic administration to rats (Drasar *et al.*, 1972) and guinea pigs (Asahina, 1972), and (*iv*) the close correlations between *in vivo* and *in vitro* metabolism by gut flora preparations both between different animals and subjects and within the same individuals prior to, during and after chronic cyclamate administration (Drasar *et al.*, 1972; Renwick and Williams, 1972b).

Whilst the findings described above provide clear evidence that the gut microflora are the site of cyclamate metabolism *in vivo*, a few studies have been published which do not support this conclusion. Incubation of cyclamate with the faeces from human converters of cyclamate by Leahy *et al.* (1967) and Davis *et al.* (1969) did not yield detectable cyclohexylamine. However, subsequent studies using human faeces (Drasar *et al.*, 1972) showed that incubation with high concentrations of cyclamate *in vitro* resulted in a loss of metabolizing capacity, which was decreased further if the nutrient medium was diluted. Studies using mixed cultures of rat intestinal organisms showed that the extent of metabolism *in vitro* could be affected by the presence in the medium of glucose

(Dalderup *et al.*, 1970) and cysteine (Tesoriero and Roxon, 1975), and by the concentration of the nutrient medium (Mallett *et al.*, 1985b).

The papers published by Kojima and Ichibagase and their co-workers following their initial discovery of cyclohexylamine excretion in 1966, have tended to be contradictory to the above conclusions and to some extent to each other. An initial study in rats and rabbits (Kojima and Ichibagase, 1968) demonstrated the presence of trace amounts of cyclohexylamine after incubation of liver samples with cyclamate. However, since the animals had been pretreated with cyclamate and no controls were reported it is impossible to interpret this observation. Subsequently Ichibagase *et al.* (1972a) studied the influence of phenylbutazone, phenobarbitone and tolbutamide on the *in vivo* and *in vitro* metabolism of cyclamate, cyclohexylamine, cyclohexanol and cyclohexanone by rabbits. However, these studies were difficult to interpret since (*i*) only two or three animals were studied with each treatment, (*ii*) the animals had not been pretreated with cyclamate to induce metabolism, and (*iii*) the conversion of the single dose of cyclamate to cyclohexylamine was 0.01% of the dose or less. The conclusion that the metabolism of sodium cyclamate in rabbits was accelerated by these enzyme inducers is therefore debatable. The following paper in this series (Ichibagase *et al.*, 1972b) studied the influence of long term treatment with cyclamate on its metabolism in rats and rabbits. Again the numbers of animals studied tended to be low, but on this occasion some of the animals pretreated with cyclamate became good converters (>1% of the dose), with considerable inter-animal variation. The authors suggested that pretreatment of rabbits with cyclohexylamine, cyclohexanol and cyclohexanone (10 mg/day) increased the metabolism of a subsequent single dose of cyclamate to these metabolites. This conclusion cannot be supported from the published data which showed no clear increase in the excretion of cyclohexylamine or its metabolites (even despite their administration). Incubation results with the livers from control and cyclamate pretreated rats and rabbits were reported to show the presence of small amounts of cyclohexylamine, cyclohexanol and cyclohexanone prior to treatment, a decrease in all three in cyclamate pretreated rats, and a decrease in cyclohexylamine but an increase in the deaminated products in pretreated rabbits. The authors concluded from this that cyclamate is metabolized in the intestine of the rat, but by the liver of rabbits, and that this is accompanied by a greater formation of cyclohexanol and cyclohexanone (a conclusion which is contradicted by the *in vivo* data in the same paper). Studies on the influence of antibiotics on cyclamate metabolism (Suenaga *et al.*, 1972) were difficult to interpret since many of the results were obtained on animals excreting less than 0.01% of the single dose as cyclohexylamine. The claimed difference between rats and rabbits following pretreatment was largely based on two rabbits which excreted less than 0.01% of the dose as cyclohexylamine prior to being given neomycin and four rats which excreted up to 1% as cyclohexylamine before they were given the antibiotic. The suppression of cyclohexylamine excretion in rats but not rabbits by neomycin, thus reflects the induction of microbial metabolism in the former but not the latter species. It is not possible to conclude from these various studies if the consistent excretion of approximately 0.01% of the dose of cyclamate as cyclohexylamine by rabbits (whether or not they were pretreated with enzyme inducers (Ichibagase *et al.*, 1972a) or antibiotics (Suenaga *et al.*, 1972)) represents tissue metabolism or trace amounts of cyclohexylamine salts in the dose material. However, what is clear is that the large induced excretion of cyclohexylamine reported by others and due to the gut flora is of infinitely greater toxicological significance.

3. The Strains of Bacteria Implicated in the Metabolism of Cyclamate to Cyclohexylamine

A number of investigators have isolated strains of bacteria from different sources which possess cyclamate metabolizing ability (Table 8.1). Clearly the activity does not reside in only one type of organism which makes the extremely wide inter- and intra-individual variability *in vivo* difficult to explain. A possible explanation is provided by the fascinating observation of Tokieda *et al.* (1979) of synergism between organisms in that single strains in isolation could not convert cyclamate to cyclohexylamine but combinations of two or more organisms produced cyclohexylamine. If this finding is extrapolated *in vivo* then cyclamate metabolism may depend on a number of variables, i.e. the appropriate concentrations of substrate, glucose, cysteine and other nutrients and the presence of a unique combination of intestinal organisms.

4. The Role of the Intestinal Bacteria in the Further Metabolism of Cyclohexylamine

Cyclohexylamine is metabolized *in vivo* by a number of pathways involving aliphatic hydroxylation and deamination (Fig. 8.6) (Renwick and Williams, 1972a). Although there are marked species differences in the extent of these reactions, the major urinary component is cyclohexylamine in all cases (Table 8.2). In all species over 95% of the radiolabelled dose was

Table 8.1 *Bacterial strains which metabolize cyclamate to cyclohexylamine*

Subject	Strain	Reference
Rat; faeces	*Clostridium* sp.	Drasar *et al.* (1972)
Guinea pig; faeces	*Pseudomonas* sp.	Asahina *et al.* (1972a)
	Corynebacterium sp.	Asahina *et al.* (1972a)
	Clostridium sordelli [a]	
	Campylobacter sp.	Matsui *et al.* (1981)
	Propionibacterium acnes	
	Propionibacterium acidipropionici	
Rabbit, caecal contents	*Clostridium* sp.	Drasar *et al.* (1972)
	Clostridium sp.	Tokieda *et al.* (1979)
	Enterobacterium sp.	Drasar *et al.* (1972)
	E. coli	Tokieda *et al.* (1979)
	Streptococcus faecalis	Tokieda *et al.* (1979)
	Bacillus sp.	Tokieda *et al.* (1979)
Dog; gut contents	*Clostridium perfringens*	Goldberg *et al.* (1969)
Man; faeces	*Enterococci sp.*	Drasar *et al.* (1972)

[a] in combination

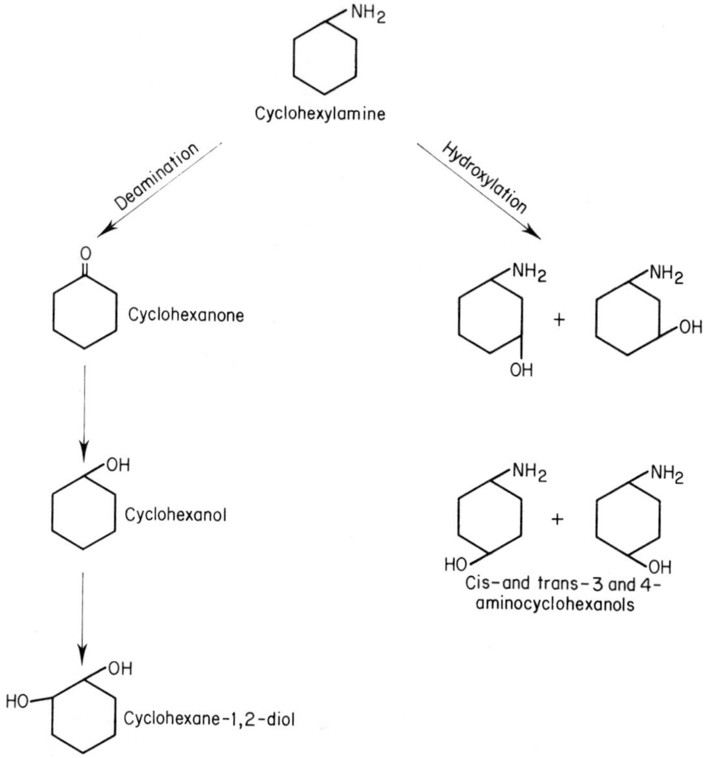

Fig 8.6 Pathways of cyclohexylamine metabolism in animals and man.

recovered in the urine and faeces, and in rats and guinea pigs less than 1% was eliminated as CO_2 (Renwick and Williams, 1972a). Formation of $^{14}CO_2$ was not detected as a metabolite of cyclamate, even in rats which had been pretreated with cyclamate and metabolized up to 40% of the dose to ^{14}C-cyclohexylamine (Renwick and Williams, 1972b). This finding is incompatible with the suggestion of Kojima and co-workers of extensive further metabolism of cyclohexanol and cyclohexanone by ring fission. Cyclohexylhydroxylamine (*N*-hydroxycyclohexylamine) has been reported as a metabolite of cyclamate by Goldberg *et al.* (1969) and of cyclohexylamine by Renwick and Williams (1972a), however quantitation in the latter study showed that it represented only 0.2% of the dose in the rabbit and was undetectable in other species, including man (Renwick and Williams, 1972a; Eichelbaum *et al.*, 1974). Dicyclohexylamine has been reported as a metabolite of cyclamate (Prosky and O'Dell, 1971),

Table 8.2 *The metabolism of ^{14}C-cyclohexylamine* in vivo

Species	Dose (mg/kg)	Sex	% ^{14}C in 0–24 hour urine			Reference
			Cyclohexylamine[a]	Hydroxylation[b]	Deamination[c]	
Wistar rat	500	F	95	6	0.1	Renwick and Williams (1972a)
Wistar rat	35	F	88	12	1–2	Roberts and Renwick (1985)
Wistar rat	35	M	78	22	1–2	Roberts and Renwick (1985)
Wistar rat	200	M	81	16	1–2	Roberts and Renwick (1985)
DA rat	200	M	93	5	1–2	Roberts and Renwick (1985)
Mouse	35	M	95	<1	1–2	Roberts and Renwick (1985)
Mouse	200	M	96	<1	1–2	Roberts and Renwick (1985)
Guinea Pig	450	F	95	3	4	Renwick and Williams (1972a)
Rabbit	100	F	61	13	15	Renwick and Williams (1972a)
Man	3	M	94	0	2	Renwick and Williams (1972a)

[a] Cyclohexylamine was given orally in aqueous solution as its hydrochloride salt.
[b] Hydroxylation: mixtures of *cis* and *trans* 3- and 4-aminocyclohexanols as free and conjugates.
[c] Deamination: mainly cyclohexanol and cyclohexane-1,2-diol as free and conjugates.

but this was not reproducible (Sonders and Wiegand, 1968; Renwick, unpublished observation) and possibly represents the presence of di-cyclohexylsulphamate in the cyclamate used in that particular study.

The major site of both hydroxylation and deamination is probably the liver, since no route of administration difference was found for the metabolism of cyclohexylamine in rats or mice (Roberts and Renwick, 1985) and rabbit liver microsomes deaminate cyclohexylamine by a cytochrome P_{450} dependent mechanism (Kurebayashi *et al.*, 1979). However, it is possible that the intestinal flora may be involved in the further metabolism of both the sulphur and cyclohexyl- moieties released following cyclamate metabolism.

The purified enzyme which hydrolyses cyclamate (cyclamate sulphamat-ase) in a strain of *Pseudomonas* (which was isolated from the faeces of cyclamate metabolizing guinea pigs) produced stoichiometrically equival-ent amounts of cyclohexylamine and sulphate (Niimura *et al.*, 1974). In whole cell suspensions of intestinal bacteria the sulphate moiety may be reduced to volatile sulphur compounds (probably H_2S) and incorporated into protein (Tesoriero and Roxon, 1975). The cyclohexylamine may undergo microbial deamination to cyclohexanone (Asahina *et al.*, 1972a; Tokieda *et al.*, 1979) which may subsequently act as a sole source of carbon for the growth of the organism *in vitro* (Asahina *et al.*, 1972a). Evidence supporting the possibility that further bacterial metabolism of cyclohexylamine may occur *in vivo* comes of two sources. Tokieda *et al.* (1979) reported suppression of cyclohexanol excretion in three out of six animals receiving cyclohexylamine in the drinking water following treatment with neomycin or metronidazole. However, the absence of any effect in half the animals makes this study difficult to interpret. Since cyclohexylamine is absorbed rapidly from the intestine (Drasar *et al.*, 1972) it is unlikely that the fate of orally administered cyclohexylamine would adequately reflect the importance of the gut flora in the further metabolism of cyclohexylamine produced in the hind gut as a result of cyclamate metabolism. Evidence supporting this possibility is given in Table 8.3, which shows that the ratio of cyclohexylamine metabolites to cyclohexylamine is higher in guinea pigs and rabbits after cyclamate administration than following cyclohexylamine. Interestingly the rat, which hydroxylates cyclohexylamine, does not show increased further metabolism of cyclohexylamine after its formation from cyclamate. Although the data are consistent with the gut flora metabolizing part of the cyclohexylamine before it is absorbed there is an equally valid explanation. The rapid absorption of cyclohexylamine after this compound is given may saturate hepatic deamination, thus reducing the extent of metabolism compared with when cyclohexylamine is slowly absorbed from the gut following its formation from cyclamate. If deamination occurs primarily in the liver, then the total absorbed cyclohexylamine 'dose' is given by cyclohexylamine plus deaminated products. Conversely, if the gut flora produce cyclohexanol and cyclohexanone prior to absorption, then this will not need to be included in calculating the total systemic dose of cyclohexylamine. However, since deamination is only a very minor route of cyclohexylamine metabolism in man and the rat (the species used in toxicity studies), the site of this reaction is not of toxicological importance.

5. *The Substrate Specificity of the Cyclamate Sulphamatase Enzyme*

Incubation of simple aliphatic sulphamates with the faeces of rats which have been pretreated with cyclamate and shown to convert cyclamate to cyclohexylamine *in vivo* resulted in rates of hydrolysis similar to that of cyclamate (Renwick, 1976) (Table 8.4). Similar data were obtained with a cell-free extract of rat faeces (McGlinchey *et al.*, 1982) and with the enzyme purified from *Pseudomonas* (Niimura *et al.*, 1974) except that phenylsulphamate was not hydrolysed by the enzyme preparation. In addition long chain N-alkylsulphamates and N,N-dialkylsulphamates were not substrates for the enzyme. The purified enzyme was also unable to hydrolyse the sulphamate anion, sulphanilamide, or cyclohexanol sulphate ester.

Attempts to develop other sulphamate sweeteners will depend on the ability of the compound to induce sulphamate hydrolysis *in vivo*, its ability to act as a substrate, and the toxicity of the amine product.

6. *Cyclamate Induced Changes in the Composition of the Gut Microflora*

Despite the marked changes in sulphamatase enzyme activity following cyclamate administration, little attention has been paid to the nature of the gut flora. Drasar *et al.* (1972) reported an increase in clostridia and bacteroides in rats given cyclamate chronically, but no difference in the faecal flora of three human volunteers, one of whom converted cyclamate to cyclohexylamine. Increased numbers of clostridia were also found in a subsequent study by the same workers (Renwick, unpublished observation) but not in the study by Bickel *et al.* (1974), in which many animals became good converters of cyclamate to cyclohexylamine. Clearly changes in bacterial numbers are not an essential part of the development of

Table 8.3 *The further metabolism of cyclohexylamine* in vivo. The results are the percentage dose in the 0–24 hour urine collected after administration of the radiolabelled compound to adult female animals. The values are for individual animals except where stated. The cyclohexylamine metabolites for rabbits are presented as the total with cyclohexanol (free plus conjugates) in parentheses and for guinea pigs as the total deaminated metabolites. The data are from A. G. Renwick (1971), PhD. Thesis, University of London (unpublished).

| Species | Compound dosed | % [14]C dose in urine | | | Ratio[c] |
		Cyclamate	Cyclohexylamine	Cyclohexylamine metabolites	
Rat[a]	^{14}C-cyclamate (50 mg/kg; po)	24.6	24.1	1.9	0.08
		27.8	39.5	4.6	0.12
		43.6	5.0	0.7	0.14
		21.6	3.2	0.7	0.22
		19.8	22.6	3.9	0.17
		16.2	37.7	5.1	0.14
Rat[b]	^{14}C-cyclohexylamine (50 mg/kg; ip) (mean of 3)	—	80.9	10.2	0.13
Rat[a]	^{14}C-cyclohexylamine (50 mg/kg; po) (mean of 3)	—	79.1	7.3	0.09

Guinea pig[a]	^{14}C-cyclamate	33.0	0.3	0.6	2.00
	(50 mg/kg; po)	18.8	2.5	0.6	0.24
		12.8	0.4	0.2	0.50
Guinea pig[b]	^{14}C-cyclohexylamine	—	73.5	13.4	0.18
	(50 mg/kg; ip)	—	90.7	7.1	0.08
		—	95.8	4.1	0.04
Guinea pig[b]	^{14}C-cyclohexylamine	—	79.9	7.4	0.09
	(50 mg/kg; po)	—	70.8	9.4	0.13
			83.8	12.8	0.15
Rabbit[a]	^{14}C-cyclamate	40.8	6.9	21.7 (8.2)	3.15 (1.19)
	(50 mg/kg; po)	73.4	0.0	0.0	—
		65.1	4.2	15.5 (6.2)	3.69 (1.48)
Rabbit[b]	^{14}C-cyclohexylamine	—	33.1	62.1 (14.5)	1.88 (0.44)
	(50 mg/kg; ip)	—	31.0	51.5 (10.4)	1.66 (0.34)
		—	51.1	35.5 (8.9)	0.70 (0.17)

[a] Cyclamate pretreated animals.
[b] Control animals.
[c] Ratio: cyclohexylamine metabolites divided by cyclohexylamine.

A. G. RENWICK

Table 8.4 *Substrate specificity of cyclamate hydrolysing enzymes*

	Relative rate		
	Pseudomonas enzyme[a]	Rat faeces[b]	Rat faecal[c] extract
N-Alkyl-and N-arylsulphamates			
Cyclohexyl-	1.0	1.0	1.0
n-Propyl-	1.7	—[d]	—
n-Amyl-	1.8	—	—
Cyclopentyl	—	0.3	0.5
n-hexyl-	1.8	—	—
Methylcyclopentyl-	—	0.6	—
Phenyl-	w	1.6	5.3
Cycloheptyl-	—	1.3	0.5
Cyclohexylmethyl-	—	0.7	—
Benzyl-	—	0.2	—
n-Octyl-	4.3	—	6.4
Cyclooctyl-	—	—	0.0
3-Phenylpropyl-	1.3	—	—
Tetrahydronaphthyl-	0.6	—	—
n-Hexadecyl-	w	—	—
n-Octadecyl-	w	—	—
N,N-dialkylsulphamates			
Di-n-propyl	w	—	—
Methyl-,cyclohexyl-	w	—	—
Other compounds			
Sulphamate ion	0	—	—
Cyclohexanol sulphate	0	—	—
Sulphanilamide	0	—	—
Saccharin	—	0	—

[a] From Niimura *et al.* (1974)
[b] From Renwick (1976) and Ball *et al.* (1977)
[c] From McGlinchey *et al.* (1982)
[d] Not determined
w Weak or uncertain activity.

cyclamate metabolizing ability. The changes in numbers detected may reflect non-specific effects on the nutritional status of the gut flora (Pfeffer *et al.*, 1985).

D. Acesulfame-K

Acesulfame-K (Fig. 8.1) is a cyclic sulfonic acid derivative that is extremely water soluble and stable under normal conditions (Arpe, 1978). It is not metabolized *in vivo* in various species, including man, following single or multiple doses (Arpe, 1978), and is not metabolized after prolonged exposure to different strains of intestinal bacteria (von Rymon Lipinski, 1985). Acesulfame-K does not show antibacterial properties (von Rymon Lipinski, 1985) but causes diarrhoea (Arpe, 1978) and caecal enlargement (COT, 1982) in rats when fed at very high dietary levels. The latter may be related to altered microbial carbohydrate metabolism (Pfeffer *et al.*, 1985).

E. Stevioside

Stevioside is a naturally occurring glycoside found in the leaves of the plant *Stevia rebaudiana* which is found in Brazil and Paraguay. The leaves contain a complex mixture of glycosides (Kinghorn and Soejarto, 1985) of which stevioside (Fig. 8.1) is the most abundant (approximately 5–10% of the leaves). Other minor constituents such as rebaudioside A (approximately 1% of the leaves) probably contribute to the sweet taste.

The toxicology of stevioside is complicated by the fact that some data have been generated on the leaf extracts whilst others involve pure stevioside and even the aglycone steviol (or *ent*-13-hydroxykaur-16-en-19-oic acid). Acute and sub-acute studies at high doses (equivalent to up to 7.0% stevioside in the diet) have shown no significant toxicity (Kinghorn and Soejarto, 1985). Long term feeding studies in rats have indicated that the no-effect level is about 550 mg/kg/day of *Stevia* leaf extract, which contained 74% stevioside and 16% rebaudioside A (Yamada *et al.*, 1985). Anecdotal reports of *Stevia* preparations being used by the indigenous Paraguayans for antifertility effects and as a remedy for diabetes have not been substantiated by various animal and human investigations. Of greatest interest within the context of the present chapter is the report that although stevioside and leaf extracts are not mutagenic, the pure aglycone (steviol) is a bacterial mutagen in the presence of metabolic activation (Pezzuto *et al.*, 1985, 1986). In view of the known ability of the intestinal bacteria to hydrolyse glycosidic bonds (Hawksworth *et al.*, 1971) it is possible that the gut flora also play a key role in the toxicological assessment of this sweetener.

In vitro incubation of stevioside with rat caecal bacteria resulted in almost quantitative conversion to steviol, which was metabolically stable under the conditions used (Wingard *et al.*, 1980). Following the oral administration of ^{3}H-stevioside to male rats approximately 70% of the dose was recovered in the faeces, 2% in the urine and 24% in the expired air as [3]H_2O, mostly between 48 and 72 hours after dosing (Nakayama *et al.*, 1986). One hour after dosing, stevioside was the main component in the gut lumen, but after 4 hours the radioactivity in the caecal contents comprised 39% stevioside, 17% steviolbioside (the free acid disaccharide of steviol) and 5% steviol. Unchanged stevioside was not detected in the caecal contents 24 hours after dosing. Steviol was the major component in faeces. The bile contained 41% of the dose over 72 hours comprising glucuronic acid and other conjugates of steviol and unidentified metabolites (Nakayama *et al.*, 1986). These data are consistent with marked hydrolysis of unabsorbed stevioside by the intestinal flora, as well as hydrolysis of steviol conjugates eliminated in the bile, and suggest the possibility of an enterohepatic circulation of the aglycone. This possibility is supported by the report that ^{14}C-steviol was completely absorbed following intra-caecal administration to rats (Wingard *et al.*, 1980). The absorbed radioactivity was recovered quantitatively in the bile in cannulated rats, confirming the enterohepatic recycling of steviol derived radioactivity.

Thus, *Stevia* extracts, stevioside and steviol pose an interesting case in the use and interpretation of toxicological data. The mutagenicity of steviol and microbial metabolism of stevioside to steviol suggest the potential for toxicity. In view of the molecular weight of steviol (315), species differences may exist between rat and man in the extent of biliary excretion of steviol and its conjugates. However, although differences in the nature and distribution of the gut bacteria occur in rat and man (see Renwick (1982)), the wide occurrence of β-glucosidase activity in different bacterial strains (Hawksworth *et al.*, 1971) suggests that these rat data should be considered to be of relevance to man. Conversely the sub-acute and long term animal toxicity studies which have fed leaf extracts, which would contain not only stevioside but other components, have not shown that this mutagenicity is expressed *in vivo*, by the development of tumours. In view of this discrepancy in the toxicological data base it is not surprising that there are differences in the regulation of *Stevia* preparations around the world, with approval for use currently restricted to Japan, Paraguay, Brazil, South Korea and The People's Republic of China (Phillips, 1987). It is ironic that if the flavour properties of the

Stevia leaf were more complex such that it resembled a 'naturally occurring spice' it would probably be more freely available.

F. Conclusions

Man's desire for sweet tastes has led not only to the accidental discovery of sweet compounds like saccharin and cyclamate but also to detailed analysis of naturally occurring sweet materials, like sucrose and stevioside. That many of these compounds are considerably sweeter than sucrose (30–300 times) allows the consumption of a highly palatable food or drink, but with fewer calories. This has resulted in a situation where low calorie products are considered as a normal part of today's lifestyle. The increased use of such compounds has resulted in an increasingly detailed and sophisticated toxicological evaluation, often at very high doses. Interactions between the sweetener and the gut flora have been reported for most of the intense sweeteners and represent key observations for saccharin, cyclamate and stevioside. In the case of saccharin there are profound perturbations in microbial metabolism at very high dietary levels which confuse the interpretation of toxicological effects seen at such doses. For cyclamate, the acceptable daily intake will be determined by its microbial metabolism to cyclohexylamine, which shows greater toxicity than the parent sweetener. Finally the regulatory status of stevioside will depend on interpretations of the relevance of *in vitro* mutagenicity data on the aglycone, released by gut flora metabolism. Clearly the intense sweeteners represent classic examples of the importance of the intestinal microflora in toxicological evaluations.

References

Anderson, R. L. (1983). Effect of saccharin ingestion on stool composition in relation to caecal enlargement and increased stool hydration. *Fd Chem. Toxicol.* **21**, 255–257.

Anderson, R. L. (1985). Some changes in gastro-intestinal metabolism and in the urine and bladders of rats in response to sodium saccharin ingestion. *Fd Chem. Toxicol.* **23**, 457–463.

Anderson, R. L. and Kirkland, J. J. (1980). The effect of sodium saccharin in the diet of caecal microflora. *Fd. Cosmet. Toxicol.* **18**, 353–355.

Anderson, R. L., Francis, W. R. and Lefever, F. R. (1987). Effect of dietary carbohydrate type and content on the response of male rats to dietary sodium saccharin. *Fd Chem. Toxicol.* **25**, 271–275.

Arnold, D. L., Moodie, C. A., Grice, H. C., Charbonneau, S. M., Stavric, B., Collins, B. T., McGuire, P. F., Zawidzka, Z. Z. and Munro, I. C. (1980).

Long-term toxicity of *ortho*-toluenesulfonamide and sodium saccharin in the rat. *Toxicol. appl. Pharmacol.* **52**, 113–152.

Arnold, D. L., Krewski, D. and Munro, I. C. (1983). Saccharin: a toxicological and historical perspective. *Toxicology* **27**, 197–256.

Arpe, H. J. (1978). Acesulfame-K, a new noncaloric sweetener. *In*: "Health and Sugar Substitutes" (ed. B. Guggenheim), pp. 178–183. S. Kager, Basel.

Asahina, M. (1972). Participation of bacteria in the metabolism of sodium cyclamate in guinea pig. *J. Fd Hyg. Soc. Jpn.* **13**, 133–136.

Asahina, M., Yamaha, T., Wattanabe, K. and Sarrazin, G. (1971). Excretion of cyclohexylamine, a metabolite of cyclamate in human urine. *Chem. Pharm. Bull. (Tokyo)* **19**, 628–632.

Asahina, M., Niimura, T., Yamaha, T. and Takahashi, T. (1972a). Formation of cyclohexylamine and cyclohexanone from cyclamate by microorganisms isolated from the feces of guinea pig. *Agr. Biol. Chem.* **36**, 711–718.

Asahina, M., Yamaha, T., Sarrazin, G. and Watanabe, K. (1972b). Conversion of cyclamate to cyclohexylamine in guinea pig. *Chem. Pharm. Bull. (Tokyo)* **20**, 102–108.

Ayres, P. H., Shinohara, Y. and Frith, C. H. (1985). Morphological observations on the epithelium of the developing urinary bladder of the mouse and rat. *J. Urol.* **133**, 506–512.

Ball, L. M., Renwick, A. G. and Williams, R. T. (1977). The fate of [^{14}C]saccharin in man, rat and rabbit and of 2-sulphamoyl-[^{14}C]-benzoic acid in the rat. *Xenobiotica* **7**, 189–203.

Bickel, M. H., Burkhard, B., Meier-Strasser, E. and Van den Broek-Boot, M. (1974). Entero-bacterial formation of cyclohexylamine in rats ingesting cyclamate. *Xenobiotica* **4**, 425–439.

Bopp, B. A., Sonders, R. C. and Kesterson, J. W. (1986). Toxicological aspects of cyclamate and cyclohexylamine. *Critical Rev. Toxicol.* **16**, 213–306.

Boutwell, R. K. and Bosch, D. K. (1959). The tumour-promoting action of phenol and related compounds for mouse skin. *Cancer Res.* **19**, 413–424.

Carlson, A. J., Eldridge, C. J., Martin, H. P. and Foran, F. L. (1923). Studies on the physiological action of saccharin. *J. Metab. Res.* **3**, 451–477.

Cohen, S. M., Arai, M., Jacobs, J. B. and Friedell, G. H. (1979). Promoting effect of saccharin and D,L-tryptophan in urinary bladder carcinogenesis. *Cancer Res.* **39**, 1207–1217.

Collings, A. J. (1971). The metabolism of sodium cyclamate. *In*: "Sweetness and Sweeteners" (eds G. G. Birch, L. F. Green and C. M. Coulson), pp. 51–68. Elsevier Applied Science Publishers Ltd., London.

COT (1982). "Food Additives and Contaminants Committee Report on the Review of Sweeteners in Food." FAC/REP/34. Her Majesty's Stationery Office, London.

Dalderup, L. M., Keller, G. H. M. and Schouten, F. (1970). Cyclamate and cyclohexylamine. *Lancet* **1**, 845.

Davis, T. R. A., Adler, N. and Opsahl, J. C. (1969). Excretion of cyclohexylamine in subjects ingesting sodium cyclamate. *Toxicol. appl. Pharmacol.* **15**, 106–116.

Drasar, B. S., Renwick, A. G. and Williams, R. T. (1972). The role of the gut flora in the metabolism of cyclamate. *Biochem. J.* **129**, 881–890.

Dunning, W. F. and Curtis, M. R. (1958). The role of indole in incidence of 2-acetylaminofluorene-induced bladder cancer in rats. *Proc. Soc. Exp. Biol. Med.* **99**, 91–95.

Eichelbaum, M., Hengstmann, J. H., Rost, H. D., Brecht, T. and Dengler, H. J. (1974). Pharmacokinetics, cardiovascular and metabolic actions of cyclohexylamine in man. *Arch. Toxikol.* **31**, 243–263.

Friedman, L., Richardson, H. L. Richardson, M. E., Lethco, E. J., Wallace, W. C. and Sauro, M. N. (1972). Toxic response of rats to cyclamates in chow and semisynthetic diets. *J. Natl Cancer. Inst.* **49**, 751–764.

Fukushima, S., Arai, M., Nakanowatari, J., Hibino, T., Okuda, M. and Ito, N. (1983a). Differences in susceptibility to sodium saccharin among various strains of rats and other animal species. *Gann* **74**, 8–20.

Fukushima, S., Hagiwara, A., Ogiso, T., Shibata, M. and Ito, N. (1983b). Promoting effects of various chemicals in rat urinary bladder carcinogenesis initiated by N-nitroso-n-butyl-(4-hydroxybutyl)amine. *Fd Chem. Toxicol.* **21**, 59–68.

Goldberg, L., Parekh, C., Patti, A. and Soike, K. (1969). Cyclamate degradation in mammals and *in vitro. Toxicol. appl. Pharmacol.* **14**, 654.

Hawksworth, G., Drasar, B. S. and Hill, M. J. (1971). Intestinal bacteria and the hydrolysis of glycosidic bonds. *J. Med. Microbiol.* **4**, 451–459.

Ichibagase, H., Kojima, S., Inoue, K. and Suenaga, A. (1972a). Studies on synthetic sweetening agents. XV. Metabolism of sodium cyclamate (4). Influences of phenylbutazone, phenobarbitol, and tolbutamide on metabolism of sodium cyclamate in rabbits. *Chem. Pharm. Bull. (Tokyo)* **20**, 175–180.

Ichibagase, H., Kojima, S., Suenaga, A. and Inoue, K. (1972b). Studies on synthetic sweetening agents. XVI. Metabolism of sodium cyclamate (5). The metabolism of sodium cyclamate in rabbits and rats after prolonged administration of sodium cyclamate. *Chem. Pharm. Bull. (Tokyo)* **20**, 1093–1101.

JECFA (1977). "Summary of Toxicological Data of Certain Food Additives. Twenty-first Report of the Joint FAO/WHO Expert Committee on Food Additives." WHO Technical Report Series No. 617. WHO, Geneva.

Kakizoe, T., Esumi, H., Kawachi, T., Sugimura, T., Takeuchi, T. and Umezawa, H. (1977). Further studies on the effect of leupeptin, a protease inhibitor, on induction of bladder tumors in rats by N-butyl-N-(4-hydroxybutyl)nitrosamine. *J. Natl Cancer Inst.* **59**, 1503–1508.

Kinghorn, A. D. and Soejarto, D. D. (1985). Current status of stevioside as a sweetening agent for human use. *In:* "Economic and Medicinal Plant Research"; Volume 1, (eds H. Wagner, H. Hikino and N. R. Farnsworth), pp. 2–52. Academic Press, New York.

Kojima, S. and Ichibagase, H. (1966). Studies on synthetic sweeteners. VIII. Cyclohexylamine, a metabolite of sodium cyclamate. *Chem. Pharm. Bull. (Tokyo)* **14**, 971–974.

Kojima, S. and Ichibagase, H. (1968). Studies on synthetic sweetening agents. XIII. Metabolism of sodium cyclamate (2). Detection of metabolites of sodium cyclamate in rabbit and rat by gas-liquid chromatography. *Chem. Pharm. Bull. (Tokyo)* **16**, 1851–1854.

Kurebayashi, H., Tanaka, A. and Yamaha, T. (1979). Oxidative deamination of cyclohexylamine and its homologs by rabbit liver microsomes. *Biochem. Pharmacol.* **28**, 1719–1726.

Lawrie, C. A. and Renwick, A. G. (1987). The effect of saccharin ingestion on the excretion of microbial amino acid metabolites in rat and man. *Toxicol. appl. Pharmacol.* (in the press).

Lawrie, C. A., Renwick, A. G. and Sims, J. (1985). The urinary excretion of bacterial amino-acid metabolites by rats fed saccharin in the diet. *Fd Chem. Toxicol.* **23**, 445–450.

Lawson, T. A. and Hertzog, P. J. (1981). The failure of chronically administered saccharin to stimulate bladder epithelial DNA synthesis in F_0 rats. *Cancer Lett.* **11**, 221–224.

Leahy, J. S., Taylor, T. and Rudd, C. J. (1967). Cyclohexylamine excretors among human volunteers given cyclamate. *Fd Cosmet. Toxicol.* **5**, 595–596.

Linke, H. A. B. and Kohn, J. S. (1984). Inhibitory effect of saccharin on glycolytic enzymes in cell-free extracts of *Streptococcus mutans*. *Caries Res.* **18**, 12–16.

Litchfield, M. H. and Swan, A. A. B. (1971). Cyclohexylamine production and physiological measurements in subjects ingesting sodium cyclamate. *Toxicol. appl. Pharmacol.* **18**, 535–541.

Lok, E., Iverson, F. and Clayson, D. B. (1982). The inhibition of urease and proteases by sodium saccharin. *Cancer Lett.* **16**, 163–169.

Lutz, W. K. and Schlatter, C. (1977). Saccharin does not bind to DNA of liver or bladder in the rat. *Chem. Biol. Interact.* **19**, 253–257.

Mallett, A. K., Rowland, I. C. and Bearne, C. A. (1985a). Modification of rat caecal microbial biotransformation activities by dietary saccharin. *Toxicol.* **36**, 253–262.

Mallett, A. K., Rowland, I. C., Bearne, C. A., Purchase, R. and Gangolli, S. D. (1985b). Metabolic adaptation of rat faecal microflora to cyclamate *in vitro*. *Fd Chem. Toxicol.* **23**, 1029–1034.

Matsui, M., Tanimura, A. and Kurata, H. (1981). Identification of cyclamate-converting bacteria (studies on the metabolism of food additives by microorganisms inhabiting the gastrointestinal tract 6). *J. Fd Hyg. Soc. Jpn.* **22**, 215–222.

McGlinchey, G., Coakley, C. B., Gestauties-Tansey, V., Gault, J. and Spillane, W. J. (1982). *In vivo* and *in vitro* studies with sulfamate sweeteners. *J. Pharm. Sci.* **71**, 661–665.

Miller, J. P., Crawford, L. E. M., Sonders, R. C. and Cardinal, E. V. (1966). Distribution and excretion of ^{14}C-cyclamate sodium in animals. *Biochem. Biophys. Res. Commun.* **25**, 153–157.

Morgan, R. W. and Wong, O. (1985). A review of epidemiological studies on artificial sweeteners and bladder cancer. *Fd Chem. Toxicol.* **23**, 529–533.

Naim, M., Brand, J. G. and Kare, M. R. (1982). Effect of unpalatable diets, food restriction and saccharin-adulterated diet on tryptic, chymotryptic and amylolytic activity in pancreas, intestine and feces of rats. *J. Nutr.* **112**, 2104–2115.

Naim, M., Zechman, J. M., Brand, J. G., Kare, M. R. and Sandovsky, V. (1985). Effects of sodium saccharin on the activity of trypsin, chymotrypsin, and amylase and upon bacteria in small intestinal contents of rats. *Proc. Soc. Exp. Biol. Med.* **178**, 392–401.

Nakayama, K., Kasahara, D. and Yamamoto, F. (1986). Absorption, distribution, metabolism and excretion of stevioside in rats. *J. Fd Hyg. Soc. Jpn.* **27**, 1–8.

Niimura, T., Tokieda, T. and Yamaha, T. (1974). Partial purification and some properties of cyclamate sulfamatase. *J. Biochem.* **75**, 407–417.

Nishio, Y., Kakizoe, T., Ohtani, M., Sato, S., Sugimura, T. and Fukushima, S. (1986). L-Isoleucine and L-leucine tumor promoters of bladder cancer in rats. *Science* **231**, 843–845.

Oser, B. L. (1985). Highlights in the history of saccharin toxicology. *Fd Chem. Toxicol.* **23**, 535–542.

Oser, B. L., Carson, S., Vogin, E. E. and Sonders, R. C. (1968). Conversion of cyclamate to cyclohexylamine in rats. *Nature* **220**, 178–179.

Oyasu, R., Kitajima, T., Hopp, M. L. and Sumie, H. (1972). Enhancement of urinary bladder tumorigenesis in hamsters by coadministration of 2-acetylaminofluorene and indole. *Cancer Res.* **32**, 2027–2033.

Pezzuto, J. M., Compadre, C. M., Swanson, S. M., Nanayakkara, N. P. D. and Kinghorn, A. D. (1985). Metabolically activated steviol, the aglycone of stevioside is mutagenic. *Proc. Natl Acad. Sci. USA* **82**, 2478–2482.

Pezzuto, J. M., Nanayakkara, N. P. D., Compadre, C. M., Swanson, S. M., Kinghorn, A. D., Guethner, T. M., Sparnins, V. L. and Lam, L. K. T. (1986). Characterisation of bacterial mutagenicity mediated by 13-hydroxy-*ent*-kaurenoic acid (steviol) and several structurally-related derivatives and evaluation of potential to induce glutathione S-transferase in mice. *Mutat. Res.* **169**, 93–103.

Pfeffer, M., Ziesenitz, S. C. and Siebert, G. (1985). Acesulfame K, cyclamate and saccharin inhibit the anaerobic fermentation of glucose by intestinal bacteria. *Ernahrungs.* **24**, 231–235.

Phillips, K. C. (1987). Stevia: steps in developing a new sweetener. *In*: "Development in Sweeteners-3" (ed. T. H. Grenby). Elsevier Applied Science, London (in the press).

Price, J. M., Biava, C. G., Oser, B. L., Vogin, E. E., Steinfeld, J. and Ley, H. L. (1970). Bladder tumors in rats fed cyclohexylamine or high doses of a mixture of cyclamate and saccharin. *Science* **167**, 1131–1132.

Prosky, L. and O'Dell, R. G. (1971). *In vivo* conversion of ^{14}C-labelled cyclamate to cyclohexylamine. *J. Pharm. Sci.* **60**, 1341–1343.

Radomski, J. L., Glass, E. M. and Deichmann, W. B. (1971). Transitional cell hyperplasia in the bladders of dogs fed D,L-tryptophan. *Cancer Res.* **31**, 1690–1694.

Radomski, J. L., Radomski, T. and McDonald, W. E. (1977). Carcinogenic interaction between D,L-tryptophan and 4-aminobiphenyl or 2-naphthylamine in dogs. *J. Natl Cancer Inst.* **58**, 1831–1834.

Renwick, A. G. (1976). Microbial metabolism of drugs. *In*: "Drug Metabolism — From Microbes to Man" (eds D. V. Parke and R. L. Smith), pp. 169–189. Taylor and Francis, London.

Renwick, A. G. (1982). First-pass metabolism within the lumen of the gastrointestinal tract. *In*: "Presystemic Drug Elimination" (eds C. F. George, D. G. Shand and A. G. Renwick), pp. 3–28. Butterworths, London.

Renwick, A. G. (1983). The fate of non-nutritive sweeteners in the body. *In*: "Developments in Sweeteners-2" (eds T. H. Grenby, K. J. Parker and M. G. Lindley), pp. 179–224. Elsevier Applied Science Publishers Ltd., London.

Renwick, A. G. (1985). The disposition of saccharin in animals and man — a review. *Fd Chem. Toxicol.* **23**, 429–435.

Renwick, A. G. (1986). The metabolism of intense sweeteners. *Xenobiotica* **16**, 1057–1071.

Renwick, A. G. and Williams, R. T. (1969). Gut bacteria and the metabolism of cyclamate in the rat. *Biochem. J.* **114**, 78.

Renwick, A. G. and Williams, R. T. (1972a). The metabolites of cyclohexylamine in man and certain animals. *Biochem. J.* **129**, 857–867.

Renwick, A. G. and Williams, R. T. (1972b). The fate of cyclamate in man and other species. *Biochem. J.* **129**, 869–879.

Roberts, A. and Renwick, A. G. (1985). The metabolism of [^{14}C]-cyclohexylamine in mice and two strains of rat. *Xenobiotica* **15**, 477–483.

Ross, M. H. and Bras, G. (1973). Influence of protein under- and over-nutrition on spontaneous tumor prevalence in the rat. *J. Nutr.* **103**, 944–964.

Schoenig, G. P., Goldenthal, E. I., Geil, R. G., Frith, C. H., Richter, W. R. and Carlborg, F. W. (1985). Evaluation of the dose response and *in utero* exposure to saccharin in the rat. *Fd Chem. Toxicol.* **23**, 475–490.

Sims, J. and Renwick, A. G. (1983). The effects of saccharin on the metabolism of dietary tryptophan to indole, a known cocarcinogen for the urinary bladder of the rat. *Toxicol. appl. Pharmacol.* **67**, 132–151.

Sims, J. and Renwick, A. G. (1985). The microbial metabolism of tryptophan in rats fed a diet containing 7.5% saccharin in a two-generation protocol. *Fd Chem. Toxicol.* **23**, 437–444.

Sonders, R. C. and Wiegand, R. G. (1968). Absorption and excretion of cyclamate in animals and man. *Toxicol. appl. Pharmacol.* **13**, 291.

Sonders, R. C., Netwal, J. C. and Wiegand, R. G. (1969). Site of conversion of cyclamate to cyclohexylamine. *Pharmacologist* **11**, 241.

Suenaga, A., Kojima, S. and Ichibagase, H. (1972). Studies on sweetening agents XVII. Metabolism of sodium cyclamate (6). Influence of neomycin and sulfaguanidine on metabolism of sodium cyclamate. *Chem. Pharm. Bull. (Tokyo)* **20**, 1357–1361.

Sweatman, T. W. and Renwick, A. G. (1979). Saccharin metabolism and tumourigenicity. *Science* **205**, 1019–1010.

Sweatman, T. W. and Renwick, A. G. (1980). The tissue distribution and pharmacokinetics of saccharin in the rat. *Toxicol. appl. Pharmacol.* **55**, 18–31.

Taylor, J. D., Richards, R. K. and Davin, J. C. (1951). Excretion and distribution of radioactive S^{35}-cyclamate sodium (sucarylsodium) in animals. *Proc. Soc. Exp. Biol. Med.* **78**, 530–533.

Taylor, J. M., Weinberger, M. A. and Friedman, L. (1980). Chronic toxicity and carcinogenicity to the urinary bladder of sodium saccharin in the *in utero* exposed rat. *Toxicol. appl. Pharmacol.* **54**, 57–75.

Tesoriero, A. A. and Roxon, J. J. (1975). [^{35}S]Cyclamate metabolism; incorporation of ^{35}S into proteins of intestinal bacteria *in vitro* and production of volatile ^{35}S-containing compounds. *Xenobiotica* **5**, 25–31.

Tokieda, T., Niimura, T., Yamaha, T., Hasegawa, T. and Suzuki, T. (1979). Anaerobic deamination of cyclohexylamine by intestinal microorganisms in rabbits. *Agric. Biol. Chem.* **43**, 25–32.

von Rymon Lipinski, G. W. (1985). The intense new sweetener acesulfame K. *Fd Chem.* **16**, 259–269.

Wingard, R. E., Brown, J. P., Enderlin, F. E., Dale, J. A., Hale, R. L. and Seitz, C. T. (1980). Intestinal degradation and absorption of the glycoside sweeteners stevioside and rebaudioside A. *Experientia* **36**, 519–520.

Wynder, E. L. and Hoffman, D. (1968). Experimental tobacco carcinogenesis. *Science* **162**, 862.

Yamada, A., Ohsaki, S., Noda, T. and Shimizu, M. (1985). Chronic toxicity study of dietary stevia extracts in F344 rats. *J. Fd Hyg. Soc. Jpn.* **26**, 169–183.

9

Metabolism of Toxic Metals

I. R. ROWLAND

A. Introduction

1. *The Role of the Metabolism in Toxicity of Metals*

Many metals, such as mercury, lead, cadmium and arsenic, are potent toxicants to living organisms, including man. The chemical form of a metal can, however, have a profound influence on its rate of absorption and excretion, and on its distribution and accumulation in the tissues where ultimately it exerts its biological effects. In view of the importance of chemical form to the disposition and toxicity of metals, the study of the interconversion of the different forms of a metal in the body is clearly crucial for understanding the mechanisms of action of a metal and for evaluating the possible health effects of its various forms.

Several toxic metals and metalloids are known to undergo biotransformation in mammals, including man. The mammalian transformation reactions relating to these toxic metals, namely mercury, arsenic, selenium, lead and tin, have been reviewed recently by Mushak (1983). Of these metals, the role of the gut microflora in the biotransformation processes has been studied in detail only in the cases of mercury and arsenic compounds, and so the present review will be confined to consideration of these two groups of chemicals.

B. Mercury

1. *Chemical Forms, Exposure and Toxic Effects*

Mercury exists in its elemental (metallic) state, as monovalent (mercurous) and divalent (mercuric) inorganic compounds and as short chain alkyl-, alkoxyalkyl- and phenyl-mercury compounds. There would appear to be no involvement of the gut flora in metabolism of elemental mercury. Although alkoxy- and phenyl-mercury compounds are known to be unstable in the body, decomposing to mercuric mercury, the role of the gut flora in this reaction has not been studied. There is, however, evidence for gut bacterial metabolism of mercuric salts and methylmercury compounds.

Mercuric salts are toxicologically more important than mercurous compounds and are widely distributed in the environment. They enter the body via food and beverages, although the daily intake by this route is very low—less than 10 μg/day (Berlin, 1979). Mercuric salts are poorly absorbed from the gut and their distribution is mostly confined to the kidneys, which are the main site of toxic action on chronic exposure.

The high toxicity of methylmercury (MeHg) is due to a combination of its efficient absorption (90%) from the gut, long retention time in the body and its ability to penetrate the blood–brain barrier and accumulate in the lipid-rich neuropile of the central nervous system, where it exerts its major toxic effects (see the review by Berlin (1979)). The main route of exposure of the general population to MeHg is via food, since it is accumulated in food chains, particularly those in aquatic environments. Moderate consumption of relatively uncontaminated fish is estimated to result in a daily intake of 1–20 μg/day (Berlin, 1979). In populations whose diets consist mainly of fish, intakes of MeHg can reach 300 μg/day and may attain toxic levels in communities which consume large quantities of fish caught in badly polluted areas (Berlin, 1979). The disastrous outbreaks of mercury poisoning in Minimata and Niigata in Japan in the 1950s and 1960s (reviewed by Takeuchi, 1972) resulted from this route of high level exposure.

2. *Metabolism of Mercury Compounds by Gut Bacteria*

(a) Mercuric chloride metabolism in vitro. Incubation of suspensions of human faeces or rat caecal contents with mercuric chloride under anaerobic conditions results in the production of small quantities (5–15 ng g^{-1} faeces or gut contents) of MeHg (Edwards and McBride, 1975; Rowland *et al.*, 1977a). Sterilization of the gut contents virtually abolished MeHg formation (Rowland *et al.*, 1977a), indicating that bacteria participated in the reaction. Microbial involvement was further confirmed by studies of MeHg synthesis by pure cultures of intestinal bacteria and yeast derived from rats and humans (Rowland *et al.*, 1975; Rowland *et al.*, 1977a).

Several alternative mechanisms have been proposed for the methylation process, but it is now thought to require the presence of a carbanion (CH_3^-) rather than a carbonium ion (CH_3^+) (Bertilsson and Neujahr, 1971; Ridley *et al.*, 1977). Methylvitamin B_{12} (methylcobalamine), which is synthesized by a number of bacterial species, is the only biological methylating agent known to have the capacity to transfer carbanions, and does so *in vitro* to mercury, lead, tin, platinum, palladium and gold (Bertilsson and Neujahr, 1971; Imura *et al.*, 1971; Wood, 1974; Agnes *et al.*, 1971). However, methylation of inorganic mercury also occurs in organisms which are unable to synthesize methylcobalamine (Vonk and Sijpesteijn, 1973) and so other mechanisms for methylation must operate in these cells. Lander (1971) has suggested that methylation of mercury may involve one or more steps in the pathway of methionine biosynthesis such that the methyl group is transferred to a mercuric ion complexed to homocysteine.

(b) Mercuric mercury methylation in vivo. The bacterial methylation of mercuric mercury converts the metal from a form poorly absorbed from the gut to one which is virtually completely absorbed and so, potentially, should increase the amount of an oral dose of mercuric mercury which passes through the gut wall. Evidence that this occurs however is very limited and has been obtained only from experiments conducted in animals with abnormal gastro-intestinal conditions. Retroperistaltic intestinal blind loops are known to harbour a more abundant microflora than the normal intestine and can be produced by surgical procedures. Abdulla *et al.* (1973) measured the mercury content (total and methylmercury) of various tissues after giving 1 mg mercuric chloride per day by gastric intubation for 3 weeks to rats with jejunal blind loops and to non-surgically treated control animals. In rats with blind-loops the total mercury and MeHg content of all tissues taken, including the brain, was much higher than in control animals (Table 9.1). Although the rats with blind-loops also developed neurological symptoms, it seems unlikely that these were induced by MeHg since brain levels of mercury (0.17 μg Hg/g) were considerably below those required (5–10 μg Hg/g) before overt neurotoxicity becomes apparent (Syverson, 1982).

Conditions which permit a microflora to develop in the upper gastro-intestinal tract are not uncommon in man, e.g. achlorhydria, partial gastrectomy, Crohn's disease (Drasar and Hill, 1974), and whilst these may increase the potential for bacterial methylation, the amounts of mercuric mercury ingested are normally too small for the reaction to be of any toxicological consequence.

(c) Methylmercury Metabolism in vitro. Incubation of [203]Hg-labelled methylmercuric chloride with gut contents from the rat or mouse, or with suspensions of faeces from humans, results in extensive metabolism of

Table 9.1 *Mercury concentrations in tissues of control and blind-loop rats. The results are the mean for four blind-loop and two control rats*

| | Mercury concentration (ng g^{-1} wet weight) | | | |
| | Blind-loop rats | | Control rats | |
Tissue	Methylmercury	Total	Methylmercury	Total
Brain	80	170	ND	NR
Blood cells	120	249	5	NR
Liver	1300	5200	88	120
Kidney	2100	9600	106	206

ND, not detected; NR, not reported. After Abdulla *et al.*, 1973.

the organomercurial over a period of 1–2 days (Rowland *et al.*, 1978, 1983). A wide range of metabolites appears to be produced depending on the source of the gut contents. In incubations of ^{203}Hg-labelled MeHg with small intestine or caecal contents from Wistar rats, substantial amounts (50–70%) of radioactivity are lost from the incubation mixture, indicating the production of volatile metabolites (Rowland *et al.*, 1978). Differences in the rates of volatilization of MeHg labelled with ^{203}Hg- and ^{14}C-labelled MeHg by rat caecal contents suggested that the carbon–mercury bond was cleaved and that at least one of the volatile products was likely to be elemental mercury, Hg^0 (Rowland *et al.*, 1978). Although such a reaction is known to occur in the presence of mercury-resistant enteric bacteria (see below) it is unlikely that these organisms are responsible for MeHg volatilization in gut contents, since the time course of the reaction (1–2 days, Rowland *et al.*, (1978)) is much slower than that for volatilization by mercury-resistant bacteria (Schottel *et al.*, 1974; Summers and Silver, 1972).

There is also evidence that MeHg reacts with hydrogen sulphide produced by intestinal bacteria, leading to volatilization by the formation of *bis*-methylmercuric sulphide (CH$_3$Hg)$_2$S, which decomposes to mercuric sulphide and dimethylmercury (Rowland *et al.*, 1977b, 1978; Craig and Bartlett, 1978).

Volatilization of MeHg to elemental Hg also occurs in the presence of gut contents from mice and faecal suspensions from humans. However, in contrast to incubations of MeHg with suspensions of rat gut contents in which no mercuric mercury was detected (Rowland *et al.*, 1978), both

Table 9.2 *The effect of weaning on MeHg demethylation by mouse caecal and human faecal suspensions. The incubation mixtures were extracted with benzene as described by Cappon and Smith (1977) to determine the amount of MeHg in solution (after Rowland* et al., *1983).*

Species	Age	Diet	% MeHg in solution after 24 hours incubation
Mouse (BALB/c)	10 days	Breast milk	94
Mouse	20 days	Stock pellets	50
Mouse	3 months	Stock pellets	46
Man	2 days	Breast milk	97
Man	4.5 months	Formula milk	90
Man	10 months	Whole milk	88
Man	8 months	Solid mixed diet	29
Man	4.5 months	Solid mixed diet	18

human faeces and mouse caecal suspensions produce substantial amounts of the mercuric form from MeHg (Rowland *et al.*, 1983). Furthermore the rate of demethylation by mouse caecal contents of methylmercury glutathione (the main form of the mercurial in bile) is similar to that of methylmercuric chloride (Rowland *et al.*, 1983).

The demethylation of MeHg to mercuric mercury by the mouse and human gut flora is age-dependent. The caecal contents from adult (3 months old) mice demethylated MeHg rapidly to the mercuric form, but in 10 day-old animals this reaction was very slow. Since the rate of demethylation by the gut flora of 20 day-old mice was similar to that in adult animals (Rowland *et al.*, 1983; Table 9.2) these findings indicated that the underlying metabolic change occurred in mice during weaning at 15–18 days.

It is noteworthy that if mice are not weaned on to a solid diet, but are instead maintained on milk, there is little if any change in the rate of MeHg demethylation, which remains at the unweaned mouse rate (Rowland *et al.*, 1983). The changes during the weaning period in mice coincide with a major alteration in the bacterial composition of the gut microflora (Schaedler, 1973). It is likely that the development of demethylating activity in the human gut flora occurs in a similar fashion, since weaned and unweaned children of similar ages exhibit markedly different faecal demethylation capacities (Table 9.2).

(d) Methylmercury metabolism in vivo.   The rapid and virtually complete absorption of MeHg from the gut makes it unusual among toxic metal compounds (Miettinen, 1973; Walsh, 1982). The cumulative body burden of mercury after methylmercury exposure is determined not only by the quantity taken in, but also by its rate of elimination. The main route of excretion is via the faeces in man and laboratory animals (Clarkson, 1979). In rats and mice given MeHg, the majority of the mercury in faeces is in the mercuric form with values of 50–90% mercuric mercury in faeces being reported (Norseth and Clarkson, 1970; Norseth, 1971a; Landry *et al.*, 1979; Clarkson, 1979; Rowland *et al.*, 1980, 1983). It would appear therefore that demethylation of methylmercury is a rate-determining step in the excretion of the organomercurial from the body.

In mice given MeHg, the proportion of the body burden of mercury present in the mercuric form after 6 days was found to be about 10% (Rowland *et al.*, 1984) although this was not distributed evenly in the tissues. In brain and blood, about 5% of the mercury content was in the mercuric form whereas in liver and kidney the mercuric mercury content was 21–24%. These results largely confirm those of an earlier study (Norseth, 1971a). In rats, the distribution of inorganic mercury after MeHg exposure appears to be similar to that seen in mice (Norseth and Clarkson, 1970; Magos and Butler, 1976; Hargreaves *et al.*, 1985). *In vitro* experiments have identified a number of potential sites for MeHg demethylation (Ishihara and Suzuki, 1976; Lefevre and Daniel, 1973). However, the studies described below using germ-free and conventional flora animals indicate a major role for the gut microflora in the *in vivo* demethylation of methylmercury.

Norseth and Clarkson (1971) first suggested that the gut microflora could be involved in the demethylation and excretion of MeHg and their suggestion has been confirmed by numerous studies, although ironically a study by Norseth himself failed to provide evidence of a role for gut bacteria (Norseth, 1971b).

MeHg gains access to the gut flora via its secretion in bile or by its presence in exfoliated intestinal cells. In adult rats, a small proportion (0.5–3% in 2 hours) of an absorbed dose of MeHg is excreted in the bile. The majority (60–80%) of the mercury in bile is found as a methylmercury–glutathione complex. In contrast only 4–5% of mercury in bile is inorganic (Ohsawa and Magos, 1974; Norseth, 1973; Klaasen, 1976; Norseth and Clarkson, 1971; Refsvik and Norseth, 1975). The methylmercury–glutathione complex or its derivatives formed by the action of pancreatic enzymes (Hirata and Takahashi, 1981) is largely reabsorbed, resulting in an enterohepatic circulation of mercury (Norseth, 1973). Conversion of MeHg in bile to the poorly absorbed inorganic forms would effectively interrupt this enterohepatic circulation and lead to increased mercury excretion in faeces. The high proportion of mercuric mercury in faeces of animals given MeHg and the low proportion of the inorganic form in bile lend support to the theory that demethylation occurs in the gut. Direct evidence for the importance of bacterial demethylation to the rate of Hg elimination and tissue distribution of Hg after MeHg exposure comes from studies in germ-free rodents and animals treated with antibiotics to suppress their gut bacteria.

In four such studies which reported mercury excretion data, all showed that the suppression or absence of the gut microflora was associated with decreased excretion of total mercury in faeces by comparison with the conventional flora control animals (Table 9.3). Three of the studies measured mercuric mercury in faeces or colon contents and showed that it was markedly decreased in the germ-free or antibiotic-treated animals (Table 9.3). Again the study of Norseth (1971b) was at variance with the rest, but this may be due to the route of administration (subcutaneous) of the MeHg. The balance study reported by Rowland *et al.* (1984) demonstrated that the decreased faecal excretion of Hg in animals treated with antibiotics was reflected in significantly higher body burdens of mercury. The half-time of mercury elimination was increased from 10 days in the conventional flora mice to more than 100 days in the antibiotic-treated animals. Furthermore the proportion of the total mercury body burden present as mercuric mercury was smaller in the animals given antibiotics. These studies (Rowland *et al.*, 1984) also showed marked diet-dependent differences in mercury excretion which could also be related to changes in gut flora metabolism; these diet effects are discussed in Chapter 15.

In general, animals in which the gut flora is absent or suppressed have higher total mercury levels in most tissues (Table 9.4), but it is the mercury concentration in the central nervous system which is of particular importance since this is the main site of toxicity of MeHg. The concentration of mercury in the brain after MeHg exposure was found to be 25–45% greater in germ-free or antibiotic-treated animals than in controls (Table 9.4). Rowland *et al.* (1980) demonstrated the significance of the elimination of the microflora on the neurotoxicity of MeHg by showing that MeHg-induced behavioural signs of neurotoxicity and the severity of the histopathological lesions in the cerebellum were much greater in antibiotic treated rats than in their conventional flora counterparts.

It should be noted that in animals lacking a gut flora, mercuric mercury is still found in faeces and in tissues, although the proportion of the total mercury in the inorganic form is usually lower. This implies that there

Table 9.3 *Studies of MeHg metabolism in germ-free antibiotic treated and conventional flora rodents*

Species	Status[a]	MeHgCl Dosing regime	Results[b]	Reference
Mouse	GF	20 μg/mouse in 1 ml drinking water	Hg in faeces decreased Hg in urine increased Hg in tissues increased	Nakamura *et al.* (1977)
Mouse	AB	60 μg i.p. per mouse	Hg and Hg^{++} in faeces decreased Hg in kidney increased Hg^{++} in kidney and liver decreased	Seko *et al.* (1981)
Mouse	AB	0.6 mg/kg p.o. ^{203}Hg labelled	Hg and Hg^{++} in faeces decreased Hg in urine decreased Hg in tissues increased	Rowland *et al.* (1984)
Rat	GF	1 mg/kg sub. cut.	Hg in blood similar Hg^{++} in faeces similar	Norseth (1971b)
Rat	AB	1 or 13 μg/rat (^{203}Hg labelled) daily for 10 days	Hg and Hg^{++} in faeces decreased Hg in urine increased Hg in tissues increased	Rowland *et al.* (1980)

[a] GF, germ-free; AB, antibiotic treated.
[b] Compared with conventional flora controls.
Hg is total mercury and Hg^{++} mercuric mercury.

Table 9.4 *The effect of germ-free status or antibiotic treatment on mercury concentration in tissues of rodents given MeHgCl.*

Species (Reference)	Ratio $\left(\frac{\text{GF or AB}}{\text{CV}}\right)$ Hg concentration in tissue			
	Brain	Blood	Liver	Kidney
Rat (Rowland *et al.*, 1980)	1.27	1.35	0.95	1.42
Mouse (Nakamura *et al.*, 1977)	1.45	ND	1.60	1.86
Mouse (Seko *et al.*, 1981)	ND	ND	1.09	1.32
Mouse (Rowland *et al.*, 1984)	1.25	2.10	1.65	1.02

GF, germ-free; AB, antibiotic; CV, conventional flora; ND, not determined.

are other (non-bacterial) sites of demethylation in the body. However the observation that antibiotic treatment of mice leads to almost complete retention of a dose of MeHg (half-time of mercury elimination greater than 100 days (Rowland *et al.*, 1984)) would suggest that non-bacterial demethylation does not play a significant role in determining the body burden of mercury after MeHg exposure.

(e) Implications of bacterial demethylation of MeHg. Dramatic differences have been found in the rate of excretion of MeHg between neonatal and weaned mice. Suckling mice absorb and retain the majority of an oral dose of MeHg (half-time of mercury elimination, $T_{\frac{1}{2}}$, greater than 100 days (Doherty and Gates, 1973)), whereas older mice excrete the mercurial much more rapidly ($T_{\frac{1}{2}}$ 6–10 days). This developmental change in rate of excretion occurs at 16–18 days after birth, coinciding with the time of weaning to a pelleted rodent diet, and has been linked to a number of possible mechanisms (reviewed by Rowland *et al.*, 1983). The most likely of these are a change in the rate of biliary secretion of MeHg into the gut at weaning (Ballatori and Clarkson, 1982) and an increase in the demethylation activity of the gut microflora. The latter has been demonstrated *in vitro* (see above) and *in vivo* where it has been shown that the mercuric mercury excretion is much greater in 20 day-old mice than in 4 or 10 day-old animals (Rowland *et al.*, 1983). Since faecal

suspensions from unweaned human babies also exhibit little ability to demethylate MeHg (Table 9.2) it seems likely that the latter also would absorb and retain more of an oral dose of MeHg than adults. Thus the lack of bacterial demethylating activity in the gut may make babies and unweaned infants more susceptible to MeHg neurotoxicity than adults.

It is also tempting to speculate that the wide range of mercury elimination rates seen in humans (Shahristani and Shihbab, 1974) may be related to the variations in the composition of the gut flora between individuals. In addition, if the major differences in gut flora that have been reported in populations in different parts of the world (Drasar and Hill, 1974) are reflected in their MeHg demethylation rates it is conceivable that there are inter-regional as well as inter-individual differences in susceptibility to MeHg poisoning.

(f) Mercury metabolism by mercury-resistant enteric bacteria. Bacteria resistant to the toxic effects of inorganic and organic mercury compounds have been isolated from heavily contaminated terrestrial and aquatic environments (Walker and Colwell, 1974) and from clinical sources (Nakahara *et al.*, 1977; Novick and Roth, 1968; Schottel *et al.*, 1974). Mercury resistance has been found in a wide range of enteric organisms, including *Escherichia*, *Proteus*, *Klebsiella*, *Staphylococcus* and *Pseudomonas* (Schottel *et al.*, 1974). Mercury resistant (Hg[r]) strains of bacteria are often resistant to other heavy metals, e.g. arsenic, lead and cadmium, and also to antibiotics. In both cases the resistance is determined by plasmids (Novick and Roth, 1968; Summers and Silver, 1972).

All Hg[r] plasmids confer resistance to mercuric mercury, but plasmid-mediated resistance to phenylmercuric acetate (PMA), *p*-hydroxymercuribenzoate, MeHg and ethylmercury has also been reported (see the review by Robinson and Tuovinen, 1984). Resistance to alkylmercurials however has not been reported in enterobacteria or staphylococci.

The mechanism of resistance to the mercury compounds appears to be via their biotransformation to elemental mercury which is lost from solution. Since the kinetics and enzymology of these reactions and the inducibility of the enzymes involved have recently been reviewed in detail by Robinson and Tuovinen (1984), they will not be considered further here. However it is relevant to consider the possible biochemical and toxicological consequences of the presence of Hg[r] bacteria in the gut microflora. Two main questions arise: (*i*) What are the selective pressures which increase or maintain numbers of Hg[r] bacteria in the gut? (*ii*) Does the presence of large numbers of Hg[r] bacteria in the gut increase the metabolism of ingested mercurials? Unfortunately, these areas have been little studied. The increased frequency of occurrence of Hg[r] bacteria in clinical specimens appears to coincide with the increased frequency of isolation of antibiotic resistant organisms. Hence it seems possible that exposure of individuals to antibiotics may select for Hg^r bacteria as well as those resistant to antibiotics. However the converse, namely that exposure to mercury compounds selects for Hg^r and antibiotic-resistant bacteria, may not be true. A study in Iraq (Groves *et al.*, 1975) revealed no difference in incidence of Hg^r staphylococci in people exposed or not exposed to methylmercury-coated grain. Intragastric administration of mercuric chloride (2 mg/day) to rats did not increase the numbers or proportion of Hg^r *E. coli* in faeces (Rowland and Davies, 1981, unpublished observations). When rats were given intragastrically large numbers of an *E. coli* strain carrying a plasmid (pUB 932) which confers resistance to Hg and tetracycline, the numbers of Hg^r *E. coli* recovered in faeces increased during the dosing period, but declined rapidly when dosing stopped. Oral administration of 2 mg HgCl$_2$ per day did not prevent the decline, although when the animals were given tetracycline in drinking water, Hg^r *E. coli* persisted in the faeces (Davies *et al.*, 1982). It would appear therefore that exposure of the host animal to mercury compounds does not affect carriage of Hg^r plasmids by members of the host microbial flora.

There is also evidence that the presence of large numbers of Hg^r bacteria in the gut does not increase the volatilization of mercuric mercury by the flora. Incubation with ^{203}HgCl$_2$ of faecal suspensions from rats given, p.o., Hg^r *E. coli* (at levels which increased the population of Hg^r *E. coli* in faeces) resulted in low rates of volatilization of ^{203}Hg similar to those seen in the presence of faeces from untreated rats (Rowland and Davies, 1981, unpublished observation). Furthermore, the ability of a pure culture of an Hg^r *E. coli* to volatilize Hg from solution was inhibited by the presence of rat faeces (Rowland and Davies, 1981, unpublished observation). The results suggest that faecal components bind HgCl$_2$, making it unavailable for metabolism by Hg^r bacteria.

C. Arsenic

1. *Chemical Forms, Exposure and Toxic Effects*

Arsenic is distributed in the environment and in food in a variety of chemical forms, notably as inorganic salts (arsenate and arsenite) and as organo-arsenicals such as monomethylarsonic acid (MMA) and dimethylarsinic acid (DMA).

In drinking water and wine arsenic is present predominantly in the inorganic forms, the exact ratio of arsenate to arsenite being affected by the prevailing redox potential of the solution (Clement and Faust, 1973; Crecelius, 1977). In fish and shellfish, arsenic appears to be present in organic forms (reviewed by Penrose, 1974).

Although chronic effects, including skin cancer, have been attributed to arsenic exposure via drinking water in certain parts of the world (Tseng, 1977), occupational exposure accounts for most incidences of acute arsenic poisoning today, and may be associated with lung cancer in some industrial workers (Vahter, 1983).

The toxicity of arsenic is dependent on its chemical form. A number of studies in laboratory animals, fish and *in vitro* cell systems have shown that arsenite (AsIII) is more toxic than arsenate (AsV) (Byron *et al.*, 1967; Nakamuro and Sayato, 1981). The organoarsenicals MMA and DMA are in turn less toxic than both the inorganic salts.

2.   In vitro *Metabolism of Arsenicals by the Gut Flora*

When incubated with suspensions of rat small intestine or caecal contents under anaerobic conditions, sodium(^{74}As) arsenate was found to be reduced and, in the presence of caecal contents, methylated (Rowland and Davies, 1981). Arsenate was rapidly reduced to arsenite by caecal contents over a period of 20 hours. MMA was formed more slowly and, after a lag of about 25 hours, DMA began to be produced. The involvement of bacteria in these metabolic changes was demonstrated by showing that reduction and methylation were absent or markedly decreased in the presence of sterilized caecal contents or gut contents from germ-free rats. The rate of arsenate metabolism by gut contents was modified by a number of factors. For example, the addition of bile acids (cholic, taurocholic, deoxycholic acids) increased the reduction to arsenite by caecal and intestinal contents without affecting methylation. Arsenate was almost completely reduced to arsenite in the presence of the reducing agent hydrogen sulphide and, surprisingly, the rate of arsenic methylation by caecal contents was also increased (Rowland and Davies, 1981). Other reducing agents, cysteine and thioglycollate, also reduced arsenate. It seems probable therefore that the gut flora generates reducing conditions in the intestinal tract which permits chemical reduction of arsenate to take place.

It is thought that the methylation of arsenic in bacteria from the environment is mediated by S-adenosyl methionine (McBride *et al.*, 1978). The pathway proposed involves reduction of arsenate to arsenite before methylation takes place. The pattern of the metabolism of arsenate by the gut microflora (described above) suggests that a similar pathway of reduction and sequential methylation operates in these organisms.

3. *Reduction and Methylation of Arsenic* in vivo

Arsenate is readily reduced to arsenite in biological systems and biomethylation of both pentavalent and trivalent forms of inorganic arsenic occurs in humans and experimental animals (Vahter, 1983; Mushak, 1983). In humans not exposed to high levels of arsenic, the metabolites in urine comprise about 60% DMA, 20% MMA and 20% inorganic arsenic (Crecelius, 1977; Smith *et al.*, 1977; Tam *et al.*, 1979; Buchet *et al.*, 1981). In contrast DMA is the major metabolite in urine and most tissues of other animal species (Lakso and Peoples, 1975; Vahter, 1983; Odanaka *et al.*, 1980; Rowland and Davies, 1982). Since DMA and MAA are much less toxic than arsenite, biomethylation can be considered a detoxification reaction.

Despite the ability of gut micro-organisms to reduce and methylate sodium arsenate *in vitro*, the prevailing evidence from *in vivo* studies in laboratory animals and man suggests that the gut microflora does not play a major role in arsenic metabolism in the intact animal.

The rapid and virtually complete absorption of arsenate and arsenite from the mammalian gut must limit the opportunity for interaction between the large population of organisms in the large bowel and ingested inorganic arsenicals (see the review by Vahter (1983)).

Studies *in vivo* have shown that in the rat reduction and methylation of inorganic arsenic is extremely rapid (Rowland and Davies, 1982) and it seems unlikely that the rates of methylation measured in gut bacteria *in vitro* could account for such a rapid appearance of MMA and DMA in tissues *in vivo*. Furthermore, the rate of arsenate reduction and methylation after intravenous injection was almost identical to that after administration of the arsenical directly into the intestine, indicating that biotransformation of inorganic arsenic was independent of the gut microflora (Rowland and Davies, 1982).

Confirmatory evidence for the unimportance of the gut flora in arsenic metabolism comes from a study in germ-free and conventional mice (Vahter and Gustafsson, 1980) in which orally administered arsenate was methylated to the same extent in both groups. The most likely site of methylation of inorganic arsenic in mammals appears to be the liver, since Shirachi *et al.* (1981) have reported the formation of DMA from arsenate by rat liver fractions *in vitro*, while Lerman and Clarkson (1983)

have demonstrated that isolated rat hepatocytes rapidly convert arsenite
to DMA.

4. *Microbial Metabolism of other Arsenicals*

A number of organic arsenic compounds based on arsanilic acid were
used in animal and poultry feeds as growth promoting agents and for
disease control. When incubated anaerobically with hen faeces, 4-
nitrophenylarsonic acid was converted to arsanilic acid (the nitro-reduction
product), 4-nitrophenylarsenoxide and 4-aminophenylarsenoxide (Moody
and Williams, 1964). Arsanilic acid was also converted to 4-aminophenyl-
arsenoxide under similar conditions. It was suggested that the growth
promoting effects of these organoarsenicals is due to their reduction in
the gut to arsenoxide derivatives which are more toxic to parasites. It
should be noted however that *in vivo* metabolic studies have shown that
in hens only the nitroreduction products of nitrophenylarsonic acid can
be detected in faeces, and arsanilic acid itself appears metabolically stable
(Moody and Williams, 1964; Overby and Fredrickson, 1963).

D. Conclusions

In vitro studies have shown that the gut microflora can biotransform a
number of metal compounds, in some cases to more toxic compounds
(by methlyation of mercuric salts), in others to less toxic derivatives (by
demethylation of MeHg, or methylation of inorganic arsenic). However,
only in the case of MeHg demethylation is there evidence that the
microbial metabolism is of toxicological significance to the host animal.
   Other metals, including selenium and lead, have inorganic and organic
salts with different toxicities and are subject to biotransformation in
mammals (see the review by Mushak, 1983). The involvement of gut
bacteria in these biotransformation processes has not been studied. Wood
et al. (1978) have provided evidence that a wide variety of toxic elements,
such as tin, tellurium, palladium, gold, thallium and lead, can be
methylated biologically. In view of the methylating capacity of the gut
microflora with respect to mercury and arsenic, studies of the ability of
the flora to alkylate other metals and metalloids are warranted.

Acknowledgments

I am grateful to Richard Hargreaves for his many helpful comments during the preparation of this manuscript.

References

Abdulla, M., Arniesjo, B. and Ihse, I. (1973). Methylation of inorganic mercury in experimental jejunal blind-loop. *Scand. J. Gastroenterol.* **8**, 565–567.

Agnes, G., Bendle, S., Hill, H. A. O., Williams, F. R. and Williams, R. J. P. (1971). Methylation by methyl vitamin B_{12}. *Chem. Commun.* **15**, 850–851.

Ballatori, N. and Clarkson, T. W. (1972). Developmental changes in the biliary excretion of methylmercury and glutathione. *Science* **216**, 61–63.

Berlin, M. (1979). Mercury. *In*: "Handbook on Toxicology of Metals" (eds L. Friburg, G. F. Nordberg and V. B. Vouk), pp. 503–530. Elsevier, Amsterdam.

Bertilsson, L. and Neujahr, H. J. (1971). Methylation of mercury compounds by methylcobalamin. *Biochemistry* **10**, 2805–2808.

Buchet, J. P., Lauwerys, R. and Roels, H. (1981). Comparison of the urinary excretion of arsenic metabolites after a single oral dose of sodium arsenite, monomethyl-arsonate, or dimethylarsinite in man. *Int. Arch. Occup. Environ. Health* **48**, 71–79.

Byron, W. R., Bierbower, G. W., Brouwer, J. B. and Hanson, W. H. (1967). Pathologic changes in rats and dogs from two-year feeding sodium arsenite and sodium arsenate. *Toxicol. appl. Pharmacol.* **10**, 132–147.

Cappon, C. J. and Smith, J. C. (1977) Gas chromatographic determination of inorganic mercury and organomercurials in biological materials. *Anal. Chem.* **49**, 365–369.

Clarkson, T. W. (1979). Effect—general principles underlying the toxic action of metals. *In*: "Handbook on the Toxicology of Metals" (ed. L. Friburg), pp. 99–117. Elsevier, Amsterdam.

Clement, W. H. and Faust, S. D. (1973). A new convenient method for determining arsenic (+3) in natural waters. *Environ. Lett.* **5**, 155.

Craig, P. J. and Bartlett, P. D. (1978). The role of hydrogen sulphide in environmental transport of mercury. *Nature* **275**, 635–637.

Crecelius, E. A. (1977). Arsenite and arsenate levels in wine. *Bull. Environ. Contam. Toxicol.* **18**, 227–230.

Davies, M. J., Coutts, T. M. and Rowland, I. R. (1982). Survival in the gut of bacteria bearing plasmids coding for mercury and tetracycline resistance. *Eur. J. Chemother. Antibiotics* **2**, 144–147.

Doherty, R. A. and Gates, A. H. (1973). Epidemic methylmercury poisoning: Application of a mouse model. *Pediat. Res.* **7**, 319.

Drasar, B. S. and Hill, M. J. (1974). "Human Intestinal Flora". Academic Press, London.

Edwards, T. and McBride, G. C. (1975). Biosynthesis and degradation of methylmercury in human faeces. *Nature* **253**, 462–464.

Groves, P. J., Short, H., Thewaini, A. J. and Young, F. E. (1975). Epidemiology of antibiotic and heavy metal resistance in bacteria: resistance patterns in staphylococci isolated from populations in Iraq exposed and not exposed to heavy metals or antibiotics. *Antimicrob. Agents Chemother.* **7**, 622–628.

Hargreaves, R. J., Foster, J. R., Pelling, D. P., Moorhouse, S. R., Gangolli, S. D. and Rowland, I. R. (1985). Changes in the distribution of histochemically localized mercury in the CNS and in tissue levels of organic and inorganic mercury during the development of intoxication in methylmercury treated rats. *Neuropathol. appl. Neurobiol.* **11**, 383–401.

Hirata, E. and Takahaski, H. (1981). Degradation of methylmercury glutathione by the pancreatic enzymes in bile. *Toxicol. appl. Pharmacol.* **58**, 483–491.

Imura, N., Sukegawa, E., Pan, S. K., Nagao, K., Kim, J. Y., Kwan, T. and Ukita, T. (1971). Chemical methylation of inorganic mercury with methylcobalamin, a vitamin B_{12} analog. *Science* **172**, 1248–1249.

Ishihara, N. and Suzuki, T. (1976). Biotransformation of methylmercury *in vitro*. *Tohoku J. Exp. Med.* **120**, 361–363.

Kwan, T. and Utika, T. (1971). Chemical methylation of inorganic mercury with methylcobalamin, a vitamin B_{12} analog. *Science* **172**, 1248–1249.

Klaasen, C. D. (1976). Biliary excretion of metals. *Drug. Metab. Rev.* **5**, 165–196.

Lakso, J. V. and Peoples, S. A. (1975). Methylation of inorganic arsenic by mammals. *Agric. Food Chem.* **23**, 674–676.

Lander, L. (1971). Biochemical model for the biological methylation of mercury suggested from methylation studies *in vivo* with Neurospara crassa. *Nature* **230**, 452–454.

Landry, T. D., Doherty, R. A. and Gates, A. H. (1979). Effects of three diets on mercury excretion after methylmercury administration. *Bull. Environ. Contam. Toxicol.* **22**, 151–158.

Lefevre, P. A. and Daniel, J. W. (1973). Some properties of the organomercury-degrading system in mammalian liver. *FEBS Lett.* **35**, 121–123.

Lerman, S. and Clarkson, T. W. (1983). The metabolism of arsenite and arsenate by the rat. *Fund. appl. Toxicol.* **3**, 309–314.

Magos, L. and Butler, W. H. (1976). The kinetics of methylmercury administered repeatedly to rats. *Arch. Toxicol.* **35**, 25–39.

McBride, B. C., Merilees, H., Cullen, W. R. and Pickett, W. (1978). *In*: "Organometals and Organometalloids: Occurrence and Fate in the Environment" (eds F. E. Brinkman and J. M. Ballama), pp. 94–115. American Chemical Society, Washington, DC.

Miettinen, J. K. (1973). Absorption and elimination of dietary mercury (Hg^{2+}) and methylation in man. *In*: "Mercury, Mercurials and Mercaptans" (eds M. W. Miller and T. W. Clarkson), pp. 233–243. Charles C. Thomas, Springfield, IL.

Moody, J. P. and Williams, R. T. (1964). The fate of 4-nitrophenylarsonic acid in hens. *Toxicol. appl. Pharmacol.* **2**, 692–706.

Mushak, P. (1983). Mammalian biotransformation processes involving various toxic metalloids and metals. *In*: "Chemical Toxicology and Clinical Chemistry of Metals" (eds S. S. Brown and J. Savory), pp. 227–245. Academic Press, London.

Nakahara, H., Ishikawa, T., Sarai, Y., Kondo, I., Kozukue, H. and Mitsuhaski, S. (1977). Frequency of heavy-metal resistance in bacteria from inpatients in Japan. *Nature* **266**, 165–167.

Nakamura, I., Hosokawa, K. Tamura, H. and Miura, T. (1977). Reduced mercury excretion with faeces in germ-free mice after oral administration of methylmercury chloride. *Bull Environ. Contam. Toxicol.* **17**, 528–533.

Nakamura, K. and Sayato, Y. (1981). Comparative studies of chromosomal aberration induced by trivalent and pentavalent arsenic. *Mutat. Res.* **88**, 73–80.

Norseth, T. (1971a). Biotransformation of methylmercuric salts in the mouse studies by specific determination in organic mercury. *Acta Pharmacol. Toxicol.* **29**, 375–384.

Norseth, T. (1971b). Biotransformation of methyl mercuric salts in germ-free rats. *Acta Pharmacol. Toxicol.* **30**, 172–176.

Norseth, T. (1973). Biliary excretion and intestinal reabsorption of mercury in the rat after injection of methylmercuric chloride. *Acta Pharmacol. Toxicol.* **33**, 280–288.

Norseth, T. and Clarkson, T. W. (1970). Studies on the biotransformation of ^{203}Hg labelled methyl mercury chloride in rats. *Arch. Environ. Health* **21**, 717–727.

Norseth, T. and Clarkson, T. W. (1971). Intestinal transport of ^{203}Hg-labelled methylmercuric chloride. Role of biotransformation in rats. *Arch. Environ. Health* **22**, 568–572.

Novick, R. P. and Roth, C. (1968). Plasmid-linked resistance to inorganic salts in *Staphylococcus aureus*. *J. Bacteriol.* **95**, 1335–1342.

Odanaka, Y., Matano, O. and Goto, S. (1980). Biomethylation of inorganic arsenic by the rat and some laboratory animals. *Bull. Environ. Contam. Toxicol.* **24**, 452–459.

Ohsawa, M. and Magos, L. (1974). The chemical form of methylmercury complex in the bile of the rat. *Biochem. Pharmacol.* **23**, 1903–1905.

Overby, L. R. and Fredrickson, R. L. (1963). Metabolic stability of radioactive arsanilic acid in chickens. *Agric. Fd Chem.* **11**, 378–381.

Penrose, W. R. (1974). Arsenic in the marine and aquatic environments: analysis, occurrence and significance. *CRC Crit. Rev. Environ. Control* **4**, 465–482.

Refsvik, T. and Norseth, T. (1975). Methylmercuric compounds in the bile. *Acta Pharmacol. Toxicol.* **36**, 67–68.

Ridley, W. P., Dizikes, L. J. and Wood, J. M. (1977). Biomethylation of toxic elements in the environment. *Science* **197**, 329–332.

Robinson, J. B. and Tuovinen, O. H. (1984). Mechanisms of microbial resistance and detoxicification of mercury and organomercury compounds: physiological biochemistry and genetic analysis. *Microbiol. Rev.* **48**, 95–124.

Rowland, I. R. and Davies, M. J. (1981). *In vivo* metabolism of inorganic arsenic by the gastro-intestinal microflora of the rat. *J. appl. Toxicol.* **1**, 278–283.

Rowland, I. R. and Davies, M. J. (1982). Reduction and methylation of sodium arsenate in the rat. *J. appl. Toxicol.* **2**, 294–299.

Rowland, I. R., Davies, M. J. and Evans, J. G. (1980). Tissue content of mercury in rats given methylmercuric chloride orally: Influence of intestinal flora. *Arch. Environ. Health* **35**, 155–160.

Rowland, I., Davies, M. and Grasso, P. (1977a). Biosynthesis of methylmercury compounds by the intestinal flora of the rat. *Arch. Environ. Health* **32**, 24–28.

Rowland, I. R., Davies, M. J. and Grasso, P. (1977b). Volatilisation of methylmercuric chloride by hydrogen sulphide. *Nature* **265**, 718–719.

Rowland, I. R., Davies, M. J. and Grasso, P. (1978). Metabolism of methylmercuric chloride by the gastrointestinal flora of the rat. *Xenobiotica* **8**, 37–43.

Rowland, I. R., Grasso, P. and Davies, M. J. (1975). The methylation of mercuric chloride by human intestinal bacteria. *Experientia* **31**, 1064.

Rowland, I. R., Robinson, R. D. and Doherty, R. A. (1984). Effects of diet on mercury metabolism and excretion in mice given methylmercury; role of gut flora. *Arch. Environ. Health* **39**, 401–408.

Rowland, I. R., Robinson, R. D., Doherty, R. A. and Landry, T. D. (1983). Are developmental changes in methylmercury metabolism and excretion mediated by the intestinal microflora? *In*: "Reproductive and Developmental Toxicity of Metals" (eds T. W. Clarkson, G. F. Nordberg and P. R. Sager), pp. 745–758. Plenum Press, New York.

Schaedler, R. W. (1973). The relationship between the host and its intestinal microflora. *Proc. Nutr. Soc.* **32**, 41–47.

Schottel, J., Mandal, A., Clark, D., Silver, S. and Hedges, R. W. (1974). Volatilisation of mercury and organomercurials determined by inducible R-factor systems in enteric bacteria. *Nature* **251**, 335–337.

Seko, Y., Miura, T., Takashi, M. and Koyama, T. (1981). Methylmercury decomposition in mice treated with antibiotics. *Acta Pharmacol. Toxicol.* **49**, 259–265.

Shahristani, H. and Shihbab, K. M. (1974). Variation of biological half-life of methylmercury in man. *Arch. Environ. Health* **28**, 324–344.

Shirachi, D. Y., Lakso, J. V. and Rose, L. J. (1981). Methylation of sodium arsenate by the rat liver *in vitro*. *Proc. West Pharmacol. Soc.* **24**, 159–160.

Smith, T. J., Crecelius, E. A. and Reading, J. C. (1977). Airborne arsenic exposure and excretion of methylated arsenic compounds. *Environ. Health Perspect.* **19**, 89–93.

Summers, A. O. and Silver, S. (1972). Mercury resistance in a plasmid-bearing strain of *Escherichia coli*. *J. Bacteriol.* **112**, 1228–1236.

Syverson, T. L. M. (1982). Effects of methyl mercury on rat brain protein synthesis. PhD Thesis, University of Trondheim, NTH-Trykk Trondheim.

Takeuchi, T. (1972). Biological reactions and pathological changes in human beings and animals caused by organic mercury contamination. *In*: "Environmental Mercury Contamination" (eds R. Harting and B. D. Dinman), pp. 247–289. Ann Arbor Science Publishers, Ann Arbor.

Tam, G. K. H., Charbonneau, S. M., Bryce, F., Pomroy, C. and Sardi, E. (1979). Metabolism of inorganic arsenic (^{74}As) in human following oral ingestion. *Toxicol. appl. Pharmacol.* **50**, 319–322.

Tseng, W.-P. (1977). Biotransformation of trivalent and pentavalent inorganic arsenic in mice and rats. *Environ. Res.* **25**, 286–293.

Vahter, M. (1983). Metabolism of inorganic arsenic in relation to chemical form and animal species. Thesis, Stockholm, 1983.

Vahter, M. and Gustafsson, B. (1980). Biotransformation of inorganic arsenic in germfree and conventional mice. *In*: "Proceedings 3rd Symposium on Trace Elements, Arsenic" (ed. M. Anke, H.-J. Schneider and C. Brückner), pp. 123–129. Abteilung Wissenschaftliche Publikationen der Friederich-Schiller-Universität, Jena.

Vonk, J. W. and Sijpesteijn, A. K. (1973). Studies on the methylation of mercuric chloride by pure cultures of bacteria and fungi. *Antonie van Leeuwenhoek* **39**, 505–513.

Walker, J. D. and Colwell, R. R. (1974). Mercury-resistant bacteria and petroleum degradation. *Appl. Microbiol.* **27**, 285–287.

Walsh, C. T. (1982). The influence of age on the gastrointestinal absorption of mercuric chloride and methylmercury chloride in the rat. *Environ. Res.* **27**, 412–420.

Wood, J. M. (1974). Biological cycles for toxic elements in the environment. *Science* **183**, 1049–1052.

Wood, J. M., Cheh, A., Dizikes, L. J., Ridley, W. P., Rakow, S. and Lakowicz, J. R. (1978). Mechanisms for the biomethylation of metals and metalloids. *Fed. Proc.* **37**, 16–21.

10

Bacterial Metabolism of Protein and Endogenous Nitrogen Compounds

O. M. WRONG

A. Introduction

This chapter describes some properties of the alimentary flora as if it were a single organ of complex biochemical functions. Metabolic processes of individual species of bacteria are frequently not considered, partly because they may not be known (the biochemical effects of the whole flora being in many instances greater than the sum of its known parts), but also because of the author's background as clinical physiologist rather than microbial biochemist. Useful recent reviews which concentrate on the functions of individual bacterial species involved in these metabolic pathways have been provided by Hespell and Smith (1983) and Vince (1986).

Two oversimplifications characterize published work on the metabolic effects of the alimentary flora, which this chapter perforce must follow. First is the tendency to concentrate research in man exclusively on the *large intestine*, admittedly the most densely populated part of the human alimentary tract with its bacterial population of 10^{11} per gram of contents. Second is the emphasis on *bacteria* to the almost total neglect of the fungal and protozoal denizens of the large intestine. One needs to remind oneself that the rumen of herbivorous animals provided the initial model suggesting that the human alimentary flora might have interesting biochemical properties, and that an important component of the ruminal flora is the protozoal population which is known to participate in some of the major metabolic processes occurring in that organ (Hungate, 1966; Clarke, 1977).

The most important aspects of bacterial metabolism of nitrogenous substances in the gut are the breakdown of proteins by proteolytic digestion with subsequent deamination and decarboxylation of the amino acids so formed, and the bacterial generation and metabolism of ammonia.

ROLE OF THE GUT FLORA IN TOXICITY AND CANCER
ISBN 0-12-599920-8

In absolute amounts the turnover of these substances is less than that of carbohydrates and organic acids, and they are less significant as sources of energy; their importance lies mainly in the effects they have on the intermediary metabolism of the host, and their role as potential systemic toxins.

B.   Total Nitrogen

1.   *Nitrogen Entering the Large Intestine*

Organically bound nitrogen reaches the lumen of the large intestine either by passage from the ileum or by secretion or shedding from the large bowel mucosa. A crude measure of the amount arriving through the ileocaecal valve is provided by the mean ileal effluent in ileostomized adult subjects of 0.5–4.0 g of nitrogen/day (Wrong *et al.*, 1981). These figures should be regarded as minimal estimates, for the volume of normal ileostomy effluent averages 500 ml/day, whereas intubation studies have shown an average of 1700 ml passing through the ileocaecal valve daily (Giller and Phillips, 1972; Cummings *et al.*, 1976b; Emonts *et al.*, 1979). The reason for the reduced ileal flow of ileostomized subjects is not clear, but possible factors include self-selection of a low-residue (hence low-fibre) diet, a bacterial flora in the terminal ileum which is about one hundred times as numerous as exists normally at this site (Gorbach *et al.*, 1967), and increased endogenous aldosterone secretion caused by sodium losses through the ileostomy. All three of these factors might theoretically influence the nitrogen content of ileostomy fluid, so there is a real need for measurements of ileocaecal nitrogen flow in intact man.

Bound nitrogen passing through the ileocaecal valve is derived both from dietary residues and from endogenous losses, but no measurements exist to indicate the relative contributions from these two sources. Major alterations in protein intake have been shown to influence ileostomy nitrogen losses (Gibson *et al.*, 1976b; Fernandez *et al.*, 1983) but the changes produced are relatively small; thus Fernandez *et al.* increased the protein content of an isoenergetic diet by 155% (from 40–50 to 110–120 g/day) and found that ileostomy nitrogen losses rose by only 36%. Endogenous nitrogen has often been assumed to be the major source of ileostomy nitrogen, but the evidence has been mainly of this negative type, or rests on deductions regarding the amount of nitrogen in shed epithelial cells, secreted mucus and intestinal enzymes. Animal studies, mainly on rats, have shown that mucosal cell turnover and mucus secretion throughout the length of the intestine are greatly influenced by the presence and nature of intestinal contents (Rübsamen and Hörnicke, 1982; Sakata and Engelhardt, 1983; DeRubertis *et al.*, 1984; Lupton *et al.*, 1985; Ross and Mayhew, 1985), and particularly by the amount of plant fibre passing through the gut. Almost all studies have shown increased mucosal activity, using a variety of measurements (e.g. mucosal dimensions and weight, mitotic activity, DNA and protein content, thymidine incorporation, mucus production) during feeding of cellulose, pectin, crude bran or guar gum, and these changes have affected both the small (Farness and Schneeman, 1982; Johnson *et al.*, 1984; Sigleo *et al.*, 1984; Vahouny *et al.*, 1985) and the large intestine (Cassidy *et al.*, 1981; Jacobs and Lupton, 1984). In man increased intake of plant fibre has been shown to increase faecal nitrogen loss (Cummings *et al.*, 1976a); it is likely that this effect is partly mediated by a similar increase in mucosal activity leading to greater losses of endogenous protein in the form of intestinal enzymes, mucus and shed epithelial cells, though other factors (particularly microbial incorporation of ammonia nitrogen—see section E 2(*b*)) may also be involved. The relative contributions of the small and large intestine to this observed effect of fibre on faecal nitrogen in man are at present unknown. Ileostomy nitrogen losses increase when pigs are fed a high fibre diet (Atkinson *et al.*, 1977), indicating an effect in the small intestine. This effect may depend on the form of fibre used, for Sandberg *et al.* found that 16 g of wheat bran daily did not increase nitrogen loss in ileostomized humans (1981), whereas 15 g of citrus pectin produced a significant 30% increase (1983).

2. Nature of Luminal Nitrogen

The bound nitrogen present within the large intestine is mainly in protein. The evidence for this dogmatic statement is largely negative. Many other nitrogenous substances have been sought and the amounts demonstrated found to make up only a small fraction of the total nitrogen present. Small molecular weight residues from proteolytic digestion of ingested protein do not normally reach the large intestine (Crawford *et al.*, 1968; Yoshida *et al.*, 1968; Adibi and Mercer, 1973; Bayley *et al.*, 1974; Padovan *et al.*, 1975), distal ileal fluid containing very little amino acid and virtually no peptide. The ileum, but not the large intestine, is permeable to small endogenous nitrogen compounds such as urea and creatinine, and their concentrations in distal ileum are close to those in blood (Padovan *et al.*, 1975), but simple calculation shows that they cannot contribute more than 15–50% to the ileal effluent of total nitrogen; the remaining nitrogen in this fluid must consist of the endogenous proteins in secreted mucus, intestinal enzymes and shed epithelial cells, with a component of dietary protein which has escaped intestinal proteolysis.

Although the amounts involved are not known, it is clear that bound nitrogen, in the form of secreted mucus and shed epithelial cells, is continually added to the large bowel lumen along its whole length. Yet the daily amount of nitrogen lost in faeces, 0.5–2 g, is about half the amount lost in ileostomy dejecta, indicating net absorption of nitrogen between these sites. Observations on the rabbit, sheep, equine and pig have shown that the decline in luminal nitrogen is progressive, from ileocaecal valve to anus, the greatest change occurring proximally (Hogan and Phillipson, 1960; Goodall and Kay, 1965; Clarke *et al.*, 1966–67; Rérat, 1978; Glade, 1983; Dixon and Nolan, 1986). Mucosal absorption of nitrogen during transit through the large intestine is unlikely to be in the form of amino nitrogen, for proteins and peptides are not absorbed through the mucosa, and free amino acids are present in such low concentrations that they could make little contribution to nitrogen absorption (see section D). Ammonia is the one nitrogen compound in the large bowel which is readily absorbed through the mucosa (see section E3), and it is probably absorption of this substance which accounts for the progressive decline in luminal total nitrogen as intestinal contents pass through the large intestine.

The 1–2 g of bound nitrogen lost in human faeces daily is 92% non-diffusible (Wrong *et al.*, 1965); in faecal fractionation studies Stephen and Cummings (1980) found that 60% of faecal nitrogen consisted of the bound nitrogen of bacterial bodies. The small diffusible component (8%) of total faecal nitrogen is made up of small molecular weight compounds including ammonia and various amines derived from bacterial metabolism of amino acids. Free amino acids are virtually absent from faeces owing to the avidity with which they are taken up by bacteria, but analytical procedures which damage the integrity of faecal bacteria lead to a rapid increase in the concentrations of free amino acids (Owens and Padovan, 1975, 1976), a difficulty which has sometimes led to uncertainty about the amounts of free amino acid actually present.

C. Bacterial Breakdown of Proteins in the Large Intestine

Pancreatic tryptic activity persists into the large intestine (Lepkovsky *et al.*, 1966) but it is generally assumed that protein breakdown in the large intestine is mainly the result of bacterial activity. The amounts of protein degraded are not known precisely, but are substantial, consisting of most of the 3–25 g (i.e. 0.5–4.0 g of nitrogen) or more entering through the ileocaecal valve and the endogenous proteins generated in the large intestine from secreted mucus and exfoliated epithelial cells.

Proteins must be degraded to peptides and amino acids before being metabolized further by gut bacteria. Very little information is available on the proteolytic properties of intestinal bacteria, most of the published work on the gastro-intestinal flora being concerned with ruminal organisms which may have greater access to protein than those of the large intestine. Because the major bacterial species in the two sites and the environments themselves are very similar, it seems reasonable to extrapolate from knowledge of ruminal bacteria to what is likely to occur in the large intestine. Proteolysis is not a widespread activity among ruminal bacteria, but is not confined to a single species. *Bacteroides amylophilus* (Blackburn, 1968a, b; Henderson *et al.*, 1969; Mahadevan *et al.*, 1980) and *Bacteroides ruminicola* (Pittman *et al.*, 1967; Hazlewood *et al.*, 1981; Hazlewood and Edwards, 1981) are the two ruminal organisms which have been most intensively studied for proteolytic properties; both produce extracellular proteases, but they differ in their active groups, their pH optima, and their specificity for different peptide linkages. Proteolytic activity is weak or absent among the predominant human faecal organisms (Moore and Holdeman, 1974), but, as with the rumen, has been demonstrated in a wide range of strains, including *Escherichia coli*, *Proteus mirabilis*, *Streptococcus faecalis*, *Clostridium welchii*, *Bacteroides melaninogenus* and *Propionibacterium* and *Bacillus* species; proteases of serine, thiol and metal type have been demonstrated from various members of this wide range of organisms (Hespell and Smith, 1983).

Breakdown of proteins by bacterial proteases usually leads to production of large oligopeptides which in turn are cleaved into smaller peptides and free amino acids. Within the rumen some proteolytic organisms possess peptidolytic properties, which may, as in the case of *Bacteroides ruminicola*, be due to the action of intracellular peptidases associated with cellular uptake of the substrate, whereas others (e.g. *Bacteroides amylophilus*) have no peptidase activity and rely on the peptidolytic properties of other ruminal organisms for provision of their nitrogen needs. In fact, many ruminal organisms which are not proteolytic contain one or more peptidases (Hespell and Smith, 1983). Similar conditions are likely to prevail among bacteria in the large intestine, several of which have been shown to have peptidase activity, although these have not been intensively studied.

Mucins, either secreted by the large intestine or reaching the large intestine from more proximal sites in the intestinal tract, are an important substrate for large bowel bacteria. The structure of mucins varies, less being known of the details of colonic mucus than about those from some other gastro-intestinal sites. All are large complex molecules, of over 500 000 daltons, consisting mainly of protein cores with extensive polysaccharide side chains which constitute 50–85% of the total molecular mass, with abundant amounts of *N*-acetylgalactosamine, *N*-acetyl glucosamine, galactose, sialic acid, fucose, phosphate and sulphate units among the polysaccharide chains (Katz *et al.*, 1982; Smith and Podolsky, 1986). About 5% of human faecal bacteria have the ability to digest gut mucins, many of the active strains being *Bifidobacteria* or *Ruminococcus* species. Carlstedt-Duke *et al.* (1986) have isolated from rat caecum a *Peptostreptococcus*, an obligatory anaerobe, which on culture degrades mucin with the production of acetate and butyrate; of interest is their observation that the caecal enlargement which accompanies the germ-free state in this animal can be largely corrected by monocontamination with this organism. In general, the first step in bacterial degradation of mucin appears to be a rupture of the polysaccharide side-arms by means of extracellular bacterial glycosidases acting on the α- and β-linkages between the individual monosaccharide and hexosamine units of the side-arms (Hoskins and Boulding, 1981; Prizont and Konigsberg, 1981). Bacterial degradation of the protein core occurs more slowly (Variyam and Hoskins, 1981), presumably as a result of attack by the same bacteria that degrade other proteins, yielding a preponderance of threonine, aspartyl, glycine and serine units (Katz *et al.*, 1982).

Short chain fatty acid anions (SCFA), consisting predominantly of acetate, propionate and butyrate, are the major anions in large bowel contents and are derived mainly from dietary polysaccharides, particularly plant fibre and starch. However, intestinal proteins are also precursors of these substances, through the action of bacteria in degrading them to their constituent amino acids which are subsequently deaminated to SCFA or SCFA precursors. Intestinal mucins, because of their large carbohydrate component, are likely to be particularly important as protein sources of SCFA, and probably make a major contribution to the high SCFA concentrations seen in the surgically defunctional human large intestine (Rubinstein *et al.*, 1969) and in the large bowel contents of carnivorous species such as the dog (Phillipson, 1947; Banta *et al.*, 1979) which do not regularly have access to dietary carbohydrate.

D. Fate of Amino Acids in the Large Intestine

Small amounts, less than 10 mmol 1^{-1}, of amino acid are present in ileal effluent; these are residues of protein digestion which have escaped absorption in the small intestine (Adibi and Mercer, 1973; Bayley *et al.*,

1974; Padovan *et al.*, 1975). Larger amounts of amino acid arise from bacterial breakdown of proteins and peptides as already discussed.

Free amino acids in the large intestine have little nutritional significance for the host. The large intestine lacks the special absorptive machinery for their uptake which is present in the small intestine (Wrong *et al.*, 1981), except in small newborn animals (Sepúldeva and Smith, 1979) where the adult microbial flora has not yet been fully established. In adult animals free amino acids are largely consumed by the intestinal flora. Germ-free rats have appreciable caecal concentrations of amino acid, averaging about 2 mg ml^{-1}, but in the presence of the normal bacterial flora concentrations are only 10% of these values (Combe *et al.*, 1965; Combe and Sacquet, 1966). The concentrations found in normal human faeces are negligible, averaging 3% only of the values in ileal effluent (Padovan *et al.*, 1975; Owens and Padovan, 1975). From these observations one can deduce that bacterial utilization of amino acids in the large intestine is normally almost complete and keeps up with their production from bacterial hydrolysis of proteins and peptides. Bacterial utilization is not entirely destructive, for many bacteria have active transport systems for structurally related amino acids, and maintain intracellular concentrations which are greater, by as much as a thousand-fold, than their surrounding concentrations (Wilson and Miles, 1975). The intracellular patterns of amino acids within faecal bacteria closely resembles that of ileostomy effluent (Owens and Padovan, 1976), suggesting that a sizable component of these bacterial amino acids has been absorbed intact, rather than synthesized by the micro-organisms. Nevertheless, studies of ruminal bacteria (Hespell and Smith, 1983) suggest that direct cellular incorporations of intact amino acids plays less role in the nitrogen economy of alimentary bacteria than does the deamination of amino acids and the subsequent utilization for growth of the ammonia so formed.

Bacteria metabolize amino acids mainly by deamination and decarboxylation (Barker, 1981). Amino acid transamination reactions also occur in the intestine, involving α-ketoglutarate and leading to the formation of glutamate and the α-keto acid of the amino acid concerned.

1. *Deamination*

Five mechanisms of bacterial deamination are known, all producing ammonia:

(i) oxidation, with the formation of an α-keto acid,
(ii) reduction, in which a saturated acid is formed,

(iii) hydrolysis, with formation of an α-hydroxy fatty acid,

(iv) removal of the elements of ammonia, yielding an unsaturated fatty acid, and

(v) the Stickland reaction, involving two amino acids, one of which is oxidized to the corresponding keto acid, the other reduced to a saturated fatty acid.

Reductive deamination is the most widely reported mechanism among intestinal bacteria (Vince, 1986), in keeping with the intensely anaerobic and reducing environment (E_h averaging -200) within the large intestine. Oxidative deamination is also utilized by many intestinal bacteria, but requires the presence of adequate electron or hydrogen acceptors, of which the Stickland reaction, utilized by many *Clostridia*, is a special example. Other electron-acceptors used by anaerobes in oxidative deamination include α and β-keto acids, α and β-unsaturated acids, their coenzyme A thioesters, and protons (Barker, 1981). The interesting suggestion has been made that methanogenic bacteria can be utilized as electron-acceptors in reducing carbon dioxide to methane. Other potential electron-acceptors currently under investigation include nitrate- and sulphate-reducing bacteria.

Apart from ammonia, the ultimate reaction products of amino acid deamination include carbon dioxide, molecular hydrogen, and a variety of organic acids including acetic, propionic, butyric, pyruvic and succinic acids. Branched-chain fatty acids are derived from the branched chain amino acids—isocaproic and isovaleric from leucine, 2-methyl *N*-butyric from isoleucine, and isovaleric and isobutyric from valine; MacFarlane *et al.* (1986) point out that these branched-chain SCFA in large bowel contents are useful indicators of the extent of bacterial proteolysis and subsequent deamination, as they appear to arise entirely by this mechanism. Bacterial metabolism of the aromatic acids tyrosine, phenylalanine and tryptophan is of particular interest in view of the many metabolites found and their frequent high lipid solubility which suggests that they are easily absorbed from the intestine; the subject has recently been reviewed by Renwick (1986). Major products of tyrosine and phenylalanine metabolism are phenol and cresol and the appropriate aryl acetic and aryl propionic acids, formed by many *Bacteroides* and *Clostridia* species. Tryptophan metabolism by bacterial deamination and transamination leads to the formation of indolepropionic, indolelactic and indoleacetic acids, indole, skatole and indican. When increased levels of tryptophan are present in the large intestine, as in Hartnup disease and the blue-diaper syndrome (two hereditary diseases characterized by defective jejunal absorption of tryptophan), or after rectal infusion of tryptophan in normal subjects, increased amounts of indole, indican and indoleacetic acid are excreted in the urine (Asatoor *et al.*, 1963; Drummond *et al.*, 1964; Fordtran *et al.* 1964), indicating absorption of increased amounts of these bacterial tryptophan metabolites through the large bowel mucosa.

2.   *Decarboxylation*

Intestinal bacteria also metabolize amino acids by decarboxylation, with the formation of an amine and carbon dioxide. Bacterial decarboxylases are inducible intracellular enzymes, which generally require pyridoxal phosphate as a cofactor. The initial decarboxylases described by Gale (1946) were specific each for ornithine, glutamine, histidine, lysine, arginine and tyrosine, all amino acids with three polar groups, but later less specific decarboxylases were described (Haughton and King, 1961; Morris and Fillingame, 1974; Johnson, 1977). Many bacterial decarboxylases have pH optima of about 5.0 (Hayes and Hyatt, 1974), a reaction sufficiently acid to inhibit the growth of most intestinal bacteria; the release of basic amines by amino acid decarboxylation will have the effect of raising the pH of the medium to a value more favourable for bacterial growth. Decarboxylase activity is widely but not universally distributed throughout intestinal bacteria, and can be found in many strains of intestinal aerobes, *Lactobacilli*, *Bifidobacteria*, *Bacteroides*, and *Clostridia*. In one detailed study of decarboxylation of the basic amino acids lysine, arginine and ornithine, Johnson (1977) found that enterobacteria and enterococci were generally active, but *Bacteroides* species were rarely so.

The products of bacterial decarboxylation include many different amines, including the diamines cadaverine and putrescine from lysine and ornithine, simple aliphatic amines such as methylamine and ethylamine from glycine and alanine, and potentially toxic amines such as histamine from histidine, and tyramine and octopamine (a substance with a chemical structure and physiological effect very like those of noradrenaline) from tyrosine. Many of these substances are further metabolized by bacterial deamination. Cadaverine and putrescine are oxidatively deaminated and converted by ring closure to the heterocyclic secondary amines piperidine and pyrrolidine, which are usually present in large bowel contents and are absorbed and excreted in the urine (Asatoor *et al.*,1967; Milne *et al.*, 1970).

It is not clear how the sulphur-containing amino acids are normally metabolized by intestinal bacteria. Of these methionine appears to be metabolized to methanethiol (methyl mercaptan) and ethanethiol, for these compounds appear in plasma when the amino acid is fed by mouth, but not after intravenous administration (Chen *et al.*, 1970). The initial bacterial conversion is likely to be hydrolysis to methanethiol and homoserine, or reduction to methanethiol and α-aminobutyric acid (Challenger and Charlton, 1947) followed by the usual deamination or decarboxylation of the residual amino acid. This latter reaction is confirmed by the finding of large amounts of α-hydroxybutyric acid in the urine in the "oasthouse syndrome", a rare inborn metabolic disorder in which intestinal absorption of methionine is defective and large amounts reach the large bowel to be metabolised by intestinal bacteria (Smith and Strang, 1958).

E.   Ammonia

1.   *Bacterial Formation*

Ammonia occupies a central position in nitrogen metabolism in the large intestine, both as an end-product of bacterial metabolism of many dietary and endogenous substances, and as a key nitrogenous compound utilized by bacteria in their own protein synthesis. A simplification of the main pathways involved is shown in Fig. 10.1. All pathways in this diagram have been well documented but there is still much uncertainty over the relative importance of the different paths, and the precise sites in the alimentary tract where the various processes occur.

The pH of large bowel contents normally varies over the range 5.5–8.0. The pK of ammonia is approximately 9.0, so in the large intestine it must exist more than 90% in the form of *ionized ammonium*, yet through habit and convenience it is usually described as 'ammonia'. Ammonia is found in the large intestine of all mammals yet studied (Wrong *et al.*, 1965; Faichney, 1968; Hecker, 1971; Knutson *et al.*, 1977). It is difficult to measure the concentration with precision, as large bowel contents generate ammonia after removal from the body (Vince *et al.*, 1976) and the measured concentration in faecal water therefore depends on how this fluid is obtained. In man *in vivo* dialysis provides the best measure in faeces, yielding average figures of 14 mmol 1^{-1}, or 2% of total faecal nitrogen (Wrong *et al.*, 1965). Samples of faecal water obtained by high speed centrifugation or ultrafiltration of faeces have yielded higher concentrations averaging 33 or 42 mmol 1^{-1} respectively (Tarlow and Thom, 1974; Bjork *et al.*, 1976), an indication of continued ammonia generation by bacteria during processing of faeces outside the body. Colonic contents from higher in the large intestine have been shown to have ammonia concentrations similar to those of terminal faeces (Bourke *et al.*, 1966; Combe and Sacquet, 1966; Ducluzeau *et al.*, 1966).

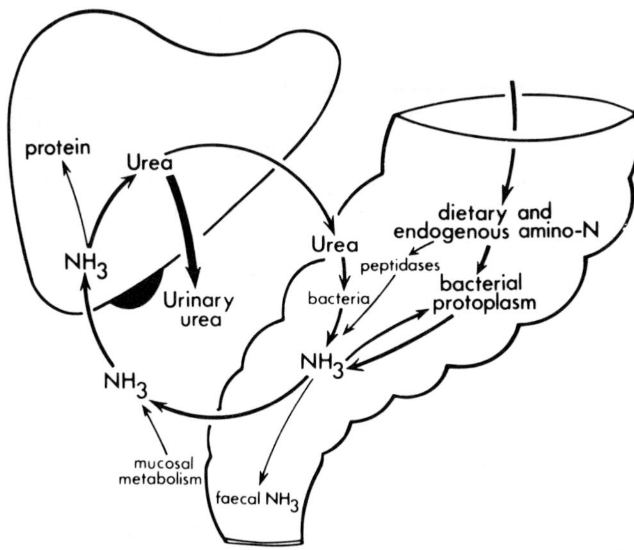

Fig 10.1 The origins and fate of ammonia in the large intestine and the enterohepatic circulation of urea nitrogen. Reprinted with permission from Wrong *et al.* (1981).

Ammonia concentrations in the alimentary tract are closely related to bacterial activity. For example, only traces are present in human saliva derived by direct intubation of salivary ducts, but within the mouth saliva rapidly generates ammonia from bacterial breakdown of nitrogenous compounds, particularly urea (Kopstein and Wrong, 1977). Concentrations in human stomach, duodenum and jejunum, all sites with low bacterial populations, are of the order of 1 mmol 1^{-1} or less (Summerskill *et al.*, 1966), but no data are available on concentrations in the intact distal ileum, a matter of interest in view of a suggestion (see section F1) that this may be the main site of bacterial urea hydrolysis in the body. The high concentration of ammonia in human faeces falls to about one third in subjects taking insoluble broad-spectrum antibiotics by mouth (Wilson *et al.*, 1968a), and in the caecum of germ-free rats the amounts present are only 10–15% of their normal values (Combe and Sacquet, 1966; Ducluzeau *et al.*, 1966). In these circumstances ammonia of non-bacterial origin could be derived from enzymatic digestion of glutamine residues by endogenous peptidases (Melville, 1935), or by diffusion of ammonia of metabolic origin from mucosal cells (Windmueller and Spaeth, 1974; Anderson *et al.*, 1976). In most circumstances bacterial metabolism does, however, appear to be the main source of ammonia within the large intestine.

In the past urea has been regarded as the main precursor of the ammonia in the large intestine (Sabbaj *et al.*, 1970; Summerskill and Wolpert, 1970; Wrong, 1971a). The chief arguments for this view were the large amount of urea known to be hydrolysed in the body as a result of the activity of intestinal bacteria (see section F1), and the knowledge that bacterial metabolism of urea involves ammonia production as the first step. In addition the urea concentration of human faecal water is very low, under 0.5 mmol 1^{-1} (Wrong *et al.*, 1965; Owens and Padovan, 1975), and steps which eliminate or reduce the bacterial flora, such as a germ-free environment (Warren and Newton, 1959; Ducluzeau *et al.*, 1966), or the use of broad spectrum antibiotics (Wilson *et al.*, 1968a,b), lead to the appearance of urea at levels similar to those of plasma, and a corresponding fall in ammonia concentration. At least superficially, these findings suggest that urea passively diffuses into the large bowel as readily as it does into other compartments of body water, and would be present there in the same concentration as in plasma were it not for bacterial degradation.

However, perfusion studies of the cleansed human large intestine have shown that it is almost impermeable to urea (Wolpert *et al.*, 1971; Bown *et al.*, 1975). Moreover, labelling of the systemic urea pool with ^{15}N has shown that little of the ammonia in large bowel contents is derived from this source. Wrong *et al.* (1984) labelled plasma urea at a constant ^{15}N enrichment over longer than the time of gastro-intestinal transit and found that the average labelling of faecal ammonia was only 8.5% of the plasma urea enrichment. Nolan *et al.* (1976) calculated from their study of isotope urea labelling that 30% of the ammonia in the caecum of a sheep was derived from plasma urea, and Forsythe and Parker (1985) found that 27% of the ammonia in rabbit caecum had this origin. These studies, although on different species, agree that circulating urea is a minor source of the luminal ammonia in both proximal and distal large intestine. They also suggest that circulating urea makes a larger, though still minor, contribution in the more proximal large intestine, a finding which tallies well with the observed impermeability of the colonic mucosa to the passage of urea, whereas the small intestine is freely permeable to this substance (Fordtran *et al.*, 1965). The greater contribution of circulating urea to caecal ammonia might be brought about by urea derived from the ileum, either hydrolysed by the bacterial flora in the terminal ileum (though the flora here is 100–1000 times less numerous than in the colon) or by the flora in the caecum after passage through the ileocaecal valve; at more distal sites in the large intestine the ammonia derived from urea would be gradually absorbed through the mucosa and progressively diluted by ammonia derived from non-urea sources. In this context it is relevant that the ^{15}N-urea labelling studies in man showed that 6.8% of faecal total nitrogen, known to consist largely of bacterial protein, was derived from the circulating urea pool, only a little less than the proportion of faecal ammonia (8.5%) from this source, indicating the close interchange between these fractions of faecal nitrogen.

Thus urea is a minor source of the ammonia in the large bowel lumen. Other small molecular weight nitrogenous substances of dietary or endogenous origin, such as creatinine and uric acid, may also yield ammonia as a result of bacterial action (see section G2), but the absolute amounts cannot be large because their concentrations in body fluid are low; by exclusion luminal ammonia must in the main be derived by deamination from the amino nitrogen of dietary and endogenous proteins. Among intestinal organisms, Gram negative anaerobes and *Clostridia* are the most active ammonia producers from non-urea sources (Vince and Burridge, 1980). An indication of the contribution of these non-urea sources to large bowel ammonia has been obtained by incubation studies of faecal homogenates under conditions favourable to survival of the anaerobic flora (Vince *et al.*, 1976); large amounts of ammonia are generated, up to 25% of the total nitrogen present (Fig. 10.2). Ammonia is evolved even more rapidly when conditions are unfavourable for bacterial survival; an extreme example occurred when all bacteria were eliminated by gamma-irradiation, yet bacterial deaminases continued to evolve ammonia as rapidly as in the presence of living bacteria.

Dietary experiments suggest that dietary protein makes a greater contribution to colonic ammonia than do endogenous sources of nitrogen. Metcalfe-Gibson *et al.* (1967) found that faecal ammonia fell to one fifth of control values when subjects consumed a protein-free diet; conversely Cummings *et al.* (1979) found a doubling of faecal ammonia, without significant change in faecal total nitrogen, when daily protein intake was increased from 63 to 136 g. These studies suggest that most of the amino nitrogen reaching the large intestine is contained in the residues of ingested dietary protein; an alternative explanation would be that endogenously-derived proteins, perhaps particularly intestinal mucins, are more resistant to bacterial breakdown than are the partially hydrolysed residues of dietary protein.

2. *Bacterial Utilization of Ammonia*

All bacteria have the ability to utilize ammonia as a nitrogen source for their own amino acid and protein requirements. This property is well displayed by gastro-intestinal bacteria, though to date most studies have been concerned with ruminal organisms.

(a) Transport	Most biological membranes are permeable to non-ionized ammonia, NH_3. Although nearly all of the 'ammonia' present in the gut is in reality the much less diffusible ammonium ion (NH_4^+), the free permeability of the NH_3 component is likely to be sufficient to fulfil bacterial requirements except under conditions of extreme ammonia limitation, which in the large intestine is unlikely to be a primary factor in preventing bacterial growth. However several bacteria, including strains of *Escherichia coli*, have been shown to possess active NH_4 transport systems (Kleiner, 1981), with which they can develop a concentration difference of NH_4 of as great as one hundredfold across their cell membranes. Some of these bacteria are capable *in vitro* of nitrogen-fixation, another bacterial adaptation to scarcity of bound nitrogen. Whether active NH_4 transport occurs in gastro-intestinal bacteria is unknown, but if so it is more likely to play a role in the rumen than in the large intestine, as feeding experiments with ammonia and urea indicate that ammonia deficiency is a factor limiting bacterial growth in the former organ (Stangel, 1967).

(b) Ammonia metabolism	Two mechanisms of bacterial assimilation of ammonia have been described, both involving the conversion of ketoglutarate to glutamate. The first and probably more important mechanism involves reductive fixation of ammonia under the action of glutamate dehydrogenase, which converts ketoglutarate directly to glutamate, with NADPH or NADH as the electron donor (Dawes and Large, 1973); the reaction is reversible and operates more efficiently at high concentrations of ammonia such as those found in the large intestine. The second mechanism involves the two enzymes glutamine synthetase and glutamate synthase which catalyse the amination of ketoglutarate to glutamine and thence to glutamate (Meers *et al.*, 1970); the reaction is irreversible, requires 1 mol of ATP for each mol of ammonia utilized, and operates even at low concentrations of ammonia (below 1.0 mM) which are unfavourable for the first reaction. The glutamate synthase activity required for the second reaction has a very limited distribution in gut bacteria (Hespell and Smith, 1983) though it may play a role in bacterial ammonia assimilation when ambient ammonia concentrations are as low as shown in the lower part of Fig. 10.2.

Ammonia is the preferred nitrogen source of most ruminal bacteria (Salter *et al.*, 1979); in the sheep rumen 50–78% of bacterial nitrogen has this origin (Pilgrim *et al.*, 1970; Mathison and Milligan, 1971). Less

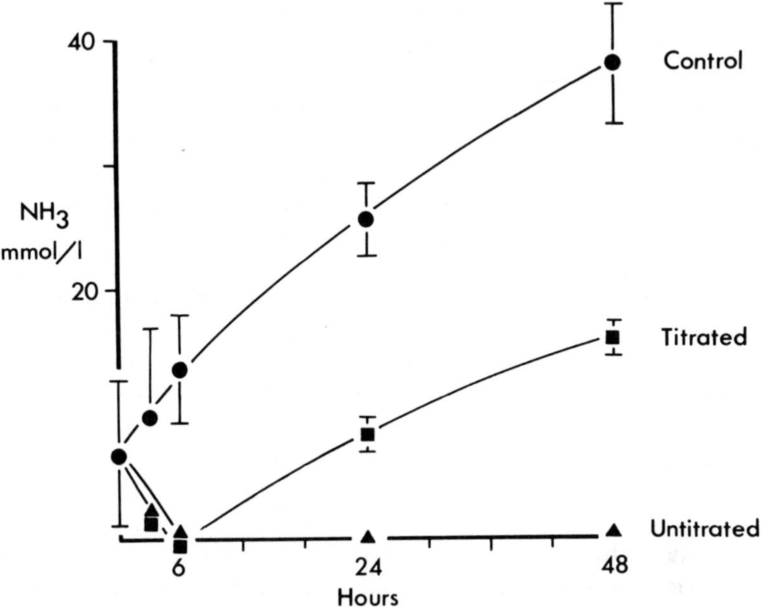

Fig 10.2 The effect of 0.09 mol 1^{-1} lactulose on ammonia generation in an anaerobic faecal incubation system. For a description see the text. Reprinted with permission from The effect of lactulose on ammonia production in a faecal incubation system, by Vince *et al. Gastroenterology*, Vol. 74, pp. 544–549. Copyright 1978 by The American Gastroenterological Association.

information is available regarding intestinal bacteria, but ambient ammonia concentrations, pH and E_h in large intestine and rumen are similar, rendering it likely that colonic bacteria make similar use of ammonia to fill their nitrogen needs. Indeed, Takahashi *et al.* (1980) found that a wide range of intestinal bacteria from pigs incorporated ammonia nitrogen into their own amino nitrogen more efficiently than nitrogen from any amino acid, the highest uptake being into aspartic acid and alanine.

Ammonia cannot be assimilated for bacterial growth unless carbon skeletons and a source of energy are both present in the medium (Vince, 1986). Carbon skeletons are provided by the organic anions produced by bacterial fermentation, mainly from dietary carbohydrate and to a lesser extent from amino acids and intestinal mucus, as described in sections C and D1. Branched-chain SCFA and straight-chained organic anions, such as acetate and lactate, are used for this purpose; in addition there is a bacterial requirement for sulphur-containing amino acids, which can sometimes be met by the provision of inorganic sulphide (Varel and

Bryant, 1974). The energy requirement of large bowel bacteria is normally also provided by fermentation of dietary carbohydrate, particularly plant fibre (Cummings, 1981) and starch which has escaped digestion in the small intestine (Anderson *et al.*, 1981; Cummings, 1983; MacFarlane and Englyst, 1986). The interplay of some of these factors influencing ammonia metabolism are shown in Fig. 10.2, in which ambient ammonia concentrations are shown in a homogenate of human faeces incubated anaerobically for 48 hours with good survival of the main bacterial strains. In the absence of added substrate ('control') bacterial production of ammonia exceeds assimilation, and ammonia concentrations rise throughout the incubation. When fermentable carbohydrate is added in the form of the disaccharide lactulose, bacterial ammonia assimilation exceeds ammonia production, and ammonia concentrations in the medium fall to negligible levels. Part of the inhibition of ammonia production is due to the low pH produced by lactulose fermentation (Vince *et al.*, 1973; Vince and Burridge, 1980); when this factor is removed by continuous titration to keep pH 5.5 or above, ammonia accumulates in the medium after the first 6 hours when the lactulose has been metabolized, and bacterial ammonia generation then exceeds ammonia assimilation. The effect of lactulose shown in this figure can be reproduced by the addition of other fermentable carbohydrates such as lactose (Lewis *et al.*, 1980) and glucose, or fermentable sugar alcohols such as sorbitol and mannitol (Vince *et al.*, 1978); fibre carbohydrates (the hemicellulose arabinogalactan and pectin) also show inhibition of net ammonia accumulation but to a much less marked extent, in keeping with their slower rate of bacterial fermentation (Vince, McNeil, Wager and Wrong in preparation).

Vince (1986) has pointed out that this effect of fermentable carbohydrate in reducing the ammonia concentration in the medium is the result of several changes in bacterial metabolism known to be induced by the presence of carbohydrate—(*i*) a decrease in the breakdown of nitrogenous substances, especially the amino acids of bacterial protoplasm, brought about by reduced production of bacterial deaminases ('catabolite repression'), and reduced activity of preformed enzymes ('catabolite inhibition') (Magasanik, 1961; Paigen and Williams, 1970; Vince and Burridge, 1980), and (*ii*) an increase in the assimilation of ammonia into bacterial protoplasm (Mason, 1974). Within the large intestine metabolizable carbohydrate exists mainly in the form of plant fibre; its effect as a bacterial substrate in increasing bacterial uptake of ammonia must reduce the availability of ammonia for mucosal absorption and increase faecal loss of nitrogen in the form of bacterial protoplasm. Increased intake of plant fibre in man is known to increase faecal nitrogen loss (Sealock *et al.*, 1941; Cummings *et al.*, 1976a; Stephen and Cummings, 1979), and this mechanism is probably largely responsible, though ammonia-trapping in a more acid medium, and intestinal hurry caused by the increased volume of colonic contents, are other factors which may play a role.

Increased faecal nitrogen caused by subsistence on a high fibre diet is paradoxical, in that such diets are usually consumed by people and animals which have restricted access to foods containing protein and digestible carbohydrate, and may be ill-able to afford an increased loss of bacterial protein in their faeces. Loss of faecal nitrogen by herbivorous animals can represent more than 50% of total nitrogen intake (Altman and Dittmer, 1968; Thornton *et al.*, 1970) and become an important factor in nitrogen balance. It is not clear whether this is also a problem for man. Burkitt *et al.* (1972) found that rural villagers in Africa, habitually eating a high-fibre diet, had mean faecal weights of 470 g/day, four times the European normal; they provided no data on faecal nitrogen, but if this increases in proportion to faecal weight, the daily loss of 4 g of nitrogen in stool would have a deleterious effect on overall nitrogen economy. Herbivorous animals have evolved two adaptations by which they combat this problem: *Coprophagy* produces a recycling of faeces through the alimentary tract, and thus permits digestion of bacterial proteins present in the faeces. A more fundamental adaptation, the *rumen*, places the main fermentation chamber in which plant fibre is degraded at the proximal rather than the distal end of the alimentary canal, so the products of bacterial metabolism are available to the digestive processes in the small intestine.

3. *Ammonia Absorption*

Ammonia is rapidly absorbed through the large bowel mucosa, but there is no evidence that active transport is involved. The rate of absorption is markedly pH-dependent, being greater at alkaline pH, a finding which suggests that absorption is predominantly in the form of unionized ammonia, NH_3 (Wolpert *et al.*, 1970; Castell and Moore, 1971; Bown *et al.*, 1975), as is characteristic of ammonia absorption through other biologic membranes (Milne *et al.*, 1958). The most convincing evidence for absorption by non-ionic diffusion was provided by Castell and Moore (1971) who found that absorption from buffered solutions infused into the large intestine was proportional both to total ammonia concentration and to pH. They calculated that the mucosa was 4–5 times as permeable to unionized NH_3 as to the ammonium ion, NH_4^+, a ratio subsequently supported by Bown *et al.* (1975) from their own data.

The pH-dependency of mucosal ammonia absorption, implied by non-ionic diffusion, suggests that the concentration of ammonia within the large bowel lumen would be inversely related to luminal pH. Down *et al.* (1972) demonstrated this relationship in human faeces, but it is much less precise than the ammonia/pH relationship of urine (Wrong and Davies, 1959), which has often been quoted as a good illustration of the influence of non-ionic diffusion on ammonia movements. Presumably in faeces the ideal relationship is to some extent obscured by the many other factors already discussed here which influence ammonia formation —the availability of amino-nitrogen for deamination, of fermentable carbohydrate for bacterial ammonia assimilation, and the activity of the various intestinal bacteria responsible for these processes. In addition the pH of the juxta-mucosal fluid layer, rather than that of large bowel contents in general, is the factor which will directly determine ammonia absorption, and there is evidence that the former is more constant and usually of lower pH than the latter (McNeil *et al.*, 1987; Rechkemmer *et al.*, 1986).

A factor which influences ammonia absorption through its effect on non-ionic diffusion is the presence of anions which themselves are subject to absorption by non-ionic diffusion. Absorption by paired non-ionic diffusion occurs when the ions of weak acids and bases are both present together, and the absorption of each non-ionized species assists the other by stabilizing the pH of the medium at a level favourable to the diffusion of both species. Within the large intestine the anions to which this principle applies are bicarbonate (which diffuses through membranes as carbon dioxide) and the anions resulting from ionization of SCFA, predominantly acetate, propionate and butyrate. Involvement of bicarbonate in paired bicarbonate/ammonia absorption by non-ionic diffusion has been demonstrated in erythrocytes (Jacobs, 1927, 1940), *Arbacia* (sea urchin) eggs (Stewart, 1931), and the mucosa of the canine urinary bladder (Rosenfeld *et al.*, 1963). Evidence that this mechanism is operative in the large intestine is twofold: normally bicarbonate is actively secreted by the mucosa of the ileum and large intestine, but net bicarbonate secretion does not occur when ammonium ion is present within the lumen (Wrong, 1971b; Parsons and Powis, 1971) presumably because back-diffusion of carbon dioxide in company with ammonia keeps pace with the mucosal secretion of bicarbonate; in addition in rat and hamster ileum the presence of bicarbonate has been shown to increase the rate of absorption of ammonia, and vice versa (Mossberg, 1967; Mossberg and Ross, 1967; Swales *et al.*, 1970). The evidence that SCFA anion participates with ammonia in absorption by paired non-ionic diffusion is less substantial owing to present uncertainties regarding the mechanisms of SCFA absorption (Fleming and Arce, 1986), but there is considerable evidence that a component of this is by non-ionic diffusion, and Hogan (1961) has found evidence of linked SCFA/ammonia absorption in the sheep rumen.

4. *Ammonia Metabolism by the Host*

Ammonia absorbed from the alimentary tract is transported to the liver in the portal vein, in which concentrations average 200 μmol 1^{-1}, about three times as high as those in peripheral blood. Concentrations in blood draining the large intestine are higher than in other tributaries of the portal vein. An important component of portal blood ammonia is that which has been formed by bacterial deamination of amino acids and amines in the large intestine, but other nitrogen compounds are degraded by intestinal bacteria with the formation of ammonia, of which endogenous urea is the one which makes the greatest contribution to portal blood ammonia. Not all the portal blood ammonia arising in the intestine is bacterial in origin, for germ-free guinea-pigs have portal blood ammonia concentrations which are 25% of the normal values (Warren and Newton, 1959), and germ-free dogs with an Eck-fistula (porto-caval anastomosis) develop systemic hyperammonaemia (Nance and Kline, 1971; Nance *et al.*, 1974). This non-bacterial ammonia is probably derived from the metabolism of intestinal mucosal cells, for both ileum and large intestine have been shown in tissue slices and vascular perfusion studies to liberate ammonia from glutamine (Windmueller and Spaeth, 1974; Anderson *et al.*, 1976). Weber and Veach (1979) have measured the contribution of these various components to total portal ammonia in the dog, and found that one half was derived from the small intestine and could be accounted for by the disappearance of glutamine from the perfusing blood; the remainder came from the large intestine of which 9% was derived from glutamine, 42% from urea, and 49% from other sources, including mucosal ammonia derived from metabolites other than glutamine and bacterial sources other than urea.

On reaching the liver most of the ammonia in the portal blood enters the Krebs–Henseleit cycle and is converted to urea. However a proportion is made use of in hepatic synthesis of non-essential amino acids, and can also be utilized in transamination reactions to form essential amino acids from keto-acid or hydroxy-acid analogues, with the exception of lysine and threonine which cannot be formed by transamination. This minor pathway of ammonia metabolism is of major importance in the nitrogen economy of some herbivorous animals, particularly ruminants, as it enables the animal to recycle ammonia derived from urea back into tissue protein, a mechanism which has become of great commercial importance in the livestock industry, where it is standard practice to feed cattle with supplements of ammonia or urea (largely converted to ammonia in the rumen) in order to increase carcase protein (Stangel, 1967). In man this pathway becomes nutritionally important only under conditions of protein starvation or rapid growth (Sprinson and Rittenberg, 1949; Snyderman et al., 1962; Read et al., 1969), though experiments using ^{15}N-labelled ammonia have shown that ammonia nitrogen makes a contribution to albumin synthesis even in adults consuming an average protein intake (Richards et al., 1967). The role of this pathway in renal failure, and its possible therapeutic manipulation in this state are discussed in section F2).

5. *Porto-systemic Encephalopathy*

The increase in systemic blood ammonia concentrations which complicates liver failure (Conn and Lieberthal, 1979) is derived from the portal vein, either because the diseased liver is unable to remove ammonia from the portal blood perfusing it, or because portal hypertension has led to the development of venous collaterals which transmit portal blood directly into the systemic circulation. Most of the clinical measures found effective in lowering systemic blood ammonia have been those which reduce bacterial formation of ammonia in the large intestine—dietary protein restriction, avoidance of constipation, oral administration of unabsorbed antibiotics such as neomycin, and the use of various small molecular weight carbohydrates or carbohydrate alcohols (lactulose, lactitol, sorbitol) which are not digested by the enzymes of the small intestine but reach the large bowel to be fermented by the bacteria there. The story of the introduction of lactulose, the best studied member of this group, is instructive. Lactulose was originally introduced by Bircher et al. (1966) at the suggestion of Ingelfinger (1964–65) in the expectation that its presence in the large intestine would assist multiplication of acid-tolerant *Lactobacilli* and reduce the growth of 'putrefactive' bacteria responsible for ammonia formation. Subsequently its undoubted efficacy in reducing plasma ammonia was attributed to ammonia-trapping in the colon caused by the very acid reaction resulting from its fermentation (Bircher et al., 1971). However, measurement of faecal ammonia showed no increase in subjects taking lactulose (Zeegen et al., 1970; Agostini et al., 1972). Later it was appreciated that lactulose induces increased protein synthesis by intestinal bacteria (Vince et al., 1978) and that the reduced blood ammonia is the result of deviation of ammonia into the protoplasm of intestinal bacteria, with a corresponding increase in faecal nitrogen (Weber, 1979).

These mechanisms of action are not, of course, mutually exclusive, but are difficult to disentangle in clinical studies when they are acting simultaneously; for example trapping of ammonia in a more acid medium cannot easily be demonstrated when less ammonia is available because of a change in bacterial metabolism. All three mechanisms are likely to play some part in the effects of lactulose therapy, probably with other mechanisms including the effects of intestinal hurry and a more acid intestinal pH (Vince *et al.*, 1973) in reducing bacterial generation of ammonia.

F. Urea

1. *Degradation of Urea*

Several endogenous nitrogen compounds are degraded by intestinal bacteria, but the degradation of urea is particularly important in the host's nitrogen economy because of the enormous amounts which are involved. In healthy human subjects taking an average diet the mean degradation rate is 21% (range 5–90%) of the urea synthesis rate, or 56% (range 12–120%) of the urea pool per day (Wrong *et al.*, 1981). If one assumes that all the urea degraded is converted to ammonia, as appears to be the case, this rate of destruction represents an average daily production of 235 mmol of ammonia.

The general consensus that urea degradation is caused by bacterial activity in the alimentary tract is based on its virtual abolition in the rat by either evisceration (Chao and Tarver, 1953) or by rearing under germ-free conditions (Levenson *et al.*, 1959). These experiments obviously cannot be repeated in man, but here as in laboratory animals a reduction in urea degradation has been demonstrated during the feeding of unabsorbed broad-spectrum antibiotics (Walser and Bodenlos, 1959; Jones *et al.*, 1969). Urea degradation has been found in all mammals investigated, being even greater as a proportion of production in man than in herbivorous animals with well-developed foregut or hindgut fermentation chambers, especially during protein-starvation or pregnancy, two situations in which increased recycling of urea nitrogen into tissue protein is desirable. In ruminants the rumen appears to be the predominant site of destruction, urea reaching the rumen both by diffusion through the mucosa and in the copious saliva produced by such animals. In man and other animals without a foregut fermentation chamber (rumen or equivalent) there is little evidence of urea destruction proximal to the caecum except for hydrolysis of the urea in saliva (Kopstein and Wrong, 1977), which in these species is small in amount and so contributes little to total urea destruction; by exclusion the large intestine is generally regarded as the main site of destruction.

Further evidence of urea degradation in the large bowel is the virtual absence of urea from the faeces of normal subjects (Wrong *et al.*, 1965; Owens and Padovan, 1975), though it is present at close to blood levels in most other alimentary secretions including ileostomy effluent (Cummings *et al.*, 1976b; Gibson *et al.*, 1976a). When normal subjects are given unabsorbed antibiotics their faecal urea concentrations rise to plasma levels, with a fall in faecal ammonia (Wilson *et al.*, 1968a). In renal failure, when plasma urea concentrations are raised because of failure in renal excretion, faecal urea and ammonia concentrations are both increased, though the former to only a small fraction of the plasma level (Wilson *et al.*, 1968b).

Ureases which hydrolyse urea to ammonia and carbon dioxide are produced by many large bowel organisms, both aerobes and anaerobes, particularly non-sporing anaerobes, *Peptostreptococcus productus* and *Proteus* species. *P. productus* appears to be the predominant urease-producing organisms in most subjects (Vince, 1986). Bacterial ureases differ among themselves in molecular weight, pH and temperature optima, V_{max} and Michaelis constants. The pH optima of most is about 7.0, and Vince *et al.* (1973) found that urea hydrolysis by *Proteus mirabilis* was inhibited at pH values below 5.3; however the pH optimum for the urease of *Lactobacillus fermentum* is 4.0. Control of urease formation differs greatly between various groups of organisms, for *Proteus vulgaris* and some bifidobacteria continue to form urease under many different conditions, whereas in *Peptostreptococcus productus* the enzyme is repressed by ammonia and some other nitrogen compounds. Bacterial ureases can be inhibited by many analogues of urea (Reithel, 1971), one of the most promising clinically being acetohydroxamate (Fishbein *et al.*, 1965), which has been shown to inhibit urea hydrolysis by faecal incubates (Swales *et al.*, 1972) and to reduce ammonia output from the large intestine when given by mouth to intubated normal subjects (Wolpert *et al.*, 1970).

The chief unresolved problem regarding urea destruction is the exact site in the intestine where this occurs. The simple and most obvious explanations do not seem to apply. Thus, calculation of the amount of urea entering the large intestine through the ileocaecal valve, from the known volume and composition of ileal effluent, shows that the urea from this source cannot account for more than 10% of the destruction rate. The other straightforward explanation, that the urea degraded has diffused passively from the blood stream into the lumen of the large intestine, seems to be invalidated by the demonstration that the human colonic mucosa is almost impermeable to urea (Billich and Levitan, 1969;

Wolpert *et al.*, 1971; Bown *et al.*, 1975); caution is required in accepting this conclusion as these studies were performed after the colon had been cleansed of its normal content, and some substances normally present within the large intestine (bile acid anions, and hydroxy- and fatty-acid anions) have been shown to markedly increase mucosal permeability to small molecules, including urea (Dobbins and Binder, 1976; Gaginella *et al.*, 1977). In their study of mucosal urea permeability Wolpert *et al.* (1971) found that urea infused into the circulation made a greater contribution to ammonia in the large bowel than urea infused directly into the colonic lumen, and suggested from this observation that the site of urea hydrolysis might be the mucosa itself or the immediately adjacent juxta-mucosal layer of the colonic lumen. Gibson *et al.* (1976a), from a study of urea breakdown in subjects with a defunctioned large intestine, agreed that these were possibilities, but made the alternative suggestion that urea breakdown might occur mainly in the distal ileum, where the mucosa is known to have a high permeability to urea, though the bacterial population there is 10^5 times less numerous than within the large intestine. Hydrolysis either within the mucosal cell or in the juxta-mucosal zone of the large intestine both pose theoretical difficulties. If the former, how does bacterial urease, a protein of large molecular size, permeate into the mucosal cell, a barrier which is almost impermeable to the much smaller urea molecule? If the latter, how does urea from the circulation permeate into the juxta-mucosal layer despite its inability to penetrate to the main gut lumen? These problems remain unresolved; similar theoretical difficulties have been encountered by those attempting to explain urea diffusion and hydrolysis in association with the rumen mucosa (Houpt and Houpt, 1968).

2. *Urea Degradation in Renal Failure*

The degradation of endogenous urea is of interest to renal physicians both because of its possible role in uraemic toxicity and because of the theoretical possibility that the process might be modified to the advantage of the patient. On first principles the urea degradation rate might be expected to rise in parallel with the plasma urea concentration, but this does not happen in man; urea degradation rates are increased, but less so than the rise in plasma urea, and the correlation between the two variables is poor (Walser, 1974; Varcoe *et al.*, 1975). Portal blood ammonia concentrations, one indication of the rate of intestinal urea destruction, are increased in the experimental uraemia caused by partial nephrectomy in the rat (Imler and Schlienger, 1979) and in the pig when plasma urea concentrations are increased by urea feeding (Rérat *et al.*,

1979). Few observations have been made on portal ammonia in human subjects with renal failure, but Tizianello *et al.* (1980) studied four subjects with moderate renal insufficiency (plasma urea 6.8–19.1 mmol 1^{-1}) and found no increase. From studies of uraemic rats Migone *et al.* (1982) suggested that endogenous hyperaldosteronism, a frequent consequence of renal failure, might play a role in reducing the expected rise in portal blood ammonia, perhaps by stimulating colonic mucosal hydrogen/sodium exchange, and so reducing non-ionic absorption of ammonia.

Enterohepatic urea recycling occurs in health, for most of the ammonia resulting from endogenous urea hydrolysis reaches the liver and is reconverted to urea (Fig. 10.1), with a small fraction being converted into tissue protein. Any increase in urea degradation caused by renal failure would normally lead to an increase in urea recycling, but theoretically it might be possible to assist conversion of portal ammonia to tissue proteins by providing essential keto acids for transamination to the corresponding amino acids, so producing advantageous reductions in dietary protein need and urea synthesis rate (Richards *et al.*, 1967). This possibility has been the subject of much active research over the last 20 years, and has recently been reviewed by Walser (1983). Although research continues, the approach has been less rewarding than hoped, partly because urea degradation in renal failure has been less than predicted from plasma urea levels, and partly because the contribution of urea-derived ammonia to tissue protein has been less than expected (Varcoe *et al.*, 1975).

G.   Other Nitrogen Compounds

1.   *Creatinine*

No mechanism is known whereby creatinine can be degraded by mammalian tissues, and it is usually regarded as an end-product of human metabolism. However, Jones and Burnett (1974) found that 16–66% of a ^{14}C-labelled oral load, given to subjects with renal failure and raised plasma creatinine levels, was metabolized in the body and converted to many different compounds, including glycollate, creatine and exhaled carbon dioxide (Jones and Burnett, 1975). Destruction of creatinine in the body appears to be the result of bacterial activity in the large bowel. Chadwick *et al.* (1977) found in ileal perfusion studies that about 90 mg (0.8 mmol) enters the large intestine each day, derived both from dietary and endogenous sources, yet creatinine is virtually absent from normal faeces (Padovan *et al.*, 1975). When incubated with faeces creatinine is converted, by organisms not yet characterized, initially to sarcosine and thence to methylamine (Jones and Burnett, 1972; Padovan *et al.*, 1975); this pathway probably accounts for the elevated faecal levels of methylamine found in subjects with renal failure (Owens and Padovan, 1979). A strain of *Clostridium welchii* isolated from human faeces was found by Ten Krooden and Owens (1975) to deaminate creatinine by an alternative route to 1-methylhydantoin.

1-methylguanidine, a reputed uraemic toxin, might theoretically be derived from creatinine, and van Eyk *et al.* (1968) have demonstrated that a soil organism, *Pseudomonas stutzeri*, can perform this conversion *in vitro*. Rats given creatinine convert much of it to 1-methylguanidine, but its presence in this animal cannot be entirely bacterial in origin, as it is found in the urine of even germ-free animals (Perez and Faluotico, 1973).

2. Uric Acid

The tissues of mammals other than primates metabolize uric acid to allantoin, so they are poor models for man in whom this pathway does not exist. Substantial amounts of uric acid are degraded in the large intestine of birds (Barnes, 1972; Campbell and Braun, 1986), but this is an even less suitable model, as here uric acid is the main end-product of nitrogen metabolism and urinary uric acid passing down the ureters has free access to the bacteria in the large intestine by reflux from the cloaca.

In man uric acid has usually been regarded as an end-product of nitrogen metabolism, but isotopic labelling of plasma urate shows that about one third of the amount produced does not appear in the urine and is presumably destroyed in the body (Wyngaarden and Stetten, 1953; Sorenson, 1960; Sorenson and Levinson, 1975). Excretion by other routes is a theoretical possibility, but less than 1% of the amount produced is excreted in sweat, and there is no free uric acid in stool, where in these studies much of the missing isotope label was found incorporated in bacterial bodies. Chadwick *et al.* (1977) found that 100 mg (0.6 mmol) of uric acid enters the large bowel daily from the ileum, and this probably comprises a major part of the fraction which is destroyed, being degraded by intestinal bacteria.

The intestinal organisms capable of urate metabolism include *Klebsiella aerogenes*, *Proteus vulgaris*, *Pseudomonas aeruginosa* and *Clostridia* species (Rouf and Lomprey, 1968; Vogels and van der Drift, 1976; Durre and Andreesen, 1983). Allantoin, allantoic acid, urea, ammonia and carbon dioxide have been identified among the products of degradation.

3. *Other Small Molecular-Weight Compounds*

Probably all endogenous nitrogen compounds which reach the large intestine are metabolized by intestinal bacteria; the ones documented here are known to be because the amounts involved are large, or the physiological effects of the metabolic products impressive. One substance so far not mentioned is choline, which reaches the intestine from ingested food and through the bile, often as part of the lecithin molecule. The pathways of its metabolism by intestinal bacteria are not clear, but when taken by mouth it is largely metabolized to trimethylamine and its oxide, a conversion also observed when it is incubated *in vitro* with a faecal suspension (de la Huerga and Popper, 1951). Within the body trimethylamine is partly demethylated to dimethylamine, and raised plasma levels of both substances, particularly dimethylamine, occur in renal failure and may contribute to uraemic toxicity (Simenhoff, 1975).

Acknowledgments

I am grateful to the Medical Research Council (UK) for research support in connection with this work, and to Dr A. J. Vince for many fruitful discussions.

References

Adibi, S. A. and Mercer, D. W. (1973). Protein digestion in human intestine as reflected in luminal, mucosa and plasma amino acid concentration after meals. *J. Clin. Invest,* **52**, 1586–1594.

Agostini, L., Down, P. F., Murison, J. and Wrong, O. M. (1972). Faecal ammonia and pH during lactulose administration in man; comparison with other cathartics. *Gut* **13**, 859–866.

Altman, P. L. and Dittmer, D. S. (1968). "Metabolism". Federation of American Societies for Experimental Biology, Bethesda.

Anderson, I. H., Levine, A. S. and Levitt, M. D. (1981). Incomplete absorption of the carbohydrate in all-purpose wheat flour. *New Engl. J. Med.* **304**, 891–822.

Anderson, N. M., Bennett, F. I. and Alleyne, G. A. O. (1976). Ammonia production by the small intestine of the rat. *Biochim. Biophys. Acta* **437**, 238–243.

Asatoor, A. M., Chamberlain, M. J., Emmerson, B. T., Johnson, J. R., Levi, A. J. and Milne, M. D. (1967). Metabolic effects of oral neomycin. *Clin. Sci.* **33**, 111–124.

Asatoor, A. M., Craske, J., London, D. R. and Milne, M. D. (1963). Indole production in Hartnup disease. *Lancet* **i**, 126–128.

Atkinson, R. M., Atlanson, T., Baird, B. and Crofts, R. M. J. (1977). The effect of processing potatoes or the apparent digestion by pigs of organic matter and nitrogen measured overall and at the terminal ileum. *Proc. Nutr. Soc.* **36**, 58A.

Banta, C. A., Clemens, E. T., Krinsky, M. M. and Sheffy, B. E. (1979). Sites of organic acid production and patterns of digestion movement in the gastrointestinal tract of dogs. *J. Nutr.* **109**, 1593–1600.

Barker, H. A. (1981). Amino acid degradation by anaerobic bacteria. *Ann. Rev. Biochem.* **50**, 23–40.

Barnes, E. M. (1972). The avian intestinal flora with particular reference to the possible ecological significance of the caecal anaerobic flora. *Amer. J. Clin. Nutr.* **25**, 1475–1479.

Bayley, H. S., Cho, C. Y. and Holmes, J. H. G. (1974). Examination of amino acids in ileal digesta as a measure of protein digestion. *Fed. Proc.* **33**, 94–99.

Billich, C. O. and Levitan, R. (1969). Effects of sodium concentration and osmolality on water and electrolyte absorption from the intact human colon. *J. Clin. Invest.* **48**, 1336–1347.

Bircher, J., Haemmerli, U. P., Trabert, E., Lagiarder, F. and Mocetti, T. (1971). The mechanism of action of lactulose in portal-systemic encephalopathy. *Rev. Eur. Etud. Clin. Biol.* **16**, 352–357.

Bircher, J., Müller, J., Guggenheim, P. and Haemmerli, U. P. (1966). Treatment of chronic portal-systemic encephalopathy with lactulose. *Lancet* **i**, 890–893.

Bjork, J. T., Soergel, K. H. and Wood, C. M. (1976). The composition of "free" stool water. *Gastroenterology* **70**, 864.

Blackburn, T. H. (1968a). Protease production by *Bacteroides amylophilus* strain H18. *J. Gen. Microbiol.* **53**, 27–36.

Blackburn, T. H. (1968b). The protease liberated from *Bacteroides amylophilus* strain H18 by mechanical disintegration. *J. Gen. Microbiol.* **53**, 37–51.

Bourke, E., Milne, M. D. and Stokes, G. S. (1966). Caecal pH and ammonia in experimental uraemia. *Gut* **7**, 558–561.

Bown, R. L., Gibson, J. A., Fenton, J. C. B., Snedden, W., Clark, M. L. and Sladen, G. E. (1975). Ammonia and urea transport by the excluded human colon. *Clin. Sci. Molec. Med.* **48**, 279–287.

Burkitt, D. P., Walker, A. R. P. and Painter, N. S. (1972). Effect of dietary fibre on stools and transit times and its role in the causation of disease. *Lancet* **ii**, 1408–1411.

Campbell, C. E. and Braun, E. J. (1986). Caecal degradation of uric acid in Gambel quail. *Amer. J. Physiol.* **251**, R59–R62.

Carlstedt-Duke, B., Midtvedt, T., Nord, C. E. and Gustaffson, B. E. (1986). Isolation and characterization of a mucin-degrading strain of *Peptostreptococcus* from rat intestinal tract. *Acta. Path. Microbiol. Immunol. Scand.[B]* **94**, 293–300.

Cassidy, M. M., Lightfoot, F. G., Grau, L. E., Story, J. A., Kritchevsky, D. and Vahouny, G. V. (1981). The effect of chronic intake of dietary fibers on the ultrastructural topography of rat jejunum and colon: a scanning electron microscopy study. *Amer. J. Clin. Nutr.* **34**, 218–228.

Castell, D. O. and Moore, E. W. (1971). Ammonia absorption from the human colon. *Gastroenterology* **60**, 33–42.

Chadwick, V. S., Jones, J. D., Debongnie, J-C., Gaginella, T. and Phillips, S. F. (1977). Urea, uric acid and creatinine fluxes through the small intestine of man. *Gut* **18**, A944.

Challenger, F. and Charlton, P. T. (1947). Studies on biological methylation. Part X. The fission of the mono- and di-sulfide links by moulds. *J. Chem. Soc.* **1**, 424–429.

Chao, F. C. and Tarver, H. (1953). Breakdown of urea in the rat. *Proc. Soc. Exp. Biol. Med.* **84**, 406–409.

Chen, S., Zieve, L. and Mehadevan, V. (1970). Mercaptans and dimethyl sulfide in the breath of patients with cirrhosis of the liver. Effect of feeding methionine. *J. Lab. Clin. Med.* **75**, 628–635.

Clarke, E. M. W., Ellinger, G. M. and Phillipson, A. T. (1966–1967). The influence of diet on the nitrogenous components passing to the duodenum and through the lower ileum of sheep. *Proc. Roy. Soc./[Biol]* **166**, 63–79.

Clarke, R. T. J. (1977). Protozoa in the rumen ecosystem. *In*: "Microbial Ecology of the Gut" (eds R. T. J. Clarke and T. Bauchop), pp. 251–275. Academic Press, London.

Combe, E., Penot, E., Charlier, H. and Sacquet, E. (1965). Métabolisme du rat "germ-free". *Ann. Biol. Anim. Biochim. Biophys.* **5**, 189–206.

Combe, E. and Sacquet, E. (1966). Influence de l'état exénique sur divers composés azotés contenus dans la caecum de rats albinos recévant des quantités variables de protéines. *C. R. Hebed. Séances Acad. Sci. Ser.D.* **262**, 685–688.

Conn, H. O. and Lieberthal, M. H. (1979). "The Hepatic Coma Syndromes and Lactulose". Williams and Wilkins, Baltimore.

Crawford, M. A., Patterson, J. M. and Yardley, L. (1968). Nitrogen utilization by Cape buffalo (*Syncesus coffer*) and other large mammals. *In*: "Comparative Nutrition of Wild Animals" (ed. M. A. Crawford), pp. 367–379. Symposia of Zoological Society of London, No. 21, Academic Press, London.

Cummings, J. H. (1981). Dietary fibre. *Brit. Med. Bull.* **37**, 65–70.

Cummings, J. H. (1983). Fermentation in the human large intestine: evidence and implications for health. *Lancet* **i**, 1206–1208.

Cummings, J. H., Hill, M. J., Bone, E. S., Branch, W. J. and Jenkins, D. J. A. (1979). The effect of meat protein and dietary fibre on colonic function and metabolism. *Amer. J. Clin. Nutr.* **32**, 2094–2101.

Cummings, J. H., Hill, M. J., Jenkins, D. J. A., Pearson, J. R. and Wiggins, H. S. (1976a). Changes in faecal composition and colonic function due to cereal fibre. *Amer. J. Clin. Nutr.* **29**, 1468–1479.

Cummings, J. H., Milton-Thompson, G. J., Billings, J. A. and Misiewicz, J. J. (1976b). The flow rate and composition of ileal contents during fasting and in response to a liquid meal in man. *Gut* **17**, 817–818.

Dawes, E. A. and Large, P. J. (1973). Class II reactions: synthesis of small molecules. *In*: "Biochemistry of Bacterial Growth", 2nd ed (eds J. Mandelstam and K. McQuillen), pp. 202–256. Blackwells Scientific Publications, Oxford.

DeRubertis, F. R., Craven, P. A. and Saito, R. (1984). Bile salt stimulation of colonic epithelial proliferation. *J. Clin. Invest* **74**, 1614–1624.

Dixon, R. M. and Nolan, J. V. (1986). Nitrogen and carbon flows between the caecum, blood and rumen in sheep given chopped lucerne (*Medicago Sativa*) hay. *Brit. J. Nutr.* **55**, 313–332.

Dobbins, J. W. and Binder, H. J. (1976). Effects of bile salts and fatty acids on the colonic absorption of oxalate. *Gastroenterol.* **70**, 1096–1100.

Down, P. F., Agostini, L., Murison, J., and Wrong, O. M. (1972). Interrelations of faecal ammonia, pH and bicarbonate: evidence of colonic absorption of ammonia by non-ionic diffusion. *Clin. Sci.* **43**, 101–114.

Drummond, K. N., Michael, A. F., Ulstrom, R. A. and Good, R. A. (1964). The blue diaper syndrome: familial hypercalcemia with nephrocalcinosis and indicanuria. A new familial disease, with definition of the metabolic abnormality. *Amer. J. Med.* **37**, 928–948.

Ducluzeau, R., Raibaud, P., Dickinson, A., Sacquet, E. and Mocquot, G. (1966). Hydrolyse de l'urée *in vitro* et *in vivo*, dans la caecum de rats gnotobiotiques, par différentes souches bactériennes isolées du tube digestif de rats conventionnels. *C. R. Hebd. Séances Acad. Sci. Ser.D.* **262**, 944–947.

Durre, P. and Andreesen, J. R. (1983). Purine and glycine metabolism by purinolytic Clostridia. *J. Bacteriol.* **154**, 192–199.

Emonts, P., Vidon, N., Bernier, J-J. and Rambaud, J. -C. (1979). Etude sur 24 heures des flux liquidiens intestinaux chez l'homme normal par la techniques de la perfusion lente d'un marqueur non absorbable. *Gastroenterol. Clin. Biol.* **3**, 139–146.

van Eyk, H. G., Vermaat, R. J., Leijnse-Ybema, H. J. and Leijnse, B. (1968). The conversion of creatinine by creatinase of bacterial origin. *Enzymologia* **34**, 198–202.

Faichney, G. J. (1968). Volatile fatty acids in the caecum of the sheep. *Aust. J. Biol. Sci.* **21**, 177–180.

Farness, P. L. and Schneeman, B. O. (1982). Effects of dietary cellulose, pectin and oat bran on the small intestine of the rat. *J. Nutr.* **112**, 1315–1319.

Fernandez, F., Kennedy, H., Truelove, S. and Hill, M. (1983). The effect of changes in the amount of dietary protein on the composition of ileostomy fluid. *Proc. Nutr. Soc.* **42**, 108A.

Fishbein, W. N., Carbone, B. P. and Hochstein, H. D. (1965). Acetohydroxamate: bacterial urease inhibitor with therapeutic potential in hyperammonaemic states. *Nature (Lond.)* **208**, 46–48.

Fleming, S. E. and Arce, D. S. (1986). Volatile fatty acids: their production, absorption, utilization and roles in human health. *Clin. Gastroenterol.* **15**, 787–813.

Fordtran, J. S., Rector, F. C., Ewton, M. F., Soter, N. and Kinney, J. (1965). Permeability characteristics of the human small intestine. *J. Clin. Invest.* **44**, 1935–1944.

Fordtran, J. S., Scroggie, W. B. and Polter, D. E. (1964). Colonic absorption of tryptophan metabolites in man. *J. Lab. Clin. Med.* **64**, 125–132.

Forsythe, S. J. and Parker, D. S. (1985). Ammonia-nitrogen turnover in the rabbit caecum and exchange with plasma urea-N. *Brit. J. Nutr.* **54**, 285–292.

Gaginella, T. S., Chadwick, V. S., Debongnie, J. -C., Lewis, J. C. and Phillips, S. F. (1977). Perfusion of rabbit colon with ricinoleic acid: dose-related mucosal injury, fluid secretion and increased permeability. *Gastroenterol.* **73**, 95–101.

Gale, E. F. (1946). The bacterial amino acid decarboxylases. *Adv. Enzymol.* **6**, 1–32.

Gibson, J. A., Park, N. J., Sladen, G. E. and Dawson, A. M. (1976a). The role of the colon in urea metabolism in man. *Clin. Sci. Molec. Med.* **50**, 51–59.

Gibson, J. A., Sladen, G. E. and Dawson, A. M. (1976b). Protein absorption and ammonia production: the effects of dietary protein and removal of the colon. *Brit. J. Nutr.* **35**, 61–65.

Giller, J. and Phillips, S. F. (1972). Electrolyte absorption and secretion in the human colon. *Amer. J. Dig. Dis.* **17**, 1003–1011.

Glade, M. J. (1983). Nitrogen partitioning along the equine digestive tract. *J. Anim. Sci.* **57**, 943–953.

Goodall, E. D. and Kay, R. N. B. (1965). Digestion and absorption in the large intestine of the sheep. *J. Physiol. (Lond.)* **176**, 12–23.

Gorbach, S. L., Nahas, L., Weinstein, L., Levitan, R. and Patterson, J. F. (1967). Studies of intestinal microflora. IV The microflora of ileostomy effluent; a unique microbial ecology. *Gastroenterol.* **53**, 874–880.

Haughton, B. G. and King, H. K. (1961). Induced formation of leucine decarboxylase in *Proteus vulgaris. Biochem. J.* **80**, 268–277.

Hayes, M. L. and Hyatt, A. T. (1974). The decarboxylation of amino acids by bacteria derived from human dental plaque. *Arch. Oral Biol.* **19**, 361–369.

Hazlewood, G. P. and Edwards, R. (1981). Proteolytic activities of a rumen bacterium, *Bacteroides ruminicola* R8/4. *J. Gen. Microbiol.* **125**, 11–15.

Hazlewood, G. P., Jones, G. A. and Manogan, J. L. (1981). Hydrolysis of leaf fraction 1 protein by the proteolytic rumen bacterium *Bacteroides ruminicola* R8/4. *J. Gen. Microbiol.* **123**, 223–232.

Hecker, J. F. (1971). Ammonia in the large intestine of herbivores. *Brit. J. Nutr.* **26**, 135–145.

Henderson, C., Hobson, P. N. and Summers, R. (1969). The production of amylase, protease and lipolytic enzymes by two species of anaerobic rumen bacteria. *In*: "Continuous Cultivation of Microorganisms" (ed. I. Malek), pp. 189–204. Academic Press, New York.

Hespell, R. B. and Smith, C. J. (1983). Utilization of nitrogen sources by gastrointestinal tract bacteria. *In*: "Human Intestinal Flora in Health and Disease" (ed. D. J. Hentges), pp. 167–187. Academic Press, New York.

Hogan, J. P. (1961). The absorption of ammonia through the rumen of the sheep. *Aust. J. Biol. Sci.* **14**, 448–460.

Hogan, J. P. and Phillipson, A. T. (1960). The rate of flow of digesta and their removal along the digestive tract of the sheep. *Brit. J. Nutr.* **14**, 147–155.

Hoskins, L. C. and Boulding, E. T. (1981). Mucin degradation in human colon ecosystems. Evidence for the existence and role of bacterial populations producing glycosidases as extracellular enzymes. *J. Clin. Invest.* **67**, 163–172.

Houpt, T. R. and Houpt, K. A. (1968). Transfer of urea nitrogen across the rumen wall. *Amer. J. Physiol.* **214**, 1296–1312.

de la Huerga, J. and Popper, H. J. (1951). Urinary excretion of choline metabolites following choline administration in normals and patients with hepatobiliary disease. *J. Clin. Invest.* **30**, 463–470.

Hungate, R. E. (1966). "The Rumen and its Microbes". Academic Press, New York.

Imler, M. and Schlienger, G. L. (1979). The effect of chronic uremia on portal and systemic ammonia in normal and porto-strictured rats. *J. Lab. Clin. Med.* **94**, 872–878.

Ingelfinger, F. (1964–65). Editorial Comments. "Year Book of Medicine" (eds P. B. Beeson *et al.*), pp. 591–592. Year Book Medical Publishers, Chicago.

Jacobs, M. H. (1927). The exchange of material between the erythrocyte and its surroundings. *Harvey Lect.* **22**, 146–164.

Jacobs, M. H. (1940). Some aspects of cell permeability to weak electcrolytes. *Cold Spring Harbor Symp. Quant. Biol.* **8**, 30–39.

Jacobs, L. R. and Lupton, J. R. (1984). Effect of dietary fibers on rat bowel mucosal growth and cell proliferation. *Amer. J. Physiol.* **246**, G378–G385.

Johnson, I. T., Gee, J. M. and Mahoney, R. R. (1984). Effect of dietary supplements of guar gum and cellulose on intestinal cell proliferation, enzyme levels and sugar transport in the rat. *Brit. J. Nutr.* **52**, 477–487.

Johnson, K. A. (1977). The production of secondary amines by the human gut bacteria and its possible relevance to carcinogenesis. *Med. Lab. Sci.* **34**, 131–143.

Jones, E. A., Smallwood, R. A., Craigie, A. and Rosenoer, V. M. (1969). The enterohepatic circulation of urea nitrogen. *Clin. Sci.* **37**, 825–836.

Jones, J. D. and Burnett, P. C. (1972). Implication of creatinine and gut flora in the uremic syndrome: induction of "creatinase" in colon contents of the rat by dietary creatinine. *Clin. Chem.* **18**, 280–284.

Jones, J. D. and Burnett, P. C. (1974). Creatinine metabolism in humans with decreased renal functions: creatinine deficit. *Clin. Chem.* **20**, 1204–1212.

Jones, J. D. and Burnett, P. C. (1975). Creatinine metabolism and toxicity. *Kidney Int.* **7**, S294–S298.

Katz, S., Izhar, M., Ashkenazi, S., Halpern, Z. and Mirelman, D. (1982). Isolated colonic loop in the rabbit: an *in vivo* system for studying intestinal mucus. *Digestion* **24**, 98–104.

Kleiner, D. (1981). The transport of NH_3 and NH_4^+ across biological membranes. *Biochim. Biophys. Acta.* **639**, 41–52.

Knutson, R. S., Francis, R. S., Hall, J. L., Moore, B. H. and Heisinger, J. F. (1977). Ammonia and urea distribution and urease activity in the gastrointestinal tract of rabbits (*Oryctolagus* and *Sylvilagus*). *Comp. Biochem. Physiol. [A]* **58**, 151–154.

Kopstein, J. and Wrong, O. M. (1977). The origin and fate of salivary urea and ammonia in man. *Clin. Sci. Molec. Med.* **52**, 9–17.

Lepkovsky, S., Furuta, F., Ozone, K. and Koike, T. (1966). The proteases, amylase and lipase of the pancreas and intestinal contents of germ-free and conventional rats. *Brit. J. Nutr.* **20**, 257–261.

Levenson, S. M., Crowley, L. V., Horowitz, R. E. and Malm, O. J. (1959). The metabolism of carbon-labelled urea in the germ-free rat. *J. Biol. Chem.* **234**, 2061–2062.

Lewis, H., Rojas, S., Uribe, M., Galvan, E. and Gill, S. (1980). Similar effect of lactose and lactulose on *in vitro* faecal ammonia generation and bacterial flora. *Gastroenterol.* **78**, 1206.

Lupton, J. R., Coder, D. M. and Jacobs, L. R. (1985). Influence of luminal pH on rat large bowel epithelial cell cycle. *Amer. J. Physiol.* **249**, G382–G388.

MacFarlane, G. T., Cummings, J. H. and Allison, C. (1986). Protein degradation by human large intestinal bacteria. *J. Gen. Microbiol.* **132**, 1647–1656.

MacFarlane, G. T. and Englyst, H. N. (1986). Starch utilization by the human large intestinal microflora. *J. Appl. Bacteriol.* **60**, 195–201.

McNeil, N. I., Ling, K. L. E and Wager, J. (1987). Mucosal surface pH of the large intestine of the rat and of normal and inflamed large intestine in man. *Gut,* **28**, 707–713.

Magasanik, B. (1961). Catabolite repression. *Cold Spring Harbor Symp. Quant. Biol.* **26**, 249–256.

Mahadevan, S., Erfle, J. D. and Sauer, F. D. (1980). Degradation of soluble and insoluble proteins by *Bacteroides amylophilus* protease and by rumen microorganisms. *J. Anim. Sci.* **50**, 723–728.

Mason, V. C. (1974). An explanation of the effect of lactulose in the treatment of hepatic encephalopathy. *Gastroenterol.* **66**, 1271.

Mathison, G. W. and Milligan, L. P. (1971). Nitrogen metabolism in sheep. *Brit. J. Nutr.* **25**, 351–366.

Meers, J. L., Tempest, D. W. and Brown, C. M. (1970). "Glutamine (amide): 2-oxoglutarate amino transferase oxido-reductase (NADP)"; an enzyme involved in the synthesis of glutamate by some bacteria. *J. Gen. Microbiol.* **64**, 187–194.

Melville, J. (1935). Labile glutamine residues and their bearing on the origin of the ammonia set free during the enzymatic digestion of proteins. *Biochem. J.* **29**, 179–186.

Metcalfe-Gibson, A., Ing, T. S., Kuiper, J. J., Richards, P., Ward, E. E. and Wrong, O. M. (1967). *In vivo* dialysis of faeces as a method of stool analysis. II. The influence of diet. *Clin. Sci.* **33**, 89–100.

Migone, L., Bono, F. and Zanelli, P. (1982). The place of dietetic treatment in chronic renal failure (cons). *Contrib. Nephrol.* **34**, 8–21.

Milne, M. D., Asatoor, A. M, Edwards, K. D. G. and Loughridge, L. W. (1970). The intestinal absorption defect in cystinuria. *Gut* **2**, 323–337.

Milne, M. D., Scribner, B. H. and Crawford, M. A. (1958). Non-ionic diffusion and the excretion of weak acids and bases. *Amer. J. Med.* **24**, 709–729.

Moore, W. E. C. and Holdeman, L. V. (1974). Human fecal flora: the normal flora of 20 Japanese-Hawaiians. *Appl. Microbiol.* **43**, 961–979.

Morris, D. A. and Fillingame, R. H. (1974). Regulation of amino acid decarboxylation. *Ann. Rev. Biochem.* **43**, 303–325.

Mossberg, S. M. (1967). Ammonia absorption in hamster ileum: effect of pH and total CO_2 on transport in everted sacs. *Amer. J. Physiol.* **213**. 1327–1330.

Mossberg, S. M. and Ross, G. (1967). Ammonia absorption in the small intestine: preferential transport by the ileum. *J. Clin. Invest.* **46**, 490–498.

Nance, F. C., Kaufman, H. J. and Kline, D. G. (1974). The role of urea in the hyperammonaemia of germ-free eck fistula dogs. *Gastroenterol.* **66**, 108–112.

Nance, F. C. and Kline, D. G. (1971). Eck's fistula encephalopathy in germ-free dogs. *Ann. Surg.* **174**, 856–862.

Nolan, J. V., Norton, B. W. and Leng, R. A. (1976). Further studies of the dynamics of nitrogen metabolism in sheep. *Brit. J. Nutr.* **35**, 127–147.

Owens, C. W. I. and Padovan, W. (1975). Quantitative method for estimating fecal amino acids. *Clin. Chem.* **21**, 1437–1440.

Owens, C. W. I. and Padovan, W. (1976). Limitations of ultracentrifugation and *in vivo* dialysis as methods of stool analysis. *Gut* **17**, 68–74.

Owens, C. W. I. and Padovan, W. (1979). Faecal methylamine in normal and uraemic subjects. *Clin. Sci.* **56**, 509–512.

Padovan, W., Owens, C. W. I. and Ferguson, R. (1975). Creatinine and amino acid profiles of ileal and faecal fluids. *Clin. Sci. Mol. Med.* **49**, 27P.

Paigen, K. and Williams, B. (1970). Catabolite repression and other control mechanisms in carbohydrate utilization. *Adv. Microbiol. Physiol.* **4**, 251–324.

Parsons, D. S. and Powis, G. (1971). Some properties of a preparation of rat colon perfused *in vitro* through the vascular bed. *J. Physiol. (Lond.)* **217**, 641–663.

Perez, G. and Faluotico, R. (1973). Creatinine: a precursor of methyl-guanidine. *Experientia* **29**, 1473–1474.

Phillipson, A. T. (1947). The production of fatty acids in the alimentary tract of the dog. *J. Exp. Biol.* **23**, 346–349.

Pilgrim, A. F., Gray, F. V., Weller, R. A. and Belling, C. B. (1970). Synthesis of microbial protein from ammonia in the sheep's rumen and the proportion of dietary nitrogen converted into microbial nitrogen. *Brit. J. Nutr.* **24**, 589–598.

Pittman, K. A., Lakshmanan, S. and Bryant, M. P. (1967). Oligopeptide uptake by *Bacteroides ruminicola*. *J. Bacteriol.* **93**, 1499–1508.

Prizont, R. and Konigsberg, N. (1981). Identification of bacterial glycosidases in rat cecal contents. *Dig. Dis. Sci.* **26**, 773–777.

Read, W. W. C., McLaren, D. S., Tchalian, M. and Nassar, S. (1969). Studies with ^{15}N labelled ammonia and urea in the malnourished child. *J. Clin. Invest.* **48**, 1143–1149.

Rechkemmer, G., Wahl, M., Kuschinsky, W. and von Engelhardt, W. (1986). pH-Microclimate at the luminal surface of the intestinal mucosa of guinea pig and rat. *Pflüg. Arch.* **407**, 33–40.

Reithel, F. J. (1971). Ureases. *In*: "The Enzymes", 3rd ed, Vol. IV (ed. P. D. Boyer), pp. 1–21. Academic Press, New York.

Renwick, A. G. (1986). Gut bacteria and the metabolism of aromatic amino acids. *In*: "Microbial Metabolism in the Digestive Tract" (ed. M. J. Hill), pp. 107–122. CRC Press, Boca Raton, FL.

Rérat, A. (1978). Digestion and absorption of carbohydrates and nitrogenous matters in the hindgut of the omnivorous nonruminant animal. *J. Anim. Sci.* **46**, 1808–1837.

Rérat, A., Lisoprawski, C., Vaissade, P. and Vaugelade, P. (1979). Métabolisme de l'urée dans le tube digestif du porc: données préliminaires qualitatives et quantitatives. *Bull. Acad. Vét. France* **52**, 333–346.

Richards, P., Metcalfe-Gibson, A., Ward, E. E., Wrong, O. M. and Houghton, B. J. (1967). Utilization of ammonia nitrogen for protein synthesis in man, and the effect of protein restriction and uraemia. *Lancet* **ii**, 845–849.

Rosenfeld, J. B., Aboulafia, E. D. and Schwartz, W. B. (1963). Influence of non-ionic diffusion on absorption of NH_4^+ and HCO_3^- from the bladder. *Amer. J. Physiol.* **204**, 568–572.

Ross, G. A. and Mayhew, T. M. (1985). Effects of fasting on mucosal dimensions in the duodenum, jejunum and ileum of the rat. *J. Anat.* **142**, 191–200.

Rouf, M. A. and Lomprey, R. F. (1968). Degradation of uric acid by certain aerobic bacteria. *J. Bacteriol.* **96**, 617–622.

Rubinstein, R., Howard, A. V. and Wrong, O. M. (1969). *In vivo* dialysis of faeces as a method of stool analysis. IV. The organic anion component. *Clin. Sci.* **37**, 549–564.

Rübsamen, K. and Hörnicke, H. (1982). Influence of osmolality, short chain fatty acids and deoxycholic acid on mucus secretion in the rat colon. *Pflüg. Arch.* **395**, 306–311.

Sabbaj, J., Sutter, V. L. and Finegold, S. M. (1970). Urease and deaminase activities in fecal bacteria in hepatic coma. *Antimicrob. Agents Chemother.* 181–185.

Sakata, T. and Engelhardt, W. von (1983). Stimulating effect of short chain fatty acids on the epithelial cell proliferation in rat large intestine. *Comp. Biochem. Physiol.* **74A**, 459–462.

Salter, D. N., Davenshkar, K. and Smith, R. H. (1979). The origin of nitrogen incorporated into compounds in the rumen bacteria of steers given protein- and urea-containing diets. *Brit. J. Nutr.* **41**, 197–209.

Sandberg, A., Adherinne, R., Andersson, H., Hallgren, B., and Hulten, L. (1983). The effect of citrus pectin on the absorption of nutrients in the small intestine. *Hum. Nutr: Clin. Nutr.* **37C**, 171–183.

Sandberg, A., Andersson, H., Hallgren, B., Hasselblad, K. and Isaksson, B. (1981). Experimental model for *in vivo* determination of dietary fibre and its effect on the absorption of nutrients in the small intestine. *Brit. J. Nutr.* **45**, 283–294.

Sealock, R. R., Basinski, D. H. and Murlin, J. R. (1941). Apparent digestibility of carbohydrates, fats and 'indigestible residue' in whole wheat and white breads. *J. Nutr.* **22**, 589–596.

Sepúldeva, F. V. and Smith, M. W. (1979). Different mechanisms for neutral amino acid uptake by new-born pig colon. *J. Physiol. (Lond.)* **286**, 479–490.

Sigleo, S., Jackson, M. J. and Vahouny, G. V. (1984). Effects of dietary fiber constituents on intestinal morphology and nutrient transport. *Amer. J. Physiol.* **246**, G34–G39.

Simenhoff, M. L. (1975). Metabolism and toxicity of aliphatic amines. *Kidney Int.* **7**, S314–S317.

Smith, A. C. and Podolsky, D. K. (1986). Colonic mucin glycoproteins in health and disease. *Clin. Gastroenterol.* **15**, 815–837.

Smith, A. J. and Strang, L. B. (1958). An inborn error of metabolism with the urinary excretion of α-hydroxybutyric acid and phenylpyruvic acid. *Arch. Dis. Chldh.* **33**, 109–113.

Snyderman, S. E., Holt, L. E., Dancis, S. J., Roitman, E., Boyer, A. and Balis, M. E. (1962). 'Unessential' nitrogen: a limiting factor for human growth. *J. Nutr.* **78**, 57–72.

Sorensen, L. B. (1960). Elimination of uric acid in man. *Scand. J. Clin. Lab. Invest.* **12** (Suppl 54), 1–214.

Sorensen, L. B. and Levinson, D. J. (1975). Origin and extrarenal elimination of uric acid in man. *Nephron* **14**, 7–20.

Sprinson, D. B. and Rittenberg, D. (1949). The rate of utilization of ammonia for protein synthesis. *J. Biol. Chem.* **180**, 707–714.

Stangel, H. J. (1967). History of the use of urea in ruminant feeds. *In*: "Urea as a Protein Supplement" (ed. M. H. Briggs), pp. 3–32. Pergamon, Oxford.

Stephen, A. M. and Cummings, J. H. (1979). The influence of dietary fibre on faecal nitrogen excretion in man. *Proc. Nutr. Soc.* **38**, 141A.

Stephen, A. M. and Cummings, J. H. (1980). The microbial contribution to human faecal mass. *J. Med. Microbiol.* **13**, 45–56.

Stewart, D. R. (1931). The permeability of the arbacia egg to ammonium salts. *Biol. Bull.* **60**, 171–178.

Summerskill, W. H. J., Aoyagi, T. and Evans, W.B. (1966). Ammonia in the upper gastrointestinal tract of man: quantitations and relationships. *Gut* **7**, 497–501.

Summerskill, W. H. J. and Wolpert, E. (1970). Ammonia metabolism in the gut. *Amer. J. Clin. Nutr.* **23**, 633–639.

Swales, J. D., Tange, J. D. and Evans, D. J. (1972). Intestinal ammonia in uraemia: the effect of a urease inhibitor, acetohydroxamic acid. *Clin. Sci.* **42**, 105–112.

Swales, J. D., Tange, J. D. and Wrong, O. M. (1970). The influence of pH, bicarbonate and hypertonicity on the absorption of ammonia from the rat intestine. *Clin. Sci.* **39**, 769–779.

Takahashi, M., Benno, Y. and Mitsuoka, T. (1980). Utilization of ammonia nitrogen by intestinal bacteria from pigs. *Appl. Environ. Microbiol.* **39**, 30–35.

Tarlow, M. J. and Thom, H. (1974). A comparison of stool fluid and stool dialysate obtained *in vivo*. *Gut* **15**, 608–613.

Ten Krooden, E. and Owens, C. W. I. (1975). Creatinine metabolism by *Clostridium welchii* isolated from human faeces. *Experientia* **31**, 1270.

Thornton, R. F., Bird, P. R., Somers, M. and Moir, R. J. (1970). Urea excretion in ruminants. III. The role of the hindgut (caecum and colon). *Aust. J. Agric. Res.* **21**, 345–354.

Tizianello, A., de Ferrari, G., Garibotto, G., Chiggeri, G. M., Robaudo, C., Motta, G. and Nahum, M. (1980). Ammonia and amino acid metabolism by the portal-vein-drained viscera in chronic renal insufficiency. *Proc. Eur. Dial. Transplant Assoc.* **17**, 695–699.

Vahouny, G. V., Le, T., Ifrim, I., Satchithanandam, S. and Cassidy, M. M. (1985). Stimulation of intestinal cytokinetics and mucin turnover in rat fed wheat bran or cellulose. *Amer. J. Clin. Nutr.* **41**, 895–900.

Varcoe, R., Halliday, D., Carson, E. R., Richards, P. and Tavill, A. S. (1975). Efficiency of utilization of urea nitrogen for albumin synthesis by chronically uraemic and normal man. *Clin. Sci. Molec. Med.* **48**, 379–390.

Varel, V. H. and Bryant, M. P. (1974). Nutritional features of *Bacteroides fragilis*. *Appl. Microbiol.* **18**, 251–257.

Variyam, E. P. and Hoskins, L. C. (1981). Mucin degradation in human colon ecosystems. Degradation of hog gastric mucin by fecal extracts and fecal cultures. *Gastroenterol.* **81**, 751–758.

Vince, A. J. (1986). Metabolism of ammonia, urea, and amino acids, and their significance in liver disease. *In*: "Microbiol Metabolism in the Digestive Tract" (ed. M. J. Hill), pp. 83–105. CRC Press, Boca Raton, FL.

Vince, A. and Burridge, S. M. (1980). Ammonia production by intestinal bacteria: the effects of lactose, lactulose and glucose. *J. Med. Microbiol.* **13**, 177–191.

Vince, A., Dawson, A. M., Park, N. and O'Grady, F. (1973). Ammonia production by intestinal bacteria. *Gut* **14**, 171–177.

Vince, A., Down, P. J., Murison, J., Twigg, F. J. and Wrong, O. M. (1976). Generation of ammonia from non-urea sources in a faecal incubation system. *Clin. Sci. Mol. Med.* **51**, 313–322.

Vince, A., Killingley, M. and Wrong, O. M. (1978). Effect of lactulose on ammonia production in a fecal incubation system. *Gastroenterol.* **74**, 544–549.

Vogels, G. D. and van der Drift, C. (1976). Degradation of purines and pyrimidines by microorganisms. *Bacteriol. Rev.* **40**, 403–468.

Walser, M. (1974). Urea metabolism in chronic renal failure. *J. Clin. Invest.* **53**, 1385–1392.

Walser, M. (1983). Nutrition in renal failure. *Ann. Rev. Nutr.* **3**, 125–154.

Walser, M. and Bodenlos, L. J. (1959). Urea metabolism in man. *J. Clin. Invest.* **38**, 1617–1626.

Warren, K. S. and Newton, W. L. (1959). Portal and peripheral blood ammonia concentrations in germ-free and conventional guinea pigs. *Amer. J. Physiol.* **197**, 717–720.

Weber, F. L. (1979). The effect of lactulose on urea metabolism and nitrogen excretion in cirrhotic patients. *Gastroenterol.* **77**, 518–523.

Weber, F. L. and Veach, G. H. (1979). The importance of the small intestine in gut ammonium production in the fasting dog. *Gastroenterol.* **77**, 235–240.

Wilson, D. R., Ing, T. S., Metcalfe-Gibson, A. and Wrong O. M. (1968a). *In vivo* dialysis of faeces as a method of stool analysis. III. The effect of intestinal antibiotics. *Clin. Sci.* **34**, 211–221.

Wilson, D. R., Ing, T. S., Metcalfe-Gibson, A. and Wrong, O. M. (1968b). The chemical composition of faeces in uraemia, as revealed by *in vivo* faecal dialysis. *Clin. Sci.* **35**, 197–209.

Wilson, G. S. and Miles, A. (1975). *In*: "Topley and Wilson's Principles of Bacteriology, Virology and Immunity", Chap. 3. Arnold, London.

Windmueller, H. G. and Spaeth, A. E. (1974). Uptake and metabolism of plasma glutamine by the small intestine. *J. Biol. Chem.* **249**, 5070–5079.

Wolpert, E., Phillips, S. F. and Summerskill, W. H. J. (1970). Ammonia production in the human colon. Effects of cleansing, neomycin and acetohydroxamic acid. *New Engl. J. Med.* **283**, 159–164.

Wolpert, E., Phillips, S. F. and Summerskill, W. H. J. (1971). Transport of urea and ammonia production in the human colon. *Lancet* **ii**, 1387–1390.

Wrong, O. M. (1971a). Intestinal handling of urea and ammonia. *Proc. Roy. Soc. Med.* **64**, 1025–1026.

Wrong, O. M. (1971b). The role of the human colon in homeostasis. *Sci. Basis Med. Annu. Rev.* pp. 192–215. Athlone Press, London.

Wrong, O. and Davies, H. E. F. (1959). The excretion of acid in renal disease. *Quart. J. Med.* **28**, 259–313.

Wrong, O. M., Edmonds, C. J. and Chadwick, V. S. (1981). "The Large Intestine. Its Role in Mammalian Nutrition and Homeostasis". MTP Press, Lancaster.

Wrong, O., Metcalfe-Gibson, A., Morrison, R. B. I., Ng, S. T. and Howard, A. V. (1965). *In vivo* dialysis of faeces as a method of stool analysis. I. Technique and results in normal subjects. *Clin. Sci.* **28**, 357–375.

Wrong, O. M., Vince, A. J. and Waterlow, J. C. (1984). The contribution of endogenous urea to faecal ammonia in man, determined by ^{15}N labelling of plasma urea. *Clin. Sci.* **68**, 193–199.

Wyngaarden, J. B. and Stetten, D. (1953). Ureolysis in normal man. *J. Biol. Chem.* **203**, 9–21.

Yoshida, T., Pleasants, J. R., Reddy, B. S. and Wostmann, B. S. (1968). Efficiency of digestion in germ-free and conventional rabbits. *Brit. J. Nutr.* **22**, 723–737.

Zeegen, R., Drinkwater, J. E., Fenton, J. C. B., Vince, A. and Dawson, A. M. (1970). Some observations on the effect of treatment with lactulose on patients with chronic hepatic encephalopathy. *Quart. J. Med.* **39**, 245–263.

11

Metabolism of Fats, Bile Acids and Steroids

H. EYSSEN and PH. CAENEPEEL

A. Metabolism of Fats

Intestinal lipids originate from endogenous lipids, dietary fats and microbial fatty acids. The effect of the microflora on fat absorption in mammals is controversial, although most studies indicate that the digestibility of fat might be slightly less efficient in conventional animals than in germ-free animals (Demarne *et al.*, 1970, 1982; Coates, 1984). Studies by Cummings *et al.* (1978) showed that in healthy young men high dietary intake of fat did not alter the faecal microflora, including the nuclear dehydrogenating *Clostridia*, although total faecal fatty acid and bile acid excretion was significantly higher.

In contrast to the limited effects on absorption of fat from the small intestine in healthy individuals, microbial contributions to the faecal fatty acid pattern are apparent from the significant differences observed between germ-free and conventional animals (Eyssen and Parmentier, 1979; Demarne *et al.*, 1979). Microbial biohydrogenation of unsaturated long-chain fatty acids has been studied extensively. The transformation of linoleic acid (18 : 2; 9-*cis*, 12-*cis*) proceeds via isomerization of the 12-*cis* double bond to an 11-*trans* double bond followed by biohydrogenation of the 9-*cis* double bond to yield transvaccenic acid (18 : 1; 11-*trans*). Many intestinal bacteria follow this particular pathway *in vivo* and *in vitro*, e.g. *Eubacterium lentum* (Eyssen and Verhulst, 1984), *Clostridium bifermentans*, *Clostridium sporogenes*, *Clostridium sordellii*, *Propionibacterium* and *Bacteroides* (Verhulst *et al.*, 1985, 1986, 1987). *E. lentum* and *Propionibacterium* also isomerized or saturated *cis*-double bonds in several other polyunsaturated fatty acids, e.g. in the linolenic acids (18 : 3) and in arachidonic acid (20 : 4). The effects, if any, of these *trans*-fatty acids on structure and function of the large intestine were not studied.

Biohydrogenation of (poly)unsaturated C-18 fatty acids into saturated stearic acid has been observed in the large bowel and in the rumen.

Rumen bacteria were shown to form, or to co-operate in the formation of, stearic acid from a variety of unsaturated fatty acids (Kemp *et al.*, 1984a,b). Although bacteria producing stearic acid from unsaturated precursors are probably present in the mammalian large intestine, pure cultures of these microorganisms have not yet been isolated. Conversion of oleic acid (18 : 1; 9-*cis*) into stearic acid (18 : 0) in rat caecum could also be the result of the concerted action of bacteria acting via the 10-hydroxystearic acid pathway (Eyssen and Parmentier, 1979). Hydration of oleic acid to produce 10-hydroxystearic acid seems to be a widely distributed property of the intestinal flora. *Bacteroides*, *Bifidobacterium*, *Clostridium*, *Streptococcus faecalis* and enterobacteria were shown to perform this reaction (Thomas, 1972; Pearson *et al.*, 1974). In contrast, the intestinal bacteria converting 10-hydroxystearic acid into stearic acid have not yet been identified.

Conventional rats also excrete significant amounts of the so-called 'bacterial' fatty acids, e.g. branched chain fatty acids (even- and odd-numbered, iso- and ante-iso). Demarne *et al.* (1979) showed that odd-numbered fatty acids (from 11 : 0 to 21 : 0) represented 6.5% of the total faecal fatty acids in conventional rats versus 1.5% in germ-free rats, both groups being on a lipid-free diet. Branched-chain fatty acid concentrations amounted to 12.9% of the faecal fatty acids in conventional rats versus 2.0% in germ-free rats. These bacterial fatty acids apparently do not influence the main characteristics of fatty acids from body and liver lipids (Demarne and Sacquet, 1981). Surprisingly, the co-mutagenic effects of these potentially toxic fatty acids apparently have not been studied. Nevertheless, these mostly cellular bacterial fatty acids are real fingerprints of the 400 or more microbial species living in the large intestine.

B. Microbial Transformation of Steroid Hormones

Many natural and synthetic steroids (Fig. 11.1) are conjugated with sulphuric or glucuronic acid prior to excretion in urine or in bile. In the intestine, these steroids are deconjugated by sulphatases or glucuronidases of endogenous or bacterial origin and are transformed by the microflora into a wide variety of metabolites by oxidation–reduction reactions at hydroxyl and oxo-groups, by hydroxylation or dehydroxylation, nuclear dehydrogenation, degradation of the side chain, etc. (Fig. 11.2). Thus, the enzymes of intestinal bacteria affect hormonal activity and bioavailability of steroids and their metabolites. Although most of these activities were originally demonstrated in the rat, they have subsequently been shown to occur in the human gut. Apart from altering the quantities and the pattern of steroid metabolites in the large intestine, the microflora can act in an indirect way by affecting liver metabolism of steroids. Einarsson *et al.* (1973) and Gustafsson *et al.* (1975), for example, showed that hepatic microsomal hydroxylation of steroid hormones proceeded more efficiently in liver preparations from germ-free rats than in those from conventional rat liver. Many basic studies on steroid hormone metabolites in bile and in faeces were carried out at the end of the 1960s and early in the 1970s. A review of that work was presented by Taylor (1971). The more recent data have been reviewed by Adlercreutz and Martin (1980), Gustafsson (1982), Macdonald *et al.* (1983), Bokkenheuser and Winter (1983), Simon and Gorbach (1984) and Adlercreutz *et al.* (1984).

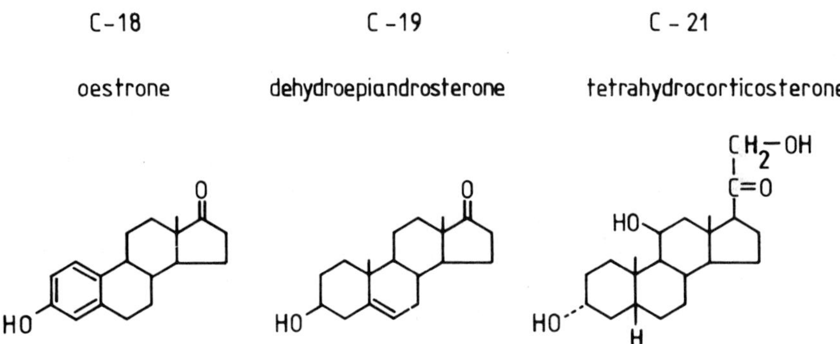

Fig 11.1. Types of steroids. Oestrone represents a phenolic C-18 steroid. Dehydroepiandrosterone represents C-19 steroids. Tetrahydrocorticosterone represents C-21 steroids from the adrenal cortex.

1. *Oxidation–Reduction and Epimerization Reactions in Ring-A*

Saturated 3-hydroxylated steroids can be oxidized by the intestinal microflora to yield the 3-oxo or the $\triangle^4$-3-oxo derivatives; conversely, 3-oxo-and $\triangle^4$-3-oxo steroids can be reduced to yield 3α- or 3β-hydroxylated steroids. According to Bokkenheuser and Winter (1983), strains of *E. lentum* convert 3α-hydroxysteroids to the 3β-hydroxy epimers, presumably via the 3-oxo intermediates. In the conditions prevailing in the intestine the predominant reactions are reductive and can be carried out by a number of intestinal bacteria, e.g. *Clostridium paraputrificum* (3α,5β-reductase), *Clostridium innocuum* (3α,5β-reductase) and *Clostridium J-1* (3β,5α-reductase), as was shown by Bokkenheuser *et al.* (1983). The intestinal microflora can therefore alter the biological activity of the hormones, e.g. by inactivation of natural or synthetic progestins such as progesterone norethindrone, dimethisterone or norgestrol (Bokkenheuser *et al.*, 1983).

Medroxyprogesterone acetate (17-acetoxy-6α-methyl-4-pregnene-3,20-dione) was readily reduced by cultures of human faecal bacteria to the saturated dihydro and tetrahydro derivatives (Martin *et al.*, 1980). Owen and Bilton (1985) incubated ring-A unsaturated 12β-hydroxyandrosta-1,4-diene-3,17-dione with suspensions of human faecal bacteria and obtained a mixture of the four possible 3,12-dihydroxy isomers of 5β-androstane-17-one with a fully reduced ring-A structure. Similarly, 12α-hydroxy-3-oxo-1,4-pregnadiene-20-carboxylic acid was converted to the corresponding 3,12-dihydroxybisnor acid by reduction of the double bonds in ring-A and the 3-oxo group.

2. Oxidation–Reduction Reactions in Ring-D

Järvenpää *et al.* (1980) studied the reduction of the 17-oxo group of phenolic steroids by incubating oestrone, oestradiol and 16α-hydroxyoestrone with pure cultures of intestinal bacteria or with suspensions of human faecal bacteria. *Alcaligenes faecalis*, *Pseudomonas aeruginosa* and *Staphylococcus aureus* reversibly converted oestrone to the biologically more active oestradiol. Reduction of oestrone to oestradiol by *Bacteroides fragilis* was irreversible, whereas *Streptococcus faecalis* converted oestradiol to oestrone. The latter microorganism also converted oestrone to 16α-hydroxyoestrone. Similar conversions were performed by *E. lentum*, *Cl. paraputrificum*, *Clostridium J-1* and *Cl. innocuum* (Winter *et al.*, 1984a). Incubates of human faeces reduced 16α-hydroxyoestrone to oestriol and 15α-hydroxyoestrone to 15α-hydroxyoestradiol, respectively (Järvenpää *et al.*, 1980).

3. Reactions in the Side Chain

Eriksson *et al.* (1969) first demonstrated that a C-21 steroid such as 3β,21-dihydroxy-5α-pregnane-20-one was 21-dehydroxylated to yield pregnane-3,20-diol when incubated with suspensions of caecal micro-organisms from conventional rats. These experiments provided an explanation for the finding that the predominant steroids in faeces from germ-free rats showed a 21-hydroxyl group, whereas only very low levels of 21-hydroxylated steroids were identified in faeces from conventional rats (Gustafsson, 1968). These reactions have now been studied in more detail and the intestinal micro-organisms which carry out the conversions have been

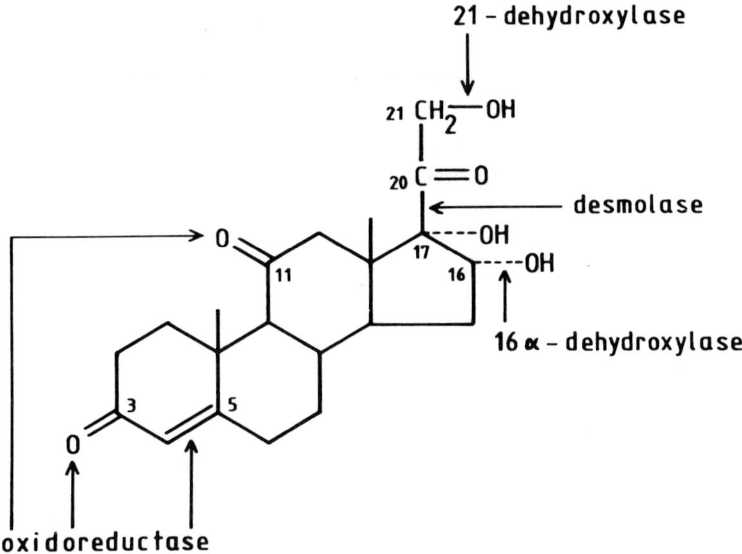

Fig 11.2 Structures of corticoids susceptible to bacterial transformations.

isolated. Bokkenheuser *et al.* (1977), Winter and Bokkenheuser (1978) and Feighner and Hylemon (1980) showed that 21-hydroxycorticoids, such as corticosterone, deoxycorticosterone and 11-dehydrocorticosterone, were 21-dehydroxylated by certain strains of *E. lentum*. The transformation was effectively prevented by a hydroxyl group at C-20.

Intestinal bacteria phenotypically similar to *E. lentum* were found to be capable of 16α-dehydroxylation of ring-D and isomerization of the side chain from the 17β- to the 17α-configuration, converting 16α-hydroxyprogesterone into isoprogesterone and 16α-hydroxypregnanolone into isopregnanolone (Bokkenheuser *et al.*, 1980, 1981; Winter *et al.*, 1982a; Glass and Burley, 1984). A 20-hydroxysteroid dehydrogenase with a narrow spectrum of activity and forming 20β-dihydrosteroids was produced by *B. fragilis* (Bokkenheuser *et al.*, 1975), and an enzyme with a similar activity but with a broader substrate specificity was found in strains of *Bifidobacterium adolescentis* isolated from the faecal flora of humans and rats (Winter *et al.*, 1982b, 1984c).

Clostridium scindens, recently isolated from human faeces, synthesizes several steroid active enzymes, among which is a desmolase which cleaves the side chain of 17-hydroxylated C-21 steroids such as cortisol and 17α-hydroxyprogesterone to yield the respective 17-oxo derivatives of the C-19 steroids formed (Bokkenheuser *et al.*, 1984; Winter *et al.*, 1984b). The same species produced a 20α-hydroxysteroid dehydrogenase, active at very low E_h (-300 mV) and reducing the 20-oxo group to a 20α-hydroxyl group regardless of the presence or absence of a 17-hydroxyl group (Winter *et al.*, 1984b). Recently, Morris *et al.* (1986) isolated from cat faeces *Eubacterium desmolans sp. nov.* This micro-organism produced steroid desmolase and 20β-hydroxysteroid dehydrogenase.

4. *Intestinal Microbial Steroid Sulphatase Activity*

The characteristics and biological roles of steroid sulphohydrolases of microbial origin were extensively reviewed by Dodgson *et al.* (1982a,b). In general, microbial steroid sulphatase and glucuronidase activities in the intestine tend to increase the enterohepatic circulation of steroids. Free oestrone is much more easily reabsorbed in the small intestine than are the 3-sulphate or 3-glucuronide derivatives (Sim and Back, 1985, 1986), and absorption of oestrone-3-sulphate from intestinal loops was found to proceed more efficiently in conventional rats than in germ-free rats (Sim *et al.*, 1983). Studies in our laboratory confirmed that orally administered oestrone-3-sulphate was more completely absorbed and less rapidly excreted by gnotobiotic rats associated with an oestrone-desulphating microflora than by gnotobiotic control rats without desulphating flora (Van Eldere *et al.*, 1987). The results of these investigations are in agreement with the observation that endogenous oestrone-3-sulphatase activity is very low in the small intestine and caecum of germ-free rats (Huijghebaert *et al.*, 1984).

The steroid-3-sulphatase producing anaerobic bacteria used in these studies on gnotobiotic rats were initially isolated from the rat for their bile salt sulphatase activity (Huijghebaert and Eyssen, 1982; Robben *et al.*, 1986) or iodothyronine sulphatase activity (de Herder *et al.*, 1985). These micro-organisms, termed *Clostridium* S_1, *Clostridium* S_2 and *strain* R_9. also hydrolysed 17β-oestradiol-3-sulphate but not oestradiol-17-sulphate or the 3-sulphates of compounds of the androstane or pregnane series. Steroid sulphohydrolases were also produced by bacteria isolated from human faeces. As is shown in Table 11.1, *Peptostreptococcus productus* and *Eubacterium cylindroides* hydrolysed oestrone-3-sulphate and 17β-oestradiol-3-sulphate but had no effect on 17β-oestradiol-17-sulphate or on the 3-sulphates of several androstane(ene) or pregnane(ene) steroids. *Peptococcus niger* produced sulphatases with a wide spectrum of activity including dehydroepiandrosterone sulphate (5-androstene-3β-ol-17-one-3-sulphate), a major steroid in human plasma; 17β-oestradiol-17-sulphate was not desulphated. These anaerobic cocci were only weakly active towards bile acid 3-sulphates.

Table 11.1 *Desulphation and deglucuronidation by pure cultures of anaerobic intestinal bacteria*

Substrates	Micro-organisms[a]					
	Clostridium S_1	Clostridium S_2	Clostridium R_9	E. cylindroides	P. niger	P. productus
Aryl sulphates						
Oestrone 3-sulphate	+	+	+	+	+	+
17β-oestradiol 3-sulphate	+	+	+	+	+	+
17β-oestradiol 17-sulphate	−	−	−	−	−	−
Oestriol 3-sulphate	tr	tr	tr	tr	tr	tr
Alkyl sulphates						
5-androstene-3β-ol-17-one 3-sulphate	−	−	−	−	+	−
5α-androstane-3β-ol-17-one 3-sulphate	−	−	−	−	+	−
5α-androstane-3α-ol-17-one 3-sulphate	−	−	−	−	+	−
5β-androstane-3α-ol-17-one 3-sulphate	nt	nt	nt	nt	+	nt
5α-pregnane-3β-ol-20-one 3-sulphate	−	−	−	−	+	−
5-pregnene-3β-ol-20-one 3-sulphate	−	−	−	−	+	−
Synthetic sulphate esters						
Paranitrocatechol sulphate	+	+	−	+	+	+
Paranitrophenol sulphate	+	+	−	+	+	+
Phenolphthalein disulphate	+	+	−	+	+	−
Glucuronide conjugates						
Oestrone 3-glucuronide	−	−	−	−	−	+
17β-oestradiol 17-glucuronide	nt	nt	nt	nt	nt	+
5α-androstane-3α-ol-17-one 3-glucuronide	−	−	−	−	−	+
5β-pregnane-3β,20-diol 3-glucuronide	nt	nt	nt	nt	nt	+
Cholic acid 3-glucuronide	nt	nt	nt	nt	nt	+
Phenolphthalein monoglucuronide	nt	nt	nt	nt	nt	+

[a] *Clostridium* species S_1, S_2 and R_9 were isolated from the rat; *Eubacterium cylindroides*, *Peptococcus niger* and *Peptostreptococcus productus* were isolated from human faeces.
tr, trace amounts, less than 15% transformed; nt, not tested; +, more than 15% transformed.

Eriksson and Gustafsson (1970) showed that caecal contents of conventional rats extensively desulphated corticosterone-21-sulphate and testosterone-17-sulphate. Similarly, Casey and MacDonald (1982) observed that deoxycorticosterone-21-sulphate was desulphated and 21-dehydroxylated in the human intestine to yield progesterone and metabolites thereof. At present, however, pure strains of steroid 17- or 21-sulphatase-producing intestinal bacteria have not yet been reported.

5. *Intestinal Microbial Steroid Glucuronidase Activity*

Extensive glucuronidation of steroids occurs in the liver, in the intestinal wall and in several other tissues (see a series of reports in Matern *et al.* (1985). The polar steroid glucuronides excreted in the bile are usually not reabsorbed well from the intestine, unless they are hydrolysed by glucuronidases produced both by the host and by the microflora. Musey *et al.* (1972), for instance, observed that biliary oestradiol-3-sulphate-17-glucuronide was deconjugated in the intestine prior to reabsorption and reconjugation at C-3 by endogenous glucuronyl transferases. Surprisingly, the effect of specific intestinal bacteria on the absorption of steroid glucuronides has not been studied extensively. Graef *et al.* (1977) reported hydrolysis of steroid glucuronides by *Escherichia coli.* Sim and Back (1985, 1986) studied the absorption of oestrone glucuronide in rats and provided evidence that efficient absorption from the small intestine required hydrolysis by mammalian or microbial enzymes, although part of the oestrone glucuronide was absorbed intact. Recently we isolated from human faeces a strain of *P. productus* producing β-glucuronidase active against, for example, oestrone-3-glucuronide, oestradiol-17-glucuronide and cholic acid-3-glucuronide (Table 11.1).

Many studies on intestinal microbial β-glucuronidases have been carried out with non-steroidal substrates, such as, for example, phenolphthalein monoglucuronide or *p*-nitrophenyl-β-D-glucuronide. A wide variety of aerobic and anaerobic intestinal bacteria have been shown to produce β-glucuronidases hydrolysing these substrates (see the review by Larsen, Chapter 4), but their activity against steroidal substrates has received scant attention.

6. *Conclusions*

It is not well understood why so many endogenous steroids and their microbially formed derivatives undergo enterohepatic circulation.

Although bacterial reduction may increase the biological activities of oestrogens, most steroid derivatives formed are devoid of significant hormonal activity and the hormonal function is usually not restored by the host. That these compounds possess biological activities (e.g. toxicity or carcinogenicity) different from the precursor molecules seems to be the exception rather than the rule, and very little is known about the tumour-promoting potential of these products of bacterial transformations in the intestine. However, epidemiological and metabolic studies suggest that gut bacterial metabolism of oestrogens might play an important role in the aetiology of breast cancer (see the review by Hill, Chapter 18).

C. Metabolism of Neutral Sterols

In studies on germ-free and conventional rats Wostmann *et al.* (1966) and Ukai *et al.* (1976) observed that the synthesis and catabolism of cholesterol were markedly accelerated in conventional animals. In addition, intestinal bacteria seem to interfere with the absorption of cholesterol from the intestine (see the review by Van Eldere and Eyssen (1984)).

Oxidation–reduction reactions at the 3-hydroxyl group and hydrogenation of the $\triangle^5$-double bond of cholesterol and other $\triangle^5$-sterols are well known microbial activities in the mammalian caecum and colon. Intestinal bacteria convert cholesterol (5-cholestene-3β-ol) to coprostanol (5β-cholestane-3β-ol) or coprostanone (5β-cholestane-3-oxo). A cholesterol-reducing micro-organism was isolated from rat faeces by Eyssen *et al.* (1973). This strictly anaerobic unnamed *Eubacterium* species ATCC 21408 required high levels of cholesterol or unsaturated plant sterols in the culture medium and reduction proceeded via a $\triangle^4$-3-oxo intermediate (Parmentier and Eyssen, 1974). Related *Eubacterium* species, some of which could be grown in the absence of sterols, were isolated from the faeces of man, the baboon and the rat by Sadzikowski *et al.* (1977), Mott *et al.* (1980) and Brinkley *et al.* (1982). Growth of the cholesterol-reducing *Eubacterium* and formation of coprostanol were inhibited at pH values below 6.5 as were obtained in the caecum of rats fed a diet rich in lactose (Eyssen *et al.*, 1974). A similar mechanism could explain, at least partly, the inhibitory effect that certain types of diet, e.g. high intake of milk, have on the conversion of cholesterol to coprostanol in the human colon.

Although the pattern of the faecal neutral sterols were determined in several studies on the correlations between diet, colon cancer and microbial production of co-mutagens in the intestine, hard data supporting the hypothesis that production of coprostanol, epicoprostanol or coprostanone might be causally related to colon cancer in man are not available. Cholesterol was shown to potentiate the carcinogenic activity of dimethylhydrazine in rats; animals fed a cholesterol-free chemically defined diet survived longer and had a lower incidence of metastases than control rats fed the cholesterol-containing diet (Cruse *et al.*, 1978). In contrast, Raicht *et al.* (1980) reported a protective effect of plant sterols against *N*-methyl-*N*-nitrosourea induced colon tumours in rats. Conversions involving the steroid nucleus as well as the side chain of cholesterol and β-sitosterol were reported to take place during incubation with *Pseudomonas* sp. NCIB 10590, or with *E. coli*, under aerobic conditions (Owen *et al.*, 1978, 1983b, 1985). Whether similar reactions occur in the deeply anaerobic colonic contents remains to be established. The epoxide of cholesterol was shown to possess *in vitro* cell transforming activity and was tumorigenic in animals (Kelsey and Pienta, 1979). By hydrolysis, cholesterol epoxide yields cholestane-3β,5α,6β-triol, and both compounds are found in human faeces (Rosemarin *et al.*, 1983).

D. Metabolism of Acidic Steroids

Primary bile acids synthesized in the liver are partially converted into *secondary bile acids* by microbial enzymes in the intestine (Fig. 11.3). The major transformations are deconjugation, oxidation–reduction reactions at the hydroxyl groups, dehydroxylation, desulphation, deglucuronidation, and nuclear dehydrogenation. These microbial activities give rise to a large number of metabolites, some of which are reabsorbed and further transformed in the liver yielding either the original primary bile acids or the *tertiary bile acids* of hybrid origin. Studies on microbial transformations of bile acids were recently reviewed by Macdonald *et al.* (1983), Hylemon and Glass (1983), and Eyssen and Van Eldere (1984).

1. *Deconjugation, Dehydrogenation, Epimerization and Dehydroxylation*

Glycine or taurine conjugated bile acids are more than 80% deconjugated by a variety of bacteria in the colon, e.g. *Bacteroides*, *Clostridium*, *Eubacterium*, *Bifidobacterium*, *Lactobacillus*, *Streptococcus* and several more species.

Bile acid dehydrogenases are produced by many bacteria, and the oxidation–reduction reactions at the hydroxyl groups give rise to a variety of metabolites, since the oxo-groups formed can be reduced by the same or by other bacteria to yield the β- as well as the α-hydroxylated epimers.

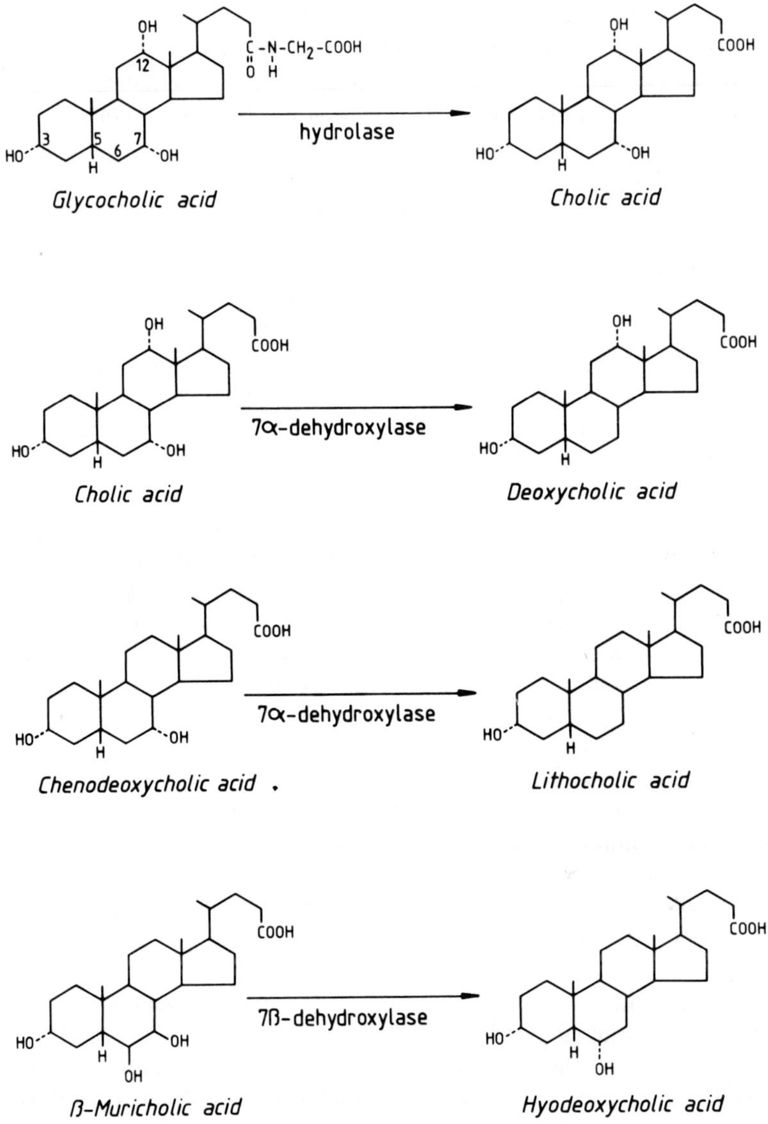

Fig 11.3 Examples of transformation of bile acids by enzymes of intestinal bacteria.

The conditions prevailing in the human colon promote reduction. The activity is found in the major population groups of the intestinal ecosystem, e.g. *Bacteroides*, *Eubacterium*, *Clostridium*, *Bifidobacterium*, *Lactobacillus*, *Peptococcus*, *Fusobacterium* and *E. coli*.

The 7β-hydroxyl group of ursodeoxycholic acid is susceptible to 7β-hydroxysteroid dehydrogenases elaborated by *Clostridium absonum*, *Peptostreptococcus productus* and *Eubacterium aerofaciens* (Macdonald and Roach, 1981; Hirano and Masuda, 1982). Interconversion of chenodeoxycholic and ursodeoxycholic acid has been observed in cultures of faecal bacteria and might proceed via formation of a 7-oxo intermediate (Fedorowski *et al.*, 1979; Hirano *et al.*, 1981b; Edenharder and Knaflic, 1981; Macdonald *et al.*, 1982; Edenharder, 1984).

Conversion of 12-oxo bile acids to the respective 12β-hydroxyl derivatives was shown to be performed by cultures of *Cl. paraputrificum*, *Clostridium tertium* and *Clostridium difficile* (Edenharder and Schneider, 1985). Similarly, the 6-hydroxyl groups of the muricholic acids in the gut of mice and rats can be epimerized by bacterial enzymes converting β-muricholate (3α,6β,7β-trihydroxy) into Ω-muricholate (3α,6α,7β-trihydroxy), and micro-organisms, performing these reactions have been described (Sacquet *et al.*, 1979; Eyssen *et al.*, 1983; Robben *et al.*, 1986).

A $\triangle^4$-double bond can be introduced in ring-A by so-called nuclear dehydrogenating bacteria, yielding products with a 3-oxo-4-ene structure. Several *Clostridium* species, e.g. strains of *Cl. paraputrificum*, *Cl. tertium* and *Cl. butyricum*, performed this reaction *in vitro* under anaerobic conditions and with added menadione as the electron acceptor (Owen, 1985). The 3-oxo-4-ene products are rarely detected in faeces, presumably because their appearance is only transient.

Bile acids can be dehydroxylated by the intestinal microflora. Dehydroxylation at C-3 has been demonstrated in cultures of faecal bacteria (Kelsey *et al.*, 1980; Borriello and Owen, 1982), but pure cultures of intestinal bacteria performing this reaction have not been described. 12-Dehydroxylation of cholate to chenodeoxycholate has been reported to occur transiently in freshly isolated cultures of human intestinal *Bacteroides* species (Edenharder, 1984). The 7α-hydroxyl group is prone to dehydroxylation by microbial enzymes and production of deoxycholic acid from cholic acid, and of lithocholic acid from chenodeoxycholic acid, is a common microbial activity in the mammalian intestine. Several strictly anaerobic bacteria, the majority of which belong to the genus *Clostridium* or *Eubacterium*, can perform the reaction (Midtvedt, 1967; Hirano *et al.*, 1981a). Intestinal strains of *Eubacterium* were reported to convert ursodeoxycholic acid into lithocholic acid by 7β-dehydroxylation (Hirano and Masuda, 1982; White *et al.*, 1982). However, as mentioned before, ursodeoxycholate can be epimerized to chenodeoxycholate which is a good substrate for the 7α-dehydroxylating bacteria. None of the 7-dehydroxylating bacteria discussed so far has been shown to be capable of 7-dehydroxylation of β-muricholic acid (3α,6β,7β-trihydroxy), α-muricholic acid (3α,6β,7α-trihydroxy) or Ω-muricholic acid (3α,6α,7β-trihydroxy) to yield hyodeoxycholic acid (3α,6α-dihydroxy) which is the predominating faecal bile acid in conventional rats. Recently such a micro-organism was isolated from rat faeces by Eyssen *et al.* (1985a).

The occurrence of 7-dehydroxylation of chenodeoxy- and ursodeoxy-cholic acid in the human colon is a matter of concern because the lithocholate formed is significantly more toxic than the parent compounds (Palmer, 1972). Lithocholic acid was reported to act as a co-mutagen and to be a potent promotor of colonic cancer (see below). Lithocholic acid and lithocholate-3-sulphate can be further converted by intestinal bacteria to isolithocholate or its 3β-palmitoyl derivative, and to 5β-cholanic acid and $\triangle^3$-cholenic acid by so far unidentified micro-organisms (Kelsey *et al.*, 1980; Borriello and Owen, 1982). It also should be noted that Owen and Bilton (1983) and Owen *et al.* (1983a) showed that *Pseudomonas* sp. NCIB 10590 converted cholic and chenodeoxycholic acid under anaerobic conditions yielding a number of neutral and acidic C-24, C-22 and C-19 metabolites, some of which possessed a 4,6-dienone structure. Whether similar reactions can be carried out by micro-organisms belonging to the indigenous intestinal microflora is not known, and the mutagenic potential of these types of derivatives remains to be investigated.

Although less toxic than lithocholic acid, high levels of deoxycholic acid can cause histological damage to the intestinal mucosa and promote colonic motility in rabbits; in the same test cholic acid was not toxic (Falconer *et al.*, 1980). In rats, deoxycholic acid caused mucosal injury and increased permeability of the mucosa of the small intestine while cholic acid or deoxycholic acid-3-sulphate had no such effects (Ammon *et al.*, 1985).

2. *Desulphation and Deglucuronidation*

In healthy man, absorbed lithocholate is extensively sulphated in the liver yielding lithocholate-3-sulphate (Palmer, 1972). Sulphation of bile acids is not well understood and is species- and sex-dependent. Mice produce cholate-7-sulphate, which undergoes little or no desulphation by the microflora (Eyssen *et al.*, 1976). In the rat, bile acids are sulphated at the 3-hydroxyl group, allo-bile salts are preferred substrates and sulphation is more pronounced in female rats (Parmentier *et al.*, 1981). Hence, hepatic enzymes catalysing the formation of bile acid sulphate esters are, at least partly, under hormonal control. This was confirmed in recent studies showing that androgens suppress hepatic glycolithocholic sulpho-transferase activity in male rats and that oestrogenic compounds stimulate this activity (Kane *et al.*, 1984; Kirkpatrick *et al.*, 1985).

Sulphation detoxifies lithocholic acid and promotes the excretion via the biliary and urinary routes. Sulphated lithocholic, chenodeoxycholic and cholic acids are poorly absorbed from the small intestine and are eliminated via the colon (Eyssen *et al.*, 1985b; Walker *et al.*, 1986). By using a perfusion system in rats, Breuer *et al.* (1983) observed that, in the colon, 5 mM unsulphated deoxycholate or chenodeoxycholate changed net water and sodium absorption to secretion and caused mucosal damage. Comparable concentrations of the 3-sulphated bile salts had no deleterious effects.

In the large intestine bile acid sulphatase producing bacteria retoxify sulphated lithocholic acid. Bile acid desulphating micro-organisms have not been isolated from human faeces, but Huijghebaert and Eyssen (1982) and Huijghebaert *et al.* (1982, 1984) studied an unnamed *Clostridium* S_1, isolated from rat caecal contents, which desulphated the 3-sulphates of lithocholic acid and the other common 5β bile acids. Neither the 7- or 12-sulphates of 5β bile acids nor the 3α-sulphates of 5α allo-bile acids were hydrolysed. Robben *et al.* (1986) isolated a related *Clostridium* S_2 from rat caecal contents. Strain S_2 desulphated the 3-sulphates of both the 5β and the 5α bile acids. Gnotobiotic rats associated with these micro-organisms excreted labelled lithocholate-3-sulphate and cholate-3-sulphate significantly more slowly via the faeces than did gnotobiotic rats without the desulphating micro-organisms (Eyssen *et al.*, 1985b).

Conjugation with glucuronic acid increases the water solubility of the bile acids and promotes their biliary and urinary excretion in man (Raedsch *et al.*, 1985). The fate of these glucuronides in the intestine is not well known. So far, the frequency of occurrence of bile acid glucuronidase producing bacteria in the intestinal microflora apparently has not been studied. As mentioned earlier, we recently observed that *Peptostreptococcus productus* hydrolysed cholate-3-glucuronide and several steroid-glucuronides (Table 11.1).

3. Co-mutagenic Activity of Bile Acids

Substantial epidemiological evidence suggests a strong correlation between high incidence rates of colon cancer and high intake of meat and animal fats. In contrast, populations using low fat and high fibre diets have a low incidence of colon cancer. This subject was comprehensibly reviewed by Rowland *et al.* (1985). Population groups at high risk of developing colon cancer were reported to excrete larger amounts of secondary bile acids in the faeces (Hill and Aries, 1971; Reddy and Wynder, 1973; Reddy, 1981a,b). In contrast, case-control studies yielded controversial or negative results (Murray *et al.*, 1980; Mudd *et al.*, 1980; Breuer *et al.*, 1985). In a study on healthy man (Cummings *et al.*, 1978), faecal bile acid excretion was higher (320 mg/day) while on a high fat diet than on a low fat diet (139 mg/day). In spite of these discrepancies, most investigators agree that secondary bile acids such as lithocholic or deoxycholic acids are present in high concentrations in stools of high-risk populations.

Hill (1974) hypothesized that colorectal cancer might be caused by high concentrations of faecal sterol or bile acid derivatives produced by anaerobic bacteria, such as the nuclear-dehydrogenating, lecithinase-negative *Clostridia*, converting 3-oxo bile acids into the respective 3-oxo-4-ene derivatives. It has not been shown that these reactions occur *in vivo*, but the appearance of the unsaturated and labile compounds might be transient. Epidemiological studies confirmed that the numbers of nuclear dehydrogenating anaerobic bacteria in the colon were higher in populations at high risk of developing colon cancer (Hill *et al.*, 1975; Borriello *et al.*, 1983).

Many investigations have been carried out to evaluate the mutagenicity or co-mutagenicity of microbial metabolites of bile acids. The subject has been reviewed by Wilkins and Van Tassel (1983), by Reddy (1984) and by McMichael and Potter (1985). Lithocholate was shown to enhance the mutagenicity of 2-aminoanthracene and benzopyrene in the Ames mutagenicity test, to transform hamster embryo cells *in vitro*, and to induce DNA strand breaks (Silverman and Andrews, 1977; Kawalek and Andrews, 1977; Friedman, 1981; Kelsey and Pienta, 1981; Kulkarni *et al.*, 1982). In addition, human intestinal bacteria were shown to convert lithocholic acid-3-sulphate to several non-polar products, the co-mutagenic activity of which remains to be studied (Kelsey *et al.*, 1980; Borriello and Owen, 1982). Secondary bile acids can act as tumour promoters *in vivo* when associated with carcinogenic substances (Narisawa *et al.*, 1974; Reddy *et al.*, 1976, 1977a,b, 1978; Cohen *et al.*, 1980; Reddy, 1981a). Recent data suggest that unsaturated bile acids are not potent mutagens, although they might possess co-mutagenic activities (McKillop *et al.*, 1983; Wilpart *et al.*, 1983). Whether cholecystectomy promotes colon carcinogenesis remains unclear (Narisawa *et al.*, 1985). As was stated by McMichael and Potter (1985), bile acids have been shown to have a range of effects on bowel mucosal cells: hyperplasia, metabolic alterations, cell membrane disruptions and stimulation of DNA-synthesis. By these mechanisms, secondary bile acids such as lithocholic acid, deoxycholic acid and their microbially formed metabolites might affect the frequency and the rate of progression of colon carcinogenesis.

In studies on rats dietary components, such as lactose or certain dietary fibres, were shown to affect the microbial metabolic activities in rat caecum (Wise *et al.*, 1984, 1986). It is not clear, however, whether dietary fibres significantly modify intestinal microbial bile acid and steroid metabolism. Low dietary fibre intake and low faecal bulk prolong the transit time and contribute to an increase in the concentration of microbially formed metabolites, e.g. the bile acids. Hence, apart from a possible direct influence on the bacterial ecology in the colon, dietary fibres dilute co-mutagens and shorten their contact with the intestinal mucosa. So far, however, the complex nature of our food, and of our individual response to it, does not allow us to define how the different dietary components affect the ecology and the metabolic activities of the intestinal microflora.

References

Adlercreutz, H. and Martin, F. (1980). Biliary excretion and intestinal metabolism of progesterone and estrogens in man. *J. Steroid Biochem.* **13**, 231–244.

Adlercreutz, H., Pulkkinen, M. O., Hämäläinen, E. K. and Korpelà, J. T. (1984). Studies on the role of intestinal bacteria in metabolism of synthetic and natural steroid hormones. *J. Steroid Biochem.* **20**, 217–229.

Ammon, H. V., Tapper, E. J., Komorowski, R. A., Charaf, U. K., Loeffler, R. F., Lewand, D. and Walter, L. G. (1985). Effects of sulfodeoxycholate on rat and rabbit small intestine. *Am. J. Physiol.* **248**, G485–G493.

Bokkenheuser, V. D. and Winter, J. (1983). Biotransformation of steroids. *In*: "Human Intestinal Microflora in Health and Disease" (ed. D. J. Hentges), pp. 215–239. Academic Press, New York.

Bokkenheuser, V. D., Suzuki, J. P., Polovsky, S. B., Winter, J. and Kelly, W. G. (1975). Metabolism of deoxycorticosterone by human faecal flora. *Appl. Microbiol.* **30**, 82–90.

Bokkenheuser, V. D., Winter, J., Dehazya, P. and Kelly, W. G. (1977). Isolation and characterization of human fecal bacteria capable of 21-dehydroxylating corticoids. *Appl. Environ. Microbiol.* **34**, 571–575.

Bokkenheuser, V. D., Winter, J., O'Rourke, S. and Ritchie, A. E. (1980). Isolation and characterization of fecal bacteria capable of 16α-dehydroxylating corticoids. *Appl. Environ. Microbiol.* **40**, 803–808.

Bokkenheuser, V. D., Winter, J., Hylemon, P. B., Ayengar, N. K. N. and Mosbach, E.H. (1981). Dehydroxylation of 16α-hydroxyprogesterone by fecal flora of man and rat. *J. Lipid Res.* **22**, 95–102.

Bokkenheuser, V. D., Winter, J., Cohen, B. I., O'Rourke, S. and Mosbach, E. H. (1983). Inactivation of contraceptive steroid hormones by human intestinal clostridia. *J. Clin. Microbiol.* **18**, 500–504.

Bokkenheuser, V. D., Morris, G. N., Ritchie, A. E., Holdeman, L. V. and Winter, J. (1984). Biosynthesis of androgen from cortisol by a species of *Clostridium* recovered from human fecal flora. *J. Infect. Dis.* **149**, 489–494.

Borriello, S. P., Drasar, B. S., Tomkins, A. and Hill, M. J. (1983). Relative carriage rates of nuclear dehydrogenating clostridia in two populations of different colorectal cancer risk. *J. Clin. Pathol.* **36**, 93–95.

Borriello, S. P. and Owen, R. W. (1982). The metabolism of lithocholic acid and lithocholic acid-3-α-sulfate by human fecal bacteria. *Lipids* **17**, 477–482.

Breuer, N. F., Rampton, D. S., Tammar, A., Murphy, G. M. and Dowling R. H. (1983). Effect of colonic perfusion with sulfated and nonsulfated bile acids on mucosal structure and function in the rat. *Gastroenterol*, **84**, 969–977.

Breuer, N. F., Dommes, P., Jaekel, S. and Goebell, H. (1985). Fecal bile acid excretion pattern in colonic cancer patients. *Dig. Dis. Sci.* **30**, 852–859.

Brinkley, A. W., Gottesman, A. R. and Mott, G. E. (1982). Isolation and characterization of new strains of cholesterol-reducing bacteria from baboons. *Appl. Environm. Microbiol..* **43**, 86–89.

Casey, M. L. and MacDonald, P. C. (1982). Metabolism of deoxycorticosterone and deoxycorticosterone sulfate in men and women. *J. Clin. Invest.* **70**, 312–319.

Coates, M. E. (1984). Fatty acids. *In*: "The Germ-Free Animal in Biomedical Research" (eds M. E. Coates and B. E. Gustafsson), pp. 285–289. Laboratory Animals Ltd., London.

Cohen, B. I., Raicht, R. F., Deschner, E. E., Takahashi, M., Sarwal, A. N. and Fazzini, E. (1980). Effect of cholic acid feeding on N-methyl-N-nitrosourea-induced colon tumors and cell kinetics in rats. *J. Natl Cancer Inst.* **64**, 573–578.

Cruse, J. P., Lewin, M. R., Ferulano, G. P. and Clark, C. G. (1978). Co-carcinogenic effects of dietary cholesterol in experimental colon cancer. *Nature* **276**, 822–824.

Cummings, J. H., Wiggins, H. S., Jenkins, D. J. A., Houston, H., Jivraj, T., Drasar, B. S. and Hill, M. J. (1978). Influence of diets high and low in animal fat on bowel habit, gastrointestinal transit time, fecal microflora, bile acid, and fat excretion. *J. Clin. Invest.* **61**, 953–963.

de Herder, W. W., Hazenberg, M. P., Otten, M. H., Pennock-Schröder, A. M. and Visser, T. J. (1985). Hydrolysis of iodothyronine sulfates by sulfatase activity of anaerobic bacteria from the rat intestinal flora. *FEMS Microbiol. Lett.* **27**, 79–83.

Demarne, Y. and Sacquet, E. (1981). Comparative study of fatty acids from body and liver lipids in germ free and conventional growing rats. *Nutr. Rep. Intern.* **23**, 1095–1104.

Demarne, Y., Sacquet, E., Flanzy, J., Garnier, H. and François, A.-C. (1970). Utilisation digestive apparente des acides gras chez le rat axénique et le rat holoxénique. *Ann. Biol. anim. Bioch. Biophys.* **10**, 369–384.

Demarne, Y., Sacquet, E., Lecourtier, M.-J. and Flanzy, J. (1979). Comparative study of endogenous fecal fatty acids in germ-free and conventional rats. *Am. J. Clin. Nutr.* **32**, 2027–2032.

Demarne, Y., Corring, T., Pihet, A. and Sacquet, E. (1982). Fat absorption in germ-free and conventional rats artificially deprived of bile secretion. *Gut* **23**, 49–57.

Dodgson, K. S., White, G. F. and Fitzgerald, J. W. (1982a). "Sulfatases of Microbial Origin, Vol. I." CRC Press Inc., Boca Raton, FL.

Dodgson, K. S., White, F. G. and Fitzgerald, J. W. (1982b). "Sulfatases of Microbial Origin, Vol. II." CRC Press Inc., Boca Raton, FL.

Edenharder, R. (1984). Dehydroxylation of cholic acid at C_{12} and epimerization at C_5 and C_7 by *Bacteroides* species. *J. Steroid Biochem.* **21**, 413–420.

Edenharder, R. and Knaflic, T. (1981). Epimerization of chenodeoxycholic acid to ursodeoxycholic acid by human intestinal lecithinase-lipase-negative *Clostridia*. *J. Lipid Res.* **22**, 652–658.

Edenharder, R. and Schneider, J. (1985). 12β-Dehydrogenation of bile acids by *Clostridium paraputrificum*, *C. tertium*, and *C. difficile* and epimerization at carbon-12 of deoxycholic acid by cocultivation with 12α-dehydrogenating *Eubacterium lentum*. *Appl. Environ. Microbiol.* **49**, 964–968.

Einarsson, K., Gustafsson, J. -Å. and Gustafsson, B. E. (1973). Differences between germ-free and conventional rats in liver microsomal metabolism of steroids. *J. Biol. Chem.* **248**, 3623–3630.

Eriksson, H. and Gustafsson, J. -Å. (1970). Steroids in germfree and conventional rats. Sulpho- and glucuronohydrolase activities of caecal contents from conventional rats. *Eur. J. Biochem.* **13**, 198–202.

Eriksson, H., Gustafsson, J. -Å. and Sjövall, J. (1969). Steroids in germ-free and conventional rats. 21-Dehydroxylation by intestinal microorganisms. *Eur. J. Biochem.* **9**, 550–554.

Eyssen, H. J. and Parmentier, G. G. (1979). Influence of the microflora of the rat on the metabolism of fatty acids, sterols and bile salts in the intestinal tract. *Zbl. Bakt.*, Suppl, 7, 39–44.

Eyssen, H. and Van Eldere, J. (1984). Metabolism of bile acids. *In*: "The Germ-Free Animal in Biomedical Research" (eds M. E. Coates, and B. E. Gustafsson), pp. 291–316. Laboratory Animals Ltd., London.

Eyssen, H. J. and Verhulst, A. (1984). Biotransformation of linoleic acid and bile acids by *Eubacterium lentum*. *Appl. Environ. Microbiol.* **47**, 39–43.

Eyssen, H. J., Parmentier, G. G., Compernolle F. C., De Pauw, G. and Piessens-Denef, M. (1973). Biohydrogenation of sterols by *Eubacterium* ATCC 21,408 – *Nova* species. *Eur. J. Biochem.* **36**, 411–421.

Eyssen, H., De Pauw, G. and Parmentier, G. (1974). Effect of lactose on $\triangle^5$-steroid-reducing activity of intestinal bacteria in gnotobiotic rats. *J. Nutr.* **104**, 605–612.

Eyssen, H. J., Parmentier, G. G. and Mertens, J. A. (1976). Sulfated bile acids in germ-free and conventional mice. *Eur. J. Biochem.* **66**, 507–514.

Eyssen, H., De Pauw, G., Stragier, J. and Verhulst, A. (1983). Cooperative formation of Ω-muricholic acid by intestinal microorganisms. *Appl. Environ. Microbiol.* **45**, 141–147.

Eyssen, H., De Pauw, G. and Van Eldere, J. (1985a). Formation of hyodeoxycholate from β-muricholate in gnotobiotic rats associated with *Clostridium* HDCA-1. *In*: "Germfree Research: Microflora Control and Its Application to the Biomedical Sciences" (ed. B. S. Wostmann), pp. 103–106. Alan R. Liss, Inc., New York.

Eyssen, H., Van Eldere, J., Parmentier, G., Huijghebaert, S. and Mertens, J. (1985b). Influence of microbial bile salt desulfation upon the fecal excretion of bile salts in gnotobiotic rats. *J. Steroid Biochem.* **22**, 547–554.

Falconer, J. D., Smith, A. N. and Eastwood, M. A. (1980). The effects of bile acids on colonic motility in the rabbit. *Q. J. Exp. Physiol.* **65**, 135–144.

Fedorowski, T., Salen, G., Tint, G. S. and Mosbach, E. (1979). Transformation of chenodeoxycholic acid and ursodeoxycholic acid by human intestinal bacteria. *Gastroenterol.* **77**, 1068–1073.

Feighner, S. D. and Hylemon, P. B. (1980). Characterization of a corticosteroid 21-dehydroxylase from the intestinal anaerobic bacterium, *Eubacterium lentum*. *J. Lipid Res.* **21**, 585–593.

Friedman, E. A. (1981). Differential response of premalignant epithelial cell classes to phorbol ester tumor promotors and to deoxycholic acid. *Cancer Res.* **41**, 4588–4599.

Glass, T. L. and Burley, C. Z. (1984). Biotransformation of 16-dehydroprogesterone by the intestinal anaerobic bacterium, *Eubacterium* sp. 144, *J. Steroid Biochem.* **21**, 65–72.

Graef, V., Furuya, E. and Nishikaze, O. (1977). Hydrolysis of steroid glucuronides with β-glucuronidase preparations from bovine liver, *Helix pomatia*, and *E. coli. Clin. Chem.* **23**, 532–535.

Gustafsson, B. E. (1982). The physiological importance of the colonic microflora. *Scand. J. Gastroenterol.*, Suppl. 77, 117–131.

Gustafsson, B. E., Einarsson, K. and Gustafsson, J. -Å. (1975). Influence of cholesterol feeding on liver microsomal metabolism of steroids and bile acids in conventional and germ-free rats. *J. Biol. Chem.* **250**, 8496–8502.

Gustafsson, J. -Å. (1968). Steroids in germfree and conventional rats. Identification of C19 and C21 steroids in feces from conventional rats. *Eur. J. Biochem.* **6**, 248–255.

Hill, M. J. (1974). Steroid nuclear dehydrogenation and colon cancer. *Am. J. Clin. Nutr.* **27**, 1475–1480.

Hill, M. J. and Aries, V. C. (1971). Faecal steroid composition and its relationship to cancer of the large bowel. *J. Pathol.* **104**, 129–139.

Hill, M. J., Drasar, B. S., Williams, R. E. O., Meade, T. W., Cox, A. G., Simpson, J. E. P. and Morson, B. C. (1975). Faecal bile-acids and clostridia in patients with cancer of the large bowel. *Lancet* i, 535–539.

Hirano, S. and Masuda, N. (1982). Characterization of NADP-dependent 7β-hydroxysteroid dehydrogenases from *Peptostreptococcus productus* and *Eubacterium aerofaciens. Appl. Environ. Microbiol.* **43**, 1057–1063.

Hirano, S., Nakama, R., Tamaki, M., Masuda, N. and Oda, H. (1981a). Isolation and characterization of thirteen intestinal microorganisms capable of 7α-dehydroxylating bile acids. *Appl. Environ. Microbiol.* **41**, 737–745.

Hirano, S., Masuda, N. and Oda, H. (1981b). In vitro transformation of chenodeoxycholic acid and ursodeoxycholic acid by human intestinal flora, with particular reference to the mutual conversion between the two bile acids. *J. Lipid Res.* **22**, 735–743.

Huijghebaert, S. M. and Eyssen, H. J. (1982). Specificity of bile salt sulfatase activity from *Clostridium* sp. strain S_1. *Appl. Environ. Microbiol.* **44**, 1030–1034.

Huijghebaert, S. M., Mertens, J. A. and Eyssen, H. J. (1982). Isolation of a bile salt sulfatase-producing *Clostridium* strain from rat intestinal microflora. *Appl. Environ. Microbiol.* **43**, 185–192.

Huijghebaert, S. M., Sim, S. M., Back, D. J. and Eyssen, H. J. (1984). Distribution of estrone sulfatase activity in the intestine of germfree and conventional rats. *J. Steroid Biochem.* **20**, 1175–1179.

Hylemon, P. B. and Glass, T. L. (1983). Biotransformation of bile acids and cholesterol by the intestinal microflora. *In*: "Human Intestinal Microflora in Health and Disease" (ed. D. J. Hentges), pp. 189–213. Academic Press, New York.

Järvenpää, P., Kosunen, T., Fotsis, T. and Adlercreutz, H. (1980). *In vitro* metabolism of estrogens by isolated intestinal micro-organisms and by human faecal microflora. *J. Steroid Biochem.* **13**, 345–349.

Kane III, R. E., Chen, L. J. and Thaler, M. M. (1984). Regulation of bile salt sulfotransferase isoenzymes by gonadal hormones. *Hepatology* **4**, 1195–1199.

Kawalek, J. C. and Andrews, A. W. (1977). The effect of bile acids on the metabolism of benzo(a)pyrene (BaP) and 2-aminoanthracene (2-AA) to mutagenic products. *Fed. Proc. Am. Soc. Exp. Biol.* **36**, 844 (abstract).

Kelsey, M. I. and Pienta, R. J. (1979). Transformation of hamster embryo cells by cholesterol-α-epoxide and lithocholic acid. *Cancer Lett.* **6**, 143–149.

Kelsey, M. I. and Pienta, R. J. (1981). Transformation of hamster embryo cells by neutral sterols and bile acids. *Toxicol. Lett.* **9**, 177–182.

Kelsey, M. I., Molina, J. E., Huang, S. -K. S. and Hwang, K. -K. (1980). The identification of microbial metabolites of sulfolithocholic acid. *J. Lipid Res.* **21**, 751–759.

Kemp, P., Lander, D. J. and Gunstone, F. D. (1984a). The hydrogenation of some *cis-* and *trans*-octadecenoic acids to stearic acid by a rumen *Fusocillus* sp. *Br. J. Nutr.* **52**, 165–170.

Kemp, P., Lander, D. J. and Holman, R. T. (1984b). The hydrogenation of the series of methylene-interrupted *cis,cis*-octadecadienoic acids by pure cultures of six rumen bacteria. *Br. J. Nutr.* **52**, 171–177.

Kirkpatrick, R. B., Wildermann, N. M. and Killenberg, P. G. (1985). Androgens and estrogens affect hepatic bile acid sulfotransferase in male rats. *Am. J. Physiol.* **248**, G639–G642.

Kulkarni, M. S., Cox, B. A. and Yielding, K. L. (1982). Requirements for induction of DNA strand breaks by lithocholic acid. *Cancer Res.* **42**, 2792–2795.

Macdonald, I. A. and Roach, P. D. (1981). Bile salt induction of 7α- and 7β-hydroxysteroid dehydrogenase in *Clostridium absonum. Biochim. Biophys. Acta* **665**, 262–269.

Macdonald, I. A., Rochon, Y. P., Hutchison, D. M. and Holdeman, L. V. (1982). Formation of ursodeoxycholic acid from chenodeoxycholic acid by a 7β-hydroxysteroid dehydrogenase-elaborating *Eubacterium aerofaciens* strain cocultured with 7α-hydroxysteroid dehydrogenase-elaborating organisms. *Appl. Environ. Microbiol.* **44**, 1187–1195.

Macdonald, I. A., Bokkenheuser, V. D., Winter, J., McLernon, A. M. and Mosbach, E. H. (1983). Degradation of steroids in the human gut. *J. Lipid Res.* **24**, 675–700.

Martin, F., Järvenpää, P., Kosunen, K., Somers, C., Lindstrom, B. and Adlercreutz, H. (1980). Ring-A reduction of medroxyprogesterone acetate [17α-acetoxy-6α-methyl-4-pregnene-3,20-dione (MPA)] in biological systems. *J. Steroid Biochem.* **12**, 491–497.

Matern, S., Back, K. W. and Gerok, W. (1985). "Advances in Glucuronide Conjugation". MTP Press Ltd., Lancaster.

McKillop, C. A., Owen, R. W., Bilton, R. F. and Haslam, E. A. (1983). Mutagenicity testing of steroids obtained from bile acids and cholesterol. *Carcinogenesis* **4**, 1179–1183.

McMichael, A. J. and Potter, J. D. (1985). Host factors in carcinogenesis: certain bile-acid metabolic profiles that selectively increase the risk of proximal colon cancer. *J. Natl Cancer Inst.* **75**, 185–191.

Midtvedt, T. (1967). Properties of anaerobic gram-positive rods capable of 7α-dehydroxylating bile acids. *Acta Path. Microbiol. Scand.* **71**, 147–160.

Morris, G. N., Winter, J., Cato, E. P., Ritchie, A. E. and Bokkenheuser, V.

D. (1986). *Eubacterium desmolans* sp. nov., a steroid desmolase-producing species from cat fecal flora. *Int. J. Syst. Bacteriol.* **36**, 183–186.

Mott, G. E., Brinkley, A. W. and Mersinger, C. L. (1980). Biochemical characterization of cholesterol-reducing *Eubacterium*. *Appl. Environ. Microbiol.* **40**, 1017–1022.

Mudd, D. G., McKelvey, S. T. D., Norwood, W., Elmore, D. T. and Roy, A. D. (1980). Faecal bile acid concentrations of patients with carcinoma or increased risk of carcinoma in the large bowel. *Gut* **21**, 587–590.

Murray, W. R., Blackwood, A., Trotter, J. M., Calman, K. C. and MacKay, C. (1980). Faecal bile acids and clostridia in the aetiology of colorectal cancer. *Br. J. Cancer* **41**, 923–928.

Musey, P. I., Green, R. N. and Hobkirk, R. (1972). The role of an enterohepatic system in the metabolism of 17β-estradiol-17-glucosiduronate in the human female. *J. Clin. Endocrinol. Metab.* **35**, 448–457.

Narisawa, T., Magadia, N. E., Weisburger, J. H. and Wynder, E. L. (1974). Promoting effect of bile acids on colon carcinogenesis after intrarectal instillation of N-methyl-N'-nitro-N-nitrosoguanidine in rats. *J. Natl Cancer Inst.* **53**, 1093–1097.

Narisawa, T., Sano, M., Sato, M., Takahashi, T., Tanida, N. and Shimoyama, T. (1985). The correlation between cholecystectomy and fecal bile acids, and large-bowel cancer induced with 1,2-dimethylhydrazine in mice. *Dis. Colon Rectum* **28**, 27–30.

Owen, R. W. (1985). Biotransformation of bile acids by clostridia. *J. Med. Microbiol.* **20**, 233–238.

Owen, R. W. and Bilton, R. F. (1983). The degradation of cholic acid by *Pseudomonas* sp. N.C.I.B. 10590 under anaerobic conditions. *Biochem. J.* **216**, 641–654.

Owen, R. W. and Bilton, R. F. (1985). Metabolism of unsaturated bile acids and androstanes by human faecal bacteria. *J. Steroid Biochem.* **22**, 817–822.

Owen, R. W., Tenneson, M. E., Bilton, R. F. and Mason, A. N. (1978). The degradation of cholesterol by *Escherichia coli* isolated from human faeces. *Biochem. Soc. Trans.* **6**, 377–379.

Owen, R. W., Hill, M. J. and Bilton, R. F. (1983a). Biotransformation of chenodeoxycholic acid by *Pseudomonas* species NCIB 10590 under anaerobic conditions. *J. Lipid Res.* **24**, 1109–1118.

Owen, R. W., Mason, A. N. and Bilton, R. F. (1983b). The degradation of cholesterol by *Pseudomonas* sp. NCIB 10590 under aerobic conditions. *J. Lipid Res.* **24**, 1500–1511.

Owen, R. W., Mason, A. N. and Bilton, R. F. (1985). The degradation of β-sitosterol by *Pseudomonas* sp. NCIB 10590 under aerobic conditions. *J. Steroid Biochem.* **23**, 327–332.

Palmer, R. H. (1972). Bile acids, liver injury, and liver disease. *Arch. Intern. Med.* **130**, 606–617.

Parmentier, G. and Eyssen, H. (1974). Mechanism of biohydrogenation of cholesterol to coprostanol by *Eubacterium* ATCC 21408. *Biochim. Biophys. Acta* **348**, 279–284.

Parmentier, G. G., Smets, L. M. -J., Janssen, G. A. and Eyssen, H. J. (1981). Effects of cholesterol feeding on the bile acids of male and female germ-free rats. *Eur. J. Biochem.* **116**, 365–372.

Pearson, J. R., Wiggins, H. S. and Drasar, B. S. (1974). Conversion of long-chain unsaturated fatty acids to hydroxy acids by human intestinal bacteria. *J. Med. Microbiol.* **7**, 265–275.

Raedsch, R., Stiehl, A., Gundert-Remy, U. and Kommerell, B. (1985). Hepatic secretion of sulphated and glucuronidated bile acids in man. *In*: "Enterohepatic Circulation of Bile Acids and Sterol Metabolism." Falk Symposium 42, pp. 225–229. MTP Press Ltd., Lancaster.

Raicht, R. F., Cohen, C. I., Fazzini, E. P., Sarwal, A. N. and Takahashi, M. (1980). Protective effect of plant sterols against chemically induced colon tumors in rats. *Cancer Res.* **40**, 403–405.

Reddy, B. S. (1981a). Bile salts and other constituents of the colon as tumor promotors. *Banbury Rep.* **7**, 345–364.

Reddy, B. S. (1981b). Diet and excretion of bile acids. *Cancer Res.* **41**, 3766–3768.

Reddy, B. S. (1984). The germ-free animal as a tool in cancer research. *In*: "The Germ-Free Animal in Biomedical Research." (eds M. E Coates, and B. E. Gustafsson), pp. 387–400. Laboratory Animals Ltd., London.

Reddy, B. S. and Wynder, E. L. (1973). Large bowel carcinogenesis: fecal constituents of populations with diverse incidence rates of colon cancer. *J. Natl Cancer Inst.* **50**, 1437–1442.

Reddy, B. S., Narisawa, T., Weisburger, J. H. and Wynder, E. L. (1976). Promoting effect of deoxycholic acid on colonic adenocarcinomas in germfree rats. *J. Natl Cancer Inst.* **56**, 441–442.

Reddy, B. S., Martin, C. W. and Wynder, E. L. (1977a). Fecal bile acids and cholesterol metabolites of patients with ulcerative colitis, a high-risk group for development of colon cancer. *Cancer Res.* **37**, 1697–1701.

Reddy, B. S., Watanabe, K., Weisburger, J. H. and Wynder, E. L. (1977b). Promoting effect of bile acids in colon carcinogenesis in germ-free and conventional F344 rats. *Cancer Res.* **37**, 3238–3242.

Reddy, B. S., Weisburger, J. H. and Wynder, E. L. (1978). Colon cancer: bile salts as tumor promotors. *In*: "Carcinogenesis, Vol. 2. Mechanisms of Tumor Promotion and Cocarcinogenesis." (eds T. J. Slaga, A. Sivak, and R. K. Boutwell), pp. 453–464. Raven Press, New York.

Robben, J., Parmentier, G. and Eyssen, H. (1986). Isolation of a rat intestinal *Clostridium* strain producing 5α- and 5β-bile salt 3α-sulfatase activity. *Appl. Environ. Microbiol.* **51**, 32–38.

Rosemarin, J., Vargo, D. and Floch, M. H. (1983). Cholesterol → epoxide → triol: a possible important pathway of cholesterol metabolism. *Am. J. Clin. Nutr.* **37**, 730 (Abstract).

Rowland, I. R., Mallett, A. K. and Wise, A. (1985). The effect of diet on the mammalian gut flora and its metabolic activities. *CRC Critical Rev. Toxicol.* **16**, 31–103.

Sacquet, E. C., Raibaud, P. M., Mejean, C., Riottot, M. J., Leprince, C. and Leglise, P. C. (1979). Bacterial formation of Ω-muricholic acid in rats. *Appl. Environ. Microbiol.* **37**, 1127–1131.

Sadzikowski, M. R., Sperry, J. F. and Wilkins, T. D. (1977). Cholesterol-reducing bacterium from human feces. *Appl. Environ. Microbiol.* **34**, 355–362.

Silverman, S. J. and Andrews, A. W. (1977). Bile acids: co-mutagenic activity in the *Salmonella*-mammalian-microsome mutagenicity test: brief communication. *J. Natl Cancer Inst.* **59**, 1557–1559.

Sim, S. M. and Back, D. J. (1985). Intestinal absorption of oestrone, oestrone glucuronide and oestrone sulphate in the rat *in situ* – I. Importance of hydrolytic enzymes on conjugate absorption. *J. Steroid Biochem.* **22**, 781–788.

Sim, S. M. and Back, D. J. (1986). Intestinal absorption of oestrone, oestrone glucuronide and oestrone sulphate in the rat *in situ* – II. Studies with the Doluisio technique. *J. Steroid Biochem.* **24**, 1085–1089.

Sim, S. M. Huijghebaert, S., Back, D. J. and Eyssen, H. J. (1983). Gastrointestinal absorption of estrone sulfate in germfree and conventional rats. *J. Steroid Biochem.* **18**, 499–503.

Simon, G. L. and Gorbach, S. L. (1984). Intestinal flora in health and disease. *Gastroenterol.* **86**, 174–193.

Taylor, W. (1971). The excretion of steroid hormone metabolites in bile and feces. *Vitam. Hormon.* **29**, 201–285.

Thomas, P. J. (1972). Identification of some enteric bacteria which convert oleic acid to hydroxystearic acid in vitro. *Gastroenterol.* **62**, 430–435.

Ukai, M., Tomura, A. and Ito, M. (1976). Cholesterol synthesis in germfree and conventional rats. *J. Nutr.* **106**, 1175–1183.

Van Eldere, J. and Eyssen, H. (1984). Metabolism of cholesterol. *In*: "The Germ-Free Animal in Biomedical Research." (eds M. E. Coates, and B. E. Gustafsson), pp. 317–332. Laboratory Animals Ltd., London.

Van Eldere, J., Parmentier, G., Robben, J. and Eyssen, H. (1987). Influence of an estrone-desulfating intestinal flora on the enterohepatic circulation of estrone-sulfate in rats. *J. Steroid Biochem.* **26**, 235–239.

Verhulst, A., Semjen, G., Meerts, U., Janssen, G., Parmentier, G., Asselberghs, S., Van Hespen, H. and Eyssen, H. (1985). Biohydrogenation of linoleic acid by *Clostridium sporogenes, Clostridium bifermentans, Clostridium sordellii* and *Bacteroides* sp. *FEMS Microbiol. Ecol.* **31**, 255–259.

Verhulst, A., Parmentier, G., Janssen, G., Asselberghs, S. and Eyssen, H. (1986). Biotransformation of unsaturated long-chain fatty acids by *Eubacterium lentum. Appl. Environ. Microbiol.* **51**, 532–538.

Verhulst, A., Janssen, G., Parmentier, G. and Eyssen, H. (1987). Isomerization of polyunsaturated long chain fatty acids by *Propionibacteria. System. Appl. Microbiol.* **9**, 12–15.

Walker, S., Stiehl, A., Raedsch, R., Klöters, P. and Kommerell, B. (1986). Colonic absorption of sulfated and nonsulfated bile acids in rat. *Digestion* **33**, 1–6.

White, B. A., Fricke, R. J. and Hylemon, P. B. (1982). 7β-Dehydroxylation of ursodeoxycholic acid by whole cells and cell extracts of the intestinal anaerobic bacterium, *Eubacterium* species V.P.I. 12708. *J. Lipid Res.* **23**, 145–153.

Wilkins, T. D. and Van Tassell, R. L. (1983). Production of intestinal mutagens. *In*: "Human Intestinal Microflora in Health and Disease" (ed. D. J. Hentges), pp. 265–288. Academic Press, New York.

Wilpart, M., Mainguet, R., Maskens, A. and Roberfroid, M. (1983). Structure–activity relationship amongst biliary bile acids showing co-mutagenic activity towards 1,2-dimethylhydrazine. *Carcinogenesis* **4**, 1239–1241.

Winter J. and Bokkenheuser, V. D. (1978). 21-Dehydroxylation of corticoids by anaerobic bacteria isolated from human fecal flora. *J. Steroid Biochem.* **9**, 379–384.

Winter, J., O'Rourke, S., Bokkenheuser, V. D., Hylemon, P. B. and Glass, T. L. (1982a). 16α-Dehydration of corticoids by bacteria isolated from rat fecal flora. *J. Steroid Biochem.* **16**, 231–237.

Winter, J., Cerone-McLernon, A., O'Rourke, S., Ponticorvo, L. and Bokkenheuser, V. D. (1982b). Formation of 20β-dihydrosteroids by anaerobic bacteria. *J. Steroid Biochem.* **17**, 661-667.

Winter, J., O'Rourke-Locascio, S., Bokkenheuser, V. D., Mosbach, E. H. and Cohen, B. I. (1984a). Reduction of 17-keto steroids by anaerobic micro-organisms isolated from human fecal flora. *Biochim. Biophys. Acta* **795**, 208–211.

Winter, J., Morris, G. N., O'Rourke-Locascio, S., Bokkenheuser, V. D., Mosbach, E. H., Cohen, B. I. and Hylemon, P. B. (1984b). Mode of action of steroid desmolase and reductase synthesized by *Clostridium "scindens"* (formerly *Clostridium* strain 19). *J. Lipid Res.* **25**, 1124–1131.

Winter, J., Shackleton, C. H. L., O'Rourke, S. and Bokkenheuser, V. D. (1984c). Bacterial formation of aldosterone metabolites. *J. Steroid Biochem.* **21**, 563–569.

Wise, A., Rowland, I. R. and Mallett, A. K. (1984). Dietary lactose and the metabolic activity of the caecal microfloras of weanling and adult rats. *Fd Chem. Toxic.* **22**, 113–117.

Wise, A., Mallett, A. K. and Rowland, I. R. (1986). Effect of mixtures of dietary fibres on the enzyme activity of the rat caecal microflora. *Toxicology* **38**, 241–248.

Wostmann, B. S., Wiech, N. L. and Kung, E. (1966). Catabolism and elimination of cholesterol in germfree rats. *J. Lipid Res.* **7**, 77–82.

12

Metabolism of Carbohydrates

MARIE E. COATES

A. Introduction

In the nutrition of the monogastric animal, carbohydrates can be roughly classified as 'available', which means they are readily digested and utilized as an energy source, or 'non-available', which means they are resistant to the mammalian digestive system, and contribute little or nothing to the animal's nutrition. This chapter is concerned with those of the former category that have special significance relative to the gut microflora. The non-available forms of carbohydrate are considered in chapter 13.

B. Starches

Hydrolysis of starch is mainly accomplished by the action of pancreatic amylase. In mammals there is little or no microbial digestion of dietary starches in the proximal part of the gastro-intestinal tract. In birds some breakdown of starch occurs in the crop through the action of bacterial amylase, and strains of amylolytic lactobacilli have been shown to be responsible (Ivorec Szylit *et al.*, 1974; Szylit *et al.*, 1980). Although starches are in general efficiently digested by the host's pancreatic amylases, some escape digestion to reach the lower ileum and large intestine where they are subject to fermentation by the microflora. It has been estimated that in man up to 20% of the dietary starch enters the colon (Stephen *et al.*, 1983), providing an available carbohydrate substrate for bacterial growth. Since microbial bodies contribute significantly to faecal mass (Stephen and Cummings, 1980) it is to be expected that in subjects on high carbohydrate diets more starch would reach the colon, resulting in increased bacterial proliferation there and a consequent increase in faecal bulk. This postulate has been advanced to explain the large faecal bulk observed in some African and Asian populations eating diets high in starch but with a relatively low fibre content (van der Westhuizen *et al.*, 1972; Shetty and Kurpad, 1986).

A small proportion of the starch which reaches the lower gut is not susceptible to breakdown by pancreatic amylase and has been termed 'resistant starch' (Englyst and Cummings, 1985). Most dietary starches consist of a mixture of about 20% amylose and 80% amylopectin. During the course of baking, freezing or storage a part of the starch undergoes modification and becomes highly resistant to hydrolysis by α-amylase, *in vivo* or *in vitro*. The phenomenon appears to be associated with the amylose fraction. Resistant starch was recovered in the faeces of human subjects and of mice given diets containing a high-amylose maize starch (amylomaize), but was absent when the diet contained ordinary commercial maize meal (Wolf *et al.*, 1977).

That resistant starch is subject to breakdown by the colonic microflora is evident from experiments with germ-free rats, which were much less able than their conventional counterparts to digest a diet containing amylomaize starch (Sacquet *et al.*, 1983). In later studies on conventional rats white wheat bread was almost completely digested, but when an antibiotic was included in the diet to suppress microbial activity in the lower gut digestibility was reduced and resistant starch was present in the faeces (Björk *et al.*, 1986).

In the experiments of Sacquet *et al.* (1983) plasma cholesterol was significantly lowered in rats given amylomaize starch, and as the effect was observed both in germ-free and conventional animals it can be concluded that it is independent of microbial action. Involvement of the microflora was, however, apparent in other aspects of cholesterol metabolism. Cholesterol concentration in the liver was increased in germ-free and decreased in conventional rats by feeding amylomaize starch. The total bile acids in the lower gut were decreased in germ-free but increased in conventional animals, and bacterial transformations of cholesterol and bile acids were suppressed. The mechanisms of these changes are not clear, but microbial fermentation of amylomaize starch in the caecum leading to increased acidity and consequent disturbance of the microbial equilibrium has been suggested as a likely cause.

Because of its refractoriness to digestion by mammalian enzymes many authors have proposed that resistant starch should be classified as a component of dietary fibre (see chapter 13).

C. Lactose

Lactose is a disaccharide which is broken down by the enzyme lactase to the monosaccharides, glucose and galactose. Lactase is abundantly produced by suckling mammals but, with the exception of some human populations (notably Caucasians), production ceases soon after weaning. In a-lactasic individuals the accumulation of lactose in the gastro-intestinal tract leads to osmotic diarrhoea, and microbial fermentation of the lactose results in symptoms of bloat, flatulence and abdominal cramps (Mathan, 1986). Studies in rats and chicks indicate that the products of microbial fermentation are available to the host. Germ-free and conventional rats were weaned at 14 days of age on to a chemically-defined, water-soluble diet containing lactose. The conventional rats survived to 60 days but the germ-free rats did not, and hence it was concluded that bacterial lactase in the gut of the conventional animals had enabled them to utilize the dietary lactose (Reddy *et al.*, 1968). A similar conclusion was reached from studies in chicks. Virtually no lactase was detected in the gut of germ-free chicks but significant amounts were present in the large intestinal contents of the corresponding conventional birds, which grew better and survived longer than their germ-free counterparts on a diet containing most of its carbohydrate as lactose (Siddons and Coates, 1972).

It has been suggested that yoghurt, which is a source of bacterial β-galactosidase, might assist the digestion of lactose in lactase-deficient subjects (Speck, 1983; Alm, 1982). Because of its lack of endogenous lactase the chick was used by Cole *et al.* (1984) to investigate this possibility. In birds given 10% lactose in the diet body weights were depressed, there was gas formation in the caecum and a lower pH of the caecal contents. None of the effects was reversed by supplements of yoghurt in the drinking water, nor were the counts of lactose-utilizing organisms in the caecum altered. The caecal contents of birds given yoghurt showed much lower activities of β-glucuronidase, but this was not dependent on the presence of viable bacteria as it also occurred with supplements of heated yoghurt. Nevertheless the authors suggested that yoghurt in the human diet might confer some advantage as β-glucuronidase activity is raised in patients with large bowel cancer. In experiments with weaned rats given diets containing lactose, yoghurt or milk there was no evidence that the yoghurt bacteria were improving the host's utilization of lactose, although milk and yoghurt both induced higher activities of β-galactosidase in the lower small intestine. Relatively low counts of *Lact. bulgaricus* were recorded in the gut of rats fed exclusively on yoghurt, and yoghurt bacilli failed to colonize the gut of rats fed on a stock diet with daily doses of yoghurt. These findings led to the conclusion that in human subjects it was unlikely that yoghurt bacteria could become a significant part of the gut microflora, especially when yoghurt formed only a part of the normal diet (Garvie *et al.*, 1984).

Lactose reaching the lower gut is fermented by the microflora resulting in a lower pH value, a condition that might be expected to induce disturbances of the normal microecological equilibrium (Eyssen *et al.*, 1974). The effects of dietary lactose on the metabolic activity of the caecal microflora was studied in weanling and adult rats by measuring the activities of the six microbial enzymes, azoreductase, β-glucosidase, β-glucuronidase, nitrate reductase, nitroreductase and urease. The activities were, in general, higher in weanlings than in adults, and the responses to increasing proportions of dietary lactose were not always comparable in the two age groups. For instance, although total activities of nitrate reductase and urease increased in both weanlings and adults, those of azoreductase and nitroreductase decreased only in weanlings (Wise *et al.*, 1984). Changes in the alimentary microflora occur during development of the young animal (Smith, 1965), which may explain the differences in activity and in response to lactose between the two age groups. Wostmann *et al.* (1977) reported that feeding an autoclaved diet containing lactose brought about a change in the faecal bile acid pattern of conventional rats, indicating a shift in numbers or activities of micro-organisms responsible for the transformation of ω-muricholic acid to hyodeoxycholic acid. However, no such change was observed when the diet was sterilized by gamma-radiation, and it seems likely that materials formed during the heat process, possibly Maillard reaction products, were responsible, rather than lactose *per se*.

D. Lactulose

Lactulose, 4-*O*-β-D-galactopyranosyl-D-fructofuranose, is produced by the action of lime water on lactose. It is resistant to the action of intestinal disaccharidases (Dahlqvist and Gryboski, 1965), but energy balance studies in rats and miniature pigs showed that considerable digestion of lactulose occurred, presumably as a result of microbial fermentation (Bird *et al.*, 1985).

Lactulose is not present in raw milk but is formed when milk is heated. In heat-sterilized liquid milk formulae for infant feeding lactulose has been reported to constitute 1–5% of the total carbohydrate (Bernhart *et al.*, 1965). The presence of lactulose in infant feeds encourages the development of *Bifidobacterium bifidum* which is the predominant organism in the microflora of breast-fed infants. In the experiments of Grütte and Haenel (1968) new-born babies received human milk for a few days after birth and were then transferred to different infant formulae. Inclusion of 1.2–1.5% lactulose in the diet induced an increase in the *B. bifidum* population in the colon accompanied by a low pH, high E_h

and low concentration of ammonia. The proliferation of anaerobic Gram-negative bacteria was inhibited and the faecal flora became similar to that of breast-fed infants. Whether or not the establishment of such a flora confers benefit on the infant remains a matter of debate.

Lactulose is used clinically as a laxative and in the treatment of portal systemic encephalopathy. Its beneficial effect in both conditions appears to be related, at least in part, to the induction of a low colonic pH. In experiments with isolated segments of guinea pig intestine peristaltic contractions of the circular muscle were increased by infusion with lactic, acetic or hydrochloric acids. It was suggested that lactulose may relieve constipation because the acids formed as a result of microbial fermentation in the colon stimulate propulsion of the faecal mass, and that the same mechanism might also contribute to the diarrhoea observed in lactase deficiency (Bennett and Eley, 1976).

Portal systemic encephalopathy is a disorder of the central nervous system secondary to severe hepatic cirrhosis. Impaired liver function allows the concentration of ammonia in systemic blood to rise, with consequent toxic effects on the brain. Ammonia is generated in the colon by the action of bacteria on amino acids, urea and other nitrogenous compounds. It might be expected that acid conditions in the colon would neutralize ammonia and increase its excretion, but no increase in faecal ammonia after lactulose has been demonstrated (Zeegen *et al.*, 1970; Agostini *et al.*, 1972). Studies on the kinetics of urea metabolism and nitrogen excretion in cirrhotic patients suggest that lactulose decreases urea production by increasing faecal output of total nitrogen. Since ammonia excretion was not increased it was postulated that precursors of ammonia might have contributed to the extra output. Increased excretion of nitrogen led to a decrease in urea production and a fall in the urea pool. Degradation of urea consequently decreased (Weber, 1979). Some of these findings are compatible with those of *in vitro* studies by Vince *et al.* (1978). In incubated stool samples, lactulose apparently altered bacterial metabolism so that utilization of ammonia increased and ammonia production decreased. Several possible explanations were advanced. The presence of a readily fermentable source of carbon and energy would reduce the need for deamination of nitrogenous compounds to fulfil these requirements. The availability of an abundant substrate would encourage bacterial proliferation and assimilation of ammonia as a nitrogen source. Low pH values such as are induced in the colon by lactulose appeared to bring about a general reduction in bacterial metabolism, including that of ammonia-producing bacteria. This is consistent with the reduced degradation of urea observed by Weber (1979) in human subjects.

E. Polyols

The polyols lactitol (4-*O*-β-D-galactopyranosol-D-sorbitol) and maltitol (4-*O*-α-D-glucopyranosol-D-sorbitol) are used in the food industry as sweetening agents with low carcinogenicity. Lactitol is not absorbed by the human small intestine, nor hydrolysed to any significant extent by mammalian enzymes (Patil *et al.*, 1987). It is, however, subject to metabolism by colonic bacteria (Saijonmaa *et al.*, 1978). In studies with rats and pigs values for the digestible and metabolizable energy of lactitol were high (Bird *et al.*, 1985), from which it can be inferred that microbial degradation of lactitol had occurred and that the resulting products were utilized by the host.

Maltitol is slowly hydrolysed by intestinal maltase to glucose and sorbitol (Dahlqvist and Telenius, 1965). Comparisons of its metabolism by germ-free and conventional rats indicated that maltitol and the sorbitol released from it were degraded by intestinal micro-organisms, but maltitol was also absorbed and hydrolysed by the host tissues (Lian Loh *et al.*, 1982).

References

Agostini, L., Down, P. F., Murison, J. and Wrong, O. M. (1972). Faecal ammonia and pH during lactulose administration in man: comparison with other cathartics. *Gut* **13**, 859–866.

Alm, L. (1982). Effect of fermentation on lactose, glucose and galactose content of milk and suitability of milk products for lactose intolerant individuals. *J. Dairy Sci.*, **65**, 346–352.

Bennett, A. and Eley, K. G. (1976). Intestinal pH and propulsion: an explanation of diarrhoea in lactase deficiency and laxation by lactulose. *J. Pharmacy Pharmacol.* **28**, 192–195.

Bernhart, F. W., Gagliardi, E. D., Tomarelli, R. M. and Stribley, R. C. (1965). Lactulose in modified milk products for infant nutrition. *J. Dairy Sci.*, **48**, 399–400.

Bird, S. P., Hewitt, D. and Gurr, M. I. (1985). Digestible and metabolizable energy values of lactitol and lactulose for the rat and miniature pig. *Proc. Nutr. Soc.* **44**, 40A.

Björk, I., Nyman, M., Pedersen, B., Siljestrom, M., Asp, N. -G. and Eggum, B. O. (1986). On the digestibility of starch in wheat bread: studies *in vitro* and *in vivo*. *J. Cereal Sci.* **4**, 1–11.

Cole, C. B., Anderson, P. H., Phillips, S. M., Fuller, R. and Hewitt, D. (1984). The effect of yoghurt on the growth, lactose-utilizing gut organisms and β-glucuronidase activity of caecal contents of a lactose-fed, lactase-deficient animal. *Food Microbiol.* **1**, 217–222.

Dahlqvist, A. and Gryboski, J. S. (1965). Inability of the human small-intestinal lactase to hydrolyse lactulose. *Biochim. Biophys. Acta,* **110**, 635–636.

Dahlqvist, A. and Telenius, U. (1965). The utilization of a presumably low-cariogenic carbohydrate derivative. *Acta Physiol. Scand.* **63**, 156–163.

Englyst, H. N. and Cummings, J. H. (1985). Digestion of the polysaccharides of some cereal foods in the human small intestine. *Am. J. Clin. Nutr.* **42**, 778–787.

Eyssen, H., De Pauw, G. and Parmentier, G. (1974). Effect of lactose on Δ^5-steroid-reducing activity of intestinal bacteria is gnotobiotic rats. *J. Nutr.* **104**, 605–612.

Garvie, E. I., Cole, C. B., Fuller, R. and Hewitt, D. (1984). The effect of yoghurt on some components of the gut microflora and on the metabolism of lactose in the rat. *J. Appl. Bacteriol.* **56**, 237–245.

Grütte, F. K. and Haenel, H. (1968). Lactose and lactulose in infant feeding. *Ernährungsforschung* **13**, 285–295.

Ivorec-Szylit, O., Raibaud, P. and Schellenberg, P. (1974). The breakdown of starch at different levels in the digestive tract of the axenic, gnotoxenic and holoxenic chicken. *In*: "Germfree Research: Biological Effect of Gnotobotic Environments" (ed. J. B. Heneghan), pp. 225–231. Academic Press, New York.

Lian Loh, R., Birch, G. C. and Coates, M. E. (1982). Metabolism of maltitol in the rat. *Brit. J. Nutr.* **48**, 477–481.

Mathan, V. I. (1986). Lactose intolerance. *In*: "Proceedings of the XIIIth International Congress of Nutrition" (eds T.G. Taylor and N.K. Jenkins), pp. 749–751. John Libbey, London, Paris.

Patil, D. H., Grimble, G. K. and Silk, D. B. A. (1987). Lactitol, a new hydrogenated lactose derivative: intestinal absorption and laxative threshold in normal human subjects. *Brit. J. Nutr.* **57**, 195–199.

Reddy, B. S., Pleasants, J. R. and Wostmann, B. S. (1968). Effect of dietary lactose on intestinal disaccharidases in germfree and conventional rats. *J. Nutr.* **95**, 413–419.

Sacquet, E., Leprince, C. and Riottot, M. (1983). Effect of amylomaize starch on cholesterol and bile acid metabolism in germfree (axenic) and conventional (holoxenic) rats. *Rep. Nutr. Dév.* **23**, 783–792.

Saijonmaa, T., Heikonen, M., Kreula, M. and Linko, P. (1978). Preparation and characterization of milk sugar alcohol, lactitol. *Milchwissenschaft* **33**, 733–736.

Shetty, P. S. and Kurpad, A. V. (1986). Increasing starch intake in the human diet increases faecal bulking. *Am. J. Clin. Nutr.* **43**, 210–212.

Siddons, R. C. and Coates, M. E. (1972). The influence of the intestinal microflora on disaccharidase activities in the chick. *Brit. J. Nutr.* **27**, 101–112.

Smith, H. W. (1965). The development of the flora in the alimentary tract of young animals. *J. Path. Bacteriol.* **90**, 495–513.

Speck, M. L. (1983). Evidence of value of live starter culture in yoghurt. *Cultured Dairy Products J.* **18**, 25–26.

Stephen, A. M. and Cummings, J. H. (1980). The microbial contribution to human faecal mass. *J. Med. Microbiol.* **13**, 45–56.

Stephen, A. M., Haddad, A. L. and Phillips, S. F. (1983). Passage of carbohydrate into the colon. *Gastroenterol.* **85**, 589–595.

Szylit, O., Champ, M., Ait-Abdelkader, N. and Raibaud, P. (1980). Rôle de cinq souches de *Lactobacillus* sur la dégradation des glucides chez le poulet monoxénique. *Repr. Nutr. Dév.* **20**, 1701–1706.

Vince, A., Killingley, M. and Wrong, O. M. (1978). Effect of lactulose on ammonia production in a faecal incubation system. *Gastroenterol.* **74**, 544–549.

Weber, F. L. (1979). The effect of lactulose on urea metabolism and N excretion in cirrhotic patients. *Gastroenterol.* **77**, 518–523.

van der Westhuizen, J., Mbizvo, M. and Jones, J. J. (1972). Unrefined carbohydrate and glucose tolerance. *Lancet* **ii**, 719.

Wise, A., Rowland, I. R. and Mallett, A. K. (1984). Dietary lactose and the metabolic activity of the caecal microfloras of weanling and adult rats. *Food Chem. Toxicol.* **22**, 113–117.

Wolf, M. J., Khoo, U. and Inglett, G. E. (1977). Partial digestibility of cooked amylomaize starch in humans and mice. *Die Stärke* **29**, 401–405.

Wostmann, B. S., Beaver, M., Chang, L. and Madsen, D. (1977). Effect of autoclaving of a lactose-containing diet on cholesterol and bile acid metabolism of conventional and germ-free rats. *Am. J. Clin. Nutr.* **30**, 1999–2005.

Zeegen, R., Drinkwater, J. E., Fenton, J. C. B., Vince, A. and Dawson, A. M. (1970). Some observations on the effects of treatment with lactulose on patients with chronic hepatic encephalopathy. *Quart. J. Med.* **39**, 245–263.

13

The Effects of Dietary Fibre Utilization on the Colonic Microflora

ROBERT E. McCARTHY and ABIGAIL A. SALYERS

A. Introduction

Dietary fibre is digested extensively in the human colon by the bacteria that reside there. This fact must be taken into account at some level in any investigation of the physiological effects of dietary fibre. Taking account of the microbial flora of the colon and its interaction with dietary fibre is not an easy matter because of the complexity of the colonic ecosystem. There are many ways of describing and evaluating the colonic microflora. Two of the most widely used are (*i*) the taxonomic approach, in which the relative levels of different species and groups of bacteria are measured, and (*ii*) digestibility experiments, in which fibre is incubated with faecal specimens and digestion monitored either as the appearance of short chain fatty acids or as disappearance of substrate. Both types of approaches have their limitations. The taxonomic approach establishes the identity and relative levels of the organisms present in colon contents, but not their metabolic activities. The digestibility studies demonstrate an activity of the mixed microbial population but yield no information about the contribution of individual groups and species.

Given the complexity of dietary fibre and of the colonic microflora, no single experimental approach can account for all aspects of the fibre–flora interaction or of the effect of fibre digestion on the host. Thus, it is important to assess each attempt to measure the complex interactions not only in terms of what is measured but also in terms of what it ignores. This can only be done if the investigator is aware of the features and capabilities of the microbial community in the colon.

The purpose of this chapter is to survey some of the different aspects of the microbial flora and its activities, with particular reference to how they affect or are affected by dietary fibre. Also, some experimental approaches which have been undertaken to gain a better understanding of this complex interaction will be described.

ROLE OF THE CUT FLORA IN TOXICITY AND CANCER
ISBN 0–12–599920–8

1. Characteristics of the Colonic Microflora

The microbial community that is found in the normal human colon is one of the most complex microbial ecosystems known. It accounts for about one third of the volume of colon contents and consists of at least 400 distinct species of bacteria (Moore *et al.*, 1978). Although fungi and protozoa can be isolated from human faeces, their numbers are very low. Bacteria appear to be the predominant micro-organisms. It is probably the case that most of the numerically predominant species of colonic bacteria have now been cultivated and described, but there may still be important groups of colonic micro-organisms that have not yet been isolated.

All of the numerically predominant species of colon bacteria are obligate anaerobes which ferment carbohydrates and produce short chain fatty acids (acetate, propionate, butyrate), lactate, succinate and gases (CO_2, H_2). The five major genera of colon anaerobes and some of their characteristics are given in Table 13.1. These genera account for about 60% of all colon isolates. Some of these genera are represented by a number of different species. To date, *Bacteroides* is the genus that has been most thoroughly characterized taxonomically. There are at least five distinct species of *Bacteroides* among the numerically predominant species. These species have diverged genetically to such an extent that the highest DNA–DNA cross homology is 40% (Johnson, 1978). In some cases, the DNA–DNA cross homology values are less than 10%. Analyses of 16S ribosomal RNA sequences have shown that the *Bacteroides–Fusobacterium* group is quite distant genetically from more familiar gram-negative bacteria such as *Escherichia*, *Salmonella*, *Pseudomonas*, and the photosynthetic bacteria (Paster *et al.*, 1985; Weisburg *et al.*, 1985). Similarly, the bifidobacteria form a genetically distinct group and *Eubacterium*, together with clostridia and the gram-positive anaerobic cocci, form yet another distinct evolutionary group (Stackebrandt and Woese, 1981). These genetic analyses confirm the initial conclusion of the taxonomists that appreciable genetic diversity is represented in the colonic ecosystem.

2. Complexity and Stability of the Colonic Microflora

It is not clear why the colonic microflora is so complex. One hypothesis is that the human colon contains many different microenvironments, such as mucosal crypts, the mucin layer, the surface of plant cell fragments and areas within plant cell fragments that have been created by prior digestion of the plant cell matrix. According to this view, the complexity

Table 13.1 *Characteristics of the numerically predominant species of colon bacteria*

Genus	Percentate of total flora[a]	Major fermentation products[b]	Other products or activities

Gram-negative rods
 Bacteroides
	20–25	Acetate
		 Propionate
		 Succinate
			Fecal mutagens[c]
			 polysaccharide
			   degraders[d]
			 bile acid
			   transformation[e]

Fusobacterium	5–10	Butyrate Acetate Formate	Bile acid transformation[e]
Gram-positive rods *Eubacterium*	20–25	Acetate Butyrate Lactate	
Bifidobacterium	10–15	Acetate Lactate	Polysaccharide[d] degraders
Gram-positive cocci *Peptostreptococcus*	5–10	Acetate Succinate Lactate	Bile acid transformation[e]

[a] Ranges obtained by summing percentages of different species given by Moore and Holdeman (1974).
[b] From Holdeman *et al.* (1977).
[c] From Wilkins and Van Tassell (1983).
[d] From Salyers *et al.* (1977b), Salyers and Leedle (1983).
[e] From Hylemon and Glass (1983).

of the colonic microflora results from evolutionary adaptation of different species and groups of colon bacteria to occupy these microenvironments or niches. An alternative hypothesis is that the colonic environment can support the growth of many different types of micro-organisms and that the composition of the colonic microflora is determined by the mixture of organisms that is ingested by the young child as its intestinal tract is being colonized. According to this view, the complexity of the colonic microflora simply reflects the diversity of organisms that are present in the environment.

At present, there is no definitive evidence to support or rule out either of these hypotheses. However, the microenvironment hypothesis is the more attractive of the two because it seems to give a more satisfactory account of why the human colonic microflora is so stable and why people in different parts of the world, eating very different diets, seem to have basically the same colonic microflora. If the microenvironment hypothesis is correct, it should not be possible to maintain the colonic ecosystem, in its full complexity, in a glass vessel fed with liquid medium. A successful demonstration of a continuous culture or fed batch culture system that maintains the complexity of the colonic microflora would be strong evidence against this hypothesis. So far no one has developed such a system, although Freter and his colleagues have made some progress in this direction (see below).

Available evidence supports the assertion that the colonic microflora of the healthy human, once established, is stable and does not vary appreciably with age or diet (Finegold and Sutter, 1978). However, the stability of the colonic microflora has not been unequivocally established. Because of the complexity of the microflora and the technical difficulties involved in isolating and identifying the predominant species of anaerobes, determinations of the species composition of the colonic microflora of a large number of subjects ingesting different diets is beyond the capacity and resources of most laboratories. A few attempts have been made to determine whether diet affects the species composition of the colonic microflora (Hentges *et al.*, 1977; Finegold and Sutter, 1978; Bornside, 1978). When the results of these studies are taken together, no consistent, statistically significant differences emerge. However, experimental variation in these studies is quite high. Given the technical limitations of classical microbiological techniques for enumeration and identification and the sizeable experimental errors involved, it is unlikely that currently available techniques could reliably detect changes of less than an order of magnitude in the concentration of individual groups or species.

Studies that have focused on particular groups of organisms have found some variation from person to person. For example, some people have much higher concentrations of methane producing bacteria than others (Miller and Wolin, 1982). Within the same person, these populations of methanogens appear to be stable with time, but no studies have been made of the effect of changes in diet. Also, some people harbour low numbers of bacteria which can utilize microcrystalline cellulose (Betian *et al.*, 1977). Bacteria which have very long generation times, such as cellulolytic bacteria or methanogens, may be particularly vulnerable to changes in diet which reduce residence time in the colon.

The question of whether the composition of the colonic microflora is affected by the hosts' diet is an important one for people who are interested in dietary fibre. A stable colonic microflora is an important factor in maintaining the health of the host, as can be seen clearly from the adverse effects sometimes associated with orally administered antibiotics (Finegold *et al.*, 1983). There is good evidence that increasing the amount of fibre in the diet increases the total number of bacteria that are excreted in faeces (Stephen and Cummings, 1980). Although the available evidence supports the assertion that this increase in numbers is obtained without altering the species composition of the flora significantly, there may be some cases in which an alteration of the colonic microflora could result from changes in the diet.

B. Flow of Carbon and Nitrogen in the Colonic Ecosystem

A schematic illustration of the different groups of bacteria that are thought to be associated with carbohydrate utilization in the colon is shown in Fig. 13.1. Polysaccharides, either from the host's diet or from the host itself, are probably the main source of carbohydrate for colon bacteria because most small molecular weight carbohydrate is absorbed higher up in the gastro-intestinal tract. Some colon bacteria are capable of utilizing dietary and host polysaccharides (Table 13.2). Utilization of polysaccharides by colon bacteria is discussed in detail below. Many carbohydrate-requiring colon bacteria cannot utilize polysaccharides (Table 13.2). These bacteria must either subsist on small molecular weight carbohydrate that escapes digestion in the small intestine or scavenge low molecular weight carbohydrate which is lost during polysaccharide digestion by the polysaccharide-degrading colon bacteria.

The main fermentation products that are detected in colon contents or in faeces are acetate, propionate and butyrate (Cummings and Branch, 1986). Little succinate or lactate is detected. Thus, there may be succinate-utilizing and lactate-utilizing bacteria in the colon. Alternatively, some factors in the colonic environment may cause bacteria which can produce succinate or lactate when they are grown in laboratory medium to produce much lower amounts of these compounds in the colon. It is known, for example, that in the case of *Bacteroides*, growth rate and composition of the growth medium can affect the ratio of end products (Kotarski and Salyers, 1981; Macy *et al.*, 1978). Also, when carbohydrate-fermenting bacteria are cocultured with methane-producing bacteria, the methanogens use hydrogen as fast as it is produced by the carbohydrate-fermenters, and in so doing shift the flow of reducing equivalents in the carbohydrate fermenter from production of succinate (or lactate) to production of hydrogen (Wolin and Miller, 1983).

Many people have methanogens in their colons. In some cases the concentration of methanogens is high enough for methane to be detectable in the person's breath. The primary methanogen in the human colon is *Methanobrevibacter smithii*, a methanogen which makes methane from hydrogen and carbon dioxide (Miller and Wolin, 1982). Another methanogen, which is found in lower concentrations in the human colon,

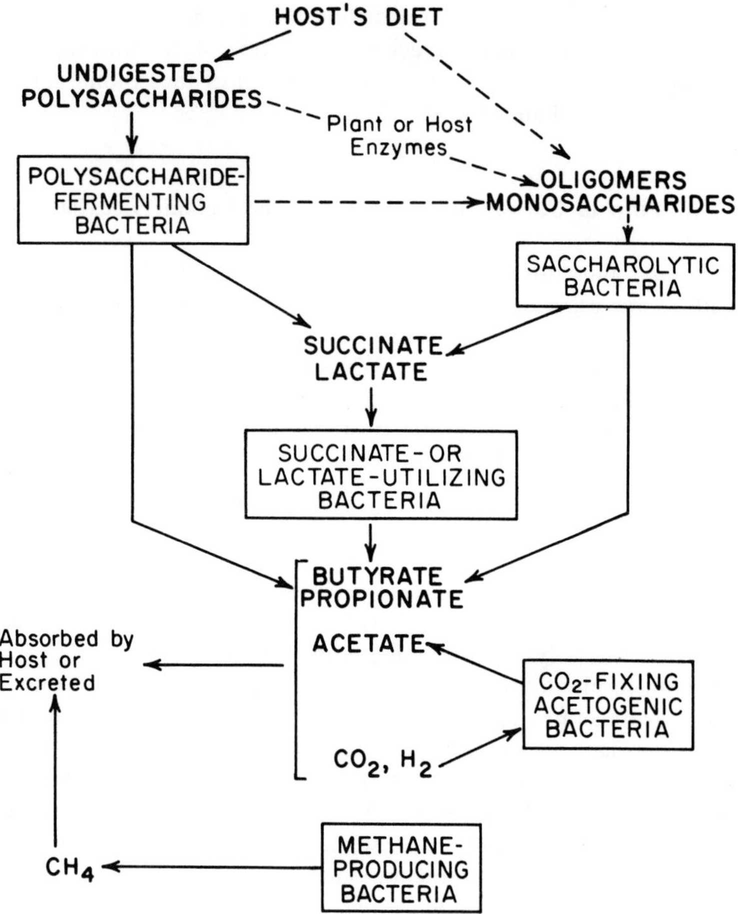

Fig 13.1. Schematic diagram of the fate of carbohydrate in the host's diet when it encounters the colonic microflora. Boxes indicate metabolic groups of colonic bacteria. Arrows between them indicate probable interactions. Dashed lines indicate steps which probably occur but which have not been demonstrated experimentally.

is *Methanosphaera stadtmaniae* (Miller and Wolin, 1985). This methanogen makes methane from methanol and hydrogen. A possible source of methanol in the colon is the demethoxylation of pectin by pectinolytic bacteria.

An acetogenic bacterium, *Eubacterium limosum*, which can make acetate from hydrogen and carbon dioxide (Genthner *et al.*, 1981) has

Table 13.2 *Carbohydrate utilization by the main groups of colon bacteria (Salyers et al., 1977a,b).*

Group	Mucin MPS[a]		Cellulose	Hemi-cellulose[b]	Pectin	Starch	Mono-/di-saccharides
Bacteroides							
vulgatus	−[c]	−	−	+[c]	+	+	+
thetaiotaomicron	−	+	−	+	+	+	+
uniformis	−	−	−	+	−	+	+
distasonis	−	−	−	−	−	−	+
3452	−	+	−	+	+	−	+
B5–21	−	+	−	+	+	+	+
Bifidobacterium							
adolescentis	−	−	−	+	−	+	+
longum	−	−	−	+	−	−	+
infantis	−	−	−	+	−	−	+
Eubacterium							
aerofaciens	−	−	−	−	−	−	+
biforme	−	−	−	−	−	−	+
eligens	−	−	−	−	+	−	+
rectale	−	−	−	−	−	+	+
Fusobacterium							
prauznitzii	−	−	−	−	−	+	+
Peptostreptococcus							
productus	−	−	−	−	−	−	+

[a] MPS: mucopolysaccharides (chondroitin sulfate, hyaluronic acid, heparin).
[b] Hemicellulose: arabinogalactan, xylan, galactomannan.
[c] + means that most strains utilize one or more of this group of substrates;
− means no strains utilize this group of substrates.

been isolated from human faeces (Barker and Haas, 1944). However, the extent of its contribution to acetate formation in the human colon remains to be established. Other such bacteria may exist but have not yet been cultivated and described. These acetogenic bacteria could potentially compete with methanogens for hydrogen and carbon dioxide.

Figure 13.1 shows the presumed flow of carbon due to carbohydrate fermentation. It is almost certainly the case that carbon from protein breakdown also contributes to maintenance of the colonic ecosystem, but virtually nothing is known about this process. None of the major species of colon bacteria are proteolytic to the extent that they can utilize protein as a sole source of carbon and energy. However, it is possible that at least some of the carbohydrate-fermenting species can utilize protein if a source of carbohydrate is available to provide energy. For example, amino acids could be incorporated directly into cell protein or the amino group removed to serve as a source of nitrogen. *Bacteroides* will not only incorporate exogenous amino acids such as leucine or isoleucine into cell protein, but also incorporates the deaminated amino acid carbon skeleton into membrane phospholipids (Smith and Salyers, 1981).

Some colonic bacterial species may be able to utilize protein as a source of carbon and energy. Ammonia, acetate, butyrate and branch chain fatty acids are typical end products of such a fermentation. Fermentation of the aromatic amino acids also results in productions of indole and other phenolics. The extent to which protein fermentation occurs in the human colon is not known, but branched chain fatty acids are detectable in human faeces. Moreover, proteolytic activity is easily detectable in the bacterial fraction of human faeces (Macfarlane *et al.*, 1986).

Further work is needed to determine which species are involved in protein turnover and what is the contribution of protein turnover to the flow of carbon and nitrogen through the colonic ecosystem. Although a significant amount of proteolysis may occur in the colon and may provide an important source of nitrogen for colon bacteria, it should be noted that protein is not the only possible nitrogen source. Amino sugars (from mucins) and urea are examples of other potential nitrogen sources, but no information is currently available which demonstrates whether these are significant sources of nitrogen for colon bacteria.

C. Utilization of Polysaccharides by Colon Bacteria

Dietary fibre is unquestionably an important source of carbon and energy for saccharolytic colon bacteria (Vercellotti *et al.*, 1977, 1978). It has long been assumed that since dietary fibre is not digested by enzymes active in the small intestine, it passes through the upper part of the digestive tract without appreciable modification and enters the colon intact. Confirmation of this comes from a recent study of ileostomy patients by Englyst and Cummings (1985). Nearly all of the ingested cellulose and hemicellulose were recovered in ileal contents. Once dietary fibre enters the colon it is extensively digested by the colon bacteria (Van Soest, 1978; Ehle *et al.*, 1982). At least half of the ingested cellulose and hemicellulose and most of the ingested pectin disappears during passage through the colon (Van Soest, 1978). People who eat high fibre diets excrete more bacteria and have higher concentrations of volatile fatty acids in their faeces (Kelsay, 1978; Stephen and Cummings, 1980).

One widely accepted definition of dietary fibre is that it is the sum of cellulose and hemicellulose. Pectin and soluble gums are sometimes included as well. Some species of colonic bacteria are capable of fermenting hemicelluloses, plant gums and pectins. In fact, some species of colonic *Bacteroides* can ferment nearly all of the components of dietary fibre excluding cellulose (Salyers *et al.*, 1977a). To date, none of the numerically predominant species of colon bacteria have been shown to be capable of fermenting cellulose (Table 13.1). Betian *et al.* (1977) isolated cellulolytic bacteria from human faeces by enrichment culture. However, they found these bacteria only in some people and at very low concentrations. Given the extent to which celluloses in human foods are consistently found to be digested in nutritional studies, it seems reasonable to expect that the cellulose degrading bacteria would be present in relatively high concentrations.

There are two possible explanations of this apparent paradox. One explanation is that the bacteria which are responsible for cellulose digestion cannot be cultivated by any of the procedures normally used to cultivate colon anaerobes or facultative bacteria. A second explanation is that the wrong types of celluloses have been used in the bacteriological screening and enrichment studies. Betian *et al.* (1977) used microcrystalline cellulose, whereas the celluloses in human foods are hydrated celluloses. Further experiments using hydrated celluloses, or even mixed cellulose–hemicellulose complexes such as those found in plant cell walls, are needed to establish the identity of the cellulose degraders in the colon. In this connection, it is interesting to note that many colon bacteria can utilize cellobiose (the disaccharide repeating unit of cellulose). Some of these bacteria might be able to degrade hydrated cellulose or cellodextrins.

Although dietary fibre is clearly a major source of carbohydrate for some colon bacteria, it is probably not the only source. Many numerically predominant colon bacteria such as *Fusobacterium prauznitzii*,

Peptostreptococcus productus, and some *Eubacterium* species are unable to utilize cellulose, hemicellulose, or pectins when grown in laboratory culture, although they grow readily on monosaccharides and disaccharides (Table 13.2). It is possible that these species utilize polysaccharides such as xyloglucan that were not included in any of the surveys of carbohydrate utilization that have been done to date. Alternatively, they may use small molecular weight carbohydrates that escape from polysaccharide-degrading bacteria. Also, some small molecular weight carbohydrate in real foods may escape breakdown and absorption in the small intestine because it is protected physically or chemically by other food components. Evidence to support the hypothesis that some small molecular weight carbohydrate enters the colon has been obtained from the studies of ileal contents from accident victims (Vercellotti *et al.*, 1978), although the amount is probably low.

Another possible source of carbohydrate for colon bacteria is starch. Recently, Englyst and Cummings (1986) have shown that appreciable amounts of starch, particularly retrograded ('resistant') starch, escapes digestion by mammalian amylases. Results of previous studies had also indicated that some starch reaches the colon, and therefore should be included in the category of dietary fibre, as plant polysaccharides which are not digested to any great extent by host digestive enzymes (Anderson *et al.*, 1981; Levine and Levitt, 1981). The hypothesis that starch might be a major source of carbon and energy for some colon bacteria is an attractive one because many of the species that are found in high number in the colon are starch-fermenters. These observations raise once again the prickly question of how dietary fibre is to be defined. If it is defined as polysaccharides that are not digested in the small intestine and that have a physiological effect due to bacterial fermentation in the colon, clearly starch that escapes digestion in the colon must be considered dietary fibre.

Host products such as mucins and mucopolysaccharides must also be included as possible sources of carbon and energy for some colonic organisms. Some of the numerically predominant species of colonic *Bacteroides* can ferment mucopolysaccharides (Table 13.2), even when they are bound up in the sterically hindered complex of proteoglycan (Kuritza and Salyers, 1983). However, the amount of mucopolysaccharide from sloughed mucosal cells or from dietary meat that enters the colon daily is probably small compared to the amount of dietary plant polysaccharides or intestinal mucin glycoproteins.

Many species of colon bacteria can ferment the monosaccharide components of mucins (fucose, hexosamines), but none of the major species of colon bacteria can utilize bovine submaxillary mucin or porcine gastric mucin as a sole source of carbohydrate. Mucin-degrading activity can be detected in faeces (Hoskins and Boulding, 1981). Some mucin-degrading bacteria have been isolated from human faeces by enrichment procedures, but their numbers are low and they do not degrade the mucin very extensively when they are grown in laboratory medium (Roberton and Stanley, 1982). It is possible that only a small number of colon bacteria are capable of utilizing mucin. Alternatively, a consortium of bacteria may be needed to degrade the complex branched carbohydrate moeity of colonic mucin (Hoskins and Boulding, 1981). The extent to which intestinal mucin contributes to maintenance of the colonic flora remains to be established. The fact that people who are ingesting totally absorbable diets nonetheless maintain a sizeable colonic microflora seems to support the hypothesis that host products do contribute to the maintenance of the microflora. An interesting, but to date unproven, hypothesis is that dietary polysaccharides are preferentially utilized by some bacteria that could attack mucin. If so, bacterial digestion of the protective mucin layer that lines the colon could be reduced by a high fibre diet.

It has been estimated that the amount of carbohydrate needed for maintenance of the bacterial mass found in the colon is between 30 and 45 g per day (Salyers and Leedle, 1983). Some attempts have been made to estimate the amount of dietary fibre in a typical western diet. Bingham *et al.* (1985) estimated the dietary fibre intake, for persons living in Britain, to average about 13 g per day. From analyses of ileal contents, it would appear that the mucin and mucopolysaccharides could contribute 2 to 4 g dry weight of carbohydrate per day (Vercellotti *et al.*, 1977; Englyst and Cummings, 1986). This leaves at least 10 to 15 g of carbohydrate per day unaccounted for. It remains to be seen whether the difference reflects the contributions of starch or low molecular weight carbohydrate to maintaining the colonic microflora.

D. End Products of Bacterial Fermentation and Their Fate in the Host

1. *Short Chain Fatty Acids*

The major non-gaseous end products which result from the bacterial fermentation of carbohydrates in the large intestine are the short chain fatty acids. The three predominant fatty acids are acetate, propionate and butyrate. Their average molar ratios are 60 : 25 : 15 respectively (Cummings and Branch, 1986).

A substantial portion of the short chain fatty acids are absorbed by the host (McNeil *et al.*, 1978). Uptake of short chain fatty acids is dependent not only on the concentration of these compounds in the colon, but also on other factors such as secretion of bicarbonate, pH, pCO_2, and transport of sodium and water. Also, the short chain fatty acids are probably absorbed both in the anionic and undissociated acid forms (Cummings and Branch, 1986).

There is evidence for selective uptake of the fatty acids at different body sites. Butyrate seems to be taken up preferentially by the mucosal cells and may stimulate their growth (Roediger, 1980). It has been observed previously that the surface area of the colonic mucosa in germ-free rodents is substantially less than in conventional animals (Abrams, 1983). It is possible that the differences between germ-free and conventional animals are due in part to the effect of butyrate on mucosal cell growth, but this hypothesis has not yet been tested experimentally. In some animals, such as dogs, the difference in mucosal surface area between germ-free and conventional animals, is not seen (Wostmann, 1981). Thus, the apparent stimulation of mucosal growth by colon bacteria could be limited to rodents.

Propionate that is absorbed from the colon seems to be taken up preferentially by the liver (McNeil *et al.*, 1978). Acetate is the main fatty acid found in the peripheral circulation (Pomare *et al.*, 1985). Thus, the entire body is affected by the colonic fermentation.

When Pomare *et al.* (1985) fed subjects who had fasted for 16 hours a test meal containing lactulose (a disaccharide of galactose and fructose which goes essentially undigested in the small intestine) or pectin, they detected a rise in venous blood acetate levels which began 2 to 4 hours after lactulose ingestion and about 6 hours after pectin ingestion. Rise and fall of blood acetate levels after pectin ingestion were much slower than those observed after ingestion of lactulose, as expected from the fact that lactulose is fermented much more rapidly than pectin. This difference reflects the fact that the physical properties of the carbohydrate may be important in determining the rate of short chain fatty acid production and absorption in the colon. It also raises the question of whether soluble polysaccharides like pectin, which are rapidly fermented by bacteria in laboratory medium, are in fact fermented as rapidly in the colon. The common assumption that virtually all fermentation of carbohydrate occurs in the ascending colon may not be correct. Certainly, there is no direct evidence from studies with humans to support or refute it. Pomare *et al.* were able to detect changes in blood acetate levels because they fed fasted subjects a single meal. In the normal person, who is eating several times a day, blood acetate levels probably remain fairly constant.

Microbial fermentation of dietary material in the colon can also be monitored by measuring breath hydrogen. Pomare *et al.* (1985) found that breath hydrogen levels paralleled blood acetate levels fairly closely. However, this was not the case for levels of breath methane. Thus, carbohydrate breakdown in the colon can be monitored fairly accurately by quantitating the level of breath hydrogen.

The finding that breath hydrogen levels parallel blood acetate levels whereas breath methane levels do not is not too surprising in view of the fact that acetate and hydrogen are the primary products of polysaccharide fermentation, whereas methane production involves the interaction of a second group of organisms with the polysaccharide degraders. The coupling between methane production and polysaccharide fermentation may not always be a tight one.

Since short chain fatty acids are absorbed by the host, they may contribute to the host's energy metabolism or have other, as yet undetermined effects on host physiology. Clearly, it is incorrect to consider dietary fibre as non-caloric, but it remains to be demonstrated whether the caloric distribution of dietary fibre is substantial enough to be counted. It is unlikely that this contribution exceeds a few percent of total caloric intake, but this will depend on the diet (McNeil, 1984).

2. *Other Bacterial Products*

Bacteria carry out a number of reactions which have no known role in their metabolism but which may affect the host. For example, colon bacteria modify bile acids, sterols and steroids (Bokkenheuser and Winter, 1983; Hylemon and Glass, 1983). These modifications are predominantly reductions, hydroxylations or dehydroxylations, but ring scission can also occur.

A very interesting and potentially important group of bacterial products are the faecal pentaenes. These substances, which are mutagenic on the Ames test, are excreted by some people (Wilkins and Van Tassell, 1983). The incidence of mutagen-excreters in a population is correlated with colon cancer risk, but no cause and effect relationship has been established. It is not yet clear whether these mutagenic substances are also carcinogenic. The faecal pentaenes are produced by some species of *Bacteroides* when the bacteria are incubated with an extract from faeces. The identity of the precursor has not been established. Nor is it known why only some people excrete mutagen, whereas everyone has high concentrations of the mutagen-producing species of *Bacteroides* in their colon. This subject is discussed in more detail in chapter 17.

3. *Faeces vs. Colon Contents*

Because of the difficulty of obtaining human colon contents, particularly from healthy individuals, most investigations of processes that occur in the human colon must rely on faecal specimens as a substitute for colon contents. Faecal specimens probably provide a reasonably accurate replica of the lumen of the colon, at least with respect to the organisms which are found there (Moore *et al.*, 1978). Some lysis of bacteria may occur in the colon but the extent of this is not known. Concentrations of short chain fatty acids, and probably other compounds as well, may not be the same in faeces as they are in colon contents. The water content of colon contents is at least twice as high as that of faeces. Also, colon bacteria may be metabolically more active in the ascending colon, although this has not been confirmed experimentally. Enzyme activities of bacteria in faeces may be very similar to those of bacteria higher up in the colon, because proteins are not turned over rapidly once they are produced and most colon bacteria do not have the opportunity to go through many generations. Faecal specimens are not very useful for investigations of adherent bacteria because only those which have been sloughed off will be represented in faeces.

E. Mechanisms which may Control the Gut Microflora

The mechanisms which operate so as to regulate the population levels of each indigenous species of the colonic microflora are probably several in number and act synergistically in that regulation. One mechanism that has been postulated as being important is the role of competition among species for limiting nutrients (Freter *et al.*, 1983a). The number of potential sources of carbon and energy in the colon is large but the amount of each particular substrate is probably low. It is clear from the data in Table 13.2 that some of the numerically predominant bacteria can utilize only one or a few potential carbon and energy sources, at least *in vitro*. In these cases, the number of organisms may be limited by the amount of these substrates which enter the colon.

It is likely that a food chain exists among the colonic flora, as is the case for many complex ecosystems, and the degradation products of one group of organisms feed another group of organisms. If so, the levels of species which depend on products of other bacteria will be controlled by the levels of those products. Cross-feeding of carbon and nitrogen has been documented in the case of rumen bacteria. One well established example of this sort is the cross-feeding of hydrogen. Some methanogens can utilize the carbon dioxide and hydrogen which are produced by a carbohydrate-fermenting bacteria, when the two are co-cultured (Wolin, 1979; Wolin and Miller, 1983). A second example involves cross-feeding of carbohydrate. When *Selomonas ruminatium* and *Bacteroides succinogenes* are grown on cellulose, both grow to about the same level. *B. succinogenes* is cellulolytic whereas *Selomonas ruminatium* is not. Clearly, the hydrolysis products of *B. succinogenes* can be used by *S. ruminatium* for growth (Scheifinger and Wolin, 1973). Cross-feeding of nitrogen and other growth factors may also occur.

It is intuitively appealing to speculate that the organisms of the gut have evolved, over time, the capacity to out-compete other organisms for the sources of carbon and nitrogen that are available in the colon. This may explain why some potentially pathogenic organisms are not able to become established in the colon unless the resident microflora has been perturbed. If there is a perturbation, either naturally or experimentally induced, and if an invading transient organism is capable of utilizing an available substrate or occupying a vacated niche, it may become established and cause disease (Savage, 1977; 1980).

Freter and co-workers have attempted to model colonic control mechanisms using continuous-flow cultures as *in vitro* models of the ecology of the large intestine. In a series of experiments, Freter *et al.* (1983c) were able to reproduce bacterial population levels in anaerobic continuous-flow culture vessels similar to those in conventional animals for at least some of the bacterial species indigenous to the conventional mouse caecum. Thick layers of bacteria were found adhering to the wall of the glass culture vessels similar to the numbers of bacteria seen in electron micrographs of the colon adhering to the gut wall. Also, a very complex nutrient source, veal infusion broth, had to be used in the continuous-flow culture vessels to provide the substances required for maintaining the ecological balance. Polysaccharides which resemble those of intestinal mucus may be present in this complex bacteriological medium. Which, if any, of the potential sources of carbon and energy in the infusion broth was limiting is not known. The mathematical model of Freter *et al.* (1983b) predicts that if two or more bacterial populations compete for the same substrate, the less efficient utilizer of the substrate can coexist with the more efficient utilizer if it has the capacity to colonize an area of the wall and if its growth rate does not fall below the lowest rate of shedding from the adherent mass.

Competition for limiting substrates may not be the only factor that determines which species colonize the colon. Toxic metabolites may also influence microbial growth. One such toxic metabolite is hydrogen sulphide, which is known to inhibit growth of some colonic organisms (Freter *et al.*, 1983a). Likewise, short chain fatty acids or bile salts may delay multiplication of an invading bacterium until it has been washed out (Freter *et al.*, 1983a).

F. Summary

There is little doubt that dietary fibre, perhaps more than any other dietary component, has an effect on the colonic microflora and ultimately on the host. The fibre–flora interaction is one of great complexity due to the tremendous diversity of microbial species which reside in the colon, and can potentially participate in the degradation of fibre. Certainly, fibre contributes to the overall flow of carbon and energy through the colonic ecosystem. The degradation of fibre by the colonic microflora and the release of the end products for eventual absorption and metabolism could have as yet undetermined consequences for the host.

Further experimental work on the basic physiology of various colonic organisms, which participate in the degradation of dietary polysaccharides, could unveil key insights into the colonic ecosystem. For example, it may be possible to use bacterial activities, present in faecal samples, as indicators of the colonic environment. These activities could be used essentially as metabolic probes so as to ascertain which groups or species of bacteria participate in the catabolism of a particular dietary component (McCarthy and Salyers, 1986). Also, studies to establish what effects certain components of dietary fibre have on the colonic microflora may prove fruitful. However, this will only be possible if well characterized and chemically defined substrates are used. The prospects for addressing many of these issues are good and will contribute to our understanding of this very complicated interaction between flora and fibre.

Acknowledgements

This work was supported by Public Health Service grant AI 17876 from the National Institutes of Health. We thank Sharon Kirk for typing this manuscript.

References

Abrams, G. D. (1983). Impact of the intestinal microflora on intestinal structure and function. *In*: "Human Intestinal Microflora in Health and Disease" (ed. D. Hentges), pp. 291–310. Academic Press, New York.

Anderson, I. H., Levine, A. S. and Levitt, M. D. (1981). Incomplete absorption of the carbohydrate in all-purpose wheat flour. *New Engl. J. Med.*, **304**, 891–892.

Barker, H. A. and Haas, V. (1944). Butyribacterium, a new genus of gram-positive, non-sporulating anaerobic bacteria of intestinal origin. *J. Bacteriol.* **47**, 301–305.

Betian, H. G., Linehan, B. A., Bryant, M. P. and Holdeman, L. V. (1977). Isolation of a cellulolytic *Bacteroides* from human faeces. *Appl. Environ. Microbiol.* **331**, 1009–1010.

Bingham, S. A., Williams, D. R. R. and Cummings, J. H. (1985). Dietary fibre consumption in Britain: new estimates and their relation to large bowel cancer mortality. *Br. J. Cancer* **52**, 399–402.

Bokkenheuser, V. D. and Winter, J. (1983). Biotransformation of steroids. *In*: "Human Intestinal Microflora in Health and Disease" (ed. D. Hentges), pp. 215–239. Academic Press, New York.

Bornside, G. H. (1978). Stability of human fecal flora. *Amer. J. Clin. Nutr.* **31**, S141–S144.

Cummings, J. H. and Branch, W. J. (1986). Fermentation and the production of short-chain fatty acids in the human large intestine. *In*: "Dietary Fiber: Basic and Clinical Aspects" (eds G. V. Vahouny and D. Kritchevsky), pp. 131–149. Plenum Press, New York and London.

Ehle, F. R., Robertson, J. B. and Van Soest, P. J. (1982). Influence of dietary fibers on fermentation in the human large intestine. *J. Nutr.* **112**, 158–166.

Englyst, H. N. and Cummings, J. H. (1985). Digestion of the polysaccharides of some cereal foods in the human small intestine. *Am. J. Clin. Nutr.* **42**, 778–787.

Englyst, H. N. and Cummings, J. H. (1986). Digestion of the carbohydrates of banana in the human small intestine. *Am. J. Clin. Nutr.* **44**, 42–50.

Finegold, S. M. and Sutter, V. L. (1978). Fecal flora in different populations with special reference to diet. *Am. J. Clin. Nutr.* **32**, S116–S122.

Finegold, S. M., Mathisen, G. E. and George W. L. (1983). Changes in human intestinal flora related to the administration of antimicrobial agents. *In*: "Human Intestinal Microflora in Health and Disease" (ed. D. Hentges), pp. 355–446. Academic Press, new York.

Freter, R., Brickner, H., Botney, M., Cleven, D. and Aranki, A. (1983a). Mechanisms that control bacterial populations in continuous-flow culture models of mouse large intestinal flora. *Infect. Immun.* **39**, 676–685.

Freter, R., Brickner, H., Fekete, J., Vickerman, M. M. and Carey, K. E. (1983b). Survival and implantation of *Escherichia coli* in the intestinal tract. *Infect. Immun.* **39**, 686–703.

Freter, R., Stauffer, E., Cleven, D., Holdeman, L. V. and Moore, W. E. C. (1983c). Continuous-flow cultures as *in vitro* models of the ecology of the large intestinal flora. *Infect. Immun.* **39**, 666–675.

Genthner, B. R., Davis, C. L. and Bryant, M. P. (1981). Features of rumen and sewage sludge strains of Eubacterium limosum, a methanol- and H_2-CO_2-utilizing species. *Appl. Environ. Microbiol.* **42**, 12–19.

Hentges, D. J., Maier, B., Burton, G. C., Flynn, M. A. and Tsutakawa, R. K. (1977). Effect of a high beef diet on the fecal bacterial flora of humans. *Cancer Res.* **37**, 568–571.

Hentges, D. J. (1983). "Human Intestinal Microflora in Health and Disease", p. 568. Academic Press, New York.

Holdeman, L. V., Cato, E. P. and Moore, W. E. C. (1977). "Anaerobe Laboratory Manual" (4th ed.). Anaerobe Lab., Virginia Polytechnic Institute and State University, Blacksburg.

Hoskins, L. C. and Boulding, E. T. (1981). Mucin degradation in human colon ecosystems. *J. Clin. Invest.* **67**, 163–172.

Hylemon, P. B. and Glass, T. L. (1983). Biotransformation of bile acids and cholesterol by the intestinal microflora. *In*: "Human Intestinal Microflora in Health and Disease" (ed. D. Hentges), pp. 189–214. Academic Press, New York.

Johnson, J. L. (1978). Taxonomy of the Bacteroides. *Interntl J. Syst. Bacteriol.* April, 245–256.

Kelsay, J. L. (1978). A review of research on effects of fiber intake on man. *Am. J. Clin. Nutr.* **31**, 142–159.

Kotarski, S. F. and Salyers, K. A. (1981). Effect of long generation times on growth of *Bacteroides thetaiotaomicron* in carbohydrate-limited continuous culture. *J. Bacteriol.* **146**, 853–860.

Kuritza, A. P. and Salyers, A. A. (1983). Digestion of proteoglycan by *Bacteroides thetaiotaomicron*. *J. Bacteriol.* **153**, 1180–1186.

Levine, A. S. and Levitt, M. D. (1981). Malabsorption of starch moeity of oats, corn and potatoes. *Gastroenterol.* **82**, 1209.

Macfarlane, G. T., Cummings, J. H. and Allison, C. (1986). Protein degradation by human intestinal bacteria. *J. Gen. Microbiol.* **132**, 1647–1656.

Macy, J. M., Ljungdal, L. G. and Gottschalk, G. (1978). Pathway of succinate and propionate formation in *Bacteroides fragilis*. *J. Bacteriol.* **134**, 84–91.

McCarthy, R. E. and Salyers, A. A. (1986). Evidence that polygalacturonic acid may not be a major source of carbon and energy for some colonic *Bacteroides* species. *Appl. Environ. Microbiol.* **52**, 9–16.

McNeil, D. H., Cummings, J. H. and James, W. P. T. (1978). Short chain fatty acid absorption by the human large intestine. *Gut* **19**, 819–822.

McNeil, N. I. (1984). The contribution of the large intestine to energy supplies in man. *Am. J. Clin. Nutr.* **39**, 338–342.

Miller, T. L. and Wolin, M. J. (1982). Enumeration of *Methanobrevibacter smithii* in human faeces. *Arch. Microbiol.* **131**, 14–18.

Miller, T. L. and Wolin, M. J. (1985). *Methanosphaera stadtmaniae* gen. nov. sp. nov.: a species that forms methane by reducing methanol with hydrogen. *Arch. Microbiol.* **141**, 116–122.

Moore, W. E. C. and Holdeman, L. V. (1974). Human fecal flora, the normal flora of 20 Japanese-Hawaiians. *Appl. Microbiol.* **27**, 961–979.

Moore, W. E. C., Cato, E. P. and Holdeman, L. V. (1978). Some current concepts in intestinal bacteriology. *Am. J. Clin. Nutr.* **31**, S33–S42.

Paster, B. J., Ludwig, W., Weisburg, W. G., Stachebrandt, E., Hespell, R. B., Hahn, C. M., Reichenbach, H., Stetter, K. O. and Woese, C. R. (1985). A phylogenetic grouping of the *Bacteroides*, *Cytophages*, and certain *Flavobacteria* System. *Appl. Microbiol.* **6**, 34–42.

Pomare, E. W., Branch, W. J. and Cummings, J. H. (1985). Carbohydrate fermentation in the human colon and its relation to acetate concentrations in venous blood. *J. Clin. Invest.* **75**, 1448–1454.

Roberton, A. M. and Stanley, R. A. (1982). *In vitro* utilization of mucin by *Bacteroides fragilis*. *Appl. Environ. Microbiol.* **43**, 325–330.

Roediger, W. E. W. (1980). Role of anaerobic bacteria in the metabolic welfare of the colonic mucosa in man. *Gut*, **21**, 793–798.

Salyers, A. A., Vercellotti, J. R., West, S. E. H. and Wilkins, T. D. (1977a). Fermentation of mucin and plant polysaccharide by strains of *Bacteroides* from the human colon. *Appl. Environ. Microbiol.* **33**, 319–322.

Salyers, A. A., West, S. E. H., Vercellotti, J. R. and Wilkins, T. D. (1977b). Fermentation of mucins and plant polysaccharides by anaerobic bacteria from the human colon. *Appl. Environ. Microbiol.* **34**, 529–533.

Salyers, A. A. and Leedle, J. A. Z. (1983). Carbohydrate metabolism in the human colon. *In*: "The Human Intestinal Microflora in Health and Disease" (ed. D. Hentges), pp. 129–146. Academic Press, New York.

Savage, D. C. (1977). Interactions between the host and its microbes. *In*: "Microbial Ecology of the Gut" (eds R. T. J. Clarke and T. Bauchop), pp. 277–310. Academic Press, London.

Savage, D. C. (1980). Colonisation by and survival of pathogenic bacteria on intestinal mucosal surfaces. *In*: "Adsorption of Microorganisms to Surfaces" (eds G. Bitton and K. C. Marshall), pp. 176–206. Wiley, New York.

Scheifinger, C. C. and Wolin, M. J. (1973). Propionate formation from cellulose and soluble sugars by combined cultures of *Bacteroides succinogenes* and *Selemonas ruminantium*. *Appl. Microbiol.* **26**, 789–795.

Smith, R. D. and Salyers, A. A. (1981). Incorporation of leucine into phospholipids of *Bacteroides thetaiotaomicron*. *J. Bacteriol.* **145**, 8–13.

Stackebrandt, E. and Woese, C. R. (1981). The evolution of procaryotes. *In*: "Molecular and Cellular Aspects of Microbial Evolution". (eds M.J. Carlile, J. R. Collins and B. Moseley), pp. 1–31. Cambridge University Press.

Stephen, A. M. and Cummings, J. H. (1980). Mechanism of action of dietary fibre in the human colon. *Nature* **284**, 283–284.

Van Soest, P. J. (1978). Dietary fibers: Their definition and nutritional aspects. *Am. J. Clin. Nutr.* **31**, S12–S20.

Vercellotti, J. R., Salyers, A. A., Bullard, W. S. and Wilkins, T. D. (1977). Breakdown of mucin and plant polysaccharides in the human colon. *Can. J. Biochem.* **55**, 1190–1196.

Vercellotti, J. R., Salyers, A. A. and Wilkins, T. D. (1978). Complex carbohydrate breakdown in the human colon. *Am. J. Clin. Nutr.* **31**, S86–S89.

Weisburg, W. G., Oyaizu, Y., Oyaizu, H. and Woese, C. R. (1985). Natural relationship between *Bacteroides* and *Flavobacteria*. *J. Bacteriol.* **164**, 230–236.

Wilkins, T. D. and R. L. Van Tassell (1983). Production of intestinal mutagens. *In*: "Human Intestinal Microflora in Health and Disease" (ed. D. Hentges), pp. 265–288. Academic Press, New York.

Wolin, M. J. (1979). The rumen fermentation: A model for microbial interactions in anaerobic ecosystems. *Adv. Microb. Ecol.* **3**, 49–77.

Wolin, M. J. and Miller, T. L. (1983). Carbohydrate fermentation. *In*: "Human Intestinal Microflora in Health and Disease" (ed. D. Hentges), pp. 147–165. Academic Press, New York.

Wostmann, B. S. (1981). The germfree animal in nutritional studies. *Ann. Rev. Nutr.* **1**, 257–279.

14

Mammalian Lignans and Phyto-oestrogens Recent Studies on their Formation, Metabolism and Biological Role in Health and Disease

K.D.R. SETCHELL and H. ADLERCREUTZ

A. Introduction

The Western-type diet, high in fat and protein and low in complex carbohydrate and fibre, has been associated with many diseases, including coronary heart disease, colon cancer and hormone-dependent cancers like mammary, endometrium and prostate cancers (Trowell and Burkitt, 1983; Palmer, 1985). The mechanism by which diet influences the development of these diseases has been discussed to a limited extent. Meanwhile it has become clear that the intestinal bacterial metabolism of macro- and micro-nutritients, xenobiotics etc., present in food, and of endogenous substances such as bile acids and oestrogens, plays a significant and central role. The influence of bacterial metabolism may occur in a positive or a negative direction with regard to the development of disease, and may depend upon the composition of the microflora, its environment and many other factors. Studies on the role of intestinal bacterial metabolism of hormones, bile acids and sterols and the mechanisms by which diet influences disease has been the focus of much interest during the last few decades. This review will describe and discuss the potential role with regard to disease of two classes of diphenols, the lignans and isoflavonic phyto-oestrogens, which in the last decade have been detected and identified in biological fluids of man. The scope of this review will be restricted to mammalian lignans and to recent results in the field of isoflavonic phyto-oestrogens, the latter having been reviewed recently by Price and Fenwick (1985).

ROLE OF THE GUT FLORA IN TOXICITY AND CANCER
ISBN 0-12-599920-8

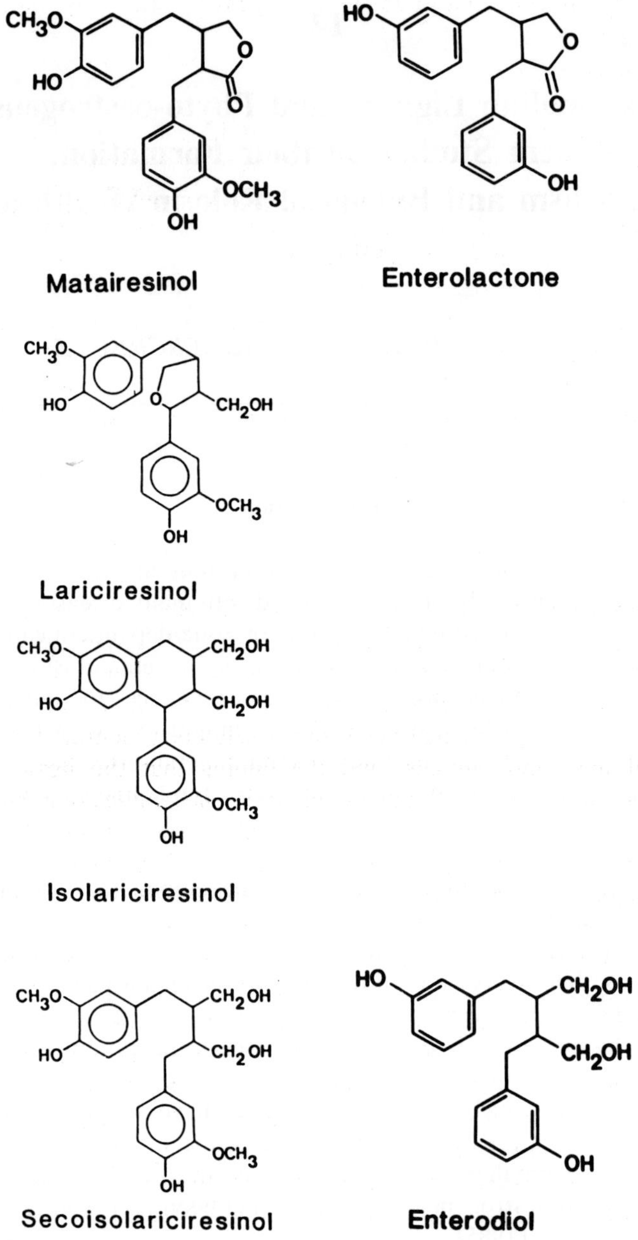

Fig 14.1. Chemical structures of mammalian lignans identified in human urine.

B.   Identification of Phyto-oestrogens in Man and Animals

1. *Lignans*

For more than a decade before their identification, a number of unusual compounds were consistently observed in urinary steroid profiles analysed by gas liquid chromatography and mass spectrometry (GLC–MS). The mass spectra of these compounds, although showing some similarities, differed significantly from spectra typical of urinary steroid hormone metabolites. It was the serendipitous observation of a cyclic pattern in the urinary excretion of these compounds, firstly in the vervet monkey (Setchell *et al.*, 1980a) and later in women (Setchell and Adlercreutz, 1979; Setchell *et al.*, 1980b, 1980c), which prompted a concerted effort to elucidate the structures of what we believed at that time to be new endogenous hormones.

With the application of infra-red, ultra-violet, and nuclear magnetic resonance spectroscopic techniques, to complement data derived from thin layer chromatography, GLC and GLC–MS analysis, these new compounds were shown to belong to the chemical class referred to as lignans (Setchell *et al.*, 1980c, 1981a; Cooley *et al.*, 1984). By definition lignans are compounds possessing a 2,3-dibenzylbutane structure, and such compounds are known to exist as minor constituents of many plants where they form the building blocks for the formation of lignin in the plant cell wall. Lignans had never previously been identified in biological fluids of man and animals, and the finding that the lignans thus far identified differ from all known plant lignans in lacking *para*-oxygen substitution is unique, while the finding that they are racemic is remarkable (Stitch *et al.*, 1980b; Groen and Leemhuis, 1980; Cooley *et al.*, 1981).

The major urinary lignan identified (Fig. 14.1) was shown to have the structure (±)*trans*-2,3-bis-(3-hydroxybenzyl)-γ-butyrolactone (originally designated HBBL), for which we adopted the trivial name enterolactone (Setchell *et al.*, 1981b). At the same time as we identified this compound, Stitch *et al.* (1980b) described its occurrence as a constituent of pregnancy urine, and the structure of this first mammalian lignan was published by the journal *Nature*. As a point of clarification, enterolactone was described by this latter group as *trans*-(±)-3,4-bis[(3-hydroxyphenyl)-methyl] - dihydro-2-(3H)-furanone, for which the acronym HPMF was used, although it has since been given the more correct name 2,3-bis-(3-hydroxybenzyl)butan-4-olide (Cooley *et al.*, 1984).

In addition to enterolactone a second important lignan, the reduction product 2,3-bis(3-hydroxybenzyl)butan-1,4-diol, referred to by the trivial name enterodiol, and several monomethoxy and dimethoxy isomers of enterolactone and enterodiol were identified (Setchell *et al.*, 1980c, 1981). The structure of one of these monomethoxy analogues was recently confirmed to be matairesinol (*trans*-2,3-bis-(3-hydroxymethoxy)-4-hydroxybenzyl)-γ-butyrolactone (Bannwart *et al.*, 1984a), while the dimethoxy analogue was definitively identified as secoisolariciresinol (Axelson *et al.*, 1982b), both compounds being intermediates in the pathway to the formation of enterolactone.

These series of mammalian lignans have variably been identified in the urine of man (Setchell *et al.*, 1980c, 1981a; Stitch *et al.*, 1980a, 1980b; Axelson and Setchell, 1980; Bannwart *et al.*, 1984a), monkey (Setchell *et al.*, 1980a, 1980c; Setchell and Bonney, 1981), chimpanzee (Adlercreutz *et al.*, 1986a) and rat (Axelson and Setchell, 1980, 1981), in human and bovine semen (Dehennin *et al.*, 1982), in serum (Setchell *et al.*, 1981b; Axelson and Setchell, 1981; Dehennin *et al.*, 1982), in bile (Axelson and Setchell, 1981), and in faeces (Setchell *et al.*, 1981b). More recently enterolactone, enterodiol and matairesinol were identified in cows' milk (Adlercreutz, *et al.* 1986c; Bamwart *et al.*, 1986) (see Table 14.1).

2. *Isoflavones*

The almost ubiquitous occurrence in plants of compounds possessing oestrogenic activity (Farnsworth *et al.*, 1975) has resulted in extensive studies of their effects on animals following ingestion (Price and Fenwick, 1985), and more recently in humans (Setchell *et al.*, 1984; Adlercreutz, 1984). The two main classes of phyto-oestrogens to be found in plants are the isoflavones and the coumestans (Price and Fenwick, 1985), and it is the former class which has received the most attention.

The phyto-oestrogens are heterocyclic phenols with a close similarity in structure to oestrogenic steroids. For example, the distance between the two aromatic hydroxyl groups in the nucleus of the isoflavones is almost identical to the distance between the C-3 and C-17 hydroxy groups of oestradiol, while the presence of a phenolic hydroxyl, a pre-requisite for the oestrogenic activity (Leclerq and Heuson, 1979), accounts for the biological activity of these compounds.

The most widely published example of the potential importance of phyto-oestrogens in the diet was their direct association with an infertility syndrome in sheep in Western Australia, named Clover Disease (Bennetts *et al.*, 1946). The condition, which decimated the sheep breeding industry, was characterized by a cystic condition of the ovaries, an irreversible endometriosis and a failure to conceive, and was subsequently shown to be caused by the ingestion of a species of clover, *Trifolium subterraneum*,

Table 14.1 *The trivial names and their chemical abstract index names of phyto-oestrogens referred to in the text*

Trivial name	Chemical Abstract Index names
Lignans	
Matairesinol	(3*R-trans*)-dihydro-3,4-bis[4-hydroxy-3-methoxy-phenyl)methyl]-2(3H)-furanone
Secoisolariciresinol	[*R*-(*R**,*R**)]-2,3-bis[(4-hydroxy-3-methoxy-phenyl)methyl]-1,4-butanediol
Lariciresinol (+)	[2*S*-(2β,3β,4β)]-tetrahydro-2-(4-hydroxy-3-methoxy-phenyl)-4-[(4-hydroxy-3-methoxy-phenyl)methyl]-3-furan-methanol
Isolariciresinol	[1*S*-(1α,2β,3α)]-1,2,3,4-tetrahydro-7-hydroxy-1-(4-hydroxy-3-methoxyphenyl)-6-methoxy-2,3-naphthalene-dimethanol
Enterolactone	*trans*-2,3-bis[(3-hydroxyphenyl)methyl]-butyrolactone
Enterodiol	2,3-bis[(3-hydroxyphenyl)methyl]-butane-1,4-diol
Isoflavones	
Biochanin A	5,7-dihydroxy-4′-methoxyisoflavone
Genistein	4′,5,7-trihydroxyisoflavone
Formononetin	7-hydroxy-4′-methoxyisoflavone
Daidzein	4′,7-dihydroxyisoflavone
'Intermediate E'	4′,7-dihydroxyisoflavene
'Intermediate O'	4′,7-dihydroxyisoflavanone
Equol	4′,7-dihydroxyisoflavan
O-desmethylangolensin	1-(2,4-dihydroxyphenyl)-2-(4-hydroxyphenyl)-propan-1-one
Methylequol	7-hydroxy-4′-methoxyisoflavan
'Isoequol'	3′,7-dihydroxyisoflavan

which is abundant in W. Australia and rich in isoflavonic phyto-oestrogens (Bradbury and White, 1954).

The isoflavones of most abundance in plants are formononetin (7-hydroxy-4'-methoxyisoflavone), daidzein (4',7-dihydroxyisoflavone) and genistein (4',5,7-trihydroxyisoflavone). Their structures are shown in Fig. 14.2. Although these compounds all possess biological activity and have been identified in biological fluids of man and animals, it is the bacterially modified isoflavan, equol (7-hydroxy-3-(4'-hydroxyphenyl)-chroman), which was shown to be the oestrogenic agent responsible for Clover Disease in sheep (see Lindsay and Kelly (1970)). This isoflavan is formed by the action of ruminal bacteria on formononetin present in the ingested clover (Nilsson *et al.*, 1967).

Equol was first identified in the urine of pregnant mares (Marrian and Haslewood, 1932) and later in the urine of the goat (Klyne and Wright, 1957), cow (Klyne and Wright, 1959), hen (MacRae *et al.*, 1960; Common and Ainsworth, 1961) and sheep (Braden *et al.*, 1967; Shutt and Braden, 1968). More recently equol was definitively identified in human urine for the first time, using a combination of GLC–MS and NMR spectroscopy (Axelson *et al.*, 1982a). Its presence in human urine was confirmed (Adlercreutz *et al.*, 1982), and subsequently it has been identified in the urine of the pregnant macaque (Monfort *et al.*, 1984; Thompson *et al.*, 1984) and chimpanzee (Adlercreutz *et al.*, 1986a).

With the advent of highly specific and sensitive methods for the determination of the isoflavones, including the use of mass spectrometry, it is inevitable that other phyto-oestrogens in the biosynthetic pathway to equol will be identified in biological fluids from man and animals. In this respect two intermediates in the proposed pathways in the metabolism of daidzein (Fig. 14.2), have been found in human urine, but their definitive identification awaits chemical synthesis of these compounds. A relatively abundant isomer of equol, the 3,7-dihydroxyflavan, has also been identified in bovine (Luk *et al.*, 1983) and human urine and cow milk (Bannwart *et al.*, 1987 (in press)), while equol and a new metabolite, methylequol, have been identified in cow's milk (Bannwart *et al.*, 1986). The latter is presumed to be an intermediate in the pathway between formononetin and equol, and represents a second pathway in the metabolism of formononetin by sheep (see Price and Fenwick (1985) (Fig. 14.2). In this herbivorous animal, biochanin A, genistein, formononetin, daidzein, methylequol and *O*-desmethylangolensin have been identified in the urine using GC/MS (Bannwart *et al.*, unpublished work).

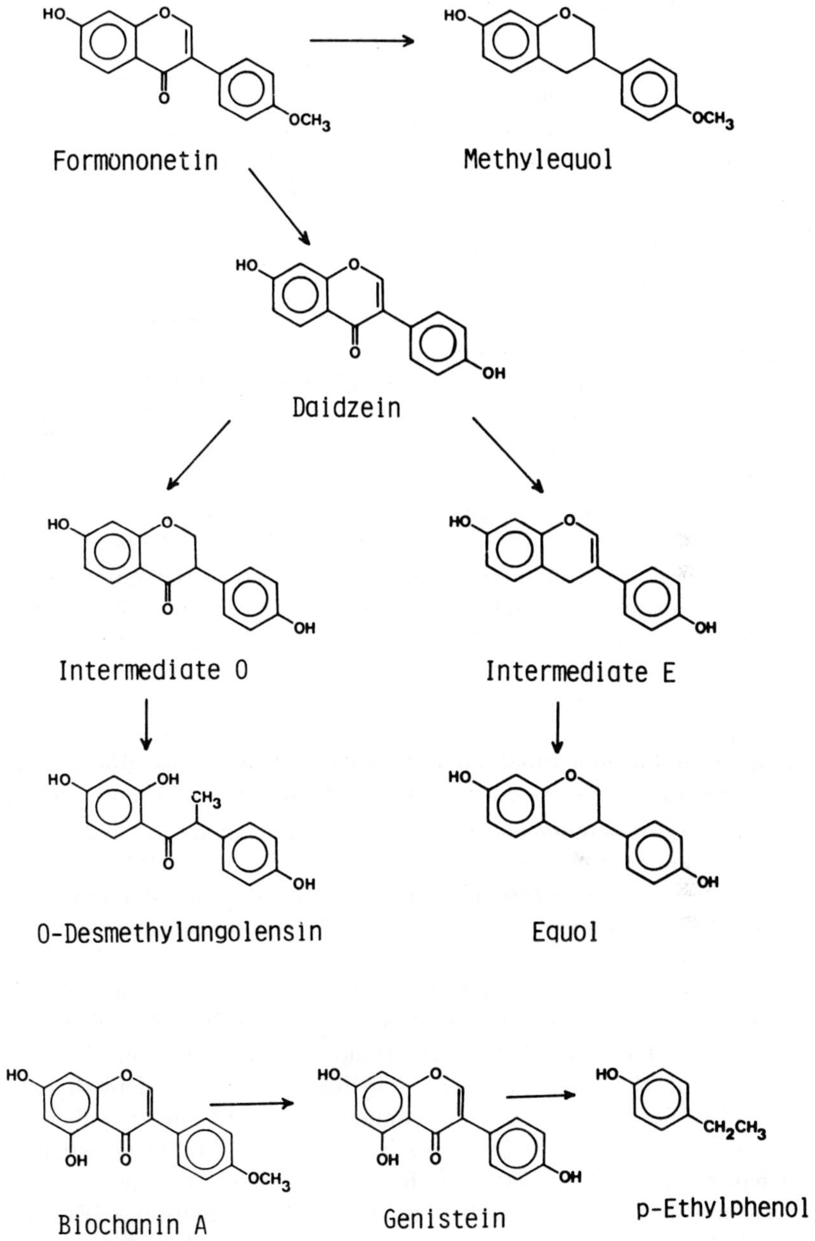

Fig 14.2. Chemical structures and metabolic pathways of dietary isoflavones in man and animals.

C. Origin and Metabolism of Lignans and Isoflavonic Phyto-oestrogens in Man

It is now well established that the human diet, particularly grain and other fibre-rich food (Adlercreutz, 1984; Adlercreutz *et al.*, 1981, 1986b, 1987b; Axelson *et al.*, 1982b; Setchell *et al.*, 1983; Borriello *et al.*, 1985), contains plant lignans, which serve as precursors for the bacterial synthesis of enterolactone and enterodiol. Evidence for this was established from animal studies in which the disappearance of mammalian lignans from biological fluids was demonstrated when rats were fed semi-synthetic diets. This model served as a useful means of pin-pointing those foodstuffs containing precursors of the lignans enterolactone and enterodiol. Prior studies using germ-free rats (Axelson and Setchell, 1981) and humans administered antibiotics (Setchell *et al.*, 1981b), had established that the production of lignans was dependent upon the presence of bacteria in the intestinal tract (Setchell *et al.*, 1982; Borriello *et al.*, 1985).

Following the observation that when linseeds (flaxseed) were ingested in relatively small amounts by rats, monkeys and man (Axelson *et al.*, 1982b; Setchell *et al.*, 1983) extremely high concentrations of enterolactone and enterodiol were excreted in the urine, work focused on isolating the precursor from raw linseeds. Using GC–MS a complex and highly polar lignan, secoisolariciresinol diglycoside, was identified as the precursor of enterolactone and its concentration in linseed was approximately 800 µg g^{-1} (Axelson *et al.*, 1982b). *In vitro* studies demonstrated the efficient conversion of secoisolariciresinol (either as the synthetic compound or in the natural form of linseeds) to enterodiol and enterolactone by human faecal flora under both anaerobic and aerobic conditions, indicating action by facultative bacteria (Borriello *et al.*, 1985). Enterolactone was also produced from matairesinol, an abundant plant lignan, after incubation with mixed faecal flora under anaerobic and aerobic conditions (Borriello *et al.*, 1985), thus confirming the earlier evidence in rats fed matairesinol that this was also a potential precursor of the mammalian lignans (Axelson *et al.*, 1982b). Conversion of secoisolariciresinol glycoside to enterodiol requires reactions involving hydrolysis of the sugar moiety, dehydroxylation and demethylation (Fig. 14.3), reactions which are commonly carried out by microbial enzymes. Formation of enterolactone from enterodiol requires oxidation, and has been demonstrated from feeding experiments (Axelson *et al.*, 1982b) and from *in vitro* incubations with human faecal flora (Borriello *et al.*, 1985), but the reverse reaction does not occur. Matairesinol which has the γ-lactone structure undergoes the comparable dehydroxylation and demethylation reactions in the pathway to enterolactone (Fig. 14.4).

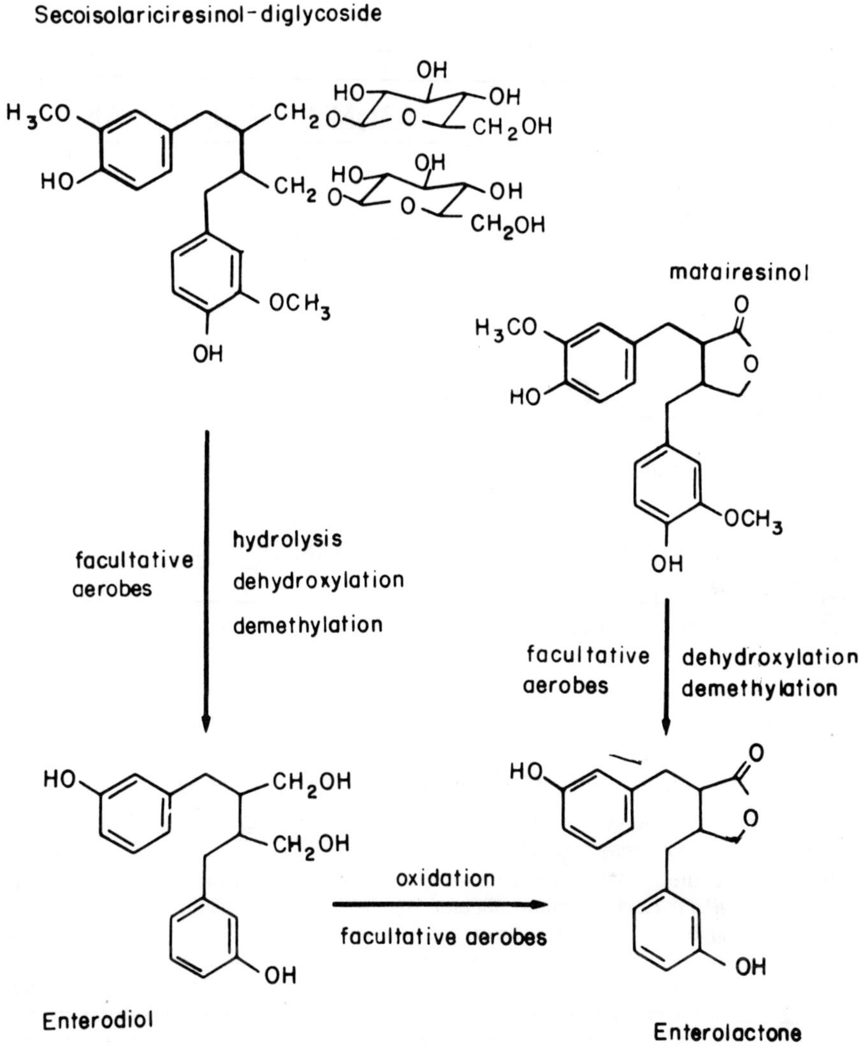

Fig 14.3. Metabolic pathways in the bacterial synthesis of the lignans enterolactone and enterodiol (from Borriello *et al.*, 1985).

Although relatively efficient bacterial conversion of these two precursors into enterolactone and enterodiol takes place, the finding of matairesinol and secoisolariciresinol in urine (Setchell *et al.*, 1980c, 1981a; Bannwart *et al.*, 1984a) indicates that these two precursors may be absorbed from

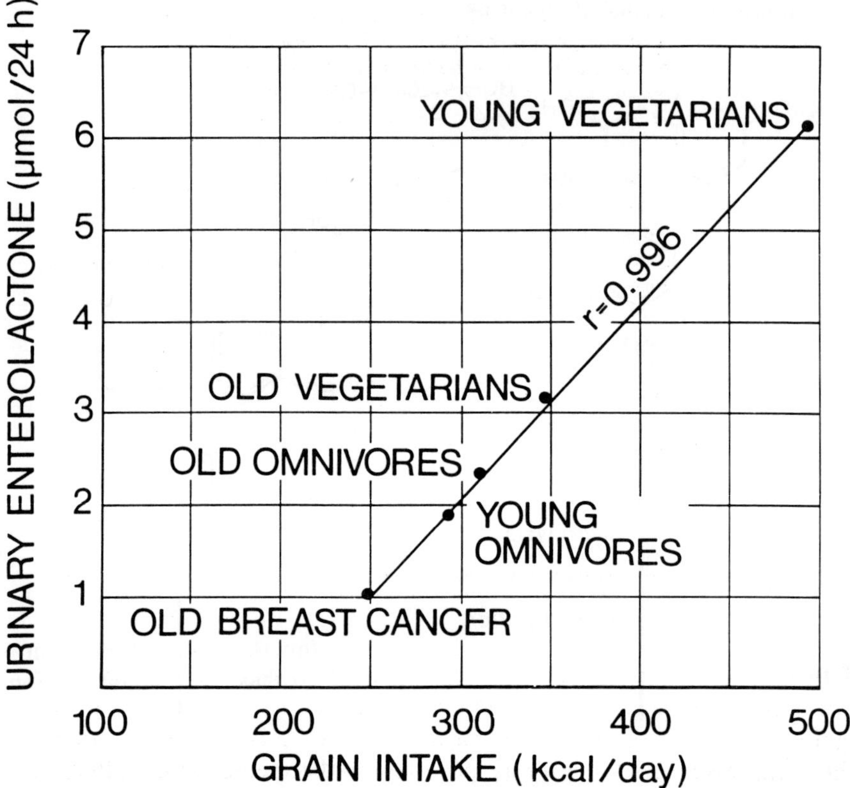

Fig. 14.4. Correlation between urinary excretion of the lignan enterolactone and dietary intake of grain products (kcal/day) in five groups of women consuming their habitual diet. Each group consists of 10 women except the old breast cancer patients ($n = 7$). Each woman collected one 72 hour urine sample four times at intervals of about 18 weeks during one year, and each point represents the geometric means of 40 values corresponding to 120 24 hour urine specimens, except for the breast cancer group (84 24 hour specimens). The samples in the young women were taken in the midfollicular phase of the menstrual cycle. Enterolactone was assayed by capillary gas chromatography (Fotsis *et al.*, 1982). The results for the postmenopausal women have been published previously (Adlercreutz *et al.*, 1982).

the gastro-intestinal tract unchanged. Our studies to date do not preclude other possible precursors to these mammalian lignans, since it is evident that many plant foodstuffs (Table 14.2) when ingested will lead to the urinary excretion of enterolactone and enterodiol (Axelson *et al.*, 1982b). In particular, grains and cereals probably account for the 'basal' levels

Table 14.2 *Total excretion of lignans in urine (μg/g foodstuff ingested) in response to the addition of different foodstuffs to rats maintained on a semisynthetic diet (Axelson et al. 1982b)*

Linseed meal	808.0 ± 45.7
Linseed Oil	17.4
Wheat bran	8.2 ± 0.5
Rye meal	6.4 ± 1.1
Buckwheat meal	4.7
Millet meal	3.7
Soya meal	2.3
Oat meal	2.1
Barley meal	2.0
Soya-bean oil	1.3
Wheat germ	0.9
Wheat flour	0.4
Corn meal	0.4
Corn oil	0.4
Fish meal	0.4

of these two lignans in man. In a study of five groups of women, the geometric mean excretion of enterolactone in urine correlated highly significantly with the geometric mean intake of dietary grain products when expressed as kilocalories per day (Adlercreutz *et al.*, 1986b). Because of the nature of their diet, subhuman primates excrete relatively high concentrations of lignans, but when the diet of chimpanzees is changed to one of a high-fat, low-grain and low-vegetable diet, urinary lignan excretion is significantly decreased (Adlercreutz *et al.*, 1987, unpublished observations).

The findings of lignans in portal venous blood and bile and the observed decrease in blood and urinary concentrations following biliary diversion in the bile fistula rat provided evidence for their enterohepatic circulation (Axelson and Setchell, 1981; Setchell *et al.*, 1982).

Good surveys on the mode of formation of phyto-oestrogen metabolites in animals have been written by Shutt (1976) and Lindner (1976). The main isoflavones occurring in plants are the glycosides of genistein and daidzein and their 4-methyl ether derivatives, biochanin A and formononetin (Farnsworth *et al.*, 1975; Price and Fenwick, 1985). When ingested by animals, phyto-oestrogens, like lignans, are modified by ruminal or intestinal bacteria, absorbed from the gastro-intestinal tract and undergo hepatic metabolism. Biochanin A and formononetin undergo demethylation, giving rise to genistein and daidzein respectively. Genistein is further metabolized to the hormonally inert p-ethylphenol, while daidzein is reduced to the isoflavan, equol (about 70%) and O-desmethylangolensin (5–20%). Further degradation of equol appears not to occur and most of the absorbed equol is conjugated in the liver with glucuronic acid before being excreted in the urine (Axelson and Setchell, 1980; Axelson *et al.*, 1984).

The metabolism of isoflavones in man seems to be similar to that in animals (Fig. 14.3). While the dietary origins of phyto-oestrogens in man may be diverse, soy-protein based foodstuffs are particularly high in the glycosides of daidzein and genistein (Walz, 1931; Setchell *et al.*, 1987a). Administration of soy protein, firstly in rats (Axelson and Setchell, 1980) and then in adults (Axelson *et al.*, 1984; Setchell *et al.*, 1984; Setchell, 1985), was shown to result in a marked increase in the urinary excretion of equol. These studies also revealed that some subjects may not be able to form equol despite a challenge from a soy protein diet (Setchell *et al.*, 1984). The reason for this is not clear, and in view of the limited number of subjects studied the proportion of non-responders in a population is uncertain. Both males and females are capable of excreting equol in urine and therefore this phenomenon is not sex-dependent. Formation of equol from daidzein is presumably influenced by the composition of intestinal microflora, and may be dependent upon factors such as transit time and redox level, which are both influenced by diet. The finding of daidzein in urine (Axelson *et al.*, 1984; Bannwart *et al.*, 1984a,b) indicates that this phyto-oestrogen, if not converted to equol by bacterial action, may also be absorbed from the gastro-intestinal tract and undergo hepatic conjugation to glucuronic acid (Axelson *et al.*, 1984) before excretion in urine. The finding of daidzein and equol in cow's milk (Bannwart *et al.*, 1986; Adlercreutz *et al.*, 1986c) suggests that equol may also be derived directly from the diet and enter the human intestinal tract and circulation without the need for intestinal bacteria, although this is probably a minor route for its origin. Very recently formononetin was identified for the first time in human urine from a breast cancer patient (Bannwart *et al.*, 1987).

D. Biological Effects of Lignans and Isoflavones

The evidence obtained thus far from the many studies of biological activity clearly indicates that both lignans and isoflavones are hormonally active. The observations regarding the origins and metabolism of these groups of compounds therefore suggest that, mediated through the action of intestinal microflora, the gastro-intestinal tract acts as a hormone-producing organ.

Lignans and the isoflavones share a common diphenolic structure, and therefore resemble the structures of the potent synthetic oestrogens, diethylstilbestrol and hexestrol. It is this structural feature which accounts for their oestrogenic activity. Our earliest studies which examined the oestrogenicity of enterolactone using a standard bioassay revealed negative results (Setchell *et al.*, 1981b), although these studies were hampered at that time by the lack of sufficient quantities of authentic compounds to determine whether this lignan was weakly oestrogenic. Subsequently, however, the lignans enterodiol and enterolactone have been found to bind weakly to rat uterine cytosol (Clark and Adlercreutz, 1986, unpublished observation), and to demonstrate weak oestrogenic activity using *in vitro* assays for pituitary cell prolactin secretion and synthesis of progesterone receptor by rat uterine cells (Jordan *et al.*, 1985).

Many weak oestrogens exhibit anti-oestrogenic properties, and although enterolactone was shown *in vivo* to reduce oestrogen-stimulated RNA synthesis in rat uterine tissue when administered 22 hours prior to oestradiol (Waters and Knowler, 1982), Jordan *et al.* (1985) could find no evidence for anti-oestrogenic activity using their *in vitro* model of prolactin stimulated rat pituitary cells.

The oestrogenic potency of the isoflavones has been well documented using a variety of *in vitro* and *in vivo* assays. Both daidzein and equol have been found to bind to oestrogen receptors (Shutt and Cox, 1972; Tang and Adams, 1980), while under some conditions they may act as anti-oestrogens. In Clover disease, ewes are made permanently infertile (Schinckel, 1948) by oestrogenic clover containing formononetin, which is converted to daidzein and equol by ruminal micro-organisms (Shutt and Cox, 1972; Shutt, 1976). The abnormalities observed in the affected ewes were similar to those observed in animals exposed neonatally to oestrogens (Adams, 1981). Equol has been found to be weakly oestrogenic (Shutt, 1976; Tang and Adams, 1980, 1981, 1982; Thompson *et al.*, 1984), although the hypothalami of the affected ewes showed a relative insensitivity to oestradiol (Findlay *et al.*, 1973; Adams, 1978). In animals with Clover disease, the uterine response to oestrogen is reduced (Tang and Adams, 1982) as is the surge in luteinizing hormone (Adams and Martin, 1983) and the degree of female sexual behaviour (Adams, 1978). It has also been shown in rats that the equol receptor complex competes with the oestradiol receptor complex for nuclear binding, and yet fails to initiate the replenishment of oestrogen receptors effectively in the cytoplasm (Tang and Adams, 1980), indicating that equol may behave as an anti-oestrogen. If equol and oestradiol were injected simultaneously, the effect on rat uterine growth was less than when oestradiol was injected alone (Tang and Adams, 1980). Furthermore, the binding of the equol–receptor complex to the nucleus was more readily extracted with KCl than the oestradiol–receptor complex. However, when equol was administered locally within the lumen of the rat uterine horn, in doses 1000-fold higher than oestradiol, no effect on uterine weight could be observed (Thompson *et al.*, 1984). The results by Tang and Adams (1980) for equol are in accord with observations obtained for enterolactone. Studies on the effect on RNA synthesis in the rat uterus (Waters and Knowler, 1982) suggest that *in vivo* enterolactone behaves like an anti–oestrogen when in the presence of oestradiol.

In a later study of ewes, two years after removal from oestrogenic Yarloop subterranian clover (*Trifolium subterraneum L*), Tang and Adams (1985) could find no difference in the nuclear binding of oestradiol or the pattern of replenishment of the cytosolic oestrogen receptors. These experiments indicate that in the absence of equol there is no defect in the oestrogen receptors in animals with Clover disease. It was suggested that the impaired response to oestrogens observed in the uterus and cervix of ovariectomized ewes with Clover disease two years after removal from clover is due to some post-receptor abnormality. The acute and long-term effects of equol must therefore be well separated from each other.

Since many plant lignans possess antimitotic activity and have been shown to be effective *in vitro* and *in vivo* against animal tumours (Hartwell, 1976; Barclay and Perdue 1976; Kaplan, 1976) and since other dietary phenolic compounds inhibit neoplasia (Wattenberg, 1983; Newmark, 1984), the mammalian lignans were tested for similar properties. Enterolactone at a concentration of about 3×10^{-4}M was found to inhibit the uptake of ^{3}H-thymidine into human lymphocytes in culture (Setchell *et al.*, 1981b), indicating either an antimitotic or cytotoxic effect. Recently such a cytotoxic effect of enterolactone at a concentration of 10^{-4}M was observed against MCF-7 and T47D breast cancer cells, but not with regard to rat primary cells (Welshons *et al.*, 1987).

Concentrations of enterolactone between 10^{-3} and 10^{-4}M have been reported to displace ouabain from its binding sites on the cardiac digitalis receptor and to inhibit Na^+/K^+ ATPase activity (Braquet *et al.*, 1986; Fagoo *et al.*, 1986). Many plant lignans, including matairesinol, which is also excreted in human urine, show Ca^{2+} antagonist activity at a concentration of about 10^{-5}M (Ichikawa *et al.*, 1986). Some of these effects however may be due to cytotoxicity.

The problem of the possible effects of these compounds in the organism seems very complicated because recently Jordan *et al.*, (1985) and Welshons *et al.* (1987) showed that enterolactone stimulates the growth of both breast cancer cell lines MCF-7 and T47D and the synthesis of progesterone receptor by the MCF-7 cells at concentrations of about 10^{-5}–10^{-6}M, and these effects were inhibited by Tamoxifen. However, no oestradiol was present in the medium. It is unlikely that such high concentrations are attained in the cells.

It has also been shown that equol increases the levels of the progesterone receptor in rat uterus and in MCF-7 cells and that it has a high dissociation rate from the oestrogen receptor *in vitro* (Thompson *et al.*, 1984). *In vivo* using an intraluminal injection technique in the rat uterine horn, equol induced a pattern of cytosol receptor depletion and replenishment similar to that of oestradiol, yet nuclear retention of the receptor–equol complex was of short duration (Thompson *et al.*, 1984).

As diphenols these compounds are weak antioxidants, and may therefore be beneficial in the intestine as inhibitors of the formation of carcinogens. One particular plant lignan, the catecholic nordihydroguaiaretic acid (NDGA), was used for a long time by the food industry as a potent antioxidant. It was later found to cause kidney toxicity in rats (Grice *et al.*, 1968; Goodman *et al.*, 1970) due to bacterial conversion to an *o*-quinone in the intestine, and this metabolite led to a cystic nephropathy. Theoretically, catecholic lignans may exist as intermediates in the pathway for enterolactone synthesis, but these have not been observed in studies to date. Plant lignans occur mainly conjugated to a carbohydrate moiety and hydrolysis of the glycosidic bonds, which may occur at gastric pH or by intestinal micro-organisms (Axelson *et al.*, 1982b), may lead to more biologically active compounds. At a local level in the intestine, it is possible that anticarcinogenic, antiviral (Markkanen *et al.*, 1981) or fungicidal properties which are typical for many plant lignans (see Rao (1978)), may be due to a direct effect before the compounds are transformed by intestinal bacteria and absorbed into the circulation.

Because of the phenolic nature of these compounds it has also been suggested that the mammalian lignans may be carcinogenic (Rowland *et al.*, 1985). On the basis of binding inhibition studies using [^{3}H] 12-*O*-tetradecanoylphorbol 13-acetate (TPA) with a mouse skin particulate fraction (Horiuchi, Fujiki and Adlercreutz, 1986, unpublished results) the mammalian lignans and phyto-oestrogens at concentrations as high as 10^{-4}M have no tumour-promoting or inhibiting effects. Furthermore, it has been shown that daidzein, genistein, formononetin and biochanin A are all non-mutagenic when screened in the *Salmonella*/mammalian microsome assay (see Price and Fenwick (1985)).

Recent studies in collaboration with Dr L. Vickery (Adlercreutz *et al.*, to be published) have shown that enterolactone is a moderate inhibitor of placental aromatase, passes freely into the cell (JEG-3 human choriocarcinoma) and shows intracellular aromatase inhibiting activity at a concentration of 10^{-6}M. Enterolactone binds to, or near, the substrate region of the active site of the P-450 enzyme and the inhibition is competitive with respect to the substrate androstenedione.

E. Physiological and Pathophysiological Effects of Phyto-oestrogens in Animals

While the results of various *in vitro* studies of biological activity of phyto-oestrogens are frequently conflicting, what is clear is that there are numerous examples in animals of direct links between the ingestion of phyto-oestrogens and physiological or pathophysiological responses. The most definitive and striking example of this was the irreversible reproductive failure seen in sheep grazing on a species of clover rich in phyto-oestrogens (Bennetts *et al.*, 1946; Shutt, 1976).

Soy-bean products, which are relatively high in the phyto-oestrogens daidzein and genistein, have been shown to produce significant uter-otrophic effects in laboratory animals (Drane *et al.*, 1975). Laboratory rat cake generally contains a significant proportion of soy-bean product and it has been suggested that soy protein may be as beneficial a growth promoter as the potent synthetic oestrogen diethylstilbestrol (Drane *et al.*, 1980). More recently evidence was obtained for a link between phyto-oestrogen ingestion and the liver disease and infertility seen in captive cheetahs (Setchell *et al.*, 1987b). In recent years the number of deaths in captive cheetahs has outnumbered live births, giving serious concern for the survival of this now endangered species. Liver disease of unknown aetiology is one of the major causes of death in captive cheetahs, while there is no evidence for this condition in the wild cheetah population.

The main hepatic lesion in captive cheetah is a vascular lesion that is characterized by partial or total occlusion of the centrilobular and sublobular hepatic veins with loosely arranged to dense fibrous connective tissue. There occurs slight to severe perivenular fibrosis and the surrounding sinusoids are usually congested with occasional extensive central haemorrhagic congestion. The parenchymal lesion varies from minor loss of liver cells to focal areas of degeneration and necrosis. The incidence of this hepatic lesion, called veno-occlusive disease of the liver, was shown to be approximately 60% in the adult captive cheetah (Setchell *et al.*, 1987b; Gosselin *et al.*, 1987). Examination of the uterus of these animals revealed a cystic endometrium with myometrial fibrosis and endometrial fibrosis, a condition which would interfere with the normal implantation or nutrition of the fertilized egg if conception occurred. This lesion was similar to those found in sheep with Clover disease induced by phyto-oestrogen ingestion. Diet is one of the obvious differences between these two populations. Captive cheetahs are generally fed a commercially prepared feline diet of horse meat with added constituents, including soy protein, while in the wild, cheetahs feed on hoofed animals. In view of these differences the normal diet of four cheetahs was changed to one consisting of chicken. Liver biopsies and blood samples for haematological and liver function tests were obtained before and after 3 months on the new diet. A significant improvement in prothrombin time and partial thromboplastin time was found after the dietary change. At the ultrastructural level hepatic mitochondria, which were abnormal in size and shape, normalized following the dietary change. These ultrastructural abnormalities and haematological changes were consistent with those observed in women taking high dose oral contraceptives (Alpert, 1976; Almen *et al.*, 1975; Dugdale and Masi, 1971). Subsequent analysis of the diet confirmed the presence of large amounts of plant oestrogens, daidzein and genistein which were derived from added soy-protein products. Dietary extracts showed a dose response related increase in uterine weight when subjected to bioassays for oestrogenicity (Setchell *et al.*, 1987b).

Since the cheetah consumes approximately 50 mg per day of phyto-oestrogen it was concluded that chronic ingestion of a diet rich in phyto-oestrogens probably explains the reproductive failure in the cheetah and may be an important factor in the aetiology of veno-occlusive disease in this captive species. It is possible that the cheetah and other exotic felids which suffer from veno-occlusive disease may be more susceptible than other animals to the exposure from phyto-oestrogens, because cats in general poorly conjugate steroids and xenobiotics in the liver (Dutton, 1980). Since conjugation is an important route for deactivation it is possible that the circulating levels of unconjugated phyto-oestrogens may be high in this species and account for the pronounced effects. It was concluded that the survival of the captive cheetah population could depend on simple change of the diet by exclusion of sources of oestrogenic agents such as soy-protein.

A further example of the effect of phyto-oestrogen ingestion on reproduction is evident in Californian quail (Leopold *et al.*, 1976). The breeding habit of this species is seasonal and dependent upon the amount of winter rainfall in the preceding spring nesting season. In a dry season the leaves of stunted desert annuals on which the quail feed are rich in the phyto-oestrogens formononetin, genistein, daidzein and biochanin A. During this dry period the higher levels of these compounds have been reported to inhibit reproduction of this species, and it has been suggested that this symbiotic relationship with these plants offers a protection against the production of young, that if born, would have an inadequate food supply for subsequent survival (Leopold *et al.*, 1976).

F. Analytical Techniques for the Determination of Lignans and Isoflavones

The physiochemical properties and behaviour in chromatographic systems of lignans and isoflavones are similar to those of steroid hormones, and it is for this reason that they were discovered during the course of urinary steroid hormone studies. The earliest techniques employed for both classes of compounds were gas–liquid chromatography, following liquid–solid extraction and liquid–gel chromatographic separation of urinary steroids (Setchell *et al.*, 1980a,b). The highly aromatic nature of these compounds provides a useful feature for their group separation from the bulk of neutral steroid hormone metabolites using either partition chromatography on Sephadex LH-20 (Setchell *et al.*, 1980a,b, 1981a), or the anion exchange gels, triethylaminohydroxypropyl-Sephadex LH-20 (TEAP-LH-20)(Axelson and Setchell, 1980, 1981) or DEAE-Sephadex (Fotsis *et al.*, 1982). In most biological fluids thus far analysed, lignans and isoflavones occur mainly as glucuronide or sulphate conjugates (Axelson and Setchell, 1980), this conjugation occurring predominantly in the liver (Setchell, 1984; Brunner *et al.*, 1986). Determination of these compounds by GLC therefore requires hydrolysis of the conjugate moiety and preparation of suitable volatile derivatives, such as the trimethylsilyl ethers (Setchell *et al.*, 1981a). These GLC techniques afford the simultaneous determination of enterolactone, enterodiol and equol. To increase sensitivity, specificity and speed, a GLC–MS with selected ion monitoring (SIM) was developed. In the early method, quantification was achieved using androstanediol as an internal standard (Setchell *et al.*, 1980b), but later when stable-labelled analogues became available (Setchell *et al.*, 1983) isotope dilution techniques were described (Dehennin *et al.*, 1982; Setchell *et al.*, 1983; Adlercreutz *et al*, 1986b) for enterolactone, enterodiol, equol, daidzein and *O*-desmethylangolensin.

A method for the analysis of unconjugated phyto-oestrogens using HPLC with u.v., electrochemical and thermospray ionization mass spectrometry detection was also developed (Setchell *et al.*, 1987a) which has proved of most value in the measurement of these compounds in food products. Since the sensitivity of this procedure is in the low pg range the technique could potentially be used for hydrolysed extracts of urine. HPLC has also been employed for the purification of enterolactone and enterodiol-glucuronides following their *in vitro* preparation by hepatic microsomal UDP-glucuronyl transferase (Brunner *et al.*, 1986). The system served to demonstrate the formation of two isomeric forms, which may reflect the diastereoisomeric glucuronides of the racemate or glucuronides at the non-equivalent phenolic rings in the molecule (Brunner *et al.*, 1986).

G. Lignans and Phyto-oestrogens in Man in Health and Disease

The earliest quantitative studies of lignans established a cyclic pattern in their urinary excretion in the vervet monkey (Setchell *et al.*, 1980a) and human (Setchell and Adlercreutz, 1979; Stitch *et al.*, 1980b; Setchell *et al.*, 1980b, 1980c). Peak excretion was observed during the luteal phase of the cycle and increases during pregnancy were also noted (Setchell and Adlercreutz, 1979; Setchell *et al.*, 1980b). The concentration of enterolactone in human and bovine semen was shown to be 2.5–25-fold higher than in peripheral blood (Dehennin *et al.*, 1982). Our early studies indicated a marked decrease in the urinary excretion of these compounds following ovariectomy, orchidectomy and adrenalectomy of rats (Axelson and Setchell, 1981; Setchell *et al.*, 1981b), while excretion was also shown to be influenced by gonadotrophin levels (Coert *et al.*, 1982). The reasons for these events is unclear, however it may reflect some hormonal control upon either the bacterial metabolism or on the efficiency of reabsorption of these compounds from the gastro-intestinal tract.

More recent studies have focused on the potential beneficial role for lignans and phyto-oestrogens in common diseases such as colon cancer and breast cancer, where there are epidemiological associations with diet. Questions regarding the potential anti-cancer or protective activity of these compounds have been raised (Setchell *et al.*, 1981b, 1982, 1984; Adlercreutz, 1984; Horwitz and Walker, 1984; Setchell, 1985), and studies of urinary excretion values in subjects consuming different diets have been carried out (Adlercreutz *et al.*, 1981, 1982, 1986b). Preliminary results were obtained for the urinary excretion of phyto-oestrogens for five groups of young women on different habitual diets (Adlercreutz *et al.*, 1986b). Three groups of women were from Boston, representing omnivorous, lactovegetarian and macrobiotic women, and an omnivorous and lactovegetarian group was studied from Helsinki (Table 14.3).

Of the five diphenols measured enterolactone was present in the highest concentration in urine, followed by daidzein and enterodiol. This is consistent with earlier studies of humans where urinary enterolactone

Table 14.3 *Urinary excretion of lignans and isoflavonic phyto-oestrogens (preliminary results) in young women on various habitual diets (geometrical means nmol in 24 hours) (according to Adlercreutz et al. (1986b))*

	Omnivores	Lactovegetarians	Macrobiotics
Boston women	($n = 9$)	($n = 9$)	($n = 12$)
Enterolactone	2050	4170	17680
Enterodiol	280	740	6260
Daidzein	320	1260	3460
Equol	69	100	868
O-desmethylangolesin	33	106	378
Helsinki women	($n = 12$)	($n = 11$)	
Enterolactone	2460	3650	
Enterodiol	203	368	
Daidzein	219	275	
Equol	102	64	
O-desmethylangolensin	25	43	

excretion was shown to be 5–10-fold greater than enterodiol (Setchell *et al.*, 1980b, 1980c). Depending on the diet, the urinary excretion of these weakly oestrogenic compounds is 10–1000-fold higher than the endogenous oestrogens. Macrobiotics excreted very high concentrations of all compounds, including enterodiol. This was also the case for the lactovegetarians from Boston. The increased excretion of enterodiol could be due to a greater intake of enterodiol precursors and/or to a decreased conversion of enterodiol to enterolactone in the intestinal tract (Axelson *et al.*, 1982b; Borriello *et al.*, 1985). The daidzein/equol ratio was much lower in the Helsinki women compared to the American women, suggesting greater conversion of daidzein to equol by gastro-intestinal bacteria or reflecting differences in the diet or microflora.

Antibiotics have a significant effect upon the urinary excretion of the lignans, by abolishing the microflora responsible for their synthesis. This effect lasts at least 6 weeks (Setchell *et al.*, 1981b; Adlercreutz *et al.*, 1986b), and probably longer, and is characterized by an increase in the relative amount of enterodiol after the abolition of enterolactone and enterodiol production. Unconjugated lignan excretion also decreases in faeces (Setchell *et al.*, 1981b).

Fig. 14.4 summarizes data from a previous study (Adlercreutz *et al.*, 1982) where the excretion of enterolactone was found to be significantly lower in the urine of postmenopausal breast cancer patients (1040 nmol in 24 hours) compared to postmenopausal controls eating a normal mixed (2300 nmol in 24 hours) or a lactovegetarian (3180 nmol in 24 hours) diet. Values for young omnivorous and vegetarian women from Boston are also given.

The results in Table 14.3 show that the omnivorous women living in Boston showed the lowest mean excretion of enterolactone (2050 nmol in 24 hours), and according to epidemiological studies this group has the highest risk for breast cancer. Both the lactovegetarians and particularly macrobiotics from Boston excrete significantly higher amounts of lignans. A similar trend was apparent for the populations in Helsinki. In a separate investigation carried out in North Karelia (unpublished), where the incidence of breast cancer is lower than in both Helsinki and Boston, the mean excretion of enterolactone in 28 young omnivorous women was found to be much higher (3020 nmol in 24 hours) than for any of the omnivorous groups from either Helsinki or Boston. More recently enterolactone excretion was measured in 12 young women with breast cancer living in the Helsinki area. The mean excretion (2045 nmol in 24 hours) was almost identical with that of the omnivorous women from Boston.

In collaboration with Dr H. Honjo, lignan excretion in the urine of Japanese subjects consuming a traditional diet was shown to be slightly higher than for Finnish women, while the level of isoflavones was ten-fold greater. These observations parallel the epidemiological data for breast cancer incidence, which is very low in areas of Japan where a traditional diet is consumed.

Non-human primates are remarkably resistant to the carcinogenic effect of oestrogens, even in combination with a potent carcinogen (see Adlercreutz et al. (1986a)). Like most sub-human primates, lignan and isoflavone excretion in chimpanzees is high and approximates that observed in human macrobiotics (Adlercreutz et al., 1986a, and unpublished results). These circumstantial findings seem to support our view that these compounds may have protective effect with regard to oestrogen-dependent cancer.

Because of methodological difficulties very little is known about the levels of unconjugated diphenols in human blood. The only one which has been measured is enterolactone. In one study, four values in English women aged 30 to 53 years varied between 0.67 and 5.6 nmol 1^{-1} (Setchell et al., 1981b). In another study of six French men, the concentration was in the range 10.3–21 nmol 1^{-1} (Dehennin et al., 1982) while in preliminary investigations of Finnish omnivorous subjects, concentrations have been found to be as high as 80 nmol 1^{-1}, which is about 100–400-fold higher than the circulating level of oestradiol.

Phyto-oestrogens may indirectly affect sex hormone metabolism by influencing the levels of sex hormone binding globulin (SHBG) and plasma non-protein bound oestrogens and androgens. Measurements of plasma SHBG and free testosterone have been carried out in groups of Finnish women (Table 14.3), including older women and breast cancer patients. In the group of 23 healthy young women statistically significant positive correlations between the urinary excretion of enterolactone, total lignan, total phyto-oestrogen and total diphenol and plasma SHBG were found. The correlation coefficients were 0.563 ($p < 0.01$), 0.562 ($p < 0.01$), 0.434 ($p < 0.05$) and 0.598 ($p < 0.01$), respectively. Furthermore, significant negative correlations between enterolactone, total lignans and total diphenols and the percentage of plasma-free oestradiol was noted, and these correlations remained even when breast cancer patients were included. In a larger group of women, including postmenopausal women ($n = 67$), positive correlations between urinary enterolactone ($p < 0.05$) and enterolactone + equol ($p < 0.001$) and plasma SHBG, and negative correlations between urinary enterolactone ($p < 0.001$) and equol ($p < 0.01$) with percentage of free oestradiol were found. The linear effect of weight and age was eliminated in these calculations. In addition, a negative correlation between urinary enterolactone and plasma free testosterone ($p < 0.001$) was found. In this connection it should be remembered that testosterone stimulates prostatic cancer growth and is the immediate precursor of oestradiol.

Previously, a positive correlation between dietary intake of total fibre and the urinary excretion of enterolactone (Adlercreutz *et al.*, 1981) was observed which has since been confirmed ($r = 0.527$; $p < 0.001$) in a separate group of women ($n = 48$). The same correlation was also found for enterodiol ($r = 0.414$; $p < 0.001$). In this context, it was also shown that increasing dietary fibre intake by the consumption of 60 g of bran per day resulted in no significant increase in lignan excretion (Setchell *et al.*, 1983). In Fig. 14.4 a positive correlation is shown between dietary intake of grain (kcal/day) and urinary enterolactone excretion. In a larger study significant positive correlations were found between intake of dietary total fibre per kilogram of body weight ($p < 0.001$), vegetable fibre ($p < 0.05$), fibre from fruits and berries ($p < 0.01$), and plasma SHBG ($p < 0.001$). These results suggest that fibre-rich food containing mammalian lignan precursors and isoflavonic phyto-oestrogens may, via the production of weakly oestrogenic mammalian lignans and equol in the intestinal tract, stimulate SHBG synthesis in the liver and may in this way reduce the concentration of free sex hormones in plasma. It is well known that oral, unlike parenterally administered, oestrogens markedly stimulate SHBG synthesis (Elkik *et al.*, 1982; Holst *et al.*, 1983), and this may explain the higher SHBG-values found in vegetarians consuming fibre-rich food.

Epidemiological studies reveal a close connection between breast and colon cancer (Drasar and Irving, 1973; Armstrong and Doll, 1975; Howell, 1976; Reddy et al., 1980) and some reproductive risk factors are common for both diseases (see Potter and McMichael (1983) and Dubin *et al.* (1984)). Colon cancer incidence and frequency of adenomatous polyps has also been found to be high following primary cancer of the breast (Agarwal *et al.*, 1984; Bremond *et al.*, 1984; Rozen *et al.*, 1986). The lack of dietary fibre containing lignan precursors may be a common denominator in the aetiology of these diseases (Adlercreutz, 1984). Dietary fibre may in different ways be protective with regard to colon cancer (Trowell and Burkitt, 1983; Trowell *et al.*, 1985) and has also been shown to interfere with the enterohepatic circulation of many endogenous compounds, including oestrogens and bile acids, both of which have been suggested to play a role in the aetiology of these diseases (see e.g. Adlercreutz, 1984).

While several workers have identified androgen and oestrogen receptors in primary colon cancers (Alford *et al.*, 1979; Sica *et al.*, 1981; Stebbings *et al.*, 1986; D'Istria *et al.*, 1986), others have disputed the presence of oestrogen receptors (Wobbes *et al.*, 1984; D'Istria *et al.*, 1986). If androgens or oestrogens have stimulatory effects on colon cancer cells, phyto-oestrogens may reduce this effect by some of the mechanisms described above. Bile acids have been implicated in the aetiology of colon cancer and it is therefore of interest that both enterolactone and enterodiol modulate *in vitro* the activities of cholesterol-7α-hydroxylase and acyl-CoA: cholesterol transferase (ACAT) in a dose-dependent fashion (Sanghvi *et al.*, 1984). Since cholesterol-7α-hydroxylase is the rate-limiting step in the synthesis of bile acids from cholesterol it is possible that lignans may lead to alterations in cholesterol catabolism.

Feminization and gynecomastia are clinical symptoms of chronic alcoholism and alterations in hepatic oestrogen metabolism are a feature of this disease (Rupp *et al.*, 1951; Brown *et al.*, 1964; Adlercreutz, 1970; Pentikainen *et al.*, 1975). In an interesting study, extracts of bourbon whisky were fed to rats and significant uterotrophic effects with depression of plasma LH levels were observed in a dose-dependent manner (Gavaler *et al.*, 1987). Following the identification of the phyto-oestrogen biochanin A it was suggested that some of the poorly understood features of alcohol liver disease might be explained by the presence of phyto-oestrogens in alcoholic beverages (Gavaler *et al.*, 1987).

H. Summary

In summary, there are several potential mechanisms by which lignans and isoflavones could influence carcinogenesis, but much of the evidence in support of these remains circumstantial. It is possible that (*i*) there is a reduction in the sensitivity of oestrogen receptors to oestradiol, as found for hypothalamic oestrogen receptors in sheep grazing clover rich in formononetin. (*ii*) The anti-oestrogenic action, which has been shown by several workers for equol and enterolactone, may inhibit the action of oestrogen-stimulated tumour growth. (*iii*) Inhibition of the aromatase enzyme in peripheral tissues could lead to lower basal oestrogen levels in populations consuming a diet rich in isoflavonic phyto-oestrogens and lignans. (*iv*) These compounds could influence sex hormone action by modulating plasma SHBG and non-protein bound sex hormone levels. (*v*) The antioxidative and/or cytotoxic properties of these compounds may have a local effect. (*vi*) The effects may be mediated through the action of these compounds on cholesterol homoeostasis.

It is clear that further studies are necessary before the possible biological role in man of lignans and isoflavonic phyto-oestrogens may be accurately defined.

The diversity in the occurrence of phyto-oestrogens in constituents of the human diet is uncertain, although collectively data indicate their occurrence to be widespread in common foodstuffs. In particular, a leaning towards a vegetarian-type diet, which has become the vogue with increasing concerns over risk factors for common diseases, will inevitably result in increased exposure to dietary oestrogens. Given the concerns over use of synthetic oestrogens it is therefore important that the potential beneficial or deleterious long-term effects of dietary oestrogens to humans be more fully investigated. Despite the deleterious effects which have been shown to occur by the exposure of animals to phyto-oestrogens, it is our belief that, based on the evidence thus far obtained, phyto-oestrogens may be one of the dietary factors affording protection against hormone-dependent disease in vegetarians and semi-vegetarians (Setchell *et al.*, 1981b, 1984; Adlercreutz, 1984).

References

Adams, N. R. (1978). Sexual behaviour responses of the ovariectomized ewe to oestradiol benzoate, and their persistent reduction after exposure to phyto-oestrogens. *J. Reprod. Fertil.* **53**, 203–208.

Adams, N. R. (1981). A changed responsiveness to oestrogen in ewes with clover disease. *J. Reprod. Fertil.*, Suppl. **30**, 223–230.

Adams, N. R. and Martin, G. B. (1983). Effects of oestradiol on plasma concentrations of luteinizing hormone in ovariectomized ewes with clover disease. *Aust. J. Biol. Sci.* **36**, 295–303.

Adlercreutz, H. (1970). Oestrogen metabolism in liver disease. *J. Endocrinol.* **46**, 29–163.

Adlercreutz, H. (1984). Does fiber-rich food containing animal lignan precursors protect against both colon and breast cancer? An extension of the "fiber hypothesis". *Gastroenterol.* **86**, 761–764.

Adlercreutz, H., Fotsis, T., Heikkinen, R., Dwyer, J. T., Goldin, B. R., Gorbach, S. L., Lawson, A. M. and Setchell, K. D. R. (1981). Diet and urinary excretion of lignans in female subjects. *Med. Biol.* **59**, 259–261.

Adlercreutz, H., Fotsis, T., Heikkinen, R., Dwyer, J. T., Woods, M., Goldin, B. R. and Gorbach, S. L. (1982). Excretion of the lignans enterolactone and enterodiol and of equol in omnivorous and vegetarian women and in women with breast cancer. *Lancet* **ii**, 1295–1299.

Adlercreutz, H., Musey, P. I., Fotsis, T., Bannwart, C., Wahala, K., Makela, T., Brunow, G. and Hase, T. (1986a). Identification of lignans and phyto-oestrogens in urine of chimpanzees. *Clin. Chim. Acta* **158**, 147–154.

Adlercreutz, H., Fotsis, T., Bannwart, C., Wahala, K., Makela, T., Brunow, G. and Hase, T. (1986b). Determination of urinary lignans and phyto-oestrogens metabolites, potential antioestrogens and anticarcinogens, in urine of women on various habitual diets. *J. Steroid Biochem.* **25**, 791–797.

Adlercreutz, H., Fotsis, T., Bannwart, C., Makela, T., Wahala, K., Brunow, G. and Hase, T. (1986c). Assay of lignans and phyto-oestrogens in urine of women and in cow milk by GC/MS (SIM). *In*: "Advances in Mass Spectrometry – 1985. Proceedings of the 10th International Mass Spectrometry Conference" (ed. J. F. J. Todd), pp. 1293–1294. John Wiley, Chichester, Sussex.

Adlercreutz, H., Hockerstedt, K., Bannwart, C., Bloigu, S., Hamalainen, E., Fotsis, T. and Ollus, A. (1987). Effects of dietary components, including lignans and phyto-oestrogens, on enterohepatic circulation and liver metabolism of oestrogens and on sex hormone binding globulin (SHBG). *J. Steroid Biochem.* (in the press).

Agarwal, N., Ulahannan, M. J., Mandile, M. A., Cayten, C. G. and Pitchumoni, C. S. (1984). Increased risk of colo-rectal cancer following breast cancer. *Am. J. Gastroenterol.* **79**, 822.

Alford, T. C., Do, H. -M., Geelkhoed, G. W., Tsangaris, N. T. and Lippman, M. E. (1979). Steroid hormone receptors in human colon cancers. *Cancer* **43**, 980–984.

Almen, T., Hartel, M., Nylander, G. and Olivercrona, H. (1975). The effect of oestrogen on the vascular endothelium and its possible relation to thrombosis. *Surg. Gynecol. Obstet.* **140**, 938–940.

Alpert, L. I. (1976). Veno-occlusive disease of the liver associated with oral contraceptives: case report and review of literature. *Hum. Pathol.* **7**, 709–718.

Armstrong, B. and Doll, R. (1975). Environmental factors and cancer incidence and mortality in different countries, with special reference to dietary practices. *Int. J. Cancer* **15**, 617–631.

Axelson, M. and Setchell, K. D. R. (1980). Conjugation of lignans in human urine. *FEBS Lett.* **122**, 49–53.

Axelson, M. and Setchell, K. D. R. (1981). The excretion of lignans in rats –

evidence for an intestinal bacterial source for this new group of compounds. *FEBS Lett.* **123**, 337–342.

Axelson, M., Kirk, D. N., Farrant, R. D., Cooley, G., Lawson, A. M. and Setchell, K. D. R. (1982a). The identification of the weak oestrogen equol [7-hydroxy-4-(4-hydroxyphenyl)-chroman] in human urine. *Biochem J.* **201**, 353–357.

Axelson, M., Sjovall, J., Gustafsson, B. E. and Setchell, K. D. R. (1982b). Origin of lignans in mammals and identification of a precursor from plants. *Nature* **298**, 659–660.

Axelson, M., Sjovall, J., Gustafsson, B. E. and Setchell, K. D. R. (1984). Soya – a dietary source of the non-steroidal oestrogen equol in human and animals. *J. Endocrinol.* **102**, 49–56.

Bannwart, C., Adlercreutz, H., Fotsis, T., Wahala, K., Hase, T. and Brunow, G. (1984a). Identification of O-desmethylangolensin, a metabolite of daidzein, and of matairesinol, one likely precursor of the animal lignan enterolactone, in human urine. *Finn. Chem. Lett.* No. 4–5, 120–125.

Bannwart, C., Fotsis, T., Heikkinen, R. and Adlercreutz, H. (1984b). Identification of the isoflavonic phyto-oestrogen daidzein in human urine. *Clin. Chim. Acta* **136**, 165–172.

Bannwart, C., Adlercreutz, H., Fotsis, T., Wahala, K., Hase, T. and Brunow, G. (1986). Identification of isoflavonic phyto-oestrogens and of lignans in human urine and in cow milk by GC/MS. *In:* "Advances in Mass Spectrometry – 1985". "Proceedings of the 10th International Mass Spectrometry" (ed. J. F. J. Todd), pp. 661–662. John Wiley, Chichester, Sussex.

Bannwart, C., Adlercreutz, H., Wähälä, K., Brunow, G. and Hase, T. (1987). Isoflavonic phytoestrogens in humans, identification and metabolism. *Eur. J. Cancer Clin. Oncol.* **23**, 1732.

Barclay, A. S., Perdue, E., Jr. (1976). Distribution of anticancer activity in higher plants. *Cancer Treat. Rep.* **60**, 1081–1113.

Bennetts, H. W., Underwood, E. J., Shier, F. L. (1946). A specific breeding problem of sheep on subterranean clover pastures in western Australia. *Aust. J. Agric. Res.* **22**, 131–138.

Bradbury, R. B., White, D. E. (1954). Oestrogens and related substances in plants. *Vitam. Horm. (NY)* **12**, 207–233.

Borriello, S. P., Setchell, K. D. R., Axelson, M. and Lawson, A. M. (1985). Production and metabolism of lignans by the human fecal flora. *J. Appl. Bacteriol.* **58**, 37–43.

Braden, A. W. H., Hart, N. K. and Lamberton, J. A. (1967). The oestrogenic activity and metabolism of certain isoflavones in sheep. *Aust. J. Agric. Res.* **18**, 335–348.

Braquet, P., Senn, N., Robin, J. -P., Esanu, A., Godfraind, T. and Garay, R. (1986). Inhibition of the erythrocyte Na^+,K^+ -pump by mammalian lignans. *Pharm. Res. Comm.* **18**, 227–239.

Bremond, A., Collet, P., Lambert, R. and Martin, J. -L. (1984). Breast cancer and polyps of the colon. *Cancer* **54**, 2568–2570.

Brown, J. B., Crean, G. P. and Ginsburg, J. (1964). Oestrogen metabolism and excretion in liver disease. *Gut* **5**, 56–59.

Brunner, G., Tegtmeier, F., Kirk, D. N., Wynn, S. and Setchell, K. D. R. (1986). Enzymatic synthesis and chromatographic purification of lignan glucuronides. *Biomed. Chromatog.* **2**, 89–92.

Coert, A., Vonk Noordegraaf, C. A., Groen, M. B. and Van der View, J. (1982). The dietary origin of the urinary lignan HPMF. *Experientia* **38**, 904–905.

Common, R. H. and Ainsworth, L. (1961). Identification of equol in the urine of the domestic fowl. *Biochim. Biophys. Acta* **53**, 403–404.

Cooley, G., Farrant, D. R., Kirk, D. N. and Wynn, S. (1981). Chemical synthesis of the first lignans to be found in humans and animals. *Tetrahedron Lett.* **22**, 349–350.

Cooley, G., Farrant, R. D., Kirk, D. N., Patel, S., Wynn, S., Buckingham, M. J., Hawkes, G. E., Hursthouse, M. B., Galas, A. M. R., Lawson, A. M. and Setchell, K. D. R. (1984). Structural analysis of the urinary lignan 2,3-bis-(3-hydroxybenzyl)butan-4-olide ('enterolactone'). A 400 MHz nuclear magnetic resonance study for the solution state and X-ray study for the crystal state. *J. Chem. Soc. Perkin Trans.* **II**, 489–497.

Dehennin, L., Reiffsteck, A., Joudet, M. and Thibier, M. (1982). Identification and quantitative estimation of a lignan in human and bovine semen. *J. Reprod. Fert.* **66**, 305–309.

D'Istria, M,, Fasano, S., Catuogno, F., Gaeta, F., Bucci, L., Benassi, G., Mazzeo, F. and Deirio, G. (1986). Androgen and progesterone receptors in colonic and rectal cancers. *Dis. Colon Rectum* **29**, 263–265.

Drane, H. M., Patterson, D. S., Roberts, B. A. and Saba, N. (1975). The chance discovery of oestrogenic activity in laboratory rat cake. *Fd Cosmet. Toxicol.* **13**, 491–492.

Drane, H. M., Patterson, D. S. P., Roberts, B. A. and Saba, N. (1980). Oestrogenic activity of soya-bean products. *Fd Cosmet. Toxicol.* **18**, 25–426.

Drasar, B. S. and Irving, D. (1973). Environmental factors and cancer of the colon and breast. *Br. J. Cancer* **27**, 167–172.

Dubin, N., Pasternack, B. S. and Strax, P. (1984). Epidemiology of breast cancer in a screened population. *Cancer Detect. Prevent.* **7**, 87–102.

Dugdale, M. and Masi, A. T. (1971). Hormonal contraception and thromboembolic disease: effects of oral contraceptives on hemostatic mechanisms. *J. Chronic Dis.* **23**, 775–790.

Dutton, G. J. (1980). The influence of sex, species and strain on glucuronidation. *In*: "Glucuronidation of Drugs and Other Compounds" (ed. G. J. Dutton), pp. 123–241. CRC Press, Boca-Raton, FL.

Elkik, F., Gompel, A., Mercier-Bodard, C., Kuttenn, F., Guyenne, P. N., Corvol, P. and Mauvais-Jarvis, P. (1982). Effects of percutaneous estradiol and conjugated oestrogens on the level of plasma proteins and triglycerides in postmenopausal women. *Am. J. Obstet. Gynec.* **143**, 888–892.

Fagoo, M., Braquet, P., Robin, J. P., Esanu, A. and Godfraind, T. (1986). Evidence that mammalian lignans show endogenous digitalis-like activities. *Biochem. Biophys. Res. Comm.* **134**, 1064–1070.

Farnsworth, N. R., Bingel, A. S., Cordell, G. A., Crane, F. A. and Fong, H. H. S. (1975). Potential value of plants as sources of new antifertility agents II. *J. Pharm. Sci.* **64**, 717–754.

Findlay, J. K., Buckmaster, J. M., Chamley, W. A., Cumming, I. A., Hearnshaw, H. and Goding, J. R. (1973). Release of luteinizing hormone by oestradiol-17β and a gonadotrophin-releasing hormone in ewes affected by clover disease. *Neuroendocriol.* **11**, 57–66.

Fotsis, T., Heikkinen, R., Adlercreutz, H., Axelson, M. and Setchell, K. D. R.

(1982). Capillary gas chromatographic method for the analysis of lignans in human urine. *Clin. Chim. Acta* **121**, 361–371.

Gavaler, J. S., Rosenblum, E. R., Van Thiel, D. H., Eagon, P. K., Pohl, C. R., Campbell, I. M. and Gavaler, J. (1987). Biologically active phyto-oestrogens are present in bourbon. *Alcoholism Clin. Exp. Res.* **11**, 399–406.

Goodman, T., Grice, H. C., Becking, G. C. and Salem, F. A. (1970). A cystic nephropathy induced by nordihydroguaiaretic acid in the rat. *Lab. Invest.* **23**, 93–107.

Gosselin, S. J., Loudy, D. L., Tarr, M. J., Balistreri, W. F., Setchell, K. D. R., Johnston, J. O., Kramer, L. W. and Dresser, B. L. (1988). The pathogenesis of hepatic vascular lesions in captive cheetah. *Vet. Path.* **25**, 48–57.

Grice, H. C., Becking, G. and Goodman, T. (1968). Toxic properties of nordihydroguaiaretic acid. *Fd Cosmet. Toxicol.* **6**, 155–161.

Groen, M. B. and Leemhuis, L. (1980). Synthesis of compound X, a non-steroidal constituent of female urine, and congeners. *Tetrahedron lett.* **21**, 5043–5046.

Hartwell, J. L. (1976). Types of anticancer agents isolated from plants. *Cancer Treat Rep.* **60**, 1031–1067.

Holst, J., Cajander, S., Carlstrom, K., Damber, M. -G. and von Schoultz, B. (1983). A comparison of liver protein induction in postmenopausal women during oral and percutaneous oestrogen replacement therapy. *Brit. J. Obstet. Gynaec.* **90**, 355–360.

Horwitz, C. and Walker, A. R. P. (1984). Lignans — additional benefits from fiber? *Nutr. Cancer* **6**, 73–76.

Howell, M. A. (1976). The association between colorectal and breast cancer. *J. Chron. Dis.* **29**, 243–261.

Ichikawa, K., Kinoshita, T. Y., Nishibe, S. and Sankawa, U. (1986). The Ca^{2+} antagonist activity of lignans. *Chem. Pharm. Bull.* **34**, 3514–3517.

Jordan, V. C., Koch, R. and Bain, R. R. (1985). Prolactin synthesis by cultured rat pituitary cells: An assay to study estrogens, antiestrogens and their metabolites in vitro. *In*: "Estrogens in the Environment II. Influences on Development" (ed. J. A. McLachlan), pp. 221–237. Elsevier, NY.

Kaplan, I. W. (1976). Condylomata acuminata. *New Orleans Med. Surg.* **94**, 388–390.

Klyne, W. and Wright, A. A. (1957). Steroids and other lipids of pregnant goat's urine. *Biochem. J.* **66**, 92–101.

Klyne, W. and Wright, A. A. (1959). Steroids and other lipids of pregnant cow's urine. *J. Endocrinol.* **18**, 32–45.

Leclerq, G. and Heuson, J. C. (1979). Physiological and pharmacological effects of estrogens in breast cancer. *Biochim. Biophys. Acta* **560**, 427–455.

Leopold, A. S., Erwin, M., Oh, J., and Browning, B. (1976). Phyto-oestrogens: adverse effects on reproduction in California quail. *Science* **191**, 98–99.

Lindner, H. R. (1976). Occurrence of anabolic agents in plants and their importance. *Environ. Qual. Saf.* **5**, 151–158.

Lindsay, D. R., and Kelly, R. W. (1970). The metabolism of phyto-oestrogens in sheep. *Austr. Vet. J.* **46**, 219–222.

Luk, K. -C., Stern, L., Weigele, M., O'Brien, R. A. and Spirt, N. (1983). Isolation and identification of "diazepam-like" compounds from bovine urine. *J. Nat. Prod.* **46**, 852–861.

MacRae, H. F., Dale, D. G. and Common, R. H. (1960). Formation *in vivo* of 16-epiestriol and 16-keto-estradiol-17β from estriol by the laying hen and occurrence of equol in hen's urine and faeces. *Can. J. Biochem. Physiol.* **38**,

523–532.

Markkanen, T., Makinen, M. L., Maunuksela, E. and Himanen, P. (1981). Podophyllotoxin lignans under experimental antiviral research. *Drugs Exp. Clin. Res.* **VII**, 711–718.

Marrian, G. F. and Haslewood, G. A. D. (1932). Equol, a new inactive phenol isolated from the ketohydroxyoestrin fraction of mare's urine. *Biochem. J.* **26**, 1227–1232.

Monfort, S. L., Thompson, M. A., Czekala, N. M., Kasman, L. H., Shackleton, C. H. L. and Lasley, B. L. (1984). Identification of a non-steroidal estrogen, equol, in the urine of pregnant macaques: Correlation with steroidal estrogen excretion. *J. Steroid Biochem.* **20**, 869–876.

Newmark, H. L. (1984). A hypothesis for dietary components as blocking agents of chemical carcinogenesis: Plant phenolics and pyrrole pigments. *Nutr. Cancer*, **6**, 58–70.

Nilsson, A., Hill, J. L. and Lloyd-Davies, H. (1967). An *in vitro* study of formononetin and Biochanin A metabolism in rumen fluid from sheep. *Biochim. Biophys. Acta* **148**, 92–98.

Palmer, S. (1985). Diet, nutrition and cancer. *Prog. Fd Nutr. Sci.* **9**, 283–341.

Pentikainen, P. J., Pentikainen, L. A., Azarnoff, D. L. and Dujovne, C. A. (1975). Plasma levels and excretion of estrogens in urine in chronic liver disease. *Gastroenterol.* **69**, 20–27.

Potter, J. D. and McMichael, J. A. (1983). Large bowel cancer in women in relation to reproductive and hormonal factors: A case-control study. *J. Natl. Cancer Soc.* **7**, 703–709.

Price, K. R. and Fenwick, G. R. (1985). Naturally occurring oestrogens in foods – A review. *Fd Add.Contam.* **2**, 73–106.

Rao, C. B. S. (1978). "The Chemistry of Lignans". Andhra University Press, Waltair, India.

Reddy, B. S., Cohen, L. A., McCoy, G. D., Hill, P., Weisburger, J. H. and Wynder, E. L. (1980). Nutrition and its relationship to cancer. *Adv. Cancer Res.* **32**, 237–245.

Rowland, I. R., Mallett, A. K. and Wise, A. (1985). The effect of diet on the mammalian gut flora and its metabolic activities. *In*: "CRC Critical Reviews in Toxicology", Vol. 16, No. 1, pp. 31–103. CRC Press Inc., Boca-Raton, FL.

Rozen, P., Fireman, Z., Figer, A. and Ron, E. (1986). Colorectal tumor screening in women with a past history of breast, uterine, or ovarian malignancies. *Cancer* **57**, 1235–1239.

Rupp, J., Cantarow, Al, Rakoff, A. E. and Paschkis, K. E. (1951). Hormone excretion in liver disease and in gynecomastia. *J. Clin. Endocrinol. Metab.* **11**, 688–699.

Sanghvi, A., Diven, W. F., Seltman, H., Warty, V., Rizk, M., Kritchevsky, D. and Setchell, K. D. R. (1984). Inhibition of rat liver cholesterol 7α-hydroxylase and acyl-CoA; cholesterol acyl transferase activities by enterodiol and enterolactone. *In*: "Proceedings of the 8th Symposium on Drugs affecting Lipid Metabolism" (eds D. Kritchevsky, R. Paoletti and W. L. Holmes). Plenum Press, New York.

Schinckel, P. G. (1948). Infertility in ewes grazing subterranean clover pastures. Observations on breeding behaviour following transfer to 'sound' country. *Austr. Vet. J.* **24**, 289–294.

Setchell, K. D. R. (1984). Hepatic conjugation of enterolactone and enterodiol:

the first mammalian lignans. *In*: "Advances in Glucuronide Conjugation" (eds S. Mattern, K. W. Bock and W. Gerok), pp. 287–291, MTP Press, Lancaster.

Setchell, K. D. R. (1985). Naturally occurring non-steroidal estrogens of dietary origin. *In*: "Estrogens in the Environment II. Influences on Development" (ed. J. A. McLachlan), pp. 69–85. Elsevier, NY.

Setchell, K. D. R. and Adlercreutz, H. (1979). The excretion of two new phenolic compounds (180/442 and 180/410) during the human menstrual cycle and in pregnancy. *J. Steroid Biochem.* **11**, xv.

Setchell, K. D. R., Bull, R. and Adlercreutz, H. (1980a). Steroid excretion during the reproductive cycle and in pregnancy of the vervet monkey (Ceropithecus aethiopus pygerythrus). *J. Steroid Biochem.* **12**, 375–384.

Setchell, K. D. R., Lawson, A. M., Axelson, M. and Adlercreutz, H. (1980b). The excretion of two new phenolic compounds during the human menstrual cycle and in pregnancy. *In*: "Endocrinological Cancer, Ovarian Function and Disease" (eds H. Adlercreutz, R. D. Bulbrook, H. V. van der Molen, A. Vermeulen and F. Sciarra) *Excerpta Med. Int. Congress Ser.* No. 515, 207–215.

Setchell, K. D. R., Lawson, A. M., Mitchell, F. L., Adlercreutz, H., Kirk, D. N. and Axelson, M. (1980c). Lignans in man and animal species. *Nature* **287**, 740–742.

Setchell, K. D. R. and Bonney, R. C. (1981). The excretion of urinary steroids by the owl monkey (*Aotus trivirgatus*) studies using open-tubular capillary column gas chromatography and mass spectrometry. *J. Steroid Biochem.* **14**, 37–43.

Setchell, K. D. R., Lawson, A. M., Conway, E., Taylor, N. F., Kirk, D. N., Cooley, G., Farrant, R. D., Wynn, S. and Axelson, M. (1981a). The definitive identification of the lignans trans-2,3-bis(3-hydroxy-benzyl)butyrolactone and 2,3-bis(3-hydroxybenzyl)butane-1,4-diol in human and animal urine. *Biochem. J.* **197**, 447–458.

Setchell, K. D. R., Lawson, A. M., Borriello, S. P., Harkness, R., Gordon, H., Morgan, D. M. L., Kirk, D. N., Adlercreutz, H., Anderson, L. C. and Axelson, M. (1981b). Lignan formation in man-microbial involvement and possible role in cancer. *Lancet* **ii**, 4–7.

Setchell, K. D. R., Lawson, A. M., Borriello, S. P., Adlercreutz, H. and Axelson, M. (1982). Formation of lignans by intestinal microflora. *In*: "Falk Symposium 31, Colonic Carcinogenesis" (eds R. A. Malt and R. C. N. Williamson), pp. 93–97. MTP Press Ltd., Lancaster.

Setchell, K. D. R., Lawson, A. M., McLaughlin, L. M., Patel, S., Kirk, D. N. and Axelson, M. (1983). Measurement of enterolactone and enterodiol, the first mammalian lignans, using stable isotope dilution and gas chromatography mass spectrometry. *Biomed. Mass Spectrom.* **10**, 227–235.

Setchell, K. D. R., Borriello, S. P., Hulme, P. and Axelson, M. (1984). Nonsteroidal estrogens of dietary origin: possible roles in hormone-dependent disease. *Am. J. Clin. Nutr.* **40**, 569–578.

Setchell, K. D. R., Welsh, M. B. and Lim, C. K. (1987a). High-Performance liquid chromatographic analysis of phytoestrogens in soy protein preparations with ultraviolet, electrochemical and thermospray mass spectrometric detection. *J. Chromatog.* **386**, 315–323.

Setchell, K. D. R., Gosselin, S. J., Welsh, M. B., Johnston, J. O., Balistreri, W. F., Kramer, L. W., Dresser, B. L. and Tarr, M. J. (1987b). Dietary estrogens – a probable cause of infertility and liver disease in captive cheetah. *Gastroenterol.* **93**, 225–233 .

Shutt, D. A. (1976). The effects of plant estrogens on animal reproduction. *Endeavour* **35**, 110–113.

Shutt, D. A. and Braden, A. W. H. (1968). The significance of equol in relation to the oestrogenic responses in sheep ingesting clover with high formononetin content. *Aust. J. Agric. Res.* **19**, 545–553.

Shutt, D. A. and Cox, R. I. (1972). Steroid and phytoestrogen binding to sheep uterine receptors in vitro. *J. Endocrinol.* **52**, 299–310.

Sica, V., Contieri, E., Nola, E., Bova, R., Papleo, G. and Puca, G. A. (1981). Estrogen and progesterone binding proteins in human colorectal cancer. A preliminary characterization of estradiol receptor. *Tumori* **67**, 307–314.

Stebbings, W. S. L., Farthing, M. J. G., Vinson, G. P., Northover, J. M. A. and Wood, R. F. M. (1986). Androgen receptors in rectal and colonic cancer. *Dis. Colon Rectum* **29**, 95–98.

Stitch, S. R., Smith, P. D., Illingworth, D., and Toumba, K. (1980a). Cyclic excretion of a non-steroidal compound in woman. *J. Endocrinol.* **85**, 23P.

Stitch, S. R., Toumba, J. K., Groen, M. B., Funke, C. W., Leemhuis, J., Vink, J. and Woods, G. F. (1980b). Excretion, isolation and structure of a new phenolic constitutent of female urine. *Nature* **287**, 738–740.

Tang, B. Y. and Adams, N. R. (1980). Effect of equol on oestrogen receptors and on synthesis of DNA and protein in the immature rat uterus. *J. Endocrinol.* **85**, 291–297.

Tang, B. Y. and Adams, N. R. (1981). Oestrogen receptors and metabolic activity in the genital tract after ovariectomy of ewes with permanent infertility caused by exposure to phyto-oestrogens. *J. Endocrinol.* **89**, 365–370.

Tang, B. Y. and Adams, N. R. (1982). Proportions of nucleic acids in the uteri of ewes with clover disease and the effect of oestrogen after ovariectomy. *Aust. J. Biol. Sci.* **35**, 527–531.

Tang, B. Y. and Adams, N. R. (1985). Apparently normal oestrogen receptor system in ovariectomized ewes with impaired response to oestrogen after prolonged grazing non estrogenic pasture. *J. Endocrinol.* **109**, 251–255.

Thompson, M. A., Lasley, B. L., Rideout, B. A. and Kasman, L. H. (1984). Characterization of the estrogenic properties of a nonsteroidal estrogen, equol, extracted from urine of pregnant Macaques. *Biol. Reprod.* **31**, 705–713.

Trowell, H. C. and Burkitt, D. P. (1983). "Western Diseases: Their Emergence and Prevention". Edward Arnold, London.

Trowell, H., Burkitt, D. and Heaton, K. (1985). "Dietary Fibre, Fibre-Depleted Foods and Diseases". Academic Press, London.

Walz, E. (1931). Isoflavon-und Saponin-Glucoside in Soja hispida. *Justus Liebigs Ann. Chem.* **498**, 118–155.

Waters, A. P. and Knowler, J. T. (1982). Effect of a lignan (HPMF) on RNA synthesis in the rat uterus. *J. Reprod. Fert.* **66**, 379–381.

Wattenberg, L. W. (1983). Inhibition of neoplasia by minor dietary constitutents. *Cancer Res. (Suppl.)* **43**, 2448s–2453s.

Welshons, W. V., Murphy, C. S., Koch, R., Calaf, G. and Jordan, V. C. (1987), Stimulation of breast cancer cells *in vitro* by the environmental estrogen enterolactone and the phytoestrogen equal. *Breast Cancer Res. Treatm.* **10**: 169–175.

Wobbes, Th., Beex, L. V. A. M. and Koenders, A. M. J. (1984). Estrogen and progestin receptors in colonic cancer? *Dis. Colon Rectum* **27**, 591–592.

15

Factors Affecting the Gut Microflora

A.K. MALLETT and I.R. ROWLAND

A. Introduction

The population of bacteria in the gastro-intestinal tract is determined and regulated by a great variety of factors, some of which are derived from the host and the chemicals to which it is exposed, while others are a consequence of the microbiota itself.

This area has been reviewed by Savage (1984) and is summarized in Fig. 15.1. From the point of view of toxicology and foreign compound metabolism, the most important of these factors are drugs, disease, age and diet. These are dealt with in detail below.

B. Drugs

1. *Antibacterial Drugs*

The treatment of man or animals with antibiotics, particularly by the oral route, often results in suppression of some, though usually not all, components of the normal gut microflora. The extent of suppression of the flora depends partly on the specificity of the antibiotic used and partly on the resistance of the bacteria in the gut.

(a) Clinical consequences of antibiotic treatment.   Once established, the microbial community of the gut is remarkably stable and is a major factor in preventing the establishment of potentially pathogenic, exogenous organisms in the gut, i.e. the normal flora contributes to the colonization resistance of the gut (Van der Waaij and Berghuis de Vries, 1974). Because many antibacterial drugs perturb the gut ecosystem, this colonization resistance can be diminished or lost allowing potential pathogens to colonize ecological niches in the gut (Savage, 1980). For

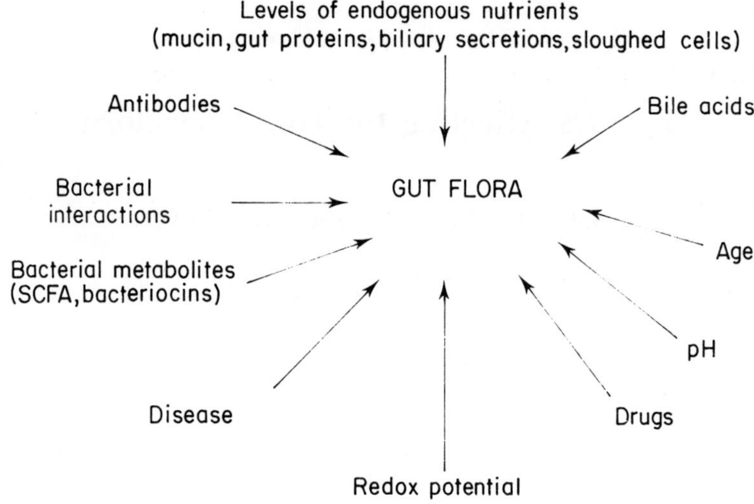

Fig 15.1. Some factors affecting the flora.

example, the susceptibility of mice to *Salmonella* infection is greatly increased by administration of streptomycin (Miller and Bohnhoff, 1962), and similar effects of antibiotic treatment have been observed in humans. The strictly anaerobic components of the microflora appear to be the most crucial to the maintenance of colonization resistance (van der Waaij, 1979).

In situations where extended prophylactic antibiotic treatment to prevent infections is necessary, for example in the case of leukopenic patients (who have greatly reduced natural defence mechanisms), it is obviously important to maintain high colonization resistance. This has led van der Waaij and colleagues to screen a number of antibiotics which selectively suppress potentially pathogenic faculative anaerobes while leaving the strict anerobes unaffected (van der Waaij *et al.*, 1982).

Supplementation of animal feeds with subtherapeutic levels of antibiotics has been used extensively since it increases growth rate, especially in chickens and pigs. There is some evidence that the mechanism involves inhibition of bacteria responsible for growth depression (reviewed by Coates and Fuller (1978)). Such indiscriminate exposure of animals to antibiotics such as penicillin and tetracycline, however, exerts a selective pressure in the gut environment which allows proliferation of drug-resistant strains of bacteria, particularly *E. coli* (reviewed by Savage (1980)). In most cases the drug resistance is encoded on plasmids which may be transferred to other bacteria in the absence of selection pressure by antibiotics. Humans treated with antibiotics can exhibit increased frequency of carriage of antibiotic-resistant organisms in the gut. The implications of antibiotic-induced, transferable drug resistance in intestinal bacteria for human health and treatment of disease are obvious and much discussed (Savage, 1980) and have led to severe restrictions on the use of antibiotics in animal feeds.

(b) Toxicological Consequences of Antibiotic Treatment. In view of the involvement of the gut microflora in the activation and detoxification of many foreign compounds, it is probable that treatment of individuals with antibiotics which suppress the flora would influence the toxicological sequelae of exposure to such chemicals. However, we are not aware of any published studies in this area.

2. *Other Drugs*

Drugs which affect the physiology of the gastro-intestinal tract can influence the microbial population. The most important of these are the H_2 – blocking agents, such as cimetidine and ranitidine which inhibit gastric acid secretion. Several studies have shown that peptic ulcer patients given cimetidine have elevated stomach pH and higher numbers of bacteria (Stockbrugger *et al.*, 1982; Reed *et al.*, 1982). The major toxicological concern has been the possibility, under these conditions, of bacterial nitrate reduction to nitrite and nitrosamine formation as is the case with hypochlorhydric individuals (see Section C). Patients given cimetidine were, in fact, found to have increased nitrite and *N*-nitrosamine concentrations (Reed *et al.*, 1981; Stockbrugger *et al.*, 1982). However, a study of the effects of cimetidine in eight healthy volunteers showed no significant increase in bacteria, nitrite or nitroso compound concentration, and only minor effects on pH (Milton-Thompson *et al.*, 1982). Thus the long term effects of treatment with H_2 blockers, particularly the possibility that patients may develop gastric cancer (as people with chronic achlorhydria are prone to do), are uncertain.

C. Disease

A wide variety of disorders of the gastro-intestinal tract are accompanied by bacterial colonization of the stomach, duodenum, jejunum or proximal ileum – regions which in the healthy person are virtually sterile. The bacteriology of these disorders, which include blind-loop syndrome, small intestinal diverticula, Crohn's disease and various gastric operations, has been comprehensively reviewed by Simon and Gorbach (1981). The presence of bacteria in the upper regions of the intestinal tract can have profound clinical and toxicological consequences. A common clinical manifestation of bacterial colonization of the small intestine is fat malabsorption (Donaldson, 1970). This is thought to be due to bacterial deconjugation of bile salts which leads to impairment of micelle formation. Bacterial overgrowth in the small bowel is also often accompanied by vitamin B_{12} deficiency, leading to megaloblastic anaemia. The bacteria have been shown to bind the vitamin preventing its absorption from the gut (Donaldson, 1962).

Toxicologically, one of the most important gastro-intestinal syndromes is hypochlorhydria, i.e. reduced capacity to secrete gastric acid, leading to elevated pH and colonization of the stomach by bacteria. Hypochlorhydria is associated with a wide variety of disease states, such as pernicious anaemia, hypogammaglobulinaemia, gastric ulcer, and atrophic gastritis, and often occurs after gastric surgery and in people treated with anti-ulcer drugs such as cimetidine (Ruddell *et al.*, 1976; Schlag *et al.*, 1982; Dolby *et al.*, 1984; Stockbrugger *et al.*, 1984; Reed *et al.*, 1981). Elevated gastric pH is also common in the elderly (Reed *et al.*, 1981), and a recent study suggests that it occurs in a significant proportion of a young and healthy western population (Mueller *et al.*, 1986).

The microbial colonization of the hypochlorhydric stomach leads to the possibility of bacterial metabolism of ingested chemicals, and particular attention has been focused on the reduction of ingested nitrate to nitrite and the subsequent bacterially-catalysed formation of *N*-nitroso compounds, many of which are known to be potent carcinogens. Gastric nitrate levels in hyochlorhydrics can reach levels of 100 μM or more (Dolby *et al.*, 1984) by comparison to levels of 1–20 μM found in the acid stomach (Walters *et al.*, 1976; Milton-Thompson *et al.*, 1982).

In a survey of gastric pH, nitrite, nitrosamines and bacterial flora in a large number of people with various gastro-intestinal disorders, Reed *et al.* (1981) found a significant relationship between pH and *N*-nitrosamine concentration ranging from 0.1 μmol 1^{-1} at pH 1–1.5 to a mean of 1.2 μmol 1^{-1} at pH 6.5–9 (in pernicious anaemia patients). Patients with atrophic gastritis have also been found to have elevated nitrite and nitrosamine levels in gastric juice (Schlag *et al.*, 1982).

There is evidence of increased risk of gastric dysplasia and gastric cancer in patients with pernicious anaemia, hypogammaglobinaemia, atrophic gastritis and gastric resection (Jones *et al.*, 1978; Siurala *et al.*, 1959; Hermans *et al.*, 1976; Mosbech and Videbaek 1950), and it has been suggested that the aetiology of the disease is related to increased nitroso compound formation due to the colonization of the stomach by nitrate-reducing bacteria which raise nitrite levels in the gastric juice (Correa *et al.*, 1975).

D. Age

The mammalian gut is sterile at birth but is rapidly colonized by micro-organisms from the mother's vagina and skin and from the environment and food. Some of these organisms are unable to colonize the gut, but others become established and a succession of types occurs governed by many factors, including pH, peristalsis, redox potential, diet and the bacterial community itself (Savage, 1984).

In most animals, the initial colonization of the gut is by lactic acid bacteria such as *Lactobacillus* spp. and *Bifidobacterium* spp. which quickly reach high numbers. Shortly after birth, facultative anaerobes such as *Streptococcus* spp. and *E. coli* can be detected in faeces along with the lactic acid bacteria (Savage, 1977). After this initial colonization, the bacterial population remains fairly stable during suckling, although qualitative changes do occur (Drasar and Barrow, 1985). However, the introduction of solid food causes major qualitative and quantitative alterations in flora as the strict anaerobes such as *Bacteroides* gain ascendancy with a concomitant decline in levels of the facultative organisms (Savage, 1977).

It would be expected, therefore, that age-related changes in the metabolic activity in the gut flora would be apparent coincident with the changes in numbers and types of organism in the gut of the developing infant. In turn, this could lead to difference in susceptibility of an infant, at different stages in development, to compounds dependent on microbial metabolism for activation or detoxication. However, this area has received very little attention, with the exception of some studies on methylmercury metabolism, where dramatic differences have been found in the rate of excretion of mercury in neonatal and weaned mice and humans. When suckling mice were given an oral dose of methylmercuric chloride, they absorbed and retained the majority of the dose with a half-time of mercury elimination greater than 100 days (Doherty and Gates, 1973). Older mice, given a similar dose of the organomercurial, excreted mercury much more rapidly (half time of mercury elimination, approximately 6 days). This developmental change in the rate of mercury excretion occurred abruptly at the 16–18th postnatal days, coinciding with the time of weaning to a pelleted rodent diet.

There are a number of possible mechanisms which may explain these developmental changes in rate of mercury excretion (Rowland *et al.*,

1983c), but there is good evidence that an age-related increase in demethylation of methylmercury by the gut microflora plays an important role. Demethylation converts methyl mercury from a form which is rapidly absorbed to an inorganic state which is poorly absorbed from the gut (see Chapter 9). Thus a low rate of demethylation in suckling mice would be associated with a high rate of absorption of the organomercurial. It was apparent that the *in vivo* formation of mercuric mercury after methylmercury exposure was much higher in weaned (20 day old) mice than in preweanling animals of 4 or 10 days (Rowland *et al.*, 1983c). Incubation of caecal contents from 10 day or 20 day old mice with methylmercuric chloride revealed that only bacteria from the older (weaned) mice were capable of demethylation. It is interesting also that mice weaned onto a milk diet rather than a pelleted rodent diet did not develop the ability to demethylate methylmercury *in vivo*, lacked a gut flora capable of demethylation and absorbed and retained virtually all of an oral dose of methylmercury (Rowland *et al.*, 1984).

In preliminary studies, faecal preparations from neonatal humans were found to be incapable of demethylating methylmercury, but the capacity for the reaction developed rapidly on weaning (Rowland *et al.*, 1983c). Thus the human neonate probably behaves like the suckling mouse in absorbing and retaining the majority of methylmercury ingested, suggesting that they are more susceptible to the toxic effects of methylmercury than adults.

E. Diet

A wide range of natural and xenobiotic chemical structures are transformed by intestinal bacterial enzymes to products which exhibit modified toxicological and pharmacological potency (Rowland *et al.*, 1985). Bacterial metabolism may be influenced by dietary factors, in particular indigestible plant cell-wall materials (Rowland *et al.*, 1985), suggesting that food components may play a pivotal role in determining the disposition of microbial substrates within the large intestine. Such diet–gut flora interactions may explain the proposed protective role of dietary fibre on chemically-induced toxicity (Ershoff, 1974; Omaye, 1986) and cancer of the large intestine (Spiller and Freeman, 1982; Reddy *et al.*, 1983), although in many instances such explanations are speculative. Recently, however, experimental studies employing laboratory animals have produced a number of examples of diet modifying the metabolism and toxicity of xenobiotic compounds. These are summarized in Table 15.1, and some examples are discussed in more detail below.

1. *Pectins and Other Indigestible Plant Cell Wall Carbohydrates*

The pectins are structurally based on a polymer of galacturonic acid residues with additional rhamnose and arabinose substituents, in which a variable proportion of the uronic carboxyl groups are esterified with methanol (Adrian, 1976). Pectins are extensively degraded within the gut and present a ready source of fermentable carbohydrate to gastro-intestinal micro-organisms (De Wilde, 1980; Holloway *et al.*, 1983). The increase in available energy within the gut may result in changes in bacterial species diversity or metabolic capability, with consequent alterations in the metabolism of foreign or host-derived compounds. Experimental studies in rodents have provided a number of examples of dietary pectin increasing bacterially-mediated toxicity *in vivo* (Table 15.2).

(a) Nitrate reductase.   High-methoxyl pectin significantly increases bacterial nitrate reductase activity present in rat intestinal or caecal contents (Mallett *et al.*, 1983) when added to a purified diet at 5% (w/w), with an associated increase in nitrate toxicity *in vivo*. Wise *et al.* (1981) reported that rats fed a pectin-containing diet were highly susceptible to nitrate-induced methaemoglobinaemia, whereas animals fed a fibre-free control diet were unaffected. Animals fed the pectin-containing diet typically showed a 10-fold increase in blood methaemoglobin 6 hours after nitrate administration relative to that observed in the control diet group (Wise *et al.*, 1981).

Bacterial reduction of nitrate to nitrite is also associated with the formation of genotoxic *N*-nitroso compounds, a reaction catalysed by several common gut micro-organisms (Hill and Hawksworth, 1971; Suzuki and Mitsuoka, 1984). In the experiment shown in Fig. 15.2, a mutagenic product was detected using *Salmonella* TA100 with S-9 activation when dimethylamine and nitrate were incubated anaerobically with caecal contents from rats fed a pectin-supplemented diet, but not a fibre-free diet. Under similar conditions *in vitro*, the formation of nitroso-L-proline form nitrate and proline was 15-fold greater in preparations from rats fed the pectin-containing diet than in the control group (Fig. 15.2). No product formation was observed if either nitrate or amine precursors were omitted from the incubation mixture. The pH of the assays was unchanged at the end of the incubation, suggesting that increased nitrate reductase activity (29 versus 6 μmol h^{-1} g^{-1} caecal contents) rather than acid catalysed nitrosation was responsible for the formation of nitroso-products.

(b) Nitroreductase.   Pectin ingestion alters the activity of bacterial enzymes responsible for the reduction of aromatic and heterocyclic

Table 15.1 *Modification of intestinal bacterial enzyme activities by major dietary components*

Diet details[a]	Time on diet	Species	Enzyme[b]	Observation[c]	Reference
Non-starch polysaccharides – purified					
1. Cellulose (5,15%)	12 days	Rat	GN	Decreased/mg faecal N by 15% cellulose, but 24 hour output unaltered	Shiau and Chang (1983)
			MU	Activity/mg N unaffected	
2. Cellulose (0–40%)	3 weeks	Rat	AR GS NR GN NT	Activities/caecum decreased with increasing cellulose concentration	Mallet *et al.* (1986)
3. Cellulose (5,15%) substituted for sucrose	20–120 days	Rat	β-N-acetyl glucosamidase β-galactosidase	Activities/mg protein generally decreased in high cellulose group at all time points	Prizont (1984)
4. Cellulose (4.5,9%)	8 weeks	Rat	GN	Decreased per mg faecal protein in high treatment group	Freeman (1986)
			GS	Unchanged	
5. Pectin (citrus; 6.5%)	?	Rat	GN	Activity/g faecal protein increased	Bauer *et al.* (1979)
6. Pectin (high or low methoxyl; 5%)	?	Rat	GN	Activity/g faecal protein unaltered (no obvious explanation for discrepancy with above study)	Bauer *et al.* (1981)

	Treatment	Duration	Species	Enzyme	Effect	Reference
7.	Pectin (citrus; 15 g/day) as supplement to normal mixed diet	18 days	Man	GN	Activity/mg faecal protein generally increased, but large variation in individual response	Ross and Leklem (1981)
8.	Pectin (high methoxyl; 5%)	15 or 45 days	Rat	AR, NR, NT	Activity/g caecal content unaltered Activity/g caecal content increased 4–12-fold	Wise *et al.* (1981)
9.	Pectin (high methoxyl; 5%)	50 days	Rat	NR	Reduction of *p*-nitrobenzoic acid/caecum increased, but metabolism of four other nitroaromatics unchanged	Rowland *et al.* (1983b)
10.	Pectin (high methoxyl; 5%)	30 days	Rat		All activities expressed/g	Rowland *et al.* (1983a)
				AR	Decreased	
				GN	Increased (two-fold)	
				GS	Decreased (~50%)	
				NR	Unchanged	
				NT	Increased (six-fold)	
		30 days	Mouse	AR, GS, GN	Unchanged	
				NR	Decreased (~50%)	
				NT	Increased (seven-fold)	
		30 days	Hamster	AR, GN, NR, NT	Unaltered	
				GS	Decreased (~50%)	

Table 15.1 *continued*

Diet details[a]		Time on diet	Species	Enzyme[b]	Observation[c]	Reference
11.	Pectin (5,15%)	12 days	Rat	GN	Activity/mg faecal N and total 24 hour faecal output decreased (15% of control) (discrepancy with other studies may reflect method of expressing activity)	Shiau and Chang (1983)
				MU	Activity/mg N in faeces unchanged. Activity/24 hour faecal output decreased by 5% pectin; unaffected at higher treatment level	
12.	Pectin (citrus; 5,10%)	28 days	Rat	NR GN	Activity/g caecal contents increased (2–3-fold)	DeBethizy *et al.* (1983)
13.	Pectin (citrus; 5%)	28 days	Rat	NR	Activity/mg caecal contexts increased	Goldstein *et al.* (1984)
14.	Pectin (citrus; 5,10%)	?	Rat	AR	Activity/g decreased, but total activity/ caecum increased (two-fold)	DeBethizy and Goldstein (1985)
15.	Pectin (apple, high methoxyl; 18 g/day) as supplement in normal mixed diet	21 days	Man	EA	Activity/g faeces and ammonia concentration increased	Mallett *et al.* (1988)
				GS GN	Activity/g faeces decreased (~50%)	
				NR NT	Activity/g faeces unchanged	

No.	Substrate	Duration	Species	Enzyme	Effect	Reference
16.	Pectin (apple, high methoxyl, 18 g/day) as supplement in normal mixed diet	21 days	Man	GS GN NR NT	Activity/10^{10} bacteria unchanged	Mallet *et al.* (1987)
	Pectin (apple, high methoxyl, 5%)		Rat (human flora)	GS	Activity increased 10^{10} bacteria	
				GN NR NT	Activity unchanged	
			Rat (CV flora)	GS GN NR	Activity unchanged/10^{10} bacteria	
				NT	Activity increased (five-fold)	
17.	Pectin (4.5,9%)	8 weeks	Rat	GS	Activity/mg faecal protein increased by approx. 40%	Freeman (1986)
				GN	Increased 4–6-fold	
18.	Guar-gum (5,10%)	?	Rat	GN	Activity/g faecal protein decreased	Bauer *et al.* (1981)
19.	Guar-gum (5,15%)	12 days	Rat	GN	Decreased/mg faecal N by 15% guar gum	Shiau and Chang (1983)
				MU	Decreased by 85% in high-dose group	
20.	Guar-gum (5%)	28 days	Rat	AR GN GS NR NT U	Increased/total caecal contents	Mallett *et al.* (1984c)

Table 15.1 *continued*

Diet details[a]		Time on diet	Species	Enzyme[b]	Observation[c]	Reference
21.	Carrageenan (type unspecified; 5,15%)	12 days	Rat	GN	Decreased/mg faecal N; total output decreased by 15% carrageenan	Shiau and Chang (1983)
				MU	Activity unchanged	
22.	Carrageenan (*iota*, 5%)	50 days	Rat	NR	Reduction of five nitro-aromatic substrates/ caecum greatly decreased (1–5% of control)	Rowland *et al.* (1983a)
23.	Carrageenan (*iota*, 5%)	30 days	Rat	AR GN GS NR NT	Activity/g caecal contents and per total caecum decreased	Mallett *et al.* (1985b)
		30 days	Mouse	AR GN GS NR	Activity/g and per total caecum decreased	
				NT	Unchanged/g caecal contents; increased per total caecum	
		30 days	Hamster	AR	Decreased/g caecal contents; unchanged per total caecum	
				GN NT	Increased/g and per total caecum	
				GS	Unchanged	
				NR	Decreased/g and per total caecum	

No.	Substrate	Duration	Species	Enzyme	Effect	Reference
24.	Agar-agar (5%)	28 days	Rat	AR GN GS NR NT U	Generally decreased/caecum	Mallett *et al.* (1984c)
25.	Gum Acacia (5%) Locust Bean Gum (5%) Carboxymethyl cellulose (5%)	28 days	Rat	AR GN GS NR NT	Generally increased/caecum	Mallett *et al.* (1984c)
26.	Hemicellulose (4.5;9%)	8 weeks	Rat	GS	Activity/mg faecal protein increased two-fold	Freeman (1986)
				GN	Decreased by 40%	

Non-starch polysaccharides—plant cell wall products, mixtures

No.	Substrate	Duration	Species	Enzyme	Effect	Reference
1.	Wheat bran (20%)	?	Rat	GN	No effect/g faecal protein	Bauer *et al.* (1979)
2.	Maize bran (20%) Soya bean bran (20%) Wheat bran (20%)	24 weeks	Mouse	GN	Decreased/g faeces by 30–90%	London *et al.* (1981)
3.	Wheat bran (5;15, 30%)	30 days	Rat	GN	Unchanged/g caecal contents	Mallett *et al.* (1986)
				GS	Increased at all dietary levels	
				NR NT	Generally decreased for all diets	

Table 15.1 *continued*

Diet details[a]		Time on diet	Species	Enzyme[b]	Observation[c]	Reference
4.	Carrot fibre (20%)	?	Rat	GN	Unchanged/g faecal protein	Bauer *et al.* (1979)
5.	Carrot fibre (10%)	28 days	Rat	AR	Decreased/g caecal contents	Rowland *et al.* (1983d)
				GS	Increased by ~50%	
				NR	Unchanged	
				GN		
	Cabbage fibre (10%)	28 days	Rat	AR	Unchanged/g caecal contents	Rowland *et al.* (1983d)
				GS		
				NR		
				GN		
Carbohydrates						
1.	Lactose (25,50%)	10 days	Rats (weaning)	GS	Unaffected/caecum	Wise *et al.* (1984)
				GN		
				AR	Decrease by 50% lactose	
				NR		
				NT	Generally increased	
				U		
			Rats (adult)	AR	Unaffected/caecum	
				GN		
				NR		
				GS	Slightly increased	
				NT	Increased (3–8-fold)	
				U		
2.	Rice starch (38%, substituted for maize starch)	21 days	Rat	EA	Unchanged/g caecal contents	Mallett and Rowland (1987, unpublished observations)
				GN		
				NT		
				GS	Decreased (by 40–60%)	
				NR		

	Diet	Duration	Species	Enzyme	Effect	Reference
	Amylomaize starch (38%, substituted for maize starch)	21 days	Rat	GS, NT	Unaffected/caecal contents	Mallett and Rowland (unpublished observations)
				EA, GN, NR	Decreased	
4.	Potato starch (38%, substituted for maize starch)			EA, GS, GN, NR	Decreased/g caecal contents	Mallett and Rowland (unpublished observations)
				NT	Not affected	
Protein						
1.	Lactalbumin (0–40%)	10 days	Rat	AR, NR	Unaffected/caecum	Wise *et al.* (1983)
				GS, GN, U	Generally increased with increasing dietary protein	
				NT	Lower activity at higher protein levels	
Fat						
1.	Corn oil, lard (5,20% in purified diet)	30 weeks	Rat	GN	Increased/mg protein and per mg dry weight contents in 20% groups	Reddy *et al.* (1977)
2.	Animal fat (62 or 152 g/day in balanced diet)	4 weeks	Man	GN	Unchanged per g faeces	Cummings *et al.* (1978)
3.	Beef fat, Cocoa butter, Olive oil, Safflower oil (35% in purified diet)	30 days	Rat	AR, GS, NT	Decreased/total caecum in comparison to low fat diet (1% safflower oil)	Mallett *et al.* (1984a,b)
				GN	Increased two-fold by beef fat and olive oil	

Table 15.1 *continued*

Diet details[a]	Time on diet	Species	Enzyme[b]	Observation[c]	Reference
Meat					
1. Beef Pork Lamb Chicken	4 days	Man	GN	Increased/mg protein, dry wt and total output (approx. three-fold) by comparison to a meat-free diet N.B. May reflect change in fat and fibre intake, rather than protein source	Reddy *et al.* (1974)
2. Beef (autoclaved, lean, 72%, w/w in purified diet)	24–40 days	Rat	AR GN NR	Increased/mg faecal protein (2–3-fold) relative to grain-based diet	Goldin and Gorbach (1976)
			GS	Decreased by 80%	
3. Red meat (eliminated from diet)	4 weeks	Man	GN NR AR	Unchanged/mg faecal protein	Goldin *et al.* (1980)
			7αDH	Decreased by 50–70% by comparison to 'red-meat diet'	
4. Beef (protein intake increased 5–10%, fat intake increased 30%)	4 weeks	Man	GN	Increased/mg dry wt faeces (1.5–3-fold) by comparison to free choice diet	Reddy *et al.* (1980)
			7αDH CDH	Unchanged	

[a] All dietary additions were in a purified diet base unless otherwise stated.
[b] Abbreviations used are AR, azoreductase; CDH, cholesterol dehydrogenase; 7αDH, 7αdehydrogenase; EA, ammonia production from endogeous substrates; GN, β-glucuronidase; GS, β-glucosidase; NR, nitro reductase; NT, nitrate reductase; U, urcase; MU, mucinase; ?, not given; CV, conventional flora.

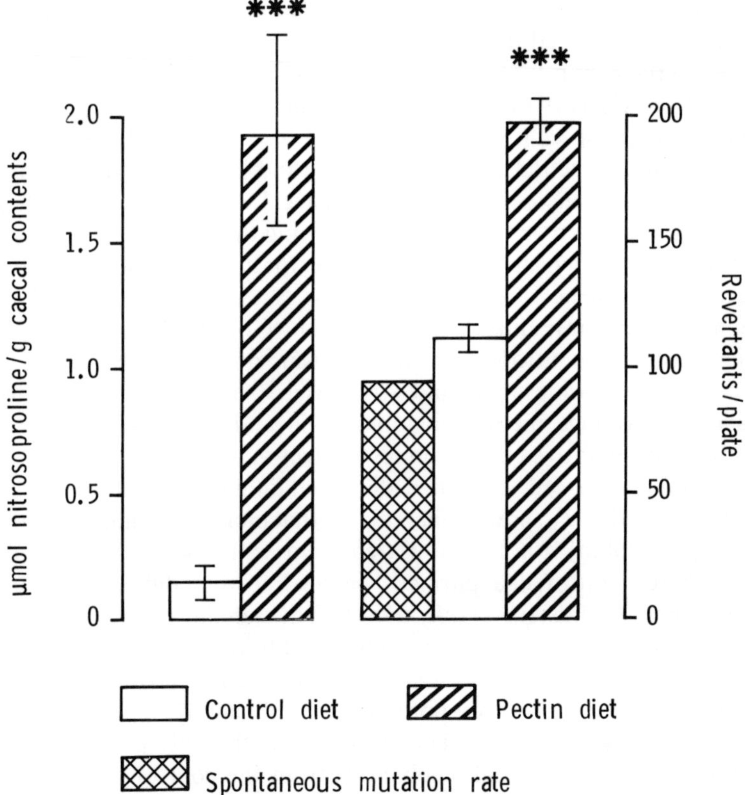

Fig 15.2. Enhanced formation of *N*-nitroso compounds *in vitro* by caecal content preparations from rats fed pectin. A 10% suspension of caecal contents from rats fed a control, fibre-free diet or that diet containing 5% high methoxyl pectin were incubated anaerobically at 37°C for 18 hours with 0.2 M sodium nitrate and 0.05 M dimethylamine or 0.05 M L-proline (5μCiL-[U-^{14}C] proline/assay) in a final volume of 4.0 ml 0.1 M potassium phosphate buffer, pH 7.4.

nitrocompounds to amines, many of which possess toxic, mutagenic or carcinogenic properties (Rowland *et al.*, 1985).

One group of compounds of interest in this respect are dinitrotoluenes, important industrial intermediates which produce hepatic tumours in several animal studies (Rickert *et al.*, 1984). 2,6-dinitrotoluene binds covalently to hepatic DNA (Long and Rickert, 1982) and is genotoxic in hepatocyte DNA repair assays (Mirsalis *et al.*, 1982), both reactions having an absolute dependence on the gut microflora before an expression of toxicity is observed. DeBethizy *et al.* (1983) reported increased hepatic macromolecular covalent binding in animals treated with [^{3}H]-2,6-dinitrotoluene and fed diets containing 5% or 10% high methoxyl pectin relative to the pectin-free control diet. Two commercially available cereal-based rations (NIH-07, Purina 5002) containing pectin in addition to other fermentable plant cell wall components also increased dinitrotoluene binding to liver fractions. Nitroreductase (and β-glucuronidase) activities were significantly increased 2–3-fold in caecal contents from rats fed the pectin-supplemented or stock diets, suggesting that diet-related alterations in bacterial metabolism were responsible for the increased hepatoxicity of 2,6-dinitrotoluene.

Generally similar findings were reported by Goldstein *et al.* (1984) on the influence of diet on nitrobenzene metabolism and toxicity. Nitrobenzene is again subject to widespread industrial usage, but is well known for its capacity to produce methaemoglobinaemia and other blood dyscrasias, as well as degenerative changes in testis, liver and spleen function (Rickert *et al.*, 1983). Rats fed a purified diet containing 5% pectin or a cereal based diet (NIH-07) showed marked methaemoglobinaemia (30–40% of total haemoglobin) 4 hours after treatment with 200 mg kg^{-1} nitrobenzene, whereas rats fed a purified, pectin-free diet did not respond to nitrobenzene (Goldstein *et al.*, 1984). The administration of a larger challenge of nitrobenzene exaggerated the differences in methaemoglobinaemia between the various dietary groups. The reductive metabolism of nitrobenzene *in vitro* differed both qualitatively and quantitatively for the different dietary treatments. Thus aniline was the only product found at low concentration in caecal incubations from the control group, but was present at 3 or 10-fold excess in incubations from the pectin or cereal based diet groups, along with detectable amounts of azoxybenzene and nitrosobenzene (Goldstein *et al.*, 1984). Since bacterial reduction is required for the development of nitrobenzene-induced methaemoglobinaemia (Reddy *et al.*, 1976), the observed effects of diet on erythrocyte function noted in this work are likely to be associated with the plant cell-wall components present in the diets.

(c) β-Glucuronidase.   Pectin and other fermentable fibres increase bacterial β-glucuronidase activity in the rodent (Bauer *et al.*, 1981) and human (Ross and Leklem, 1981) hindgut floras. One potential consequence of this diet-induced change is the increased retention of potentially toxic agents within the body (Chadwick *et al.*, 1978; De Bethizy *et al.*, 1983) due to the pivotal role of β-glucuronidase in enterohepatic recirculation (Rowland and Walker, 1983). Modification of bacterial β-glucuronidase by diet could also play a part in influencing the metabolism and tumourigenicity of carcinogens which undergo hepatic conjugation and biliary excretion (see section 4 for more details).

Table 15.2 *Modification of bacterial metabolite formation by dietary components*

Dietary component	Bacterial enzyme altered	Bacterial substrate	Host response
Pectin	Azo reductase	Amaranth	Plasma naphthionic acid increased
	Nitrate reductase	Nitrate	Methaemoglobin
	Nitro reductase	2,6-dinitrotoluene	Macromolecular covalent binding
		Nitrobenzene	Methaemoglobinaemia
Rutin	β-glycosidase	Rutin	Release of mutagenic product
Saccharin	Tryptophanase	Tryptophan	Indole/cresol intoxication (?)

(d) Azoreductase. A further reductive function of the gut microflora which is susceptible to dietary modification is azoreductase activity, as exemplified by metabolism of the food colour amaranth. Male rats fed a purified diet containing 15% cellulose exhibited an approximate 20-fold increase in blood naphthionic acid concentration 12 hours after amaranth administration relative to a control, fibre-free group (DeBethizy and Goldstein, 1985). Anaerobic incubation of caecal contents *in vitro* from rats fed the pectin containing diet showed a decreased rate of amaranth reduction relative to control animals, although the total azoreductase activity per caecum was twofold greater in the pectin-fed animals, presumably due to caecal enlargement. These results again suggest a strong modifying effect of pectin ingestion on the metabolism of foreign compounds by bacterial enzymes in the large intestine.

(e) Methylmercury demethylase. By comparison to inorganic salts of mercury, methylmercury is rapidly absorbed after ingestion. A proportion of the absorbed dose is secreted back into the intestine via the bile leading to an enterohepatic circulation (Norseth and Clarkson, 1971). There is good evidence from *in vitro* and *in vivo* studies that the gut microflora can demethylate methylmercury to inorganic forms and thereby interrupt the enterohepatic cycle and increase mercury excretion, thus lowering mercury body burden and tissue levels (see Chapter 9). Landry *et al.* (1979) reported differences in methylmercury retention and tissue concentration in mice fed different diets. Rowland *et al.* (1984) provided evidence that diet-induced differences in the rate of methylmercury

excretion are a consequence of diet-dependent changes in demethylation of the organomercurial by the gut microflora. It was found that in methylmercury-treated mice, the percentage of the total Hg body burden present as inorganic Hg (Hg^{++}) was higher (35.5%) in those animals fed a purified diet (which showed a high rate of mercury excretion) than in mice fed a stock diet (Hg^{++} 10.4% of total Hg). Treatment of the mice with antibiotics decreased both the rate of mercury excretion and the percentage of mercury present as Hg^{++}, and at the same time abolished the dietary differences in mercury excretion.

Recently the effect of various dietary fibres on methylmercury excretion in mice has been studied (Rowland et al., 1986). Dietary wheat bran was found to increase mercury excretion after methylmercury exposure and to decrease the total mercury concentration in the brain and blood. Again the proportion of mercury found in the inorganic form in several tissues was higher in the bran-fed animals than in those fed a fibre-free diet, and the theory that bran induced increased demethylation of organomercury in the gut was invoked.

In both of these studies the increased mercury excretion was reflected in lower concentration of mercury in the brain. Since the central nervous system is the target tissue of methylmercury the results suggest that the neurotoxic effects of the organomercurial may be modified by diet-induced alterations in gut flora metabolism.

2. Glycosidic Plant Flavonoids

Flavonoids are polyphenolic compounds, common in plant materials, which are conjugated with L-rhamnose, D-glucose, glucorhamnose, galactose or arabinose to form the appropriate glycosidic derivative (Kühnau, 1976). A large number of these materials are common dietary constituents, but because of their hydrophilic nature and high molecular weight are poorly absorbed from the small intestine. Within the large intestine, however, such structures may be extensively hydrolysed by bacterial enzymes (Table 15.2) and the aglycone subjected to subsequent ring fission and degradation (Griffiths, 1975; Baba et al., 1983; Chapter 5).

Flavones are one of the most widespread subgroups of flavonoids found in vegetable matter, and about thirty of these have been identified as possessing mutagenic activity in mammalian and microbial cells (Mac-Gregor, 1986). The hindgut microflora contains a number of constitutive β-glycosidase enzymes (Hawksworth et al., 1971; Prizont and Konigsberg, 1981) capable of hydrolysing flavone glycosides to products possessing genotoxic activity (Tamura *et al.*, 1980). MacDonald *et al.* (1983) showed that preparations of faecal micro-organisms from cultures grown in the presence of rutin or quercitrin exhibited greatly enhanced formation of the aglycone quercetin, as assessed from the expression of mutagenic activity towards *Salmonella typhimurium* TA98, indicating substrate induction of β-glycosidase activity *in vitro*. Subsequent studies showed that strains of *Streptococcus* sp. isolated from human faeces possessed the necessary enzyme after incubation with rutin *in vitro* (MacDonald *et al.*, 1984). We have found that bacterial β-glycosidase activity present in rat caecal contents is also induced following the administration of a purified, fibre-free diet containing 0.5–2.5% (w/w) rutin (Fig. 15.3), showing an 8-fold increase at the highest treatment level. Mutagen release by bacterial enzymes *in vivo* could therefore be increased by rutin ingestion in a manner analogous to that reported *in vitro* (MacDonald *et al.*, 1983; 1984).

As well as being genotoxins, flavonoid aglycones may induce (Wattenburg and Leong, 1970) or inhibit (Sousa and Marletta, 1985) the metabolic activity of certain mammalian enzymes, in particular the mixed function oxidase system localized in the endoplasmic reticulum, with associated alterations in formation of pharmacologically or toxicologically active products. In the experiment reported in Table 15.3, hepatic postmitochondrial fraction prepared from rats fed a purified diet or that diet containing 1% (w/w) rutin exhibited marked differencees in mutagen activating capacity (when compared with control preparations). Thus the cooked food mutagens IQ (2-amino-3-methylimidazo[4,5-*f*]quinoline), MeIQ (2-amino-3,4-dimethylimidazo[4,5-*f*]quinoline) and MeIQ$_x$ (2-amino-3,8-dimethylimidazo[4,5-*f*]quinoxaline) were approximately twice as active when incubated with liver factions from rutin-fed rats. Such effects are presumably mediated *via* the gastro-intestinal flora, since rutin requires bacterial hydrolysis to quercetin before it can be absorbed from the gut and influence foreign compound metabolism in the liver.

3. *Non-Nutritive Sweeteners*

The synthetic, non-nutritive sweeteners cyclamate and saccharin were widely used by food manufacturers over a number of years until questions relating to long-term safety resulted in the compounds being withdrawn from use in many countries. Saccharin increased the incidence of bladder tumours in laboratory animals exposed to high levels over two generations and promoted the genotoxic action of known bladder carcinogens (Arnold *et al.*, 1983). Experimental studies with cyclamate suggested the increased

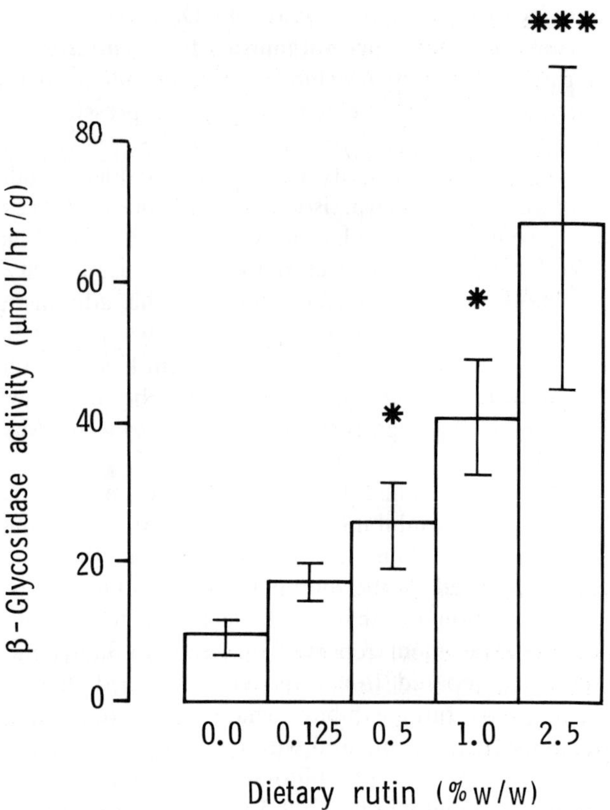

Fig 15.3. Induction of β-glycosidase activity in caecal contents from rats fed differing amounts of dietary rutin. β-glycosidase activity was determined using *p*-nitrophenyl-β-D-glucopyranoside as described by Mallett *et al.* (1985a). The data are presented as the mean ± SEM for groups of five rats fed diets for 14 days. Statistical analysis relative to the 0% rutin group: *P<0.05; ***P<0.001.

occurrence of bladder tumours in rats given high doses as well as conversion to cyclohexylamine *in vivo*, a compound reported to induce testicular atrophy in certain rodents following extended exposure. Both cyclamate and saccharin alter directly, or indirectly, certain metabolic characteristics of the gut flora which may be associated with the toxicity of these materials, although evidence for a role of bacterial metabolites in host toxicity remains largely speculative (Table 15.2). This work is discussed in detail in Chapter 8.

Table 15.3 *Activation of the cooked food mutagens IQ, MeIQ and MeIQ$_x$ by liver fractions from rats fed a purified or rutin-containing diet.* The mutagens IQ (20 ng), MeIQ (10 ng) and MeIQ$_x$(25 ng) were incubated with *S. typhimurium* TA98, liver fraction and cofactors for 30 minutes before plating onto Vogel Bonner medium. The data are given as the mean ± SEM, n = 12 (statistical analysis (ANOVA): *$P<0.05$; ***$P<0.001$)

Mutagen	His$^+$ revertants per plate	
	Control diet	1% Rutin diet
IQ	426 ± 62	850 ± 40***
MeIQ	938 ± 129	1772 ± 66***
MeIQ$_x$	211 ± 32	472 ± 23*

4. Diet and Gut Flora Interaction in Cancer

It is intended in this review to concentrate on those studies which provide evidence that dietary modification of the microflora and/or its metabolic activities can alter the incidence of tumours, either spontaneous or chemically-induced.

(a) Hepatic neoplasms. Studies using germ-free and conventional flora mice have established that the presence or absence of intestinal bacteria influences the development of spontaneous and chemically-induced liver tumours in C3H mice (Mizutani and Mitsuoka, 1980). In general, tumour incidence was much higher in the conventional animals than in their germ-free counterparts, but colonization of the germ-free mice with specific intestinal bacteria modified the tumour incidence. In a subsequent paper, Mizutani *et al.* (1982) demonstrated that feeding C3H mice 10% konjac mannan (a glucomannan derived from tubers of *Amorphallus konjac*) significantly decreased the hepatic tumour incidence. Changes in faecal flora were also observed in the animals fed the glucomannan and in particular an increase in numbers of bifidobacteria was noted. In the previus study (Mizutani and Mitsuoka, 1980) the presence of *Bifidobacterium longum* suppressed the promoting effect on liver tumourigenesis of a cocktail of intestinal bacteria (*Escherichia coli*, *Streptococcus faecalis* and *Clostridium paraputrificum*). Thus there is circumstantial evidence, at least, that modification of the gut microflora by diet is

associated with changes in tumour incidence in the liver. Whether there is a causal relationship remains to be established since dietary fibre has many effects on gut function, which could influence the activity of dietary or endogenous carcinogens and tumour promoters (see Rowland *et al* (1985) for a review).

(b) Intestinal tumours. Epidemiological studies indicate that environmental factors, particularly diet, are important in the aetiology of colon cancer (Hill, 1986). Experimental studies in animals have been carried out to determine the factors involved. Various dietary components have been shown to affect the incidence of intestinal tumours induced in the rat by chemical initiators such as 1,2-dimethylhydrazine (DMH). However, the effects reported in the different studies are not always in agreement. For example, dietary fat has been shown to enhance colon carcinogenesis in some studies (Howarth and Pihl, 1985; see the review by Reddy, 1983) but not in others (Locniskar *et al.*, 1985). Similar inconsistencies have been seen in the effect of dietary fibre on colon tumourigenesis with inhibition, no effect and tumour enhancement being observed (reviewed by Kritchevsky, 1983). The type of fibre employed also markedly influences the outcome of studies of this type (Freeman *et al.*, 1984; Reddy and Mori, 1981; Reddy *et al.*, 1983; Jacobs and Lupton, 1986). The lack of unanimity in the results may reflect strains of animals used, diet composition, route of administration of carcinogen and, in the case of fibre, the particular type used.

(i) β-*glucuronidase*. Several of the hypotheses developed to explain the diet-related effects on large intestinal tumourigenesis are related to the dietary modification of colonic microbial metabolism involved in the activation or detoxication of carcinogens and promoters. The variability of the gut flora between species and strains of animals and individuals, and the susceptibility of the flora to dietary manipulation, may explain some of the discrepancies in studies mentioned above of experimental colon tumourigenesis. We have considered below the various hypotheses and the evidence that the gut flora dependent activity can be modified by dietary change.

Microbial hydrolysis of hepatic glucuronide conjugates secreted into the hindgut *via* the bile has been proposed to play an important role in the tumourigenic action of dimethylhydrazine (Takada *et al.*, 1982; Likhachev *et al.*, 1985). It is noteworthy that other carcinogens such as benzo(a)pyrene and *N*-hydroxy-*N*-2-fluorenylacetamide are also conjugated, leading to liberation of carcinogens in the gut after hydrolysis (Weisburger, 1971; Renwick and Drasar, 1976; Kinoshita and Gelboin, 1978; Nanno *et al.*, 1986). Dietary modification of bacterial β-glucuronidase activity in the gut could, therefore, explain diet-related changes in response of animals to carcinogens capable of being conjugated with glucuronic acid in the liver. The effects of dietary fibre on this microbial enzyme activity have been discussed earlier in this chapter.

Bauer *et al.* (1979) studied the effect of wheat bran (20% in a purified diet), carrot fibre (20%) and citrus pectin (6.5%) on induction of colorectal tumours by DMH in rats. No significant differences in tumour incidence were seen between the wheat bran or carrot fibre groups and the group fed a fibre-free diet. In contrast the group fed pectin had a significantly higher incidence of colorectal tumours and auditory duct tumours. The authors also showed that rats fed pectin exhibited a ninefold increase in β-glucuronidase activity in the gut by comparison to those fed carrot fibre (twofold increase), or wheat bran (no significant increase). A drawback of this study was the particularly high colorectal tumour incidence in all the groups (over 87%), so that weak effects of the diets may not have been detected. However, other studies, e.g. Jacobs and Lupton (1986), have also shown that pectin and indeed other fermentable fibres, such as guar gum, which increase β-glucuronidase activity, enhance DMH-induced colon carcinogenesis.

Numerous studies in rodents and man have shown that an increase in dietary fat is often associated with an increase in β-glucuronidase activity of gut contents or faeces (Table 15.1). Similarly an increase in DMH induced tumour incidence has been detected in several, but not all, studies in which the fat content of the diet has been increased (Reddy, 1983; Howarth and Pihl, 1985; Locniskar *et al.*, 1985). However, tumour incidence and β-glucuronidase activity have not been consistently measured in studies of this type so a correlation is difficult to prove. Additionally, other factors such as neutral and acid steroid levels in faeces have been proposed to account for the enhancing effect of dietary fat on colorectal tumourigenesis in rats.

(ii) *Bile acid metabolism.* The bacterial metabolism of acid steroids and their postulated role in the aetiology of human cancer have been comprehensively reviewed elsewhere (see Chapters 11 and 18). Briefly, it is postulated that the bacterial metabolites of bile acids, termed secondary bile acids, act as promoters of carcinogens in the gut. The predominant secondary bile acids are lithocholic acid (LCA), hyodeoxycholic acid (HDCA; derived from chenodeoxycholic acid (CDCA)) and deoxycholic acid (DCA; derived from cholic acid (CA)). In addition, it has been proposed that cholesterol and its metabolites may also be involved in the aetiology of colon cancer (Broitman *et al.*, 1977; Cruse *et al.*, 1978).

Evidence for dietary modification of acid steroid metabolism has been sought in humans and laboratory animals by monitoring levels of bacterial metabolites in faeces and by assaying faecal enzymes involved in steroid metabolism, notably 7α-dehydroxylase which converts CA to DCA and CDCA to LA. As might be expected, an increase in dietary meat protein intake in humans has no effect on faecal bile acid concentration (Cummings *et al.*, 1979). An increase in dietary fat, on the other hand, markedly enhances excretion of faecal bile acids (Cummings *et al.*, 1978). There is no evidence however that dietary fat alters the activity of bile acid metabolizing enzymes (Cummings *et al.*, 1978).

The effects of dietary fibre on faecal bile acid concentration, total excretion and metabolism by bacteria vary markedly with the type of fibre ingested. Fibres such as lignin and pectin, which can adsorb or sequester bile acids, increase total sterol excretion and faecal bile acid concentration in man (Kay and Trusswell, 1980). Oat bran also increases bile acid output in man but, because of its stool bulking properties, the concentration of steroid is not greatly altered (Kay, 1981). Wheat bran also has stool bulking properties which result in a decrease in faecal bile acid concentration in man (Kay, 1981). In some cases, this is accompanied by an increase in total bile acid excretion, but in other cases no significant increase was seen (Kay and Trusswell, 1977a,b; Cummings and Branch, 1982).

The influence of dietary fibre on bile acid metabolism by the rat hindgut flora is similarly variable. Corn bran, which is rich in highly fermentable hemicelluloses, increases both the faecal concentration and excretion of bile acids, whereas lignin, which is resistant to bacterial degradation, has no effect on concentration, although total ouput is increased (Reddy *et al.*, 1983). Presumably, the bulking properties of fibre or physical adsorption of bile acids in the gut lumen may explain these observations. In contrast, 10% alfalfa bran and cellulose increase the proportion of secondary bile acids present in rat faeces, signifying increased bacterial metabolism (Nigro *et al.*, 1979).

(iii) Low pH of lumenal contents and short chain fatty acid production. The lower pH of the intestinal contents in conventional-flora rats in comparison to germ-free animals indicates that bacterial fermentation in the gut reduces the luminal pH (Ward *et al.*, 1986). In man low faecal pH has been associated with high dietary fibre intakes (Walker *et al.*, 1979; van Dokkum *et al.*, 1983) while studies in rats have shown that dietary pectin, cellulose, guar gum and oat bran decreases the pH of the colon and caecal contents in comparison to animals fed a fibre-free diet (Jacobs and Lupton, 1986). It seems likely that the bacterial fermentation of dietary fibre and poorly absorbed carbohydrates such as lactulose to short chain fatty acids (SCFA) is responsible for this change (Cummings,

and Englyst, 1987). As might be expected the degree of reduction in faecal pH in man appears to vary with the type of dietary fibre ingested, since fibre sources differ in their susceptibility to bacterial attack. Van Dokkum *et al.* (1983) reported a significant decrease in faecal pH when volunteers consumed a vegan diet, rich in hemicellulose, in comparison to a mixed Western diet. Wheat bran, in contrast, does not appear to alter faecal pH in man (Stephen and Cummings, 1981) or the SCFA concentration in faeces (Cummings *et al.*, 1979). It is possible, however, that faecal SCFA concentration does not reflect that in the colon, the principal site of bacterial fermentation, from where it is known that these anions can be absorbed.

Some SCFA, notably butyric acid, have been shown to suppress neoplastic characteristics of tumour cells *in vitro* (see the review by Cummings and Branch (1982)), suggesting one possible mechanism for a protective effect against colon cancer. Acidification of the gut contents may also inhibit the formation or activation of carcinogens or cocarcinogens in the gut, thereby reducing the incidence of the tumours (Thornton, 1981), or may selectively influence the growth rates of malignant and normal colonic epithelial cells (see the review by Cummings and Branch (1982)). A decrease in colonic pH may also alter the absorption of tumourigenic bacterial metabolites across gut epithelia. Evidence for an ameliorating effect of low luminal pH on DMH-induced colon cancer in rats is, however, lacking. In fact Jacobs and Lupton (1986) demonstrated that the feeding of various fermentable dietary fibres, including guar gum, oat bran and pectin, increased colon tumour incidence in rats despite significantly lowering colonic pH.

Ammonia. The central position of ammonia in nitrogen metabolism in the large intestine, both as an end-product of the microbial degradation of endogenous or exogenous nitrogen compounds (amino acids, urea) or as a starting point for bacterial synthesis of cell constituents, has been discussed by Wrong (see Chapter 10). High ammonia concentrations have been associated with certain toxic events *in vivo*. For example ammonia-intoxicated mice exhibit inflammatory lesions of the colon and altered DNA synthesis (Gibson *et al.*, 1971; Visek, 1978), implying that ammonia can increase cell proliferation. This has led to theories that ammonia may enhance neoplastic transformation in the gut (Visek, 1978).

In rats the concentration of ammonia in the caecum has been shown to increase as the amount of protein in the diet increased (Wise *et al.*, 1983), although the results were significant only at the highest protein level (400 g/kg diet). Fermentable carbohydrates, including dietary fibre, have marked effects on ammonia production by gut micro-organisms *in vitro* and *in vivo*. The addition of monosaccharides and disaccharides,

Table 15.4 *Effect of dietary fibre on caecal ammonia concentration*

Fibre added	Concentration of caecal ammonia (μmol g^{-1})
None	10.0
Agar	2.9
Carrageenan	1.4
Guar gum	7.0
Gum acacia	7.1
Pectin	5.9

such as glucose, lactose and lactulose, and sugars such as sorbitol and mannitol, to anaerobic incubations of human faecal suspensions inhibits ammonia production (Vince *et al.*, 1978; Vince and Burridge, 1980), because of the low pH produced by sugar fermentation. *In vivo*, similar effects on ammonia concentration have been reported. The addition of various types of dietary fibre to a purified diet resulted in a decrease in ammonia concentration in the caecum in many cases (Table 15.4; Mallett *et al.*, 1984c). The mechanisms involved are probably more complex than for the *in vitro* inhibition of ammonia production by sugars. Vince (1986) has discussed various possible mechanisms by which fermentable fibres might influence ammonia production, such as stimulation of ammonia assimilation into bacterial protoplasm with a corresponding increase in faecal nitrogen. It should be noted however that Mallett *et al.* (1984c) reported that non-fermentable carbohydrates, e.g. agar and carrageenan, were more effective than the fermentable fibres in decreasing ammonia levels in the caecum (Table 15.4).

Faecal ammonia concentrations in man have also been shown to decrease when fibre, in the form of wheat bran, is added to the diet with a concomitant increase in faecal nitrogen concentration (Cummings and Branch, 1982). The toxicological significance of the diet-induced changes in intestinal ammonia concentrations have not been assessed. The influence of dietary fibre and protein on ammonia concentration in the gut appears to fit in with the epidemiological studies of diet and colon cancer risk. However to suggest a causal relationship between diet, ammonia levels and colon cancer would be highly speculative.

References

Adrian, J. (1976). Gums & hydrocolloids in nutrition. *World Rev. Nutr. Diet.* **25**, 189–216.

Arnold, D. L., Krewski, D. and Munro, I. C. (1983). Saccharin: a toxicological and historical perspective. *Toxicol.* **27**, 179–256.

Baba, S., Furuta, T., Fujioka, M. and Goromaru, T. (1983). Studies on drug metabolism by use of isotopes XXVII: Urinary metabolites of rutin in rats and the use of intestinal microflora in the metabolism of rutin. *J. Pharm. Sci.* **72**, 1155–1157.

Bauer, H. G., Asp, N. G., Dahlquvist, A., Fredlund, P. E., Nyman, M. and Oste, R. (1981). Effect of two kinds of pectin and guar gum on 1,2-dimethylhydrazine initiation of colon tumours and on fecal β-glucuronidase activity in the rat. *Cancer Res.* **41**, 2518–2523.

Bauer, H. G., Asp, N. G., Oste, R., Dahlquvist., A. and Fredland, P. E. (1979). Effect of dietary fibre on the induction of colorectal tumors and fecal β-glucuronidase activity in the rat. *Cancer Res.* **39**, 3752–3756.

Broitman, S. A., Vitale, J. J., Jakuba, E. V. and Gottlieb, L. S. (1977). Polyunsaturated fat, cholesterol and large bowel tumorigenesis. *Cancer* **40**, 2455–2463.

Chadwick, R. W., Copeland, M. F. and Chadwick, C. J. (1978). Enhanced pesticide metabolism, a previously unreported effect of dietary fibre in mammals. *Fd Cosmet. Toxicol.* **16**, 217–225.

Coates, M. E. and Fuller, R. (1978). The gnotobiotic animal in the study of gut microbiology. *In*: "Microbial Ecology of the Gut" (eds R. T. J. Clarke and T. Bauchop), pp. 311–346. Academic Press, London, New York.

Correa, P., Haenszel, W., Cuello, C., Tannenbaum, S. and Archer, M. (1975). A model for gastric cancer epidemiology. *Lancet* **ii**, 58–60.

Cruse, J. P., Lewin, M. R., Ferulano, G. P. and Clark, C. G. (1978). Cocarcinogenic effects of dietary cholesterol in experimental colon cancer. *Nature* **278**, 822–825.

Cummings, J. H. and Branch, W. J. (1982). Postulated mechanisms whereby fiber may protect against large bowel cancer. *In*: "Dietary Fiber in Health and Disease" (eds G. V. Vahouney and D. Kritchevsky), pp. 313–325. Plenum Press, New York, London.

Cummings, J. H. and Englyst, H. N. (1987). Fermentation in the human large intestine and the available substrates. *Am. J. Clin. Nutr.* **34**, 1243–1255.

Cummings, J. H., Hill, M. J., Jivrag, T., Houston, H., Branch, W. J. and Jenkins, D. J. A. (1979). The effect of meat protein and dietary fiber on colonic function and metabolism. *Am. J. Clin. Nutr.* **32**, 2086–2093.

Cummings, J. H., Wiggins, H. S., Jenkins, D. J. A., Houston, H., Jivraj, T., Drasar, B. S. and Hill, M. J. (1978). Influence of diets high and low in animal fat on bowel habit, gastrointestinal transit time, fecal microflora, bile acid and fat excretion. *J. Clin. Invest.* **61**, 953–963.

DeBethizy, J. D. and Goldstein, R. S. (1985). The influence of fermentable dietary fibre on the disposition and toxicity of xenobiotics. *In*: "Xenobiotic Metabolism – Nutritional Effects", pp. 37–50. American Chemical Society Symposium Series, ACS, Washington.

DeBethizy, J. D., Sherril, J. M., Rickett, D. E. and Hamm, T. E. (1983). Effects of pectin-containing diets on hepatic macromolecular covalent binding of 2,6-dinitro-[H^3]toluene in Fischer 344 rats. *Toxicol. Appl. Pharmacol.* **69**, 369.

De Wilde, R. (1980). Influence of supplementing citrus pectin to a diet with and without antibiotics on the digestibility of pectins and other nutrients. *Z. Tierphysiol.* **43**, 109–116.

Doherty, R. A. and Gates, A. H. (1973). Epidemic methylmercury poisoning: application of a mouse model. *Pediat. Res.* **7**, 319–322.

Dolby, J. M., Webster, A. D. B., Borriello, S. P., Barclay, F. E., Bartholomew, B. A. and Hill, M. J. (1984). Bacterial colonization and nitrite concentration in the achlorhydric stomachs of patients with primary hypogammaglobulinaemia or classical pernicious anaemia. *Scand. J. Gastroenterol.* **19**, 105–110.

Donaldson, R. M. (1962). Malabsorption of ^{60}Co labelled cyanocobalamin in rats with intestinal diverticula. I. Evolution of possible mechanisms. *Gastroenterol.* **43**, 271–281.

Donaldson, R. M. (1970). Small bowel bacterial overgrowth. *Adv. Intern. Med.* **16**, 191–212.

Drasar, B. S. and Barrow, P. (1985). Intestinal microbiology. "Aspects of Microbiology Vol. 10." American Society for Microbiology.

Ershoff, B. H. (1974). Antitoxic effects of plant fiber. *Am. J. Clin. Nutr.* **27**, 1395–1398.

Freeman, H. J., Spiller, G. A. and Kim, Y. S. (1984). Effect of high hemicellulose corn bran in 1,2-dimethyl hydrazine-induced rat intestinal neoplasia. *Carcinogenesis* **5**, 261–264.

Freeman, H. J. (1986). Effects of differing purified cellulose, pectin, and hemicellulose fiber diets on fecal enzymes in 1,2-dimethylhydrazine-induced rat colon carcinogenesis. *Cancer Res.* **46**, 5529–5532.

Gibson, G. E., Zimber, A., Krook, L. and Visek, W. J. (1971). Nucleic acids and brain and intestinal lesions in ammonia intoxicated mice. *Fed. Proc.* **30**, 578.

Goldin, B. R. and Gorbach, S. L. (1976). The relationship between diet and rat fecal bacterial enzymes implicated in colon cancer. *J. Natl Cancer Inst.* **57**, 371–375.

Goldin, B. R., Swenson, L., Dwyer, J., Sexton, M. and Gorbach, S. L. (1980). Effect of diet and Lactobacillus supplements on human fecal bacterial enzymes. *J. Natl Cancer Inst.* **64**, 255–262.

Goldstein, R. S., Chism, J. P., Sherrill, J. M. and Hamm, T. E. (1984). Influence of dietary pectin on intestinal microfloral metabolism and toxicity of nitrobenzene. *Toxicol. Appl. Pharmacol.* **75**, 547–553.

Griffiths, L. A. (1975). The role of the intestinal microflora in flavonoid metabolism. *In*: "Topics in Flavonoid Chemistry and Biochemistry" (eds L. Farkas, M. Gabor and F. Kallay), pp. 201–213, Akademai Kiado, Budapest.

Hawksworth, G., Drasar, B. S. and Hill, M. J. (1971). Intestinal bacteria and hydrolysis of glycosidic bonds. *J. Med. Microbiol.* **4**, 451–458.

Hermans, P. E., Diax-Buxo, J. A. and Stobo, J. D. (1976). Idiopathic late-onset immunoglobin deficiency. Clinical observations in 50 patients. *Am. J. Med.* **61**, 221–237.

Hill, M. J. (1986). "Microbes and Human Carcinogenesis". Edward Arnold, London.

Hill, M. J. and Hawksworth, G. (1971). Bacterial production of nitrosamines *in vitro* and *in vivo*. *In*: "N-Nitroso Compounds — Analysis and Formation" (eds P. Bogovski, R. Preussman, E. A. Walker and W. Davis), pp. 116–121. IARC Scientific Publication No. 3. International Agency for Research on Cancer, Lyon.

Holloway, W. D., Tasman-Jones, C. and Maher, K. (1983). Pectin digestion in humans. *Am. J. Clin. Nutr.* **37**, 253–255.

Howarth, A. E. and Pihl, E. (1985). High-fat diet promotes and causes distal shift of experimental rat colonic cancer — beer and alcohol do not. *Nutr. Cancer* **6**, 229–235.

Jacobs, L. R. and Lupton, J. R. (1986). Relationship between colonic luminal pH, cell proliferation, and colon carcinogenesis in 1,2-dimethylhydrazine treated rats fed high fiber diets. *Cancer Res.* **46**, 1727–1734.

Jones, S. M., Davies, P. W. and Savage, A. (1978). Gastric juice nitrite and gastric cancer. *Lancet* **i**, 1355.

Kay, R. M. (1981). Dietary fiber. *J. Lipid Res.* **23**, 221–242.

Kay, R. M. and Trusswell, A. S. (1977a). Effect of wheat fibre on gastrointestinal function, plasma lipids and steroid excretion in man. *Br. J. Nutr.* **37**, 227–234.

Kay, R. M. and Trusswell, A. S. (1977b). Effect of citrus pectin on blood lipids and fecal steroid excretion in man. *Am. J. Clin. Nutr.* **30**, 171–175.

Kay, R. M. and Trusswell, A. S. (1980). Dietary fibre: effects on plasma and biliary lipids in man. *In:* "Medical Aspects of Dietary Fibre", (eds G. A. Spiller and R. M. Kay), pp 153–173, Plenum Press, New York, London.

Kinoshita, N. and Gelboin, H. V. (1978). β-glucuronidase catalysed hydrolysis of benzo(a)pyrene-3-glucuronide and binding to DNA. *Science* **199**, 307–309.

Kritchevsky, D. (1983). Fiber, steroids and cancer. *Cancer Res. Suppl.* **43**, 24915–24955.

Kühnau, J. (1976). The flavonoids, a class of semi-essential food components: their role in human nutrition. *Wld Rev. Nutr. Diet* **24**, 117–191.

Landry, T. D., Doherty, R. A. and Gates, A. H. (1979). Effects of three diets on mercury excretion after methylmercury administration. *Bull. Environ. Contam. Toxicol.* **22**, 151–158.

Likhachev, A., Anisimov, V., Parvanova, L. and Pozharisski, K. (1985). Effect of exogenous β-glucuronidase on the carcinogenicity of 1,2-dimethylhydrazine in rats: evidence that carcinogenic intermediates from conjugates act through their subsequent enzymatic release. *Carcinogenesis* **6**, 679–681.

Locniskar, M., Nauss, K. M., Kaufmann, P. and Newberne, P. M. (1985). Interaction of dietary fat and route of carcinogen administration on 1,2-dimethylhydrazine-induced colon tumorigenesis in rats. *Carcinogenesis* **6**, 349–354.

London, J. F., Clapp, N. K. and Henke, M. A. (1981). Effects of dietary bran and the colon carcinogen 1,2-dimethylhydrazine on faecal β-glucuronidase activity in mice. *Fd Cosmet. Toxicol.* **19**. 707–711.

Long, R. M. and Rickert, D. E. (1982). Metabolism and excretion of 2,6-dinitro-[^{14}C] toluene *in vivo* and in isolated perfused rat livers. *Drug. Metab. Dispos.* **10**, 455–458.

MacDonald, I. A., Mader, J. A. and Bussard, R. G. (1983). The role of rutin and quercetin in stimulating flavonol glycosidase activity by cultured cell-free microbial preparations of human feces and saliva. *Mutation Res.* **122**, 95–102.

MacDonald, I. A., Bussard, R. G., Hutchison, D. M. and Holdeman, H. V. (1984). Rutin-induced-β-glucosidase activity in *Streptococcus faecium* VGH-1 and *Streptococcus sp.* strain FRP-17 isolated from human feces; formation of the mutagen quercetin from rutin. *Appl. Environ. Microbiol.* **47**, 350–355.

MacGregor, J. T. (1986). Genetic toxicology of dietary flavonoids. *In*: "Genetic Toxicology of the Diet" (ed. I. Knudsen), pp. 33–43. Alan R. Liss Inc., NY.

Mallett, A. K., Bearne, C. A., Rowland, I. R., Farthing, M. J. G., Cole, C. B.

and Fuller, R. (1987). The use of rats associated with a human faecal flora as a model for studying the effects of diet on the human gut microflora. *J. Appl. Bacteriol.* **62**, 39–46.

Mallett, A. K., Rowland, I. R. and Bearne, C. A. (1986). Influence of wheat bran on some reductive and hydrolytic activities of the rat cecal flora. *Nutr. Cancer* **8**, 125–131.

Mallett, A. K., Rowland, I. R., Bearne, C. A., Flynn, J. C., Fehilly, B. J., Udeen, S. and Farthing, M. J. G. (1988). Effect of dietary supplements of apple pectin, wheat bran or fat on the enzyme activity of the human faecal flora. *Microbial Ecol. Hlth Dis.* **1** (in the press).

Mallett, A. K., Rowland, I. R., Bearne, C. A. and Nicklin, S. (1985). Influence of dietary carrageenan on microbial biotransformation activities on the cecum of rodents and on gastrointestinal immune status in the rat. *Toxicol. Appl. Pharmacol.* **78**, 377–385.

Mallett, A. K., Rowland, I. R. and Wise, A. (1983). Interaction between pectin and rat hindgut microflora. *Appl. Environ. Microbiol.* **45**, 116–121.

Mallett, A. K., Rowland, I. R. and Wise, A. (1984a). Influence of dietary fats on the rat caecal microflora. *Proc. Nutr. Soc.* **43**, 7.

Mallett, A. K., Rowland, I. R. and Wise, A. (1984b). Dietary fat and cecal microbial activity in the rat. *Nutr. Cancer* **6**, 86–91.

Mallett, A. K., Wise, A. and Rowland, I. R. (1983). Effect of dietary cellulose on the metabolic activity of the rat caecal microflora. *Arch. Toxicol.* **52**, 311–317.

Mallett, A. K., Wise, A. and Rowland, I. R. (1984c). Hydrocolloid food additives and rat caecal microbial enzyme activities. *Fd Chem. Toxicol.* **22**, 415–418.

Miller, C. P. and Bohnhoff, M. (1962). A study of experimental *Salmonella* infection in the mouse. *J. Infect. Dis.* **111**, 107–116.

Milton-Thompson, G. J., Lightfoot, N. F., Ahmet, Z., Hunt, R. H., Barnard, J., Bavin, P. M., Brimblecombe, R. W., Darkin, D. W., Moore, P. J. and Viney, N. (1982). Intragastric acidity, bacteria, nitrite and N-nitroso compounds before, during and after cimetidine treatment. *Lancet* i, 1091–1095.

Mirsalis, J. C., Hamm, T. E., Sherrill, J. M. and Butterworth, B. E. (1982). The role of gut flora in the genotoxicity of dinitrotoluenes in rats. *Nature* **295**, 322–323.

Mizutani, T. and Mitsuoka, T. (1980). Inhibitory effect of some intestinal bacteria on liver tumorigenesis in gnotobiotic C3H/He male mice. *Cancer Lett.* **11**, 89–95.

Mizutani, T., Benno, Y. and Mitsuoka, T. (1982). Effect of dietary fiber on tumorigenesis and longevity: with special reference to the faecal microflora. *Nutr. Rep. Int.* **26**, 289–296.

Mosbech, J. and Videbaek, A. (1950). Mortality from and risk of gastric carcinoma among patients with pernicious anaemia. *Br. Med. J.* **II**, 390–394.

Mueller, R. C., Hagel, H. -J., Wild, H., Ruppin, H. and Domschke, W. (1986). Nitrate and nitrite in normal gastric juice. *Oncology* **43**, 50–53.

Nanno, M., Morotomi, M., Takayama, H., Kuroshima, T., Tanaka, R. and Mutai, M. (1986). Mutagenic activation of biliary metabolites of benzo(*a*)pyrene by β-glucuronidase-postive bacteria in human faeces. *J. Med. Microbiol.* **22**, 351–355.

Nigro, N. D., Bull, A. W., Klopfer, B. A., Dak, M. S. and Campbell, R.

L. (1979). Effects of dietary fiber on azoxymethane-induced intestinal carcinogenesis in rats. *J. Natl Cancer Inst.* **62**, 1097–1102.

Norseth, T. and Clarkson, T. W. (1971). Intestinal transport of ^{203}Hg-labelled methylmercury chloride. *Arch. Environ. Health*, **22**, 568–577.

Omaye, S. T. (1986). Effect of diet on toxicity testing. *Fed. Proc.* **45**, 133–135.

Prizont, R. (1984). Influence of high dietary cellulose on fecal glycosidases in experimental rat colon carcinogenesis. *Cancer Res.* **44**, 557–561.

Prizont, R. and Konigsberg, N. (1981). Identification of bacterial glycosidases in rat cecal contents. *Dig. Dis. Sci.* **26**, 773–777.

Reddy, B.S., Weisburger, J.H. and Wynder, E.L. (1974). Fecal bacterial β-glucuronidase: Control by diet. *Science* **183**, 416–417.

Reddy, B. S., Pohl, L. R. and Krishna, G. (1976). The requirement of the gut flora in nitrobenzene-induced methaemoglobinaemia in rats. *Biochem. Pharmacol.* **25**, 1119–1122.

Reddy, B. S., Mangat, S., Sheinfil, A., Weisburger, J. H. and Wyndon, E. L. (1977). Effect of type and amount of dietary fat and 1,2-dimethyl hydrazine on biliary bile acids, fecal bile acids and neutral sterols in rats. *Cancer Res.* **37**, 2132–2137.

Reddy, B. S., Hanson, D., Mangat, S., Mathews, L., Sbaschnig, M., Sharma, C. and Simi, B. (1980). Effect of high-fat, high-beef diet and of mode of cooking of beef in the diet on fecal bacterial enzymes and fecal bile acids and neutral sterols. *J. Nutr.* **110**, 1880–1887.

Reddy, B. S. and Mori, H. (1981). Effect of dietary wheat bran and dehydrated citrus fibre on 3,2'-dimethyl-4-aminobiphenyl-induced intestinal carcinogenesis in F344 rats. *Carcinogenesis* **2**, 21–25.

Reddy, B. S. (1983). Effect of diet on intestinal tumor production. *Environ. Sci. Res.* **29**, 91–107.

Reddy, B. S., Maeura, Y. and Wayman, M. (1983). Effect of dietary corn bran and autohydrolyzed lignin on 3,2'-dimethyl-4-aminobiphenyl-induced intestinal carcinogenesis in male F344 rats. *J. Natl Cancer Inst.* **71**, 419–423.

Reed, P. I., Haines, K., Smith, P. L. R., Walters, C. L. and House, F. R. (1982). Intragastric acidity, bacteria, nitrite and nitrosocompounds before during and after cimetidine treatment. *Lancet* **ii**, p. 39.

Reed, P. I., Smith, P. L. R., Haines, K., House, F. R., Walters, C. L. (1981). Effect of cimetidine on gastric juice N-nitrosamine concentration. *Lancet* **i**, 553–555.

Renwick, A. G. and Drasar, B. S. (1976). Environmental carcinogens and large bowel cancer. *Nature* **263**, 234–235.

Rickert, D. E., Butterworth, B. E. and Popp, J. E. (1984). Dinitrotoluene: acute toxicity, oncogenicity, genotoxicity and metabolism. *CRC Crit. Rev. Toxicol.* **13**, 217–234.

Rickert, D. E., Bond, J. A., Long, R. M. and Chism, J. P. (1983). Metabolism and excretion of nitrobenzene by rats and mice. *Toxicol. Appl. Pharmacol.* **67**, 206–214.

Ross, J. K. and Leklem, J. E. (1981). The effect of dietary citrus pectin on the excretion of human fecal neutral and acid sterols and the activity of 7a-dehydroxylase and β-glucuronidase. *Am. J. Clin. Nutr.* **34**, 2068–2077.

Rowland, R., Mallett, A. K. and Wise, A. (1983a). A comparison of the activity of five microbial enzymes in cecal content from rats, mice and hamsters and response to dietary pectin. *Toxicol. Appl. Pharmacol.* **69**, 143–148.

Rowland, I. R., Mallett, A. K., Wise, A. and Bailey, E. (1983b). Effect of dietary carrageenan and pectin on the reduction of nitro-compounds by rat caecal microflora. *Xenobiotica* **13**, 251–256.

Rowland, I. R., Mallett, A. K. and Wise, A. (1985). The effect of diet on the mammalian gut flora and its metabolic activities. *CRC Crit. Rev. Toxicol.* **16**, 31–103.

Rowland, I. R., Mallett, A. K., Flynn, J. and Hargreaves, R. J. (1986). The effect of various dietary fibres on tissue concentration and chemical form of mercury after methylmercury exposure in mice. *Arch. Toxicol.* **59**, 94–98.

Rowland, I. R., Robinson, R. D., Doherty, R. A. and Landry, R. D. (1983c). Are developmental changes in methylmercury metabolism and excretion mediated by the intestinal microflora? *In*: "Developmental and Reproductive Toxicity of Heavy Metals" (eds T. W. Clarkson, G. F. Nordberg and P. R. Sager), pp. 745–758. Plenum Press, New York.

Rowland, I. R., Robinson, R. D. and Doherty, R. A. (1984). Effects of diet on mercury metabolism and excretion in mice given methylmercury: role of the gut flora. *Arch. Environ. Hlth* **39**, 401–408.

Rowland, I. R. and Walker, R. (1983). The gastro-intestinal tract in food toxicology. *In*: "Toxic Hazards in Food" (eds D.M. Conning and A. Lansdown), pp. 183–274. Croom-Helm, London.

Rowland, I. R., Wise, A. and Mallett, A. K. (1983d). Metabolic profile of caecal microorganisms from rats fed indigestible plant cell-wall components. 2Fd Chem. Toxicol. **21**, 25–29.

Ruddell, W. S. J., Bone, E. S., Hill, M. J., Blendis, L. M. and Walters, C. L. (1976). Gastric juice nitrite. A risk factor for cancer in the hypochlorhydric stomach? *Lancet* **ii**, 1037–1039.

Savage, D. C. (1977). Microbial ecology of the gastrointestinal tract. *Ann. Rev. Microbiol.* **31**, 107–133.

Savage, D. C. (1980). Impact of antimicrobials on the microbial ecology of the gut. *In*: "Effects on Human Health of Subtherapeutic Use of Antimicrobials in Animal Feeds", Appendix D, National Academy of Sciences, Washington, DC.

Savage, D. C. (1984). Present view of the normal flora. *In*: "The Germ-Free Animal in Biomedical Research" (eds M.E. Coates and B.E. Gustafsson), pp. 119–140. Laboratory Animals Ltd, London.

Schlag, P., Böckler, R. and Peter, M. (1982). Nitrite and nitrosamines in gastric juices: risk factors for gastric cancer? *Scand J. Gastroenterol.* **17**, 145–150.

Shiau, S. -Y. and Chang, G. W. (1983). Effects of dietary fiber on fecal mucinase and β-glucuronidase in rats. *J. Nutr.* **113**, 138–144.

Simon, G. L. and Gorbach, S. L. (1981). Intestinal flora in health and disease. *In*: "Physiology of the Gastrointestinal Tract", Vol. 2 (ed. L.J. Johnson), pp. 1361–1380. Raven Press, NY.

Siurala, M., Eramaa, E. and Tapiovaara, J. (1959). Pernicious anaemia and gastric carcinoma. *Acta Med. Scand.* **164**, 431–436.

Sousa, R. L. and Marletta, M. A. (1985). Inhibition of cytochrome P-450 activity in rat liver microsomes by the naturally occurring flavonoid quercetin. *Arch. Biochem. Biophys.* **240**, 345–357.

Spiller, G. A. and Freeman, H. J. (1982). Recent advances in dietary fiber and colorectal diseases. *Am. J. Clin. Nutr.* **34**, 1145–1152.

Stephen, A. M. and Cummings, J. H. (1981). The effect of wheat fibre on fecal pH in man. *Gastroenterol.* **80**, 1294–1298.

Stockbruegger, R. W., Cotton, P. B., Eugenides, N., Bartholomew, B. A., Hill, M. J. and Walters, C. L. (1982). Intragastric nitrites, nitrosamines and bacterial overgrowth during cimetidine treatment. *Gut* **23**, 1048–1054.

Stockbruegger, R. W., Cotton, P. B., Menon, G. G., Beiby, J. O., Bartholomew, B. A., Hill, M. J. and Walters, C. L. (1984). Pernicious anaemia, intragastric bacterial overgrowth and possible consequences. *Scand. J. Gastroenterol.* **19**, 355–364.

Suzuki, K. and Mitsuoka, T. (1984). N-Nitrosamine formation by intestinal bacteria. *In*: "N-Nitrosocompounds: Occurrence, Biological Effects and Relevance to Human Cancer" (eds I. K. O'Neill, R. C. von Borstel, C. T. Miller, J. Long and H. Bartsch), pp. 275–281. IARC Scientific Publications No. 57. International Agency for Research on Cancer, Lyon.

Takada, H., Hirooka, T., Hiramatsu, Y. and Yamamoto, M. (1982). Effect of β-glucuronidase inhibitor on azoxymethane-induced colonic carcinogenesis in rats. *Cancer Res.* **39**, 3752–3756.

Tamura, G., Gold, C., Ferro-Luzzi, A. and Ames, B. N. (1980). Fecalase: A model for activation of dietary glycosides to mutagens by intestinal flora. *Proc. Natl Acad. Sci. USA* **77**, 4961–4965.

Thornton, J. R. (1981). High colonic pH promotes colorectal cancer. *Lancet* **1**, 1081–1083.

van der Waaij, D. (1979). Colonisation resistance of the digestive tract as a major lead in the selection of antibiotics for therapy. In: "New Criteria for Antimicrobial Therapy — Maintenance of Digestive Tract Colonisation Resistance" (eds D. van der Waaij and J. Verhoef), pp 271–280. Excerpta Medica, Amsterdam.

van der Waaij, D. and Berguis-de Vries, J. M. (1974). Selective elimination of Enterobacteriaceae species from the digestive tract in mice and monkeys. *J. Hyg. Camb.* **72**, 205–211.

van Dokkum, W., de Boer, B. C. J., van Fassen, A., Pikaar, N. A. and Hermus, R. J. J. (1983). Diet, faecal pH and colorectal cancer. *Br. J. Cancer* **48**, 109–110.

Vince, A. (1986). Metabolism of ammonia, urea and amino acids and their significance in liver disease. *In*: "Microbial Metabolism in the Digestive Tract" (ed. M. J. Hill), pp. 83–105. CRC Press, Boca Raton, FL.

Vince, A. and Burridge, S. M. (1980). Ammonia production by intestinal bacteria: the effects of lactose and glucose. *J. Med. Microbiol.* **13**, 177–191.

Vince, A., Killingley, M. and Wrong, O. M. (1978). Effect of lactulose on ammonia production in a fecal incubation system. *Gastroenterol.* **74**, 544–549.

Visek, W. J. (1978). Diet and cell growth modulation by ammonia. *Am. J. Clin. Nutr.* **31**, S216–220.

Walker, A. R. P., Walker, B. F. and Segel, I. (1979). Faecal pH value and its modification by dietary means in South African black and white school children. *S. Afr. Med. J.* **55**, 495–498.

Ward, F. W., Coates, M. E. and Walker, R. (1986). Nitrate reduction, gastrointestinal pH and N-nitrosation in gnotobiotic and conventional rats. *Fd Chem. Toxicol.* **24**, 17–22.

Wattenberg, L. W. and Leong, J. L. (1970). Inhibition of the carcinogenic action of benzo[a]pyrene by flavones. *Cancer Res.* **30**, 1922–1925.

Weisburger, J. H. (1971). Colon carcinogenesis, their metabolism and mode of action. *Cancer* **28**, 60–70.

Wise, A., Mallett, A. K. and Rowland, I. R. (1982). Dietary fibre, bacterial metabolism and toxicity of nitrate in the rat. *Xenobiotica* **12**, 111–118.

Wise, A., Mallett, A. K. and Rowland, I. R. (1983). Dietary protein and cecal microbial metabolism in the rat. *Nutr. Cancer* **4**, 267–272.

Wise, A., Rowland, I. R. and Mallett, A. K. (1984). Dietary lactose and the metabone activity of the caecal microfloras of weanling and adult rats. *Fd Chem. Toxicol.* **22**, 113–117.

16

Caecal Enlargement

R. WALKER

A. Introduction

Caecal enlargement in its broadest sense may be taken to mean any increase in the size of the filled caecum, whether or not accompanied by an increase in tissue mass or histological changes. In this sense, caecal enlargement is one of the most commonly reported effects in oral toxicity studies in rodents but, as has been pointed out previously (Walker, 1978), the definition is unhelpful in that it begs the question as to what yardstick should be used to measure the effect. Different, totally nutritionally adequate, laboratory rodent diets may result in different caecal sizes and there is no unique norm, so it is not surprising that statistically significant differences may be observed when a diet is varied by incorporation of a test substance; significant differences have been reported between animals receiving diets containing maize and gelatinized potato starch, both of which are well utilized (Walker, 1978). Nor is it surprising that caecal enlargement has been variously interpreted as an adaptive and as a toxic response, since it has been reported in many studies in which there have been no adverse consequences for survival or well-being, whereas in others there have been obvious pathological sequelae.

B. The Nature of the Effect

In its mildest manifestation, caecal enlargement may take the form of a modest increase in the weight of the contents of the caecum with little or no change in the weight of the tissue of the caecal wall relative to animals on a control diet and no histological abnormality. At the other extreme, the organ may be grossly enlarged with marked increases in caecal tissue mass and histological changes such as loss of muscle tone, oedematous changes in mucosa and submucosa and prominent lymphatics

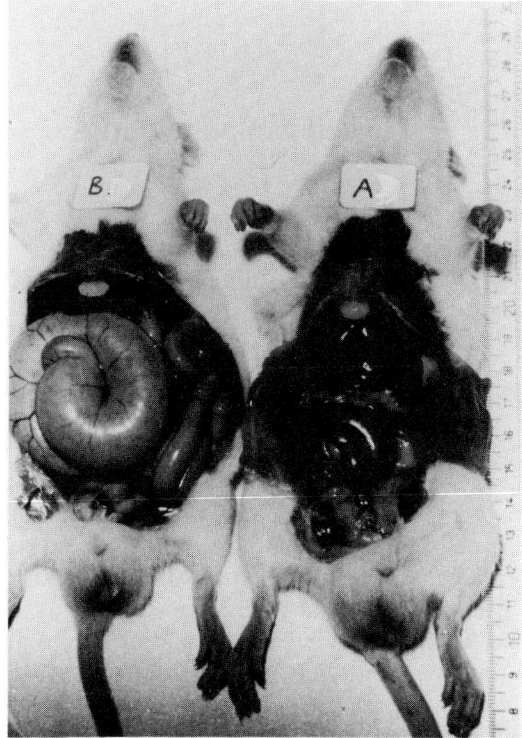

Fig 16.1. Gross caecal enlargement and abdominal distension induced by raw potato starch.
A. Control rat fed diet containing 71% maize starch
B. Rat fed diet containing 71% raw potato starch for 21 days.

(Figs 16.1 and 16.2) (Walker, 1978); in some cases changes in goblet cell counts and activity have been reported (O'Brien, 1987, personal communication). With most substances which cause caecal enlargement, there is a dose related progression in the magnitude and severity of the effect, but not all compounds cause the most severe changes, even at high dietary levels. Even when caecal enlargement is of considerable magnitude and sustained over substantial periods of time in chronic toxicity studies, there is no evidence of any increase in neoplastic lesions of the gastro-intestinal tract and it is noteworthy that it is reversible within a relatively short period after withdrawal of the causal agent. The caecal enlargement associated with the germ-free status in rodents is similarly reversible when the gut is colonized.

Where there is an increase in tissue mass of the caecal wall, this could be a result of hyperplasia, of cell hypertrophy, of increased cell life and

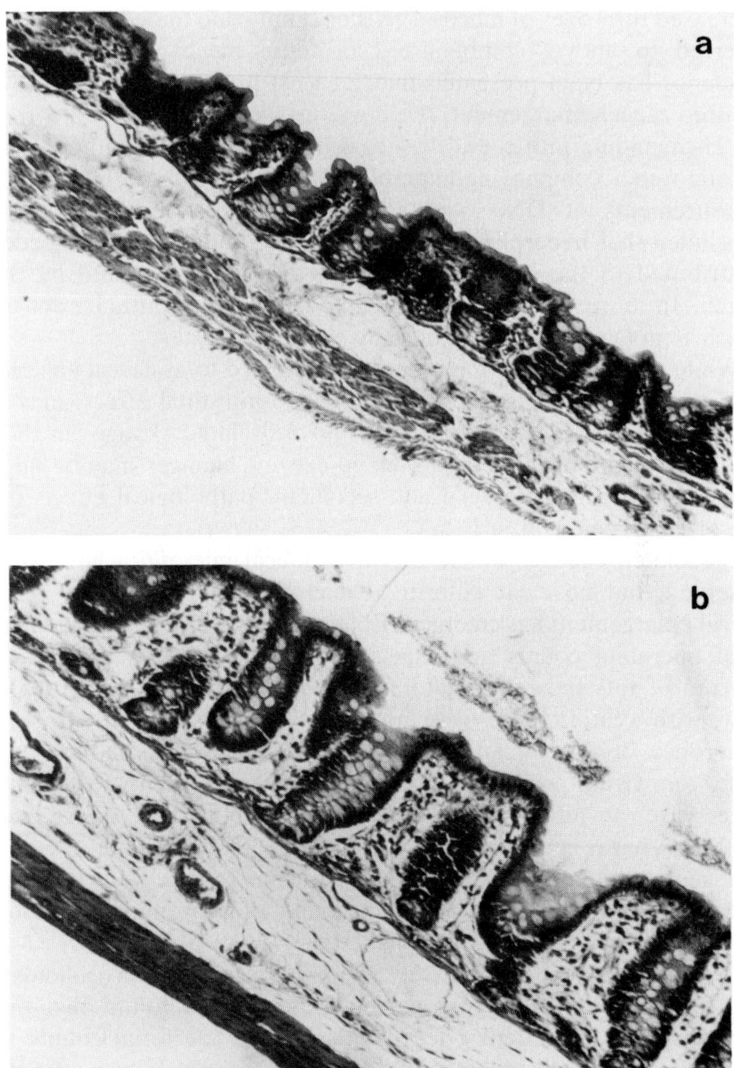

Fig 16.2 Histological sections of caecal wall (Haematoxylin and Eosin stain) of (a) normal and (b) grossly enlarged caecum.

Note loss of muscle tone, oedematous changes and prominent lymphatics associated with the grossly enlarged caecum.

decreased turn-over of mucosal cells or simply due to oedematous changes referred to above; combinations of these mechanisms may co-exist. Evidence has been presented that, at least in the case of potato starch-induced caecal enlargement, there was an increased rate of incorporation of ^{3}H-thymidine into caecal tissue, which is consistent with an increased mitotic rate accompanying hyperplasia (Walker, 1978). On this basis and measurements of DNA and water content of caecal tissues, it was concluded that hyperplasia, cell hypertrophy and a degree of oedema all contributed to the fourfold increase in tissue mass caused by this raw starch. In more mild cases, there may be no contribution from oedema which is not observed histologically.

While the phenomenon is commonly referred to as caecal enlargement, it should perhaps be noted that the gastro-intestinal effects may not be confined to this organ. There may also be related changes in the colon and even in the distal ileum. Such co-existing changes may be important in relation to the functional and secondary pathological effects of gross caecal enlargement (see below).

Associated changes in the caecal or faecal microflora have also been observed, but no clear pattern of microflora which may be related to caecal enlargement has emerged. El Harith *et al.* (1977) reported increased total microbial counts and especially lactic anaerobes in the enlarged caecum of rats fed raw potato starch, but Salminen *et al.* (1985) found that, with xylitol, there were no major changes in total aerobes, total anaerobes, aerobic or anaerobic streptococci or yeasts, although a clear shift from Gram-positive to Gram-negative populations was seen; in the latter case, an adaptation to increased metabolism of xylose occurred. With saccharin as the agent causing caecal enlargement, only slight changes in the composition of the caecal microflora were detected, but there were significant changes in metabolic profile (Anderson and Kirkland, 1980; Sims and Renwick, 1983).

In a systematic study of the effects of several hydrocolloids which caused caecal enlargement, Mallett *et al.* (1984) found that different substances had different effects both on total bacterial counts and on microbial metabolic profiles. It appears, therefore, that there is no consistent type of microbial population established which can be associated with caecal enlargement, nor does the effect depend on an ablation or eradication of the gut microflora as occurs with antibiotics or in the germ-free state. Such changes in the gut microflora as do occur appear to be dictated by the substance in question rather than the condition of an enlarged caecum. Conversely, it is not obvious that quantitative or qualitative changes in the microflora are causally related to caecal enlargement.

C. Mechanisms of Causation

The phenomenon of caecal enlargement has often been encountered in toxicological studies on food ingredients and food additives in rodents (Table 16.1), i.e. substances of low oral toxicity and which may be tolerated in the diet of experimental animals in substantial quantities. It is a common feature of the high-dose effects on the gastro-intestinal tract of poorly absorbed sugars and sugar alcohols, and of higher molecular weight polysaccharides and related polyols which are resistant to hydrolysis by endogenous carbohydrases. It is, therefore, tempting to speculate that a common mechanism may be involved in the aetiology of caecal enlargement. However, the effect is not confined to polyhydric compounds of this type; it is also caused by high dietary concentrations of structurally unrelated compounds such as azo and other food colours, saccharin and even inorganic compounds such as magnesium sulphate. Furthermore, caecal enlargement is a common effect of oral antibiotics and an unusually large caecum is a feature of germ-free rodents. Any proposed common mechanism must take account of all these observations.

A common feature of the substances which have been observed to cause caecal enlargement is that they are poorly or incompletely absorbed from the small intestine and that they are osmotically active molecules, or may be degraded by the microflora of the lower gut to yield such molecules. It may therefore be postulated that caecal enlargement is an adaptive, homeostatic response to the presence of osmotically active moieties in the hind gut; such a mechanism was proposed by Leegwater et al. (1974) to explain the aetiology of the condition. This model would also accommodate the caecal enlargement which occurs in germ-free animals since, in such animals, there is an increase in the luminal concentration of colloidal glycoproteins which are broken down by the microflora of conventional animals. It is also consistent with the fact that, frequently, large dietary concentrations of a substance (which overload the absorptive and metabolic capacity of the small intestine) are required to produce the effect, and with the reversibility of the condition on removal of the causal agent.

Where measurements have been made of the osmotic activity of caecal contents, these have usually resulted in values similar to controls without enlarged caeca, which is what might be expected if homeostasis is maintained, but does not provide evidence for osmotic effects being causally involved in effecting caecal enlargement. In one study in which osmotic activity was measured at various intervals of time after introduction of raw potato starch into the diet of rats, a transient increase was seen at three days (Walker, 1978). Raw potato starch is refractory to pancreatic

Table 16.1 *Some food ingredients, additives and other substances which cause caecal enlargement*

Substance	Reference
Carbohydrates	
Raw starches	El Harith *et al.* (1976) Walker and El Harith (1978)
Chemically modified starches	De Groot *et al.* (1974)
Lactose	Reussner *et al* (1963) Leegwater *et al.* (1974) Feron *et al* (1978)
Glucose syrup, high molecular weight fraction	Birch and Etheridge (1973) Birch *et al.* (1973)
Dextrins	Dupuis and Fournier (1963)
Sugar alcohols and other polyols	
Hydrogenated glucose syrup	Dupas *et al.* (1984)
Isomalt	Musch *et al.* (1973)
Maltitol	Hosoya (1972)
Mannitol	Salminen (1982)
Sorbitol	Morgan and Yudkin (1957) MacKenzie *et al.* (1986)
Xylitol	Hunter *et al.* (1978) Salminen (1982)
Polyethylene glycol	Loeschke *et al.* (1973)
Hydrocolloids	
Agar	Mallet *et al.* (1984)

amylase and the results suggest the following course of events: initially the starch granules reached the caecum but, being insoluble, exerted little effect on the osmotic activity; this was followed by an adaptive change in the gut microflora leading to increased hydrolysis of the starch to low molecular weight, osmotically active species and, finally, the resultant increase in osmotic activity triggered the homeostatic mechanism. While such a mechanism is plausible within the model hypothesized by Leegwater *et al.*, further experimental confirmation is required that caecal enlargement is a response to hyperosmolarity of the luminal contents.

The 'hyperosmolarity hypothesis' is not the only one which has been

Table 16.1 *Continued*

Substance	Reference
Carboxymethylcellulose	Mallet *et al.* (1984)
Carrageenan	Mallet *et al.* (1984)
Guar gum	Mallet *et al.* (1984)
Gum acacia	Mallet *et al.* (1984)
Gum tragacanth	Elsenhaus *et al.* (1981)
Locust bean gum	Mallet *et al.* (1984)
Pectin	Rowland *et al.* (1983) Mallet *et al.* (1984)
Miscellaneous food additives	
Saccharin	Anderson (1979, 1983, 1985)
Caramels	Gaunt *et al.* (1977)
Erythrosine	Butterworth *et al.* (1976)
Yellow 2G	Gaunt *et al.* (1971)
Food interaction products Maillard intermediates (Amadori compounds)	O'Brien (1987, personal communication)
3,4-dideoxy-4-sulphohexosulose (reaction product in sulphited foods)	Mendoza-Garcia (1981)
Other Magnesium sulphate	Leegwater *et al.* (1974)

proposed to explain the mechanism of caecal enlargement; the involvement of gastro-intestinal hormones has also been suggested (Salminen *et al.*, 1982, 1984). The loss of smooth muscle tone has been taken as suggestive of the presence of a kallikrein-like substance, and this and other polypeptide hormones may be involved as the molecular 'trigger' of the tissue changes associated with gross caecal enlargement. A role may also be proposed for prostaglandins which are known to modulate mucus secretion and have a cytoprotective role in the gastro-intestinal tract; the changes in goblet cell numbers and activity previously mentioned (O'Brien, 1987, personal communication) could be controlled in this way.

These various hypotheses are not necessarily mutually exclusive and may reflect a multifactorial causation. However, the central role of the presence of osmotically active material in the lumen of the gut is currently favoured.

The postulate that caecal enlargement, however regulated, is a homeostatic mechanism for controlling caecal osmolarity is an attractive one, but it must be recognized that homeostatic mechanisms can be overloaded, leading to adverse functional and pathological changes.

D. Functional Changes Associated with Caecal Enlargement

A number of functional changes have been observed associated with caecal enlargement, primarily in the flux of water and electrolytes, and notably affecting the absorption of calcium, and possibly phosphorus and magnesium. These functional changes have far-reaching consequences in relation to secondary pathological sequelae. In addition, as mentioned above, there may be significant changes in intestinal metabolism of both exogenous and endogenous compounds with toxicological consequences.

A regular feature of animals displaying caecal enlargement is an increased fluid intake and an increased excretion of water both in urine and in faeces (associated with both increased faecal mass and water content). The polyuria leads to increased electrolyte (Na, K, Cl) excretion. There appears to be an increased permeability of the intestinal wall leading to alterations in the absorption of a number of substances, and among the most notable, most thoroughly studied and most toxicologically significant is an increased absorption of calcium.

The effect of lactose in increasing calcium absorption has been recognized for more than 60 years (Bergeim, 1926) and has received most attention. Rats appear to be more sensitive to the effects than mice and there are age-related differences within a species (Fournier *et al.*, 1971). Inclusion of 25% lactose in the diet, replacing glucose, led to increased absorption and excretion of calcium, increased net calcium balance, but a decreased net balance of magnesium (Forbes, 1961). The effect has been rationalized from a nutritional point of view in that lactose in milk may serve a useful physiological purpose in facilitating calcium absorption in suckling animals with a high requirement for skeletal growth. However, facilitated calcium absorption is not confined to lactose; it appears to be a common feature of compounds causing caecal enlargement including xylose, arabinose (Fournier *et al.*, 1972), sorbitol (Fournier *et al.*, 1967), dextrin (Bergeim, 1926), and caramelized dextrose (Fournier, 1959). It has been suggested that incomplete absorption of such carbohydrates in the small intestine leads to further absorption in the lower gut and that, by a mechanism which has not been fully elucidated, carbohydrate absorption in the hind gut facilitates calcium absorption. This may be by a coupled absorptive process or simply due to the permeability of the gut wall being increased. Whatever the mechanism, the normal regulation of calcium absorption in the small intestine via effects of vitamin D (or rather its hormonally-active, hydroxylated metabolites) on the synthesis of calcium binding protein in the mucosal cells is over-ridden by the facilitated absorption in the lower gut.

The coupling of calcium to carbohydrate absorption might still apply in the case of saccharin, where, at dietary levels which cause caecal enlargement, it inhibits intestinal carbohydrases and proteases, and increases absorption of calcium, phosphorus and magnesium (Anderson, 1985). In the germ-free animal, in which facilitated calcium absorption also is observed (Reddy *et al.*, 1969), again the reduced absorptive capacity due to villous atrophy in the small intestine leads to unabsorbed carbohydrates reaching the lower gut, so similar mechanisms might apply. Antibiotics such as penicillins and chloramphenicol, which also cause caecal enlargement, have been reported to increase calcium absorption (Wiseman, 1964; Wasserman and Taylor, 1969).

Although effects of caecal enlargement on absorption of calcium, and to a lesser degree magnesium and phosphorus, have received most attention in relation to the aetiology of nephrocalcinosis in rats, absorption of other electrolytes may also be affected; for example, stimulation of sodium transport has been associated with caecal enlargement (Loeschke *et al.*, 1973).

E. Metabolic Changes

As indicated above, there may be changes in the activities of intestinal enzymes, both endogenous and microbial, associated with caecal enlargement, but it is not always clear whether these are due to the caecal enlargement *per se* or result from inhibition/induction of enzymes by the agent which causes the increase in caecal size. For example, in the case of saccharin, at the concentrations arising in the intestine resulting from administration of high dietary levels, inhibition of endogenous carbohydrases and proteases has been observed with an associated increase in protein metabolism by the gut flora and appearance of microbial metabolites such as indican in increased concentrations in urine (Sims and Renwick, 1985). Such a change is not a general feature of caecal enlargement but the reduced activity of pancreatic amylase seen in potato starch-induced caecal enlargement may occur more generally (El Harith *et al.*, 1977).

Marked differences in metabolic activity of the gut microflora may accompany caecal enlargement and related changes in microbial populations, but these are obviously secondary to the effects of the causal agent and not a systematic feature of the increased caecal size. Clearly, microbial metabolism varies from zero in the enlarged caecum of germ-free animals to considerable where the caecum is heavily populated, and in a study of the effects of different hydrocolloids on the activity of six microbial enzymes, the activities depended on the hydrocolloid rather than caecal size (Mallett *et al.*, 1984). No generalizations were possible, even among structurally related compounds other than that the terrestrial plant gums tended to increase the activity of some enzymes (not necessarily the same ones) while the sulphated polysaccharide algal gums tended to decrease microbial enzyme activity.

In some cases, such as xylitol or sorbitol, an initial osmotic diarrhoea may occur if the material is introduced at high levels into the diet, but this resolves with time as adaptive changes in the gut flora occur leading to an increased capacity to metabolize the compound. Again, this cannot be considered a general aspect of caecal enlargement but specific to the causal substance; however it can explain transient effects in short-term studies.

F. Toxicological Consequences of Caecal Enlargement

It has been pointed out that a small degree of caecal enlargement may occur without accompanying histological changes in the tissue and with no effect on survival rates; in such circumstances the changes may be considered physiological and of no toxicological significance. However, in extreme cases where the caecal size may be increased several fold, there may be both primary and secondary toxicological consequences.

In short-term studies, raw potato starch induced such gross caecal enlargement that respiratory function was impaired and deaths occurred, a situation analogous to bloat in cattle (El Harith *et al.*, 1976). Histological changes in the caecal wall were also of such nature and magnitude as to be considered pathological. Where such gross effects are seen, it is clear that homeostatic mechanisms have been overloaded and there are direct toxic results. However, the functional changes described above, particularly those involving changes in mineral absorption, may have secondary toxic sequelae even when the caecal tissue appears morphologically normal. This has proved a particular problem in long-term studies in rats where an association may be seen between caecal enlargement and renal pelvic nephrocalcinosis.

The mechanism by which nephrocalcinosis is caused in long-term studies in rodents, especially rats, has been the subject of considerable research since it occurred commonly, but with variable frequency, in control animals receiving conventional laboratory diets (Woodard, 1971; Meyer *et al.*, 1982). It emerged that the rat is particularly sensitive to the dietary levels of calcium and phosphorus and the ratio between these two; low dietary levels of magnesium exacerbated the situation. The BARR Committee (1972) recommended the mineral concentration of rat diets should be 0.5% Ca, 0.4% P, and 0.04% Mg, and it is now generally accepted that the Ca : P ratio should approximate to 1. Some workers consider the figure for magnesium to be rather low since sub-optimal levels of magnesium exacerbate the problem of nephrocalcinosis.

The above data were derived from studies in normal animals, so it is not surprising that, even when diets which comply with these standards are used, the deranged mineral absorption associated with caecal enlargement may lead to an increased incidence of nephrocalcinosis. The net result of the facilitated absorption of calcium is the same as an imbalanced diet with excess calcium. Since such secondary effects of caecal enlargement usually occur only at high dietary levels of poorly absorbed carbohydrates, polyols or other food additives, and since the rat appears to be particularly prone to nephrocalcinosis of a type not usually encountered in man, the toxicological relevance for man is questionable.

A further toxicological complication has been encountered in the safety evaluation of polyols and similar materials which cause caecal enlargement, namely an associated incidence of adrenal medullary hyperplasia. High dietary levels (20%) of the sugar alcohols sorbitol, xylitol and mannitol cause an increase in the incidence of hyperplastic changes of the adrenal medulla of rats. In the case of xylitol it appears that this may progress to neoplasia, and tumours classified as phaeochromocytomas have been described (see the review by Roe and Bär (1985)). Since adrenal medullary hyperplasia also is observed in rats given high dietary concentrations of lactose, it seems likely that this may again be a secondary consequence of deranged calcium metabolism. Brion and Dupuis (1980) reported that the adrenal medullary hypofunction in vitamin D deficient rats could be ameliorated by correcting the hypocalcaemia without administration of vitamin D; this correction could be achieved simply by incorporating lactose at a level of 20% in the diet. Roe and Bär have extended this observation to suggest that hypercalcaemia resulting from the facilitated calcium absorption associated with caecal enlargement might be the common factor leading to adrenal medullary hyperplasia.

In reviewing the data for sorbitol in 1982, the Joint FAO/WHO Expert Committee on Food Additives largely discounted observations of renal pelvic calcinosis and adrenal medullary hyperplasia as they only occurred at such high dietary levels that there was gross dietary imbalance which may have resulted in metabolic disturbance. The Committee concluded that "the adrenal medullary hyperplasia produced by high dietary levels of sorbitol and certain other nutrients might occur as a physiological consequence of the stresses induced in aging rats."

It has been argued that the deranged mineral homeostasis associated with caecal enlargement caused by saccharin at high dose levels and the resultant changed mineral composition of the urine may be factors in the production of bladder tumours by this compound. While this may be the case, it cannot be the whole story since bladder carcinogenesis is not a general feature of caecal enlargement and some more specific effect must also be involved. It has been suggested that this specific effect is the deranged protein metabolism referred to above (Sims and Renwick, 1985). The increased protein metabolism by the microflora in the lower gut consequent on the inhibitory effect of saccharin on endogenous proteases leads to an increase in the urinary excretion of the metabolite, indole, which has been shown to be a promoter of bladder carcinogenesis induced by 2-acetylaminofluorene (Oyasu *et al.*, 1972). However, the observed changes in mineral concentrations of the urine and urothelial tissue may also play a part in promoting neoplastic changes.

G. Summary and Conclusions

From the foregoing it may be concluded that:
 (i) caecal enlargement is a common feature in rodents if poorly absorbed, osmotically active materials reach the lower gut;
 (ii) moderate caecal enlargement may be considered a physiological, homeostatic response but which may be overloaded under more extreme conditions;
(iii) functional changes, particularly affecting mineral absorption and intestinal metabolism, are a common concomitant of caecal enlargement even in the absence of histological changes in the caecal tissue;
(iv) secondary pathological changes, including nephrocalcinosis and adrenal medullary hyperplasia and neoplasia, may result from deranged mineral homeostasis, especially in the rat.

References

Anderson, R. L. (1979). Response of male rats to sodium saccharin ingestion: urine composition and mineral balance. *Fd Cosmet. Toxicol.* **17**, 195–200.
Anderson, R. L. (1983). Effect of saccharin ingestion on stool composition in

relation to caecal enlargement and increased stool hydration. *Fd Chem. Toxicol.* **21**, 255–257.

Anderson, R. L. (1985). Some changes in gastro-intestinal metabolism and in the urine and bladders of rats in response to sodium saccharin ingestion. *Fd Chem. Toxicol.* **23**, 457–463.

Anderson, R. L. and Kirkland, J. J. (1980). The effect of sodium saccharin in the diet on caecal microflora, *Fd Cosmet. Toxicol.* **18**, 353–355.

BARR Committee on Animal Nutrition (1972). "Nutrient Requirements of Laboratory Animals" (revised edn). National Academy of Sciences, Washington DC.

Bergeim, O. (1926). Carbohydrates and calcium and phosphorus absorption. *J. Biol. Chem.* **70**, 35–45.

Birch, G. G. and Etheridge, I. J. (1973). Chemical and physiological properties of glucose syrup components, *Starke.* **25**, 235–238.

Birch, G. G., Etheridge, I. J. and Green, L. F. (1973). Short-term effects of feeding rats with glucose syrup fractions and dextrose, *Br. J. Nutr.* **29**, 87–93.

Brion, F. and Dupuis, Y. (1980). Calcium and monoamine regulation: Role of vitamin D nutrition, *Can. J. Physiol. Pharmacol.* **58**, 1431–1434.

Butterworth, K. R., Gaunt, I. F., Grasso, P. and Gangolli, S. D. (1976). Acute and short-term toxicity studies on Erythrosine BS in rodents, *Fd Cosmet. Toxicol.*, **14**, 525–531.

De Groot, A. P., Til, H. P., Feron, V. J., Dreef-van der Meulen, H. C. and Willems, M. I. (1974). Two-year feeding and multigeneration studies in rats on five chemically modified starches, *Fd Cosmet. Toxicol.* **12**, 651–663.

Dupas, H., Leroy, P. and D'Alayer, C. (1984). 24 months safety study of Lycasin® 80/55 on rats. Unpublished report from Roquette Freres, Lestrem, France. *In*: "Toxicological Evaluation of Certain Food Additives and Contaminants", WHO Fd Add. Ser. No. 20, pp. 191–192. WHO, Geneva.

Dupuis, Y. and Fournier, P. (1963). Lactose and the absorption of calcium and strontium, *In*: "The Transfer of Calcium and Strontium across Biological Membranes" (ed. R. H. Wasserman), pp. 277–293. Academic Press, New York, London.

El Harith, E. A., Dickerson, J. W. T. and Walker, R. (1976). Potato starch and caecal hypertrophy in the rat. *Fd Cosmet. Toxicol.* **14**, 115–121.

El Harith, E. A, Walker, R., Birch, G. G. and Sukan, G. (1977). Some factors influencing caecal enlargement induced by raw potato starch in the rat, *Fd Chem.* **2**, 279–289.

Elsenhaus, B., Blume, R. and Caspary, W. F. (1981). Long-term feeding of unavailable carbohydrate gelling agents. Influence of dietary concentration and microbiological degradation on adaptive responses in the rat. *Am. J. Clin. Nutr.* **34**, 1837–1848.

Feron, V. J., Til, H. P. and de Groot, A. P. (1978). Chronic (89-week) feeding study with hydroxypropyl distarch phosphate, starch acetate, lactose and sodium alginate in mice. *In*: "Central Institute for Nutrition and Food Research (CIVO/TNO) Report" No. 5690.

Forbes, R. M. (1961). Excretory patterns and bone deposition of zinc, calcium and magnesium in the rat as influenced by zinc deficiency, EDTA and lactose, *J. Nutr.* **74**, 194–200.

Fournier, P. (1959). Physiological qualities of caramel and dextrin prepared by the action of dry heat on glucose and starch, *C. r. Acad. Sci., Paris Ser. D* **248**, 3744–3746.

Fournier, P., Dupuis, Y, Digaud, A. and Fournier, A. (1972). Mechanisms of action of sugars on calcium absorption and retention, *C. r. Acad. Sci., Paris Ser. D* **275**, 85–88.

Fournier, P., Dupuis, Y. and Fournier, A. (1971). Effect of lactose on the absorption of alkaline earth metals and intestinal lactase activity. *Israel J. Med. Sci.* **7**, 389–391.

Fournier, P. L., Gambier, J. and Fontaine, N. (1967). Effects of prolonged ingestion of sorbitol on calcium utilization and bone formation in rats, *C. r. Acad. Sci. Paris Ser. D* **264**, 1301–1304.

Gaunt, I. F., Carpanini, F. M. B., Kiss, I. S. and Grasso, P. (1971). Short-term toxicity of Yellow 2G in rats, *Fd Cosmet. Toxicol.* **9**, 343–353.

Gaunt, I. F., Lloyd, A. G., Grasso, P., Gangolli, S. D. and Butterworth, K. R. (1977). Short-term study in the rat on two caramels produced by variations of the ammonia process. *Fd Cosmet. Toxicol.* **15**, 509–521.

Hosoya, N. (1972). Effect of sugar alcohol on the intestine, "IXth International Congress of Nutrition", Mexico City, (eds A. Chávez, H. Bourges and S. Basta) S. Karger, Basel.

Hunter, B., Colley, J., Street, A. E., Heywood, R., Prentice, D. E. and Magnusson, G. (1978). Xylitol: Tumorigenicity and toxicity study in long-term dietary administration to rats. "Huntingdon Research Centre Report", cited in MacKenzie *et al.* (1986).

Leegwater, D. C., de Groot, A. P. and van Kaimthout-Kuyper, M. (1974). The aetiology of caecal enlargement in the rat. *Fd Cosmet. Toxicol.* **12**, 687–697.

Loeschke, K., Uhlich, E. and Halbach, R. (1973). Caecal enlargement combined with sodium transport stimulation in rats fed polythylene glycol, *Proc. Soc. exp. Biol. Med.*, **142**, 96–102.

MacKenzie, K. M., Hauck, W. N., Wheeler, A. G. and Roe, F. J. C. (1986). Three-generation reproduction study of rats ingesting up to 10% sorbitol in the diet — and a brief review of the toxicological status of sorbitol, *Fd Chem. Toxicol.*, **24**, 191–200.

Mallett, A. K., Wise, A. and Rowland, I. R. (1984). Hydrocolloid food additives and rat caecal microbial enzyme activities. *Fd Chem. Toxicol.*, **22**, 415–418.

Mendoza-Garcia, M. A. (1981). Some toxicity studies on sulphite interaction products in food. Ph.D Thesis, University of Surrey, Guildford, Surrey, UK.

Meyer, O., Blom, L. and Sondergaard, D. (1982). The influence of minerals and protein on the nephrocalcinosis potential for rats of semisynthetic diets, *Lab. Anim.* **16**, 271–273.

Morgan, T. B. and Yudkin, J. (1957). The vitamin sparing action of sorbitol, *Nature* **180**, 543–545.

Musch, V. K., Siebert, G., Schiweck, H. and Steinle, G. (1973). Physiological-nutritional studies on the utilization of isomaltitol in rats. *Z. Ernahrungwiss. Suppl.* **15**, 3–16.

Oyasu, R., Kitajima, T., Hopp, M. L. and Sumie, H. (1972). Enhancement of urinary bladder tumorigenesis in hamsters by coadministration of 2-acetylaminofluorene and indole. *Cancer Res.* **32**, 2027–2033.

Reddy, B. S., Pleasants, J. R. and Wostman, B. S. (1969). Effects of intestinal microflora on calcium, phosphorus and magnesium metabolism in rats. *J. Nutr.* **99**, 353–362.

Reussner, G., Andros, J. and Thiessen, R. (1963). The utilisation of various starches and sugars in the Rat, *J. Nutr.* **80**, 291–298.

Roe, F. J. C. and Bar, A. (1985). Enzootic and epizootic adrenal medullary proliferative disease of rats: influence of dietary factors which affect calcium absorption. *Hum. Toxicol.* **4**, 27–52.

Rowland, I. R., Wise, A. and Mallett, A. K. (1983). Metabolic profile of caecal micro-organisms from rats fed indigestible plant cell-wall components, *Fd Chem. Toxicol.* **21**, 25–29.

Salminen, E., Salminen, S. and Porkka, L. (1984). The effect of xylitol on gastric emptying and secretion of gastric inhibitory polypeptides in the rat. *J. Nutr.* **114**, 2201–2203.

Salminen, S. (1982). Investigations on the toxicological and biological properties of xylitol, *Ph.D. Thesis, University of Surrey, Guildford, Surrey, UK.,* pp. 1–191.

Salminen, S., Salminen, E., Koivistoinen, P., Bridges, J. and Marks, V. (1985). Gut microflora interactions with xylitol in the mouse, rat and man. *Fd Chem. Toxicol.* **23**, 985–990.

Salminen, S., Salminen, E. and Marks, V. (1982). The effects of xylitol on the secretion of insulin and gastric inhibitory polypeptide in man and rats, *Diabetalogia* **22**, 480–482.

Sims, J. and Renwick, A. G. (1983). The effects of saccharin on the metabolism of dietary tryptophan to indole, a known cocarcinogen for the urinary bladder of the rat, *Toxicol. appl. Pharmacol.* **67**, 132–151.

Sims, J. and Renwick, A. G. (1985). The microbial metabolism of tryptophan in rats fed a diet containing 7.5% saccharin in a two-generation protocol, *Fd Chem. Toxicol.* **23**, 437–444.

Walker, R. (1978). Some observations on the phenomenon of caecal enlargement in the rat. *In:* "Chemical Toxicology of Food" (eds C. L. Galli, R. Paoletti and G. Vettorazzi), pp. 339–348. Elsevier/North Holland, Amsterdam.

Walker, R. and El Harith, E. A. (1978). Nutritional and toxicological properties of some raw and modified starches, *Ann. Nutr. Alim.* **32**, 671–679.

Wasserman, R. H. and Taylor, A. N. (1969). Some aspects of the intestinal absorption of calcium with special reference to vitamin D. *In:* "Mineral Metabolism — An Advanced Treatise" (eds Colmar and Bronner), pp. 320–403, Academic Press, New York, London.

Wiseman, G. (1964). *In:* "Absorption from the Intestine", p. 208. Academic Press, New York, London.

Woodard, J. C. (1971). Relationship between the ingredients of semi-purified diets and nutritional nephrocalcinosis of rats. *Am. J. Path.* **65**, 269–271.

17

Mutagens in Human Faeces and Cancer of the Large Bowel

S. VENITT

A. Introduction

1. *Rationale for Studying Faecal Mutagens*

In the decade since Bruce and his colleagues (1977) first reported the occurrence of mutagenic activity in extracts of human faeces, a considerable amount of time, effort, and money has been spent in the unpleasant, tedious, frustrating and often anti-social task of confirming and extending these original observations. The driving force behind this scatological excursion into genetic toxicology is part of a quest for knowledge of the cause of cancer of the large bowel, the second commonest malignancy of rich, industrialized countries. Malignant neoplasms of the intestinal tract are a major cause of death from cancer in Western Europe, North America, Australia and New Zealand. In England in 1983 15 803 people died of intestinal cancer (mainly of the colon and rectum), accounting for 12.7% of all cancer deaths. This is second only to the number of deaths from respiratory-tract cancer (34 336, 27.5%) (DHSS, 1984). However, despite numerous epidemiological and laboratory studies performed over many decades, our knowledge of the aetiology of cancer of the large bowel consists of a few broad clues rather than any hard facts. To quote a leading group of faecal genotoxicologists: "All theories regarding the cause of colon cancer suffer from the lack of solid proof" (Van Tassell *et al.*, 1982a).

Of those factors which have been studied, diet is generally considered to be an important determinant of risk of bowel cancer, though which particular aspects are critical to the development of cancer has not been established. Diets which are high in fat and meat and low in fibre are thought to confer a high risk of bowel cancer, and diets which are rich in vegetables and fibre, but low in fat and meat are thought to constitute a low risk (Correa and Haenszel, 1978; Kinlen, 1983; Zaridze, 1983; Boyle *et al.*, 1985; Armstrong and Mann, 1985). However, a recent study of colorectal cancer mortality among Maori and non-Maori New Zealanders throws some doubt on the importance of these risk factors (Smith *et al.*, 1985). The study of diet, though likely to be crucial, is unlikely to provide more than a partial explanation of the aetiology of bowel cancer, bearing in mind the existence of genetic predispositions to colon cancer (e.g. familial polyposis coli, and colon-cancer-prone families (Knudson, 1982)), and other factors such as the recently described protective effect of early age at first pregnancy on colorectal cancer in women (Potter and McMichael, 1983; Howe *et al.*, 1985). Doll and Peto (1981) have written a particularly useful review on the possible mechanisms whereby diet may affect the incidence of cancer.

Diet is a part of our external environment to which the lining of the gut is continually exposed, in the same way that the skin is exposed to sunlight, or the lungs may be exposed to tobacco smoke — a view developed by Wilkins and Van Tassell (1983) in a recent review on intestinal mutagens. By analogy with ultraviolet radiation from sunlight or carcinogens in tobacco smoke, which pose carcinogenic threats to skin and lungs respectively, certain dietary constituents or the products of their digestion, metabolism and excretion may provoke neoplastic change in the lining of the gut, an organ which provides a very large surface area for contact with material originating from the external environment. It has been suggested, therefore, that bowel cancer may be caused by carcinogens in food, or generated by interaction of constituents of gut contents with the intestinal microflora or with the metabolic machinery of the cells lining the gut, or by various combinations of these. Correa and Haenszel (1978) summarized epidemiological data for an aetiological model for large-bowel cancer which is based on the presence of a carcinogen in the intestinal contents which becomes increasingly concentrated as it travels from the ileocaecal valve to the rectum. This hypothesis (based on segment-specific tumour incidence in high and low-risk populations) sugests that carcinogenic activity should be detectable in faeces, since most tumours of the intestine arise in the colon and rectum, organs which receive prolonged exposure to faeces (Correa and Haenszel, 1978).

A simple test of the hypothesis would be to assay faecal samples (preferably taken from a variety of subjects representing groups at low risk and high risk of bowel cancer) for carcinogenic activity. However, carcinogenicity assays employing laboratory rodents – in general use for testing chemicals – are time-consuming, expensive, and most importantly, are very insensitive, requiring high doses of even quite potent carcinogens to produce statistically convincing results. Given (*i*) that cancer of the large bowel is generally a disease of middle and old age (mortality rates being a function of the fourth to the sixth powers of age) (Maskens, 1982) and (*ii*) that even in a high-risk country like England, less than 3% of the population died from large-bowel cancer in 1983 (DHSS, 1984) it is very likely that the postulated bowel carcinogens are present at very low levels, or are weak, or are both dilute and weak. It is not surprising, therefore, that a study of the carcinogenicity of human stool samples has yet to be published (or even attempted).

Because it is not feasible to look for faecal carcinogens *per se*, methods for detecting biological activity which is characteristic of carcinogens (e.g., DNA-damaging activity, mutagenicity, clastogenicity) have been used instead. Of such methods, the detection of mutagenic activity using short-term bacterial assays has proved to be the most popular, such assays being well-validated, sensitive, rapid and cheap. However, this approach is subject to several limitations (IARC, 1986).

2. *Limitations of Short-term Tests for Carcinogenicity*

The first limitation stems from evidence that the development of cancer is a multistep process. At least two steps – 'initiation' and 'promotion' – have been identified in animal experiments for a variety of tumours, including those of the large bowel (for reviews, see Berenblum (1982), Farber (1982), and Whitehead (1984)). Epidemiological studies suggest that human cancer develops in the same way (Moolgavkar and Knudson, 1981; Alderson, 1984; Carter, 1984). There is much evidence to support the idea that colon cancer develops from pre-existing adenomas – a classical example of multi-step carcinogenesis in humans (Morson *et al.*, 1983; Eide, 1986).

Initiation is a short-lived and irreversible process, involving DNA damage, mutagenic events (e.g., point mutation, chromosomal damage and rearrangement), and can be induced, therefore, by agents with genotoxic properties. Recent evidence that cellular proto-oncogenes can be activated by mutation, chromosomal translocation or gene amplification gives added weight to the idea that DNA is a critical target in the process of tumour initiation (Land *et al.*, 1983; Balmain, 1985). Tumour promotion is a longer-term process which may be reversible. The mechanisms underlying tumour promotion and the later stages of carcinogenesis are less well understood, but there is sufficient evidence to suggest that although mutational events may be involved, they are probably not essential to these later steps. Therefore short-term tests based on the detection of genotoxic activity will detect only those agents which have initiating activity, and will not pick up promoting agents which are not genotoxic. Agents are also known which although carcinogenic, appear to act by mechanisms which do not involve genetic toxicity — certain metals and their salts, and a few hormonally active compounds such as diethylstilboestrol fall into this category, and will not be detected in short-term tests which depend on genotoxic activity as an end point.

The less than perfect concordance between carcinogenicity and activity in short-term tests is another limitation which must be kept in mind when using such tests to look for potential carcinogens in faeces. For example, the best validated of all the short-term tests — the *Salmonella* test — is considered to be about 83% predictive by its originators (see Maron and Ames, 1983). Moreover, there is little evidence for a quantitative relationship between bacterial mutagenicity and carcinogenicity; a weak mutagen is not necessarily a weak carcinogen, neither is a potent mutagen necessarily a potent carcinogen (Venitt, 1980).

Another limitation to the use of short-term tests, especially bacterial assays employing reverse mutation, is that they were designed for screening pure chemicals, and are subject to a variety of artefacts when used with complex biological mixtures (Combes *et al.*, 1984; IARC, 1986).

3. *Advantages of Short-term Tests for Carcinogenicity*

As well as these limitations, short-term tests also have their advantages in the study of genotoxicity in body fluids and excreta. Tests, especially those which use bacteria, are rapid, cheap, relatively easy to perform, well validated against a very wide range of chemical classes, and adaptable. For example, they can be used for monitoring biological activity in complex fractionation procedures, where more elaborate long-term tests would be prohibitively costly in resources and time (Zimmermann and Taylor-Mayer, 1985). Thus the search for genotoxic activity in human faeces may provide valuable clues to the aetiology of cancer of the large bowel, and the knowledge gained may eventually lead to means for reducing the incidence of this disease.

4. *Previous Reviews of Faecal Mutagenicity*

Several reviews of studies of faecal mutagenesis and its relationship with bowel cancer have been published (Venitt, 1981, 1982a,b; Wilkins and Van Tassell, 1983; Reddy, 1986; Schiffman, 1986.).

5. *Tabular Summary of Faecal Mutagenicity Studies*

Table 17.1 contains brief summaries of the majority of studies of faecal mutagenicity published since 1977, the year when Bruce *et al.* (1977) produced the first evidence that human faeces contained mutagenic constituents. The reader may refer to Table 17.1 for technical details of each study in the following discussion. The work on the identification of faecal mutagens ('fecapentaenes') has not been included in this table, but is described in detail in section C.

Inspection of Table 17.1 reveals a rather bewildering array of different types of study obtained with a variety of methods and donors. Nevertheless, a pattern can be discerned. For example, there are studies of donors who represent populations at differing risks of bowel cancer; most of these studies used organic-solvent extraction combined with the *Salmonella* test, but a minority employed the more sensitive fluctuation test for assaying mutagenic activity of aqueous faecal extracts. There are also studies on the effects of dietary intervention on faecal mutagenicity. In this chapter, studies of mutagenicity of human faeces will be reviewed where possible by the type of assay employed, since each method of assay is associated with particular problems, some which are intrinsic to the assay, and others which are related to the nature of the test material.

B. Studies using the *Salmonella* Test

One way of testing the hypothesis that faecal mutagens are implicated in cancer of the large bowel is to determine the levels of faecal mutagens in groups of donors who represent populations at different risk of the disease. Most of the investigators who used this approach have employed the *Salmonella* test (Ames *et al.*, 1975; Maron and Ames, 1983) for assaying faecal extracts made with organic solvents.

1. *Description and Critical Features of the Test*

(a) Description of the test.   The standard *Salmonella* test employs the pour-plate technique: to molten 'top agar' containing a trace of histidine are added about 10^8 histidine-requiring bacteria, the test-compound solution, and S9- mix. S9-mix contains a post-mitochondrial supernatant prepared from the livers of rats treated with a mixture of polychlorinated biphenyls (Aroclor 1254) to increase the level of hepatic mixed-function cytochrome mono-oxygenases, the enzymes responsible for biological oxidations of foreign compounds. This agar mixture is poured on to an

Table 17.1 *Summary of studies of mutagenic activity in human faeces (studies relating to the isolation and identification of fecapentaenes are described in section C of the text)*

Type of study	Number of donors, nationality, health etc.	Design and sampling	Extraction method	Assay method	Control for auxotrophic growth	Result	Remarks	Reference
First report of mutagenic activity in human faeces	5 people on Western diet	Single bowel movements	Complex procedure, including ether, alkaline and acid washes, giving several different fractions.	Ames test: TA1535, 1537, 98, 100 ± Aroclor rat-liver S9.	no	Highest mutagenicity in TA100 >TA1535 >TA98, (−S9) in ether fraction washed in NaOH. Large variation in mutagenicity of consecutive samples from 1 donor. At least 1 sample from 4 other donors was positive.	Authors also show that faeces contain materials which can inhibit mutagenicity of faecal mutagens or reference mutagens.	Bruce *et al.* (1977)
Effect of dietary ascorbate on faecal mutagenicity	1 donor on Western diet	Daily stool samples taken for 7 days before ascorbate, 11 days during ascorbate, 8 days after ascorbate.	Ether extract of freeze-dried faeces	Ames test: TA100 without S9	no	Large daily variation in mutagenic activity. Means fell from >400/plate before ascorbate to about 250 during ascorbate, and did not recover by day 27.	Authors claimed on basis of HPLC/TEA that mutagen was a nitroso compound whose formation could be inhibited by dietary ascorbate. [This claim has since been withdrawn — Lee *et al.* (1981)]	Varghese *et al.* (1978)
Comparison of populations at high or low risk of bowel cancer.	42 urban whites (high risk) 82 urban blacks 108 rural blacks (low risk). All resident in S. Africa	Single bowel movements	Ether extract of freeze-dried faeces	Ames test: TA98, 100 ± Aroclor rat-liver S9	no	9/42 whites, 5/82 urban blacks, 2/108 rural blacks gave MR[a] >2, all without S9. Difference between MR in whites and either of black groups was significant.	Authors conclude that they had shown that a population at high risk of bowel cancer excreted more faecal mutagen than 2 low-risk populations.	Ehrich *et al.* (1979)
Detection of clastogenic activity in human faeces	3 donors on Western diet	Single bowel movement	Faeces homogenised with equal weight of water and extracted with chloroform : methanol 1 : 1. Organic phase dried, assayed.	Chromosomal damage in Chinese Hamster CHO cells. Effects of Cu^{2+}, Mn^{2+}, Fe^{2+}, Fe^{3+} and catalase tested.	NA	All 3 samples gave dose-related increase in chromosomal aberrations, enhanced by Cu and Mn and inhibited by Fe or catalase or catalase + Mn.	Authors suggested that faecal mutagens might be reducing thiols.	Stich and Kuhnlein (1979)

Detection of faecal mutagens in different groups of people; effect of dietary ascorbate	11 students 18 bowel cancer patients 23 retired people (normal Western diet) 11 retired people (higher levels of ascorbate, α-tocopherol, fibre in diet).	Single bowel movements. 1 donor given various dietary changes (high ascorbate, tocopherol, fibre, or extra meat, fat).	Freeze-dried faeces extracted with ether which was then washed with NaOH.	Ames test: TA100, no S9.	no	Data given only in charts. Group with high-vitamin, high fibre diet appeared to have lowest mutagenicity. In 1 donor, low fibre or high meat seemed to raise, and high vitamins to lower mutagenicity	Authors claimed on basis of HPLC/TEA that mutagen was a nitroso compound whose formation could be inhibited by dietary ascorbate. Also claimed presence of a variety of N-nitroso-compounds in faeces. [These claims have since been withdrawn — Lee et al. (1981)]	Bruce et al. (1979)
Comparison of bowel-cancer patients with haemorrhoid patients	17 colon-cancer patients 17 haemorrhoid patients	not stated	not stated	Ames test: TA100, no S9.	no	7/17 cancer patients, 9/17 haemorrhoid patients gave positive results (difference not significant).		Bruce and Dion (1980)
Increasing the yield of faecal mutagen by anaerobic incubation of faeces in vitro	2 Caucasian donors who regularly excrete mutagens, and 2 Caucasians who don't.	Single bowel movements. Samples were incubated aerobically or anaerobically at 37°C before extraction.	Ether extract of freeze-dried faeces	Ames test: TA100, no S9	no	Mutagenicity increased by factors of up to 20 fold after anaerobic incubation. This did not occur in the cold, in air, after autoclaving or after mixing with antimicrobial agents. TLC showed only a single spot corresponding with mutagenic activity.	Authors concluded that the major mutagenicity in human faeces appeared to be due to a single type of compound which may be produced by anaerobic bacteria.	Lederman et al. (1980)
Comparison of three populations at different risks of colon cancer	11 SDA[b] from New York 15 Finns from Kuopio (low-risk groups) 18 Omnivores from New York (high-risk group)	Entire faecal output over 2 days collected from each donor.	Entire sample from each donor pooled and freeze-dried. Ether extract chromatographed on silica column; ether eluate used in assay.	Ames test: TA98, 100 ± Aroclor rat-liver S9	no	0/11 SDA, 2/13 Finns, 4/18 New Yorkers gave MR >3 in at least 1 test system [no significant difference between any of the 3 groups]. Finns positive only in TA98 + S9. New Yorkers positive in TA98 − S9 and TA100 ± S9.	Results suggest presence of several different mutagenic classes. [The difference between the groups looks impressive in % terms, but the absolute numbers of positive donors in each group is too low for statistical significance].	Reddy et al. (1980a)

Cont'd

Table 17.1 (*Continued*)

Type of study	Number of donors, nationality, health etc.	Design and sampling	Extraction method	Assay method	Control for auxotrophic growth	Result	Remarks	Reference
Comparison of populations at high and low risk of colon cancer	16 SDA from New York (low risk group) 18 Omnivores from New York (high risk group) [chosen from previous study (Reddy *et al.* 1980 — see above) on basis of negative faecal mutagenicity assay]	Entire faecal output over 2 days collected from each donor	Dichloromethane extraction from aqueous NaOH. Water absorbed by Preptube, solvent evaporated, extract chromatographed on silica column; 3 fractions collected by stepwise solvent elution.	Ames test: TA98, 100 ± Aroclor rat-liver S9. Co-mutagenicity assayed with MNNG ($-$S9) and AAF ($+$S9).	no	0/16 SDA, 0/18 New Yorkers positive in standard Ames test. Fraction 3 showed co-mutagenic activity (enhanced mutagenicity, mainly of AAF + S9). Extracts from New Yorkers were more co-mutagenic than SDA extracts.	Authors suggest that co-mutagenicity is a discriminant for colon cancer.	Reddy *et al.* (1980b)
Study of faecal mutagenicity in normal donors given controlled formula diets	Expt. A: 6 men (aged 24–27) Expt. B: 6 men (aged 63–77). (All healthy and usually consuming a Western diet). Study performed in California, USA.	A: Donors fed formula diet for 108 days. 3-day pooled samples at 49–51, 52–54 and 70–72 days. B: as A, but for 47 days. 3-day pooled samples at 30–32, 42–44 and 45–47 days.	Aqueous, with centrifugation and filtration.	Fluctuation test: TA98, 100, no S9	yes: by calibration with histidine in blank assays.	Variation in mutagenicity between subjects was much greater than between different samples from the same donor. Subjects could be classified into groups with high, intermediate and low mutagenicity.	Authors concluded that 12 donors on essentially the same diet showed considerable inter-subject variation in faecal mutagen output which did not disappear even after 72 days. Same trend for faecal pH (low pH being correlated with high mutagenicity in TA100). Suggests long-term dietary habits or genetics controls bowel physiology and faecal mutagens.	Kuhnlein and Kuhnlein (1980)

Study	Subjects	Sampling	Extraction	Assay	Internal standard	Results	Conclusions	Reference
Comparison of faecal mutagens in vegetarians and non-vegetarians	6 ovolactovegetarians 11 strict vegetarians 12 non-vegetarians. All from urban Vancouver, Canada.	Single bowel movements	Aqueous: 1 g water per g wet-weight faeces, with centrifugation and filtration.	Fluctuation test: TA98, 100, no S9	yes: by calibration with histidine in blank assays.	6/6 ovo-lacto-vegetarian, 11/11 strict vegetarian, 12/12 non-vegetarian were positive in at least 1 or more doses and strains. Pooled data showed vegetarian extracts slightly but significantly less mutagenic than non-vegetarian extracts, especially in TA100.	Authors conclude that 17 vegetarians had significantly lower faecal mutagenicity than 12 non-vegetarians, supporting the theory that faecal mutagens are involved in bowel cancer. Also suggested that correlation studies between pH and mutagenic activity in TA98 and 100 indicate the presence of 2 or more major faecal mutagens.	Kuhnlein *et al.* (1981)
Dietary: lacto-vegetarians vs. omnivores	Caucasians: 8 vegetarians 11 omnivores	24 hour samples	Freeze-dried; then DMSO or ethanol	Differential survival uvr^+/uvr^- spot-test	NA	Omnivores' SR[c] significantly greater than vegetarians' which was about 1	Authors conclude that omnivores' faeces contained DNA damaging agents, vegetarians' did not [but differences very slight]	Nader *et al.* (1981)
Effect of fried beef (200 g/day for 3 weeks) added to Western diet.	6 Caucasians	24 hour samples: 1 before, 3 during, 2 after beef	Ether extraction from 1N NaOH then pentane and silica column, solvent extraction	Ames test: TA98, 100 ± Aroclor rat-liver S9. Also co-mutagenicity with AAF	no	All samples negative Co-mutagenicity increased with beef diet, then decreased.	Authors do not comment on negative result [significance of co-mutagenicity is not clear]	deVet *et al.* (1981)
Comparison of Caucasians (± bowel cancer) with Polynesians	22 Caucasian (bowel cancer) 18 healthy Caucasians 19 SDA healthy Caucasians 13 healthy Samoans 11 healthy Maoris	single bowel movements	Ether extraction	Ames test: TA100, no S9	no	2/83 samples greater than 2 × background	Authors claimed significant difference between Caucasian and Polynesian data	Ferguson and Alley (1982)

Cont'd

Type of study	Number of donors, nationality, health etc.	Design and sampling	Extraction method	Assay method	Control for auxotrophic growth	Result	Remarks	Reference
Effect of ascorbic acid and α-tocopherol on faecal mutagenicity	A: 1 Caucasian male B: 19 Caucasians (A and B on Western diets)	A: 13 day faeces from 2 weeks without vitamins, 2 weeks with vitamins, 2 weeks without vitamins. B: last 3 day faeces from 2 weeks without vitamins and 2 weeks with vitamins	Alkaline dichloromethane	Ames test: TA100, no S9	no	A: Mutagenicity significantly reduced in vit$^+$ period then rose to 40% of 1st vit$^-$ level. B: 8 donors negative, 11 donors positive, mutagenicity fell during vit$^+$.	Addition of vitamins to faeces in vitro did not affect the mutation assay. Authors suggest that antioxidants in diet may have a role in lowering exposure of body to endogenous mutagens.	Dion *et al.* (1982)
Comparison of 2 Japanese populations at different risks of bowel cancer	223 high-risk (Hawaii) 166 low-risk (N. Japan)	Single bowel movements	Freeze-dried then ether extraction.	Ames test: TA98, TA100 ± Aroclor rat-liver S9. Also rec+/− spot-test.	no	Ames test: MR of 90% samples was less than 2 in either strain. Of 10% with MR >2, significantly more found in Hawaiians than in Japanese residents.	Authors claim detection of 5 different mutagens and that high-risk Hawaiian and Japanese have more faecal mutagens than low-risk Japanese resident in Japan	Mower *et al.* (1982)
Detection of clastogenic activity in human faeces	4 people on Western diet	Single bowel movements	Multi-step aqueous/ solvent extraction resulting in a hexane fraction (neutrals, bases) and a water/ethanol fraction (acids).	Chromosomal damage in Chinese Hamster CHO cells. ± Aroclor rat-liver S9	NA	2/4 samples (acid fraction) induced dose-related increases in exchanges. 2/4 induced smaller increases just below toxic dose. S9 had no effect. Hexane fraction was inactive		Barnes and Powrie (1982)

Comparison of colon cancer patients with healthy donors	16 colon-cancer patients 35 donors without bowel symptoms and with negative haemoccult test. All from Queensland, Australia	Single bowel movements	Ether extraction of freeze-dried faeces	Ames test: TA98, TA100 $\pm$ Aroclor rat-liver S9.	no	4/16 colon-cancer samples and 7/35 control samples gave MR >2, in TA98 without S9. (p > 0.16, NS)	Authors concluded that incidence of mutagens in colon cancer patients is similar to that found in a high-risk group.	Askew *et al.* (1982)
Effect of short-term dietary modification on faecal mutagens	6 healthy Caucasians on Western diet	Days 1–7, Western baseline diet Days 8–21, low-risk ovo-lacto-vegetarian diet Days 22–35, high-risk 5 oz meat/day, refined grain. 24 hour samples: 2 baseline, 3 low- 3 high-risk.	Aqueous 1 ml water per g wet-weight faeces, with centrifugation and filtration.	Fluctuation test: TA98, 100, no S9	no	Pooled data gave dose-related increases in pos. wells for all 3 diets. Small but significant increase with baseline vs. meat, non-meat vs. meat	Authors concluded that certain aspects of bowel physiology connected with faecal mutagenicity can be altered within 2 weeks.	Kuhnlein *et al.* (1983)
Development of anaerobic methods and effects of auxotrophic feeding on fluctuation tests of faecal extracts	1 male Caucasian in good health, on Western diet	Single bowel movements collected anaerobically. 5 collections over several months.	Aqueous, 1 ml per g wet-weight faeces, with centrifugation and filtration.	Microtitre fluctuation test: TA100, aerobic and anaerobic assays.	yes: bioassay using auxotrophic bacteria	4/5 samples promoted auxotrophic growth to an extent which prevented mutagenicity assay. 1/5 sample was mutagenic if assayed aerobically, but was negative in anaerobic conditions	Authors concluded that auxotrophic growth enhancement could seriously compromise reverse-mutation fluctuation tests; presence or absence of air is also important.	Venitt and Bosworth (1983)
Study of mutagenicity of different faecal fractions	24 donors from a wide socioeconomic background; mostly Caucasians on a Western diet	Single bowel movements	Acetone, dried, 1:1 methanol/DCM[d], cellulose to silica columns, then stepwise solvent elution.	Ames test: TA98, 100 $\pm$ Aroclor rat-liver S9	no	Only acetone eluate from silica gave +ve results: 7/24 with TA98, 4/24 with TA100. S9 reduced the mutagenicity of this fraction. HPLC of active fraction suggested 1 or several related compounds.	High correlation between u.v. absorption of HPLC peak and mutagenicity.	Dion and Bruce (1983)

Cont'd

Table 17.1 (*Continued*)

Type of study	Number of donors, nationality, health etc.	Design and sampling	Extraction method	Assay method	Control for auxotrophic growth	Result	Remarks	Reference
Study of faecal mutagens from donors on a Western diet	99 healthy subjects from New York (USA) consuming a low-fibre high-fat diet.	Single bowel movements	Each sample divided in 2, 0.5 frozen, 0.5 incubated 96 hours at 37°C anaerobically. Samples lyophilised, extracted from 0.1N NaOH with ether/hexane 1 : 1. Water absorbed on Preptube, then eluate fractionated on silica column; 2 particular fractions combined and tested.	Ames test: TA98, 100 $\pm$ Aroclor rat-liver●S9	no	11/99 unincubated samples gave MR >3 in at least 1 test condition. 30/99 incubated samples gave MR >3 in at least 1 test condition. Pattern of data suggests several types of mutagen. HPLC showed several peaks which were highly mutagenic with TA98 + S9	Mutagenicity of faecal samples could be enhanced by incubation of faeces for 96 hours at 37°C under anaerobic conditions.	Reddy *et al.* (1984)
Use of nuclear abberations produced in mouse colon to detect karyotoxicity of human faecal fractions	10 healthy adults on Western diet	Single bowel movements	Faeces mixed with Na_2SO_4, Na_2CO_3 and cellulose. Mix placed on Florisil column, and eluted with solvents. 5 fractions collected.	Faecal fractions instilled *per rectum* in each of 10 C57BL/6 mice. 24 hour later, colons removed, Fulegen strained and nuclear abberations scored.	NA	3/10 donors' faeces produced significant increase ($\times 3$) in NA. Only dichloromethane fraction was active.	Authors suggest that faeces contain carcinogens, since known carcinogens produce NA in mouse colon.	Suzuki and Bruce (1984)
Comparison of Caucasians ($\pm$ bowel cancer) with Polynesians	11 Caucasian (bowel cancer) 20 healthy Caucasians 18 SDA[b] healthy Caucasians 9 healthy Samoans 9 healthy Maoris	Single bowel movements	Stool sample incubated anaerobically at 22°C for 22 hours, freeze-dried, ether-extracted, residue extracted with 80% ethanol and used in assay.	Differential killing of *E. coli* WP2 uvr+ Lex+ vs. uvr− Lex−. Assayed by colony formation after liquid incubation.	NA	Positive samples: 4/11 bowel cancer 8/20 Caucasians 2/9 Samoans 2/9 Maoris 0/18 SDA	No significant difference between Caucasians ($\pm$ bowel cancer) and Polynesians. SDA significantly lower than Caucasians.	Ferguson *et al.* (1985)

Faecal mutagens in healthy Finnish populations at different risk of bowel cancer	55 men and women from Kuopio (low-risk) 50 men and women from Helsinki ('intermediate' risk)	Single bowel movements	Stool samples incubated anaerobically at 37°C for 96 hours. Lyophilised, extracted from 0.1N NaOH with ether/hexane 1 : 1. Water absorbed on Preptube, then eluate fractionated on silica column; 2 particular fractions combined and tested.	Ames test: TA98, 100 ± Aroclor rat-liver S9	no	6/55 low-risk samples and 18/50 intermediate-risk samples gave MR >3 in at least 1 test condition (p <0.005). Mean mutants per plate for samples MR >3 not significantly different.	Authors point out that majority of donors with high faecal mutagenicity consumed diets low in whole-grain cereals and bread, suggesting a low-fibre diet. Lack of mutagenicity in some donors on low-fibre, high-fat diet may be due to inhibitors of mutagens in the gut.	Reddy *et al.* (1985)
Detection of faecal mutagenicity after ingestion of fried ground beef	1 Japanese man 1 Japanese woman 1 Caucasian man – all healthy	Donors abstained from cooked meat or fish from day 1. Meal of fried beef taken on day 4. Consecutive stool samples collected from days 3–8. No other cooked meat taken from days 5–8.	Aqueous extract treated with Blue Cotton, which was eluted with water and NH_3-methanol. Extract was evaporated, dissolved in water, and treated with Blue Cotton and passed through CM cellulose column	Ames test: TA98 + PCB-induced rat-liver S9	NA	Mutagenicity rose from almost zero on days 3 and 4, to high levels (MR 4–10, day 5) at days 5 and 6, and fell to previous low level by day 8. Extracts of the cooked meat were very mutagenic.	On the basis of HPLC studies, authors suggest that faecal mutagenicity is due to metabolites of mutagens which were present in the fried beef eaten by the donors, and was formed by pyrolysis of proteins and amino acids during cooking.	Hayatsu *et al.* (1985)
Development of modified Ames test for detecting faecal mutagens	Not reported	Single bowel movements	Aqueous extracts washed with dichloromethane	Modified Ames test: TA100; Aroclor Hamster-liver S9. Test-material placed in 9 cm^2 island in centre of plate, and ratio of these mutants to rest of plate is a measure of mutagenicity.	no	5/6 stool samples gave dose-related increases in ratio of island revertants to revertants on rest of plate. Different samples gave different slopes.	Authors claim that this method required less material to obtain a positive response than a standard pre-incubation plate assay. (The number of samples tested is not clear; no raw data are provided).	Shaw *et al.* (1985)

Cont'd

Table 17.1 (*Continued*)

Type of study	Number of donors, nationality, health etc.	Design and sampling	Extraction method	Assay method	Control for auxotrophic growth	Result	Remarks	Reference
Study of role of histidine in faecal mutagenicity assays	35 normal 10 inflammatory bowel disease 5 Crohn's disease 5 ulcerative colitis 4 carcinoma of rectum	Single bowel movements	Aqueous, 1 ml per g wet-weight faeces, with centrifugation and filtration.	Ames test: TA100, preincubation plate assay without S9	Yes: faecal histidine determined by HPLC	0/49 samples positive	Authors claimed that histidine was found only in faeces from donors with major gastro-intestinal disease	Silverman *et al.* (1986)
Baseline study of faecal genotoxicity in a single donor using 2 bacterial assays	1 healthy Caucasian man on Western diet. 6 samples collected over 5 months	Single bowel movements	Aqueous, 1 ml per 0.75 g wet-weight faeces, with centrifugation and filtration.	Microtitre fluctuation tests: TA100; *E. coli* WP2*uvr*ApKM101 aerobic and anaerobic. Also: SOS Chromotest.	Yes: faecal amino acids by HPLC. Bioassay with auxotrophic bacteria	5/6 positive in TA100, 6/6 positive in *E. coli*. Auxotrophic growth limited highest testable dose. 0/6 positive in TA100 (anaerobic); 6/6 positive in *E. coli* (anaerobic). 0/6 positive in SOS Chromotest.	Authors concluded that donor regularly excreted at least 2 kinds of water-soluble mutagens which were not detected in SOS Chromotests at 5× dose which gave positive results in fluctuation tests. Importance of allowing for auxotrophic feeding stressed.	Venitt and Bosworth (1986)
Pilot study of effect of high-fat or high-fibre diet on faecal mutagenicity	1 healthy Caucasian man on western diet.	Single bowel movements. 5 consecutive samples on normal diet; 4 consecutive samples in 2nd week of high-fat diet; 4 consecutive samples in 3rd week of high fibre diet.	Aqueous, 1 ml per 0.75 g wet-weight faeces, with centrifugation and filtration.	Mictotitre fluctuation tests: TA100; *E. coli* WP2*uvr*ApKM101	Yes: bioassay with auxotrophic bacteria	5/5 normal samples, 4/4 high-fat samples were positive in both strains; no significant difference between diets. 1/4 high-fibre samples positive in both strains. Difference in mutagenic activity between high fibre and other diets was significant.	Authors concluded that auxotrophic growth enhancement limited the usefulness of the fluctuation test, but could not account for fall in mutagenicity seen with high-fibre diet.	Venitt *et al.* (1986)

[a] MR is the mutagenicity ratio — the number of revertant colonies on treated plates divided by number of revertant colonies on control plates.
[b] SDA are Seventh-Day Adventists.
[c] SR is the survival ratio — the number of surviving colonies on treated plates divided by number of surviving colonies on control plates.
[d] DCM is dichloromethane.

agar plate containing glucose and a simple salts medium and is allowed to set. Plates are then incubated for 2 to 3 days at 37°C. The trace of histidine in the top agar allows the logarithmic division of the histidine-requiring bacteria in the presence of the test-compound and any of its metabolites generated by the S9- mix. This period of several generations of auxotrophic cell division is essential for the fixation of pro-mutagenic lesions in the DNA, and results in the formation of a lawn of histidine-requiring bacteria whose further division is prevented by exhaustion of histidine. Only that small fraction of bacteria which has reverted to histidine-independence (either spontaneously or by the action of the test chemical) will continue to divide to form discrete, visible colonies, each one of which consists of the progeny of a single mutant bacterium. The assay determines whether addition of graded doses of the test substance to a series of such plates induces a dose-related increase in mutant colonies compared with plates treated only with the appropriate volume of solvent. Parallel assays are performed both in the absence and presence of S9 in a series of tester-strains, each carrying a different mutation in the histidine operon. The strains most widely used in faecal mutagenicity studies are *S. typhimurium* TA98 (a frameshift mutant) and TA100 (a base-pair substitution mutant). A base-pair substitution tryptophan-requiring mutant of *E. coli* (WP2*uvrA*pKM101) is also used in assays of this type (Venitt, 1981; Dyrby and Ingvardsen, 1983; Venitt *et al.*, 1984).

(b) Critical features of the test. Although considered to be robust and sensitive, the *Salmonella* test can yield misleading results for a variety of reasons. Two are of particular importance when assaying faecal extracts. The first concerns the toxicity of faecal extracts. In order to detect induced mutation frequencies of the order of one in 10^6, it is necessary to ensure that the bacterial population is well in excess of this size by the end of the period of auxotrophic growth. Since the mutagen or its metabolites are likely to be most active during the first few hours of incubation, a large number of bacteria must therefore be present at the outset. If a faecal extract contains bacteriostatic or bacteriocidal constituents, it may reduce the size of the bacterial population to an extent which precludes detection of revertant colonies. Reducing the dose of the extract below the toxic level may not solve this problem, since it may also reduce the amount of mutagenic constituents below the detection level of the assay.

The second problem which may hinder the interpretation of data from *Salmonella* tests of faecal extracts is connected with the fact that although the test bacteria are entirely dependent on histidine (or in the case of *E. coli* WP2*uvrA*pKM101, on tryptophan) for growth in minimal media, they can use other biosynthetic precursors of the required amino acid to support auxotrophic growth. This is because the mutation which confers amino-acid dependence in each strain occurs at a step in the biosynthetic chain several stages before the production of the amino acid itself. Thus, growth can occur, for example, if *E. coli* WP2*uvrA*pKM101 (which carries a *trpE* mutation) is supplied with anthranilic acid or indole, or if *S. typhimurium* TA100 (which carries a *hisG* mutation) is supplied with phosphoribosyl-ATP. The occurrence in faecal extracts of these or other relevant biosynthetic intermediates may therefore increase the number of spontaneous revertants, not by mutation, but by generation of 'plate mutants'. These arise spontaneously, at a low level, at each round of cell division. The number of plate mutants is dependent on the final number of auxotrophic bacteria which grow on the plate, which is in turn dependent on the supplement of required amino acid (*or suitable amino acid precursor*) in the agar. In a mutation assay of a faecal extract of unknown composition, therefore, anything less than a doubling of the spontaneous number of revertants (i.e., the background established from plates treated only with the solvent) may be attributable to plate mutants generated by the presence of the required amino acid or its precursor rather than to the mutagenic effect of the extract. The presence of faecal amino acids or precursors at levels which produce more than a doubling of the background mutation is signalled by an abrupt thickening of the bacterial lawn which obscures any revertant colonies (see Silverman *et al.* (1986) for examples).

2. *Studies of High-risk and Low-risk Populations*

Ehrich *et al.* (1979) were the first to publish a full account of this approach. Using a single ether-extracted sample from each donor, they found that a significantly greater proportion (21%) of high-risk donors (white residents of Johannesburg) produced mutagenic faeces than age- and sex-matched low-risk urban (6%) or rural (2%) blacks. In the white group, more samples were mutagenic to TA100 than to TA98. Addition of S9 abolished the mutagenicity of faecal extracts. The pH of faeces from the black groups was significantly lower than that of the whites, a finding corroborated in later studies (Cummings, 1985; Samelson *et al.*, 1985; Walker *et al.*, 1986). The authors concluded that a population at high risk of bowel cancer excrete mutagenic faeces more frequently than did two low-risk populations.

Using similar methods (but 2-day pooled samples, and a more elaborate method of extraction), Reddy *et al.* (1980a) compared the faecal mutagenicity of three groups with different risks of bowel cancer. The percentages of mutagenic faeces were as follows: 13% in omnivorous residents of rural Finland (low risk); 0% in ovolacto-vegetarian Seventh-Day Adventists from New York (low risk); 22% in omnivorous New Yorkers (high risk). However, the *numbers* of positives in each group (0/11, 2/13, 4/18 respectively) were very low, and there is in fact no statistically significant difference between any of them ($p > 0.13$, Fisher's Exact test). The pattern of strain-specificity and requirement for metabolic activation (S9) suggested the presence of several different mutagens in the faeces of these donors.

Reddy *et al.* (1980b) extended this study by investigating the co-mutagenic properties of faecal extracts which the previous study had shown to be non-mutagenic. In this study, co-mutagenicity was determined by testing faecal extracts in the presence or absence of two potent mutagens, 2-acetylaminofluorene (AAF) with S9 or *N*-methyl-*N'*-nitro-*N*-nitrosoguanidine (MNNG) without S9, and subtracting the number of revertant colonies induced by each reference mutagen from the number induced by mutagen + faecal extract. The authors claimed on the basis of means of pooled data that New Yorkers' (high risk) faeces were more co-mutagenic than faeces from Seventh-Day Adventists (low risk), and suggested that co-mutagenicity could be used as a discriminant for colon cancer. This *enhancement* of mutagenicity of reference mutagens by faecal extracts must be contrasted with the *inhibitory* effects of faecal extracts on the mutagenicity of reference mutagens, demonstrated by Bruce *et al.* (1977) and in greater detail by Hayatsu *et al.* (1981a,b), who ascribed the inhibitory effects to oleic and linoleic acids. To add to the confusion, Silverman and Andrews (1977) showed that lithocholic acid and three of its conjugates enhanced the S9-mediated mutagenicity of 2-aminoanthra-cene. A detailed account of these conflicting findings was included in the review by Venitt (1982b), who could not resolve the problem, but urged caution in the interpretation of differences in the production of faecal mutagens by different risk groups until much more was known about enhancement or inhibition of mutagenicity by faecal extracts.

In a brief report of a preliminary study conducted in New Zealand, Ferguson and Alley (1982) determined the faecal mutagenicity of ether extracts of single samples from groups of Caucasians with or without bowel cancer, and from groups of healthy Caucasian Seventh-Day Adventists, Samoans and Maoris, the last three groups being at lower risk of bowel cancer than the former two. Of 83 samples tested, only two (both from bowel cancer patients) induced more than a doubling of the background mutation in *S. typhimurium* TA100, assayed in the absence of S9. Less than a doubling is generally considered to be indicative of a negative result, particularly so in the case of faecal extracts, bearing in mind the problem of plate mutants referred to in Section B1 (*a*). The proportion (5%) of high-risk Caucasians who produced mutagenic faeces is far lower than that found by Ehrich *et al.* (1979) in white South Africans (21%) or Reddy *et al.* (1980a) in white New Yorkers (22%), both populations considered to be at high risk of bowel cancer.

Results rather similar to those obtained by Ferguson and Alley (1982) were reported by Mower *et al.* (1982), who assayed single ether-extracted samples from 223 Hawaiian Japanese who were, on average, at four times the risk of bowel cancer than 166 Japanese residents of Japan whose faeces were also assayed. Only about 10% of the samples doubled the background mutation in at least one of the four test conditions (TA100 ± S9, TA98 ± S9). Of the 10% positive samples, significantly more were found in Japanese residents of Hawaii (high risk) than in Japanese residents of Japan (low risk), with the greatest differences seen in the frameshift mutant TA98, both in the presence and absence of S9. The authors concluded that the high-risk Japanese from Hawaii have more faecal mutagens than do the low-risk Japanese of Japan.

The marked differences in colon-cancer risk between different Scandinavian populations have intrigued epidemiologists and experimentalists for many years, and elaborate studies of these populations have been conducted (e.g. IARC, 1982). Reddy *et al.* (1985) chose two such Finnish populations from which to select age- and sex-matched groups of donors to provide faecal specimens. The high risk group (20 men, 30 women) came from Helsinki, where the age-standardized colon cancer incidence was 17.0 per 100 000, compared with 6.7 per 100 000 for the low risk group which consisted of 27 men and 28 women from rural Kuopio (the population sampled in the earlier study by Reddy *et al.* (1980a)). However, the data from the later study cannot be directly compared with those collected in the earlier one since the method of preparing the faecal extracts was different in the two investigations. In the later study (Reddy *et al.*, 1985) faeces were incubated anaerobically for 96 hours before being freeze-dried, extracted from 0.1 N NaOH and chromatographed on silica. This procedure was based on the work of Lederman *et al.* (1980), who showed that anaerobic incubation enhanced the mutagenicity of faeces collected from donors who regularly excreted mutagenic faeces and in some cases from those who did not. This was confirmed by Reddy *et al.* (1984) who showed that of 99 stool samples from 99 healthy New Yorkers living on a low-fibre, high-fat diet, 11 were mutagenic when extracted without the incubation step, the number of positives rising to 30/99 after 96 hours anaerobic incubation before extraction. Moreover, this incubation step increased the content of mutagens which required exogenous activation (S9) and which were active in both TA98 and

TA100, a finding not reported in the earlier study of Lederman *et al.* (1980).

The results of the investigation of rural and urban Finns by Reddy *et al.* (1985) (for faeces which received 96 hours anaerobic incubation) have been calculated from the percentages shown in Table 1 of that reference and are summarized in Table 17.2. There is no significant difference between the two groups in the excretion of mutagens which do not require S9 for their detection either in TA98 or TA100. There was a modest excess of positive samples detectable only in TA98 with S9 in the Helsinki group, and a highly significant excess in positive samples detectable in TA100 with S9, again in the group at higher risk of colon cancer. This contrasts with the findings of Ehrich *et al.* (1979) who found that about 21% of their high-risk white South African group produced faecal mutagens which did *not* require S9 to express their mutagenic activity (see above). There were significantly more samples which were mutagenic under at least one test condition in the Helsinki (higher risk) group than in the group from Kuopio. For those samples giving a mutation ratio greater than 3 there was no significant difference in the mean number of revertants per 200 mg dry faeces between the two groups. HPLC analysis of mutagenic extracts showed that mutagenic activity coincided with u.v.-absorption peaks eluting between 70 and 75% methanol : water gradients, with several different peaks of activity being discernible, depending on the bacterial strain and presence or absence of S9. Detailed analysis of the usual diet of the donors (by means of food tables) showed that

Table 17.2 *Numbers of stool samples from healthy donors from rural Kuopio and urban Helsinki showing mutagenic ratios greater than 3 in the Salmonella test (data calculated from Table 1 of Reddy* et al. *(1985))*

| | Samples with mutation ratios >3 | | | | |
| | TA98 | | TA100 | | Samples showing mutagenic activity in at least one test |
Population group	+ S9	−S9	+ S9	− S9	system
Kuopio (low risk)	5/55	14/55	4/55	28/55	6/55
Helsinki (intermediate risk)	12/50	19/50	14/50	28/50	18/32
p (χ^2 with Yates' correction), high risk > intermediate risk	0.079	0.241	0.012	0.744	<0.005

although there was no significant difference in the intake of total protein, fat or calories, the Kuopio group consumed significantly more dietary fibre (especially from bread) than the Helsinki group. The authors also claimed that, irrespective of which group they came from, men who consumed more than 28 g total dietary fibre per day, or women who consumed more than 24 g per day produced faeces which were not mutagenic as judged by a mutation ratio greater than 3.

3. *Studies of Cancer Patients and Controls*

Another way of establishing the relevance of faecal mutagens to human bowel cancer is to perform comparative studies of patients with bowel cancer (or preneoplastic lesions carrying a high risk of progressing to cancer) and matched controls who are known to be free of these conditions. However, this approach is beset with problems. For example, if cancer patients produce more faecal mutagens than do controls, or more cancer patients than controls produce faecal mutagens, it could be argued that this could be a result of the disease rather than related to its cause. If there is no difference between patients and controls, this might indicate that levels of faecal mutagens produced at the time of presentation of the disease are not relevant to its initiation, bearing in mind the long latency of bowel cancer and its multistep development.

Bruce and Dion (1980) drew attention to this problem in a brief report of a study in which they measured the mutagenicity of ether extracts of single stool samples in 17 colon cancer patients and 17 age-matched control patients who had haemorrhoids. There was no significant difference between the two groups, 7/17 patients and 9/17 controls producing faeces which were mutagenic to *S. typhimurium* TA100.

In a study conducted in New Zealand (already mentioned in section B2 (Ferguson and Alley, 1982)), faecal samples from 2/22 bowel cancer patients were mutagenic to TA100 without S9 (> 2 times background) compared with 0/18 from matched controls (not significant; $p > 0.2$, Fisher's Exact test).

Askew *et al.* (1982), in a study performed in Australia, found no significant difference in faecal mutagenicity between 16 colon-cancer patients and 35 matched donors without bowel symptoms and with negative haemoccult tests, 4/16 patients and 7/35 controls producing samples which were mutagenic to TA98 without S9.

Aqueous extracts of faecal samples from 35 control donors, 10 patients with inflammatory bowel disease, 5 with Crohn's disease, 5 with ulcerative colitis and 4 with carcinoma of the rectum were assayed in TA100 without S9. None of the samples was positive (Silverman *et al.*, 1986).

4. *Dietary Intervention Studies*

Although diet is accorded a central role in the aetiology of cancer of the large bowel, a causal relationship between any of the three most studied dietary variables—high meat, high fat and low fibre—has not been established conclusively (Doll and Peto, 1981; Kinlen, 1983; Armstrong and Mann, 1985). Manipulation of the diet, followed by assay of faeces for mutagenic activity, may be one way of approaching this problem. Several investigators have used this method, using either the *Salmonella* test or the fluctuation test as the method of assay.

(a) Faecal nitrosamines—do they exist?   Before considering dietary intervention studies in detail, it is necessary to discuss the still unresolved problem of the existence of faecal nitrosamines, and (if they do exist) their relevance to faecal mutagenicity and to cancer of the large bowel. This is necessary because Bruce and his colleagues (Varghese *et al.*, 1978; Bruce *et al.*, 1979; Bruce and Dion, 1980) claimed that *N*-nitroso compounds, formed by endogenous nitrosation of secondary amines by nitrite, were responsible for the mutagenic activity of organic-solvent extracts of human faeces, and that dietary supplementation with ascorbate and alpha-tocopherol (both anti-oxidants and inhibitors of nitrosation) reduced the mutagenicity of the faeces. These and other claims for the occurrence of *N*-nitroso compounds in human faeces (Wang *et al.*, 1978) were withdrawn after a very careful series of investigations established that there was no convincing evidence for the presence of nitrosamines in faeces from donors on a normal Western diet (Archer *et al.*, 1981; Eisenbrand *et al.*, 1981; Lee *et al.*, 1981; Saul *et al.*, 1981). However, this view has in turn been challenged by Suzuki and Mitsuoka (1981) who claimed, on the basis of methods known to minimize the chances of artefact formation, that Japanese individuals given a balanced Western dict (high fat, high meat) produced faeces which contained levels of several volatile nitrosamines which were about 5 to 10 times higher than those detected when the same subjects consumed a typical Japanese diet (rice, fish and vegetables). The precautions taken to prevent artefactual generation of *N*-nitrosamines were later found to have been insufficient. Using more rigorous methods these authors concluded that volatile nitrosamines do not seem likely to be present in significant amounts in human faeces (Suzuki and Mitsuoka, 1985). The un-named author of a concise review of these conflicting results summarized the position aptly: "Both the question of the presence of nitrosamines in faeces and (if they are present) of the implications for man have yet to be determined" (Anonymous, 1982). The extreme difficulty of measuring nitrosamines in

human faeces seems to have deterred further progress, at least as judged by the absence of any reference to faecal nitrosamines in a 1000-page book devoted to the occurrence, biological effects and relevance to human cancer of *N*-nitroso compounds (O'Neil *et al.*, 1984).

(b) Dietary supplementation with vitamins.   The claims of Bruce and his co-workers (Varghese *et al.*, 1978; Bruce *et al.*, 1979; Bruce and Dion, 1980) that addition of ascorbate and alpha-tocopherol to the diet reduced the level of faecal mutagens have been challenged. In a briefly-reported study using three donors, Wilkins *et al.* (1981) did not detect any changes in faecal mutagen levels following 3-week dietary supplementation with ascorbate or alpha-tocopherol (or combinations of these vitamins). These authors used HPLC and u.v.-spectrophotometry for detecting the major mutagenic fraction from organic-solvent extracted faeces. However, in a similar investigation, but using the *Salmonella* test instead of direct chemical measurement to determine the levels of faecal mutagenicity in a total of 20 donors, Dion *et al.* (1982) reported significant decreases in the mutagenicity of dichloromethane-extracted faeces from healthy donors given daily supplements of ascorbate and alpha-tocopherol. In the first experiment, a 55-year old man ate the same controlled Western diet every day for 2-week test periods, each test period being separated by a 3-week rest period on an uncontrolled Western diet. In the first test period he took a placebo capsule 4 times daily; in the second test period he took 100 mg each of ascorbate and alpha-tocopherol 4 times daily; in the third test period he took the placebo. Individual stool samples from the last 13 days of the test periods were collected and assayed for mutagenicity. There was marked variability in the mutagenicity from sample to sample in the control periods, as has been shown in many studies of human faeces (Venitt, 1982b). The mean value for mutagenicity fell to 21% of the first control value ($p < 0.001$) and rose to 40% of this value in the second control period ($p > 0.05$). A significant trend to decreasing mutagenicity with time was seen in the period when vitamins were taken. In a second experiment, one man and 18 women (22–28 years old, Caucasian) on self-selected Western diets were studied for 4 weeks. The first 2 weeks was the control period and in the second 2 weeks each donor took 400 mg of ascorbate and alpha-tocopherol daily. Stool samples were collected over the last 3 days of each period. Of the 19 donors, 11 were found to produce faeces which were mutagenic to widely varying degrees. From the figure provided in the paper, it appears that in 9 of the 11 mutagen producers there was a marked fall in faecal mutagenicity following the two-week period when the vitamin capsules were taken. The authors reported that the median level was 21% of the mutagenicity recorded before vitamin supplementation, with first and third quartiles

of 16% and 67%. Addition of vitamins to faeces after collection did not interfere with the extraction/assay procedure. Application of the HPLC/ u.v. method used by Wilkins *et al.* (1981) (*loc. cit.*) to the dichloromethane fraction used by Dion *et al.* (1982) in the study under discussion showed a fall to 45% of control values in the first experiment with the single donor, and a mean reduction to 38% for three donors in the second experiment.

This is the only fully-reported investigation of the effect of vitamin supplementation on faecal mutagenicity. The changes in faecal mutagenicity seen in some of the donors are dramatic, and as yet are not easily explainable in terms of a direct anti-oxidant effect, bearing in mind the anaerobic environment of the colon. The results are in conflict with those reported by Wilkins *et al.* (1981) who found no effect of dietary alphatocopherol and ascorbate on the output of faecal mutagens. However, the high degree of variability between individuals, the idiosyncratic response to vitamin supplementation reported by Dion *et al.*, and the fact that Wilkins *et al.* used only three donors may be a partial explanation of these discordant findings.

(c) Faecal mutagenicity, fried meat and mutagenic pyrolysates. It has been known for many years that the process of cooking produces mutagenic activity in a variety of foods, especially those with a high protein content. The pyrolysis products of proteins and amino acids are particularly well studied and several heterocyclic amines have been isolated from grilled (broiled) or fried meat and fish. These compounds are potent bacterial mutagens, and some are carcinogenic to animals (for recent reviews, see Nagao *et al.* (1985) and Sugimura (1985)). For example, fried beef is a source of 2-amino-3 8-dimethylimidazo[4,5-f]quinoxaline (MeIQ$_x$), which is a very potent frameshift mutagen which requires metabolic activation for its activity. Since a diet high in meat is thought to be associated with a high risk of large-bowel cancer, and fried meat is a known source of mutagens (and probably carcinogens), several investigators have thought it worthwhile to study the effects of meat on faecal mutagenicity. Two such studies, both of fried beef, have used the *Salmonella* test as the indicator of mutagenic activity. Another investigation of the effect of a diet rich in meat employed the fluctuation test and will be considered in section D.3.

Six healthy men and women (23–28 years old) provided 24-hour stool samples 2 weeks before starting a 3-week period during which they ate about 200 g of fried beef every day. The beef was fried 'medium-done' (brown outside, slightly pink inside). Laboratory tests indicated that the surface of the meat reached 175°C to attain this condition. Further weekly 24-hour stool samples were collected during the high-beef diet, followed by samples taken in the third and eighth week after cessation of the test diet. None of the partially-purified ether extracts from any of the donors showed any mutagenic activity in *S. typhimurium* TA98 or TA100, either in the presence or absence of S9. There was, however, an increase in the enhancing activity of faecal extracts on the S9-mediated mutagenicity of the reference mutagen 2-acetylaminofluorene (especially in TA98) which coincided with the start of the high-beef diet, and declined after cessation of the diet (deVet *et al.*, 1981). In a previous study from the same laboratory (Reddy *et al.*, (1980a), summarized in Table 17.1 and section B.2), 4 of 18 (22%) New Yorkers on a typical Western diet produced mutagenic faeces. The total lack of mutagenic activity of faecal extracts from the six donors on the high-beef diet is not too surprising, therefore; on average, 22% (1.3) of these six donors might have been expected to produce mutagenic faeces. The biological significance of the enhancing effect ('co-mutagenicity') of the extracts (previously reported in another study—Reddy *et al.* (1980b)) is not clear to this reviewer, as already discussed in Section B2 and Venitt (1982b).

With the benefit of more work on the generation of mutagens by cooking, and a study recently reported by Hayatsu *et al.* (1985a) it is possible to suggest further reasons why deVet *et al.* failed to detect mutagenic activity in faeces from people who ate nearly half a pound of fried beef every day for 3 weeks. Hayatsu *et al.* cooked ground beef patties (containing about 10% fat) to an internal temperature of 90–110°C. Two middle-aged Japanese (a man and a woman) and an American Caucasian man ate meals which contained no cooked meat or fish for 3.5 days. During the evening of the fourth day they ate 150 g (raw weight) of the cooked beef patties, and then abstained from cooked meat or fish from the fourth to the eighth day of the study. Each bowel movement from day 3 to day 8 was extracted and assayed for mutagenicity. Faeces (and samples of the cooked meat) were extracted with water which was then treated with 'Blue Cotton', a proprietary product consisting of absorbent cotton covalently linked with trisulphonated copper-phthalo-cyanine residues. This material is particularly suited to adsorbing from aqueous solution condensed aromatic compounds with 3 or more aromatic rings. The Blue Cotton was extracted twice with alkaline methanol which was evaporated, the residue being chromatographed on CM cellulose. Each fraction was assayed in *S. typhimurium* TA98 with S9. The faecal extracts contained sufficient oleic acid to inhibit mutagenicity (see Hayatsu *et al.* (1981a) and section B.2 above), but this was separated from the mutagenic activity by the CM cellulose chromatography. Faeces collected before the meal of fried beef were slightly mutagenic, but in each donor the activity rose very steeply after the meal, reaching a peak at day 5 (between 4 to 10 times the background level) and then declined to the level seen before the meal by the eighth day. Extracts of the cooked beef were highly mutagenic, 50% of the activity being accounted for by $MeIQ_x$. Analysis by HPLC of the mutagenic fractions isolated from faeces collected at the time of peak mutagenicity following the meal indicated that the mutagenic activity was probably due to metabolites of the mutagens present in the cooked meat, since the active components in the faeces showed an elution pattern which was different from the pattern given by the cooked-meat mutagens.

This study shows that faecal mutagenic activity resulting from ingestion of cooked beef is rather transient, and that its detection seems to require fairly elaborate extraction and fractionation methods in order to separate inhibitors (such as oleic acid) from mutagenic constituents. Moreover, the beef which was fed to the donors was shown to be mutagenic; the meat consumed by the volunteers in the study of de Vet *et al.* may or may not have been mutagenic. The factors which govern the generation of mutagenic activity during the cooking of meat have been studied in several laboratories, the general conclusion being that mutagen production increases with time and temperature of cooking (Övervik *et al.*, 1984; Knize *et al.*, 1985; Nagao *et al.*, 1985; Nilsson *et al.*, 1986). Other factors, such as the fat content and water content, may also be important. The precise degree of 'doneness' is clearly important when trying to interpret such studies, bearing in mind the strong dependence of mutagenicity on cooking time and temperature. Descriptions such as 'medium done' (de Vet *et al.*, 1981) or 'well done' (Hayatsu *et al.*, 1985a) or 'well done but not charred' (Knize *et al.*, 1985) may mean different things to people from different culinary backgrounds. In this regard it is instructive to inspect the excellent colour photographs provided by Övervik *et al.* (1984) to illustrate the degree of browning of lean pork associated with cooking temperature and the subsequent mutagenicity of extracts prepared from the meat. In that study, there was no significant mutagenic activity in pork cooked below a starting temperature of 200°C (pan temperature); the photographs show that at temperatures above 150°C the meat looked distinctly overcooked and unpleasant, and (as the authors suggest) would probably be rejected by most people.

The relevance to colon cancer of faecal mutagens derived from cooked meat is difficult to judge from just one well conducted study of three people. However, other investigations have shown significantly raised levels of *urinary* mutagenicity within a few hours following meals of fried meat (e.g., fried bacon or pork (Baker *et al.*, 1982); fried beef (Hayatsu *et al.*, 1985b; Sousa *et al.*, 1985)). Mutagenic activity of urine was found to decrease within 24 hours (compared with 2–3 days for faecal mutagenicity), although in some cases it remained elevated after this time. In the study by Baker *et al.* (1982) it was found that urinary mutagenicity levels were not increased in a volunteer who had eaten a meal of bacon or pork cooked in a microwave oven, emphasizing the importance of the browning process in the production of mutagens. These results show that mutagens derived from cooked meat are readily absorbed, enter the bloodstream and are excreted in urine, suggesting perhaps that sites other than intestine (e.g., stomach, liver, bladder, breast?) may be at risk from mutagenic insult. Epidemiological studies to test this idea are difficult to mount, bearing in mind the problems associated with obtaining reliable dietary information (Armstrong and Mann, 1985). Ikeda *et al.* (1983) conducted a cohort study of 7553 adult residents of Hiroshima and Nagasaki, with a follow-up period of about 11 years. Frequent consumption of broiled fish (a known source of mutagenic pyrolysates) was significantly associated with a slight excess of mortality from cancer at all sites and with stomach cancer. However, the authors did not consider their findings anything other than suggestive of an effect, and urged the need for further investigation.

Given that frying meat and fish at temperatures high enough to cause browning and charring produces mutagens and carcinogens, and that mutagens and carcinogens of diverse types have been detected in other foods and beverages (Grasso, 1984; Nagao *et al.*, 1985) it is timely to put the question posed by Burkitt (1980) in an essay on colon cancer and the high-fat, low-fibre hypothesis: "Are active carcinogens swallowed or are they formed in the colon?" He put forward the following answer: "The mucosal surface of the small intestine is over 100 times as great as that of the colon, yet both benign and malignant tumours are over 100 times as frequent in the large as in the small bowel; thus tumour risk relative to mucosal area is more than 10 000 times greater in the large than in the small bowel. Allowing for the fact that large-bowel mucosa appears more likely to undergo neoplastic change, this observation must suggest that the agents responsible for colon cancer are either formed or activated in the gut rather than being consumed in food in an active form and traversing the small intestine without modifying it." Protein and amino acid pyrolysates of the type found in fried beef are indirect mutagens, that is, they require metabolic activation in order to generate electrophilic metabolites capable of reacting with DNA. The human small-bowel mucosa contains mono-oxygenase activity (e.g., cytochrome P-450) of the type known to metabolize carcinogens (Hoensch *et al.*, 1982). These authors suggest that the presence of such enzyme systems in the small bowel affords protection from dietary carcinogens by biotransforming them to inactive compounds, thus preventing carcinogens from reaching the colon. However, the demonstration of mutagenic activity in faeces and urine following intake of indirect mutagens produced by cooking of normal foods argues against this simplistic model, and indicates that the ileal mucosa can absorb such mutagens and pass them into the bloodstream, possibly unchanged or as metabolites and, moreover, that mutagens can pass from the small bowel to the large bowel.

The colonic mucosa also possesses enzyme systems capable of metabolizing indirect mutagens and carcinogens to active derivatives. Fang and Strobel (1978) and Strobel and Fang (1981) showed that S9 prepared from the colonic mucosa of rats could metabolize 2-aminoanthracene and benzo(a)pyrene to mutagens detectable in *S. typhimurium* TA100, and that a human cell-line derived from the colon could hydroxylate benzo(a)pyrene, this mixed-function oxygenase activity being inducible with benz(a)anthracene. It is reasonable to suppose, therefore, that the normal human colonic mucosa is capable of metabolizing a variety of substrates to reactive derivatives. Whether or not compounds such as $MeIQ_x$ can be metabolized to mutagenic species in cells of the human colon remains to be determined, but there seems to be good evidence that compounds of this type can reach the colon via the faecal stream, and must therefore be of interest to those studying the influence of diet on cancer of the digestive tract.

C.   Fecapentaenes: Potent Mutagens formed in the Human Colon

1.   *Purification and Identification of Fecapentaenes*

One of the most interesting products of the fusion of modern analytical and synthetic chemistry with genetic toxicology is the isolation, identification and synthesis of a novel class of mutagens—the 'fecapentaenes'—found in human faeces. These discoveries arose directly from the original finding of Bruce *et al.* (1977) that ether extracts of human faeces contained directly-acting mutagens detectable in the *Salmonella* test. The structure of fecapentaenes was solved independently by two groups of investigators, one working in Toronto, Canada (Bruce and co-workers), the other in Blacksburg, Virginia, USA (Wilkins and co-workers). Both groups published their findings in 1982 (Bruce *et al.*, 1982; Hirai *et al.*, 1982), the term 'fecapentaene' being coined by Bruce and his colleagues, indicating that the compounds originate in the faecal stream and contain a pentaene moiety. More detailed accounts of the structural elucidation of these compounds have been published (Gupta *et al.*, 1983; Hirai *et al.*, 1985). Wilkins and Van Tassell (1983) described the frustrating work involved in isolating in a pure state a compound present in faeces in very small quantities and which is extremely labile in air, light and mildly acidic conditions.

Several factors helped in the identification of these elusive compounds. The first was that mutagenic fractions isolated by both groups of workers shared a very characteristic and intense u.v.-absorption spectrum, with maxima at 327, 340 and 358 nm (Bruce *et al.*, 1981; Wilkins *et al.*, 1980, 1981). This spectrum suggested the presence of a conjugated pentaene with a very high extinction coefficient (Bruce *et al.*, 1981; Kingston *et al.*, 1981), indicating that only very small quantities (micrograms per kilogram) of active product were present in faeces. A combination of u.v.-spectrophotometry, HPLC and *Salmonella* tests helped in keeping track of the active compounds. A second factor which aided the isolation of fecapentaenes was that both groups of workers discovered a small group of donors who regularly excreted faeces containing relatively high levels of the mutagenic fraction with the characteristic u.v. absorption. Bruce and his colleagues pooled samples from four such donors (Baptista *et al.*, 1984), whilst Wilkins's group obtained their material from a single individual (Hirai *et al.*, 1985). A key finding which both groups exploited was the substantially increased yield of mutagen which was obtained by incubating the faecal sample under anaerobic conditions for 96 hours at 37°C before extraction (Lederman *et al.*, 1980).

(a) Structure elucidation by Bruce and colleagues. Starting with about 2 kg of faeces, incubated anaerobically at 37°C for 96 hours, Bruce and his co-workers (Bruce *et al.*, 1982; Gupta *et al.*, 1983) fractionated this material with a combination of extractive chromatography with Florisil, followed by further chromatography on silica gel, Sephadex LH-10, preparative HPLC on silica gel and then reversed-phase HPLC, all performed under subdued light, under argon or nitrogen, and with antioxidant treatment with butylated hydroxytoluene (BHT). The fractions obtained from reversed-phased HPLC (about 8 or 9 peaks) were monitored with u.v.-absorbance at 340 nm and with *Salmonella* tests using TA100 and TA98. Four fractions were highly mutagenic, of which three eluted early and close to one another, and a fourth, which eluted later, was well separated from other material. The identity of the two major peaks (3 and 4) was established by nuclear magnetic resonance, HPLC/mass-spectrometry and gas chromatography of hydrogenated derivatives. Compound 4 was named fecapentaene-14, (1-(1-glycero)tetradeca-1,3,5,7,9-pentaene) having a chain-length of 14, and fraction 3 was named fecapentaene-12 (1-(1-glycero)dodeca-1,3,5,7,9-pentaene (Fig. 17.1)). It was suggested that compounds 1–3 were various geometrical isomers of fecapentaene-12. Pure fecapentaenes were highly mutagenic, yielding about 5000 revertants per 1 OD unit (about 1 microgram). The authors noted several difficulties encountered during the purification of fecapentaenes, including their extreme lability, especially in the pure

$$CH_2-O-CH=CH-CH=CH=CH-CH=CH=CH-CH=CH-CH_2-(CH_2)_n-CH_3$$
$$|$$
$$CHOH$$
$$|$$
$$CH_2OH$$

Fig 17.1. The structure of fecapentaenes as published by Gupta *et al.* (1983). For fecapentaene-12, $n = 0$ and fecapentaene-14, $n = 2$.

state, the variability of faeces from one donor to another, and the variability added by pooling faeces from several donors.

(b) Structure elucidation by Wilkins and colleagues. The group working in Blacksburg, Virginia (Hirai *et al.*, 1982, 1985) used a week's collection of faeces from a single donor. After anaerobic incubation at 37°C for 96 hours the material was freeze-dried, and extracted with hexane, the residue being extracted exhaustively with diethyl ether. The ether extract was subjected to silica-gel chromatography, followed by three successive HPLC separations, using normal phase, reversed phase and finally normal phase chromatography, resulting in two overlapping peaks as determined by u.v.-spectrophotometry. With the exception of the final step, all solvents contained the antioxidant BHT, which allowed the purification to be performed in an open laboratory. The identity of the mutagens was established by a combination of mass-spectrometry and gas-chromatography of hydrogenated compounds, and of acetylated, trimethylsilylated and methylated derivatives. The data suggested the presence of geometric isomers of the compound (hence the two overlapping peaks). Final confirmation of the structure of one of the isomers of the mutagen was made by NMR, and was designated as (*S*)-3-(1,3,5,7,9-dodecapentaenyloxy)-1,2-propanediol (Fig. 17.2), and was identical (except for stereochemistry) to the compound named as fecapentaene-12 by Bruce and his co-workers. Fecapentaenes isolated by the Blacksburg group (Hirai *et al.*, 1985) were very similar in mutagenic activity to the compounds isolated by the Toronto group (Gupta *et al.*, 1983), yielding about 2000–3000 revertants of TA100 per 1 OD unit.

(c) Collaborative study by both groups. Thus two different groups isolated faecal mutagens which were essentially identical in structure and properties. The only major discrepancy was that the Canadian workers (Gupta *et al.*, 1983) identified two different fecapentaenes (-12 and -14), whereas those working in Virginia (Hirai *et al.*, 1985) found only one (fecapentaene-12). This discrepancy was resolved in a joint publication from both groups (Baptista *et al.*, 1984). At least two stool samples were collected from donors whose faeces had been used previously in the

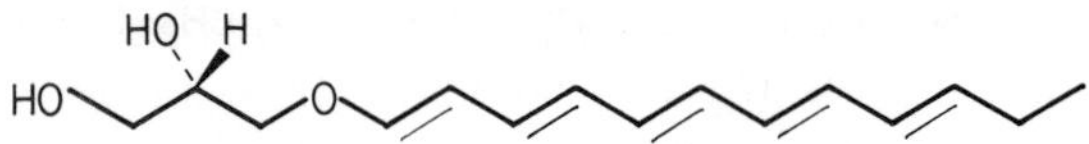

Fig 17.2.   The structure of fecapentaene-12, as published by Hirai *et al.* (1982).

studies leading to the identification of fecapentaenes by both groups. Omitting the preliminary anaerobic incubation, and using a modification of the purification method used by Gupta *et al.* (1983) and on-line HPLC u.v.-spectrophotometry, the relative proportions of fecapentaenes-12 and 14 were determined for faeces from each of the four donors. The results of this study showed that, although both types were produced by all the people studied, in some samples, fecapentaene-12 was present in large excess over fecapentaene-14 (a ratio of 20 : 1 was found in the donor who supplied faeces to the Blacksburg group), whilst other samples contained equal amounts of both compounds, or more fecapentaene-14 than fecapentaene-12. The fecapentaene-12/14 ratio appeared to be reproducible and characteristic for a particular donor.

(d) Origin of fecapentaenes.   In a series of studies performed before the identity of fecapentaenes was established, Wilkins and his colleagues had already shown that these mutagens were products of bacterial metabolism in the human colon. Mention has already been made of the observation that the level of faecal mutagenicity increased substantially following anaerobic incubation of faeces for 4 days at 37°C before extraction. This increase did not occur if antimicrobial agents were added to the faeces, or if incubation was performed in the cold, or if the faeces were heat-sterilized (Lederman *et al.*, 1980; Wilkins *et al.* 1980). During the 96 hour incubation, the pH of the incubate did not fall below 6.0. These results were highly suggestive of the involvement of bacterial metabolism in the increased output of faecal mutagens.

Subsequently, Van Tassell *et al.* (1982a) showed that bile and bile acids stimulated the production of faecal mutagen when mixed with human faeces followed by anaerobic incubation at body temperature. Bile was effective in stimulating mutagen production only with stool samples obtained from donors who regularly produced mutagenic faeces. Such faeces could be autoclaved and still retain the ability to support production of the mutagen when inoculated with a small sample of faeces from a mutagen-positive donor. Individual bile acids, with the exception of lithocholate and glycolithocholate, also stimulated faecal mutagen production. The levels of bile acids required to produce this effect were much higher than those normally found in faeces. The authors suggested that bile acids were unlikely to be precursors of the faecal mutagen because (*i*) even before identification of fecapentaenes, enough was known about their structure to predict that there was no structural similarity with bile acids; (*ii*) the amount of bile acids required to stimulate mutagen production was several orders of magnitude greater than the level of faecal mutagen; (*iii*) mutagenic activity was not obtained when bile broths were incubated with mutagen-positive faeces. On this basis, the authors stated their belief that bile acids most probably act by solubilizing a precursor, enabling bacteria to use it for production of mutagen. Alternatively, they suggested that bile supplementation resulted in selection for increased growth of bile-resistant mutagen-producing bacteria.

Further work on the production of faecal mutagens *in vitro* (Van Tassell *et al.*, 1982b) showed that of 40 anaerobic species of bacteria tested, five species of *Bacteroides* were capable of producing five- to eightfold increases in faecal mutagen when incubated anaerobically with broth which contained bile, a dilute faecal inoculum and a methanol extract of faeces from a mutagen donor. Mutagen production appeared to be constitutive and occurred over 3–4 days during the stationary phase of growth; autoclaved faeces produced results similar to those obtained with fresh faeces. Cell-free extracts of *B. thetaiotaomicron* strain ATCC 29184 produced the mutagen more rapidly than did intact cells (6–12 hours compared with 3–4 days). The authors noted that the mutagen-producing species of bacteria (*B. thetaiotaomicron, B. fragilis, B. ovatus, B. uniformis, Bacteroides* group 3452A) are among the most common in the human intestinal microflora, present both in mutagen excretors and non-excretors alike. They suggested that production of the mutagen by certain people is dependent on the presence of a precursor whose nature and origin is unknown. This work was summarized by Hirai *et al.* (1985) as follows: "... fecapentaenes-12 are produced by colonic bacteria, and certain conditions are necessary for mutagen production. These conditions include the presence of a precursor of presently unknown structure and origin, the presence of a sufficiently high concentration of bile acids, a pH above 6.0, and the presence of lysed cells of *B. thetaiotaomicron* or other related *Bacteroides* species ... These conditions, with the exception of the presence of the unknown precursor, are those that would be expected in the colon of an individual on a high-fat, low-fiber diet ...".

(e) Mode of action of fecapentaenes.   Fecapentaenes are directly-acting bacterial mutagens which are active at very low doses, and Gupta *et al.* (1983) suggested that their mutagenic potency was due to the ease with which a stabilized carbo-cation (carbonium ion) could be formed, invoking charge-delocalization as the stabilizing mechanism. This idea was elaborated in greater detail and tested in a model study performed by Gupta *et al.* (1984). They pointed out that the characteristic structural

feature of fecapentaenes is their highly unsaturated conjugated enol ether system. This is susceptible to hydrolysis by aqueous acid to an unsaturated aldehyde and glycerol. In this reaction, the acid protonates the enol ether to yield a carbo-cation, which itself is susceptible to further rearrangements and transformations. They argued that cation formation would be favoured by extended conjugation, since an increasingly conjugated system would be expected to delocalize the charge more effectively. Carbo-cations of the type postulated to form from fecapentaenes are highly electrophilic, and would be expected to react avidly with nucleophilic centres in macromolecules such as DNA, a property which is characteristic of most ultimate mutagens and carcinogens.

The authors reasoned that increasing the length of the conjugated polyenyl chain should result in a series of increasingly reactive and therefore mutagenic carbo-cations; i.e., they predicted that mutagenicity should increase concomitantly with increase in chain length. A series of methyl enol ethers of increasing polyenyl chain length (from 1 to 5 C=C bonds) was synthesized and tested for mutagenicity in TA100. In this series of analogues, the glycerol moiety of the fecapentaenes was substituted by a methyl group, on the grounds that it probably played no direct part in the postulated mechanism. In order to take account of the possibility that mutagenicity might be due to formation of aldehydes by acid hydrolysis of the methyl enol ethers, the series of corresponding aldehydes was synthesized and tested for mutagenicity. A set of *saturated* aldehydes of corresponding chain length served as a negative control for the experiment. Fecapentaene-14 and MNNG were positive controls. The results fulfilled the prediction that increasing the number of C=C bonds would be accompanied by an increase in mutagenicity. In both the enol ether series and in the unsaturated aldehyde series, analogues with 1 or 2 C=C bonds were inactive, those with 3 and 4 were active at doses ranging from 250 to 500 micrograms per plate, and those with 5 (as in fecapentaenes) were mutagenic at doses of 25 micrograms per plate (aldehyde) and 2.5 micrograms per plate (enol ether). As expected, the saturated aldehydes were not mutagenic. Of the compounds which were mutagenic, the enol ethers were consistently more active than the unsaturated aldehydes. The mutagenicity of the enol ether analogue with 5 C=C bonds was about 20% of that of fecapentaene-14, but it was much more toxic. These results showed that neither the glycerol nor the saturated moieties of fecapentaenes are necessary for their mutagenic activity. The authors suggested that these moieties may modulate the activity of fecapentaenes, for example by formation of an acetal from glycerol, or by influencing their transport across membranes. The general conclusion was that fecapentaenes act as alkylating agents via the formation of carbo-cations, and that these electrophilic intermediates react, by intramolecular or intermolecular linkage, with cellular macromolecules such as protein or DNA.

(f) Studies with synthetic fecapentaenes.   Fecapentaenes are present in human faeces at extremely low levels, and their extraction and purification is tedious, and results in a mixture of stereoisomers which is extremely labile (Hirai, 1982; Gupta *et al.*, 1983; Wilkins and Van Tassell, 1983). Clearly, a source of synthetic and less labile fecapentaenes would be of great value in detailed studies of their biological properties and their distribution in the human population. The first report of the synthesis of racemic fecapentaene-12 came from Kingston's laboratory in Virginia (Gunatilaka *et al.*, 1983). Their synthetic route yielded a racemic mixture which was identical to an authentic sample of fecapentaene-12 prepared and characterized as described by Hirai *et al.* (1982). Another synthesis of racemic fecapentaene-12 was reported by Nicolaou *et al.* (1984), who used a different synthetic route. Like the natural product, synthetic mixtures of *cis–trans* isomers of the fecapentaenes made by Gunatilaka *et al.* and Nicolaou *et al.* were found to be labile and therefore difficult to handle. Using a stereospecific synthetic route Pfaendler *et al.* (1986) described the synthesis of 1 g of a crystalline racemic stereoisomer of. fecapentaene-12, possessing the *all-trans* configuration in the olefinic portion of the molecule. This product proved to be stable for at least a month when kept under argon at room temperature. However, it decomposed completely within 30 minutes if exposed to air at room temperature.

Salmonella tests of *all-trans*-fecapentaene-12 (Göggelman *et al.*, 1986) showed it to be a potent mutagen, a dose of 5 micrograms per plate giving 8-fold and 6.5-fold increases in revertants in *S. typhimurium* TA100 and TA98 respectively. It was less mutagenic to TA102, a strain designed to detect mutations at AT basepairs rather than at GC basepairs favoured in the other commonly used strains of *S. typhimurium* and which detects a variety of oxidative mutagens (Levin *et al.*, 1982). Addition of S9 to the assay resulted in a large decrease in mutagenic activity in all three strains. A saturated derivative of *all-trans*-fecapentaene-12 was not mutagenic, in agreement with the results obtained by Gupta *et al.* (1984). The mutagenic activity of *all-trans*-fecapentaene-12 is of a similar order to that reported in earlier studies of the natural racemic mixture, strongly suggesting that *all-trans* isomer is a suitable example of a fecapentaene for studies of its biological effects in systems other than those relying on bacterial mutation.

Such studies are underway. Heat denaturation/renaturation assays of plasmid pBR322 linear DNA treated with fecapentaene-12 suggested the formation of DNA cross-links, a suggestion supported by electron microscopy studies (Harris *et al.*, 1985). In experiments using cultured human fibroblasts (Plummer *et al.*, 1986), a repair proficient line was more resistant to the cytotoxic and mutagenic effects of fecapentaene-12 at doses between 0.1 and 2 μM than a repair-deficient line (obtained from a patient with *xeroderma pigmentosum*). In both cell lines, fecapentaene-12 induced up to 10-fold increases in thioguanine-resistant mutants, indicating that this compound can induce point mutations at the hypoxanthine-guanine phosphoribosyltransferase locus in human cells and that excision-repair of fecapentaene-induced DNA adducts probably occurs. On a molar basis, fecapentaene-12 appeared to be 900 times more mutagenic than the potent mutagenic alkylating agent *N*-methyl-*N*-nitrosourea. Further studies showed that fecapentaene-12 induced dose-related increases in single-strand DNA breaks and sister-chromatid exchanges in human fibroblasts.

Pertel (1985) has advocated the use of the mini-pig as a useful species in which to study factors which govern the endogenous synthesis of fecapentaenes, having shown that certain pigs have the physiological and microbiological components necessary to synthesize fecapentaenes in their intestinal tracts.

D. Studies using the Fluctuation Test

It is evident from the foregoing review of results gained from the use of the *Salmonella* test that some investigators have had little or no success in detecting the frequency of faecal mutagen excretion claimed by others. This may mean that most peoples' faeces do not normally contain mutagens. On the other hand, it could indicate that the standard *Salmonella* test is unsuitable for detecting mutagens which are intrinsically weak or present in very low concentrations, or are mixed with constituents which kill the test bacteria or prevent them growing. Evidence that there is some truth in this latter explanation comes from the use of an alternative method of detecting mutation with amino-acid auxotrophs of the type used in the *Salmonella* test. This is known as the fluctuation test.

1. *Description and Critical Features of the Test*

(a) Description of the test. The type of fluctuation test used in studies of faecal mutagenicity was developed by Green and his colleagues (Green and Muriel, 1976; Green *et al.*, 1976) as a method for detecting low levels of mutagens or weak mutagens at non-toxic doses. The principle of the test is as follows.

A set of replicate, independent cultures of an amino-acid auxotroph is prepared with the initial viable titre set low enough to exclude relatively rare pre-existent revertants. The culture medium contains a small quantity of the required amino acid whose presence, during an overnight incubation, allows several generations of auxotrophic cell division, until the amino acid is exhausted. The next morning, selective medium, *containing no amino acid*, is added to each tube: incubation is then continued for several days, during which time only revertant (prototrophic) bacteria will be able to grow and divide. This luxuriant growth causes a drop in the pH of the medium which is detected by a colour change in an indicator dye added with the selective medium. The number of tubes which have produced revertants ('positive tubes') can thus be scored. The power of the test to detect small increases in mutation frequency increases with the degree of replication: 50 replicate cultures per test point have been found to be effective in most cases. In another form of the test, 96-well microtitration plates are used instead of tubes (Gatehouse and Delow, 1979).

In order to perform a fluctuation test, several sets of 50 tubes (or 96-well plates) are prepared: one serves as a zero-dose or solvent control (to give the background mutation), while each of the other sets receives a graded dose of the test chemical, which is added just before the period of auxotrophic growth. If required, S9 is also added at this stage, followed by incubation and challenge as described above. A statistically significant increase in positive tubes in treated sets compared with the control set shows that the treatment was mutagenic.

(b) Critical features of the test. Because of its high sensitivity to non-toxic levels of weak mutagens, the fluctuation test would appear to be ideal for detecting mutagenic activity in faecal extracts. However, this test will give a falsely positive result with any test material which allows extra growth of auxotrophic bacteria (Green and Muriel, 1976). As has already been explained (section B1 (*b*)), the material need not be histidine or tryptophan *per se*, but any precursor which the amino-acid requiring strain is capable of using for the synthesis of the required amino acid. Because the test is performed in liquid suspension rather than on agar plates, it is impossible to distinguish readily between true revertants and auxotrophs which have not been reverted (mutated) but continue to grow on the extra supply of nutrient supplied by the test material. Any faecal constituent which is capable of supporting the growth of the amino-acid auxotrophs used in fluctuation tests, and which is a constituent of the extract to be tested will render the test invalid unless steps are taken to account for this effect. Thus, simply measuring the amino acid content of extracts and applying a correction is not sufficient to control for the

effects of auxotrophic growth enhancement. This has been established in studies by Venitt and Bosworth (1983, 1986) and Venitt *et al.* (1986), who advocated the use of bioassay techniques for controlling for the confounding effect of auxotrophic growth enhancement on fluctuation tests (see section D3).

2.   *Studies of High-risk and Low-risk Populations*

Kuhnlein *et al.* (1981) used fluctuation tests to determine the mutagenicity of aqueous faecal extracts prepared from three different dietary groups: 12 omnivores, 6 ovo-lactovegetarians and 11 strict vegetarians. All samples were positive in TA100 and 28/29 were positive in TA98 at at least one dose. The range of concentrations of faecal extract (0.25–2 mg wet-weight per ml) giving positive results was about 100 times less than those used by Bruce *et al.* (1977) in assays of ether extracts with the *Salmonella* test, confirming the greater sensitivity of the fluctuation test. Using a non-parametric analysis of the pooled data obtained for each subgroup, the authors concluded that the mutagenicity of faecal extracts from non-vegetarians ranked significantly higher than the combined values obtained from the two groups of vegetarians, for both TA100 ($p < 0.01$) and TA98 ($p < 0.05$). Comparisons between the three separate diet-groups showed that non-vegetarians ranked higher than strict vegetarians or ovo-lacto vegetarians; the difference between non-vegetarians and ovo-lacto vegetarians was significant only for TA100. There was no significant difference between strict vegetarians and ovo-lactovegetarians. Correlation analysis of mutagenicity of extracts in TA98 and TA100 in relation to pH of the faecal homogenates and faecal mutagenicity suggested the presence of two or more faecal mutagens.

In a previous review of this work, the present author calculated the magnitude of the differences in mutagenicity between the various dietary groups (Venitt, 1982b). Slopes were calculated by linear regression of average number of mutants per tube against dose, giving values of mutants per microlitre of faecal extract, with the following results: strict vegetarians, range 0.12 to 1.65, mean 0.66; ovo-lacto vegetarians, range 0.3 to 3.33, mean 0.93; non-vegetarians, range 0.42 to 1.70, mean 0.92. This analysis, which assumed a linear relationship between the average number of mutants per tube and dose of faecal extract over the initial region of the dose-response curve, showed that there was not more than a 1.4-fold increment in the mutagenicity of non-vegetarian faecal extracts over faecal extracts from vegetarians. Moreover, as the authors themselves pointed out, the most mutagenic samples were found in the vegetarian diet-groups.

The authors excluded the possibility that their results could be explained by the effects of auxotrophic growth enhancement by performing reconstruction experiments with histidine and faecal extracts. They claimed that their results support the hypothesis that faecal mutagens are involved in the aetiology of colon cancer, on the basis that vegetarian diets are known to be associated with a low risk of cancer of the colon.

3. *Dietary Intervention Studies*

In a study designed to establish the variation in faecal mutagenicity among different individuals on identical diets, and between different samples from the same individual, Kuhnlein and Kuhnlein (1980) arranged two experiments in a metabolic unit in the University of California with two groups of six healthy men who were fed controlled formula diets for periods of up to 108 days. A liquid formula diet consisting of egg-albumen, malto-dextrine, corn-starch, sucrose, cottonseed oil, choline and essential vitamins and trace-elements was used. Fibre was provided in the form of raffinose and methyl cellulose. In experiment A, six men (aged between 24 and 27) were given this diet for 108 days; in experiment B, six older men (63–77 years old) were fed the diet for 47 days. Three-day pooled stool samples were collected as shown in Table 17.1. The mutagenicity of aqueous extracts was determined by the fluctuation test, using, in the first instance, a dose equivalent to 0.125 mg dry weight per ml of medium. The effects of growth-enhancement were controlled for as described in the previous study on vegetarians and non-vegetarians (see section D2 above and Kuhnlein *et al.* (1981)). The results showed that there was no statistically significant difference in mutagenicity of faecal extracts taken at three different times from the same individual, but there was considerable and statistically significant variation in mutagenicity between individuals. Three additional concentrations (0.03, 0.06 and 0.25 mg per ml) were then tested, which, together with the first dose, gave dose-response curves averaged for the three samples from each subject. In experiment A, three subjects gave consistently high levels of faecal mutagens, and three produced faeces with no detectable mutagenic activity in the dose-range tested (which was very similar to the range tested in the vegetarian/non-vegetarian study described by Kuhnlein *et al.* (1981)). In experiment B, two subjects produced mutagen levels similar to those of the high-mutagen group in experiment A, three were intermediate, and one donor produced no detectable mutagenic activity. All these results were obtained with TA100. A smaller number of samples were assayed in TA98: faecal extracts of two subjects found to be negative in TA100 were positive in TA98. There was a positive association between mutagenicity in TA100 and TA98. The variability in pH of faecal homogenates was greater between different subjects than between different samples from the same subject. Low pH seemed to correlate positively with high mutagenicity in TA100. This relationship between low pH and high mutagenicity contrasts with the observation that faeces of patients with large-bowel cancer have a higher pH than controls, and that the faecal pH of high-risk groups is higher than in low-risk groups (summarized in Cummings (1985) and Samelson *et al.* (1985); see also Walker *et al.* (1986)). It also conflicts with the results of Ehrich *et al.* (1979) who found a higher mean faecal pH and more faecal mutagenicity in a group of high-risk whites compared with groups of low-risk blacks (see section B2).

This dietary study showed that of 12 men fed on essentially the same rigorously controlled diet, eight consistently produced mutagenic faeces. The level of mutagenic activity varied from person to person, and these differences persisted even after 72 days of the dietary regime. The authors suggested that the physiological functions which determine the output of faecal mutagens are controlled by dietary habits of a duration much longer than that explored in their study, or that genetic factors might play an important part in determining the production of faecal mutagens.

Rather different conclusions were drawn by these investigators (H.V. Kuhnlein *et al.*, 1983) from a 5-week study of the effects of dietary modification on the mutagenicity of faeces from six donors. On the basis of this later investigation, the authors concluded that faecal mutagenicity can be altered in a 2-week period, and that at least some physiological factors responsible for faecal mutagenicity respond quickly to dietary changes. Five women and one man (25–35 years old) kept daily dietary records. A normal Western 'baseline' diet was eaten on days 1–7. During days 8–35, the volunteers consumed nutritionally adequate diets, without added vitamins or minerals, composed of regularly marketed foods in reasonable amounts. Upon this normal Western diet was imposed a 'low-risk' regime (days 8–21; whole-grain cereals and ovo-lacto-vegetarian items, but no meat) and a 'high-risk' regime (days 22–35; 5 oz meat daily (mainly beef) and refined grain products). Consecutive 24-hour stool specimens were collected at the end of each dietary period, two collections for the baseline period, three for the non-meat and meat periods. Aqueous extracts were prepared and assayed for mutagenicity in fluctuation tests with *S. typhimurium* TA98 and TA100. Free histidine levels were not measured in this study, however. All six subjects produced mutagenic faeces. When the data for all donors were combined and transformed by the Poisson distribution to give the average number of revertants per tube, dose-response curves resulted which were rather similar in initial slope and shape for all three dietary periods in both bacterial strains, especially at the lower doses. At higher doses, faeces from the high-meat period appeared to be more mutagenic than those from the baseline and non-meat periods, which did not differ from each other. Chi-squared analysis of the data obtained by pooling the total numbers of positive tubes at each dose and for each diet period revealed no significant differences between the baseline and non-meat periods. The high-meat period, however, produced significantly more positive tubes than the other two diet periods at the two highest doses when tested in TA100 and at the highest dose tested in TA98. At the lowest dose tested, the high-meat period produced more revertant tubes in TA98 than did the baseline diet. Analysis of the data by a non-parametric test for the significance of the direction of a change rather than its magnitude confirmed the χ^2 analysis, namely, that the high-meat diet led to a consistently higher average number of positive tubes than either the baseline or non-meat diets. Analysis of other measurements taken during the study revealed no significant relationships between mutagenicity, stool weights, frequency of bowel movements or pH of the faecal homogenates. On the basis of rank correlation analysis of their data, the authors claimed that the high-meat diet affected the spectrum of faecal mutagens as well as their overall levels.

Studies in the reviewer's laboratory (Venitt and Bosworth, 1983, 1986) have shown that the fluctuation test is very vulnerable to interference by auxotrophic growth enhancing constitutents in aqueous extracts of faeces, for the reasons discussed in section D1 (*b*). In these studies, auxotrophic growth enhancement was quantified by determining the extent to which faecal extracts could support the growth of auxotrophic bacteria. By interpolation of standard curves constructed by growing his$^-$ or trp$^-$ bacteria to their limit in graded amounts of histidine or tryptophan, 'growth windows' were calculated in terms of amino-acid equivalents. The growth-window defines the dose of faecal extract above which auxotrophic growth enhancement is likely to obscure mutagenicity and sets an upper level for the amount of faecal extract which can be assayed in a fluctuation test. Detailed study (Venitt and Bosworth, 1986) of aqueous extracts of six complete bowel movements collected from one male donor on a Western diet over a period of 5 months showed that levels of auxotrophic growth enhancement varied widely. All six samples contained enough histidine and tryptophan or their precursors to compromise the interpretation of fluctuation tests at the higher doses tested, i.e. at doses approaching or exceeding the growth window. Under aerobic conditions, 5/6 samples were mutagenic to *S. typhimurium* TA100 and 6/6 were mutagenic to *E. coli* WP2*uvr*ApKM101 when assayed in microtitre fluctuation tests. In a previous study of faecal extracts from the same donor, 4/5 contained levels of auxotrophic growth enhancers high enough to preclude mutagenicity assay. The remaining sample was mutagenic to TA100 (Venitt and Bosworth, 1983).

With these results in mind, an experiment was performed to examine the extent to which auxotrophic growth enhancement could compromise investigations of the effect of dietary manipulation on the output of faecal mutagens (Venitt *et al.*, 1986). A healthy non-smoking man, consuming a normal 'Western' diet (meat, vegetables, bread and alcohol) collected five consecutive complete bowel movements. He then added an extra 150 g of fat (from butter, cheese, milk, chocolate, peanuts, bacon, and eggs) to his daily diet for 2 weeks, and collected four further consecutive bowel movements in the second week. After 6 months on his normal diet, he added 30 g of wheat bran to his daily diet for 3 weeks, and collected four complete stool samples in the third week. Aqueous faecal extracts were prepared and assayed for auxotrophic growth-enhancement and bacterial mutagenicity (using fluctuation tests with *Salmonella typhimurium* TA100 and *Escherichia coli* WP2*uvr*ApKM101). There was no significant difference in faecal wet weight between 'normal' and 'high-fat' collections, but addition of 30 g brain to the diet was associated with a 1.8-fold increase in stool weight ($p = 0.04$), in good agreement with published data. Fluctuation tests showed that normal and high-fat samples were mutagenic to *S. typhimurium* TA100 and to *E. coli* WP2*uvr*ApKM101. There was considerable variation in mutagenic activity between consecutive bowel movements. There was no significant difference in mutagenicity between normal and high-fat samples. Faecal samples collected during the course of the high-fibre diet were significantly less mutagenic to both bacterial strains. This was especially noticeable in TA100, where only one of the four high-fibre samples was mutagenic (albeit weakly) compared with 9/9 mutagenic samples collected during the normal and high-fat diets. Changes in auxotrophic growth-enhancing activity could not account for these changes in mutagenicity, since the pattern of change in growth-enhancement was very different from that seen for mutagenicity. For example, for assays with TA100, the level of auxotrophic growth enhancement was significantly *higher*, but mutagenicity was very significantly *lower* during the high fibre diet compared with the normal or high-fat periods. The authors concluded that faecal extracts prepared from stool samples collected from this one donor during both the normal and the high-fat diet were mutagenic to about the same extent, and that addition of 30 g of wheat bran to the diet noticeably reduced this activity.

The simplest explanation for the decline in faecal mutagenicity during consumption of the high-fibre diet is that the increase in faecal weight which coincided with the addition of fibre simply diluted out a more or less constant amount of mutagenic activity. However, the simplest explanation may not be the true explanation, especially with regard to the effect of fibre on the composition of human faeces and the physiology of defaecation. This may be confirmed by reading a recent and comprehensive review by Cummings (1985) on the relationship between dietary fibre and cancer of the large bowel.

4. *Aerobic vs. anaerobic fluctuation tests*

In all the studies reviewed so far, mutation assays were performed under normal laboratory conditions, and the faecal extracts were therefore exposed to air for some considerable time, although steps may have been taken to exclude air during the extraction and preparation of extracts, for example by incubation of faeces under anaerobic conditions before extraction (see, for example, Lederman *et al.* (1980) and Ferguson *et al.* (1985)). However, in none of these studies were faecal extracts *assayed* under strictly anaerobic conditions. Since the *milieu* of faeces is anaerobic, it is possible that the mutagenic activity of faecal extracts is artefactual, being caused by oxidation of faecal constituents during extraction or assay. In order to test this possibility, Venitt and Bosworth (1983, 1986) compared the mutagenicity of samples of aqueous faecal extracts which had been prepared and assayed aerobically or anaerobically. In the first study (Venitt and Bosworth, 1983) the product of a complete bowel movement from a healthy man consuming a normal Western diet was collected and homogenized with an equal weight of degassed water under anaerobic conditions. Half of the homogenate was centrifuged, filtered and stored anaerobically. The other half was exposed to air by further homogenization in a conventional air-flow safety cabinet, centrifuged, filtered and stored with precautions to exclude air. Bioassay of this sample showed that the level of auxotrophic growth enhancement was low enough to avoid false-positive mutagenicity results due to feeding (see sections D1 (*b*) and D3). Experiments with reference mutagens showed that microtitre fluctuation tests performed with *S. typhimurium* TA100 and *E. coli* WP2*uvr*ApKM101 from start to finish in an anaerobic enclosure were feasible, reproducible, and slightly more sensitive than assays performed under aerobic conditions.

Using *S. typhimurium* TA100, positive results were obtained only in assays conducted under aerobic conditions, irrespective of whether the sample had been extracted aerobically or anaerobically. Even a brief exposure of an anaerobic sample to air, followed by assay in air produced a positive result. Conversely, an aerobic sample proved negative when assayed anaerobically. The absence of mutagenic activity in an aqueous faecal extract prepared and assayed anaerobically stood in sharp contrast to the reproducible mutagenicity of the same stool sample which had been extracted and assayed aerobically. In the absence of any other experiments, it might have been concluded that the mutagenicity of the aerobically extracted and assayed sample depended on the presence of air, and that the mutagenic constituent or constituents was or were products of oxidation. This suspicion was apparently confirmed in the experiment where an anaerobic sample already shown not to be mutagenic when assayed anaerobically became, on brief exposure to air, mutagenic when assayed aerobically. The finding that under anaerobic conditions there was no mutagenic activity in material which had been exposed to air almost from the time of its collection, and which was reproducibly mutagenic when assayed under conventional aerobic conditions was unexpected and difficult to explain. The authors speculated that the mutagenic constituent(s) may be reversibly oxidized or reduced, or that non-mutagenic, reduced compounds could be converted by aerobic bacterial metabolism to active mutagens. The results of this very small-scale study illustrate the substantial variations in experimental data which can result simply by changing the conditions of extraction and assay of material as complex as human faeces.

In a second study (Venitt and Bosworth (1986), referred to in section D3), aqueous extracts of six complete bowel movements collected anaerobically from one donor on a Western diet over a period of 5 months were assayed aerobically and anaerobically in fluctuation tests using *S. typhimurium* TA100 and *E. coli* WP2*uvr*ApKM101. Within the limits set by growth windows established by bioassay, 5/6 samples were positive in *S. typhimurium* TA100 when assayed aerobically, but none were positive when assayed anaerobically. In *E. coli* WP2*uvr*ApKM101, 6/6 samples were positive under both conditions of assay, the anaerobic dose-response curves being markedly non-linear. The authors suggested that this donor regularly excretes faeces which contain at least two classes of directly-acting mutagens: (*i*) those which are detectable in *S. typhimurium* TA100 and which are mutagenic only in the presence of air, and (*ii*) those which are detectable in *E. coli* WP2*uvrA*(pKM101) and which are active both aerobically and anaerobically. Whether or not these distinct classes of mutagenic activity can be understood in terms of different modes of DNA reaction is, for the moment, a matter of speculation. However it is worth noting that the *his*G46 histidine mutation in *S. typhimurium* TA100 is a GC base-pair substitution (Maron and Ames, 1983) (and would be expected to favour detection of reaction at GC basepairs) whilst the *trpE* mutation in *E. coli* WP2 strains is an *ochre* mutation (AT basepair substitution (Green and Muriel, 1976)) favouring detection of reaction at AT basepairs. These results, though limited in scope, suggest that faeces might contain substances which remain non-mutagenic in the highly reducing conditions within the lumen of the bowel. Should such substances reach the interior of mucosal cells lining the bowel, the aerobic conditions prevailing in these cells might be sufficient to oxidize potential mutagens to active mutagens.

E. Studies using DNA-Repair Tests in Bacteria

It is clear that both the *Salmonella* test and the fluctuation test are subject to a variety of problems when used in assays of faecal extracts. One method of avoiding these problems without losing the advantages of speed and economy afforded by the use of bacteria as test organisms is to use DNA repair instead of reverse mutation as an end-point. However, direct chemical measurement of DNA repair is technically demanding and time-consuming, and indirect methods of assaying for this manifestation of genotoxic activity have been developed.

1. *The Differential Survival Test using Bacteria*

(a) Description of the test.   Several different genetically controlled routes of DNA repair are invoked when bacteria are treated with genotoxic agents (Kenyon, 1983; Tweats *et al.*, 1984; IARC, 1986). Strains of bacteria which are mutant in one or more of these repair genes are available, and are more susceptible to the lethal effects of DNA damage than bacteria which are wild-type with respect to DNA repair. Stimulation of DNA repair, and hence production of DNA damage, can be inferred, therefore, by observing a difference in survival between two strains of bacteria which are isogenic save for genes which govern proficiency in DNA repair. There are several different ways of conducting these assays and a multiplicity of different strains have been used in them. The simplest (but not necessarily the best) method is to spread each of a pair of nutrient agar plates with an inoculum of the chosen bacterial strains, one plate receiving the repair$^+$ strain, the other the repair$^-$ strain. An equal dose of the test agent is applied to the centre of each plate (either in a well cut into the agar, or on a small paper disc), and the plates are then incubated to allow growth of the bacteria. The test is regarded as positive if the diameter of the zone of inhibition (a clear circle in the bacterial lawn) is significantly greater in the repair$^-$ strain than in the repair$^+$ strain. The assay is carried out at several doses, and S9 can be incorporated as in the *Salmonella* test. A streak of test agent, rather than a spot, is used in some versions of this test, in order to provide a longer concentration gradient across the plate. Liquid incubation assays have

also been described where the pairs of strains are separately incubated in suspension culture with graded doses of test agent, with or without S9. After incubation, aliquots are serially diluted and plated out for determination of viable counts by colony assay. A significant reduction in survival of colony-forming ability in the repair⁻ strain is taken as evidence for genotoxic activity. In a simplified version of this test, cell growth is monitored by turbidimetric measurements instead of by colony assay.

(b) Critical features of the test.   Indirect assays for DNA repair are subject to a variety of unresolved technical problems which limit their usefulness as primary screens for potential carcinogens and mutagens (Leifer *et al.*, 1981; Tweats *et al.*, 1984). Problems which must be borne in mind when evaluating data from studies of human faecal extracts include: different growth rates in DNA-repair⁺ and repair⁻ strains can give false results; anomalous results have been obtained for agents which are known to require metabolic activation for genotoxic activity but which are positive in the absence of such activation in DNA-repair tests; 'spot-tests' which depend on diffusion of test material through agar are insensitive, especially to insoluble materials and give tests which are often uninterpretable; failure to use isogenic strains can invalidate assays.

2.   *Results of Studies using the Differential Survival Test*

In a study of 8 lactovegetarians and 11 omnivores, Nader *et al.* (1981) collected a 24-hour faecal sample from each donor and prepared ethanol or dimethylsulphoxide (DMSO) extracts from the freeze-dried material. Spot-test assays were conducted in *S. typhimurium* TA1978 (excision-repair⁺) and TA1538 (excision-repair⁻), using ratios of inhibition-zone diameters as the measure of differential killing in the two strains. Analysis of pooled data showed that for omnivores, inhibition zones were significantly greater (by 30% for DMSO extracts and 41% for ethanol) in the repair-deficient strain than in the repair-proficient strain, suggesting the presence of DNA-damaging agents in these extracts. In the vegetarians, there was no significant difference in the diameters of zones between the two strains for either of the two kinds of extracts. However, the mean diameter of inhibition-zones caused by vegetarians' extracts approximated to the mean of those seen in the repair-*deficient* strain after treatment with omnivores' extracts, rather than to that in the repair-proficient strain. This effect is difficult to interpret as an *absence* of DNA-damaging activity, since this is normally signalled by zones of inhibition which are characteristic of the repair-proficient strain. The authors concluded that this anomalous result was probably due to bacterial toxicity unconnected with DNA damage, and that their data showed that faeces from subjects eating a mixed diet contained more DNA-damaging agents than faeces from vegetarians.

In the investigation of high and low risk Japanese conducted by Mower *et al.* (1982), in addition to the *Salmonella* test already described in section B2, aqueous extracts of the ether-extracted residue of single stool samples were assayed in a differential killing test. Two strains of *E. coli*, one rec^+ (repair-proficient) and the other rec^- (repair-deficient) were used in a spot test. The diameter of the inhibition zone in the repair$^+$ strain was subtracted from that in the repair$^-$ strain, and a test was scored positive if the net zone of inhibition was equal to or greater than 2 mm. By this criterion, 36/152 low-risk samples and 68/202 high risk samples were positive ($p = 0.0545$, corrected χ^2). This level of significance was maintained after adjustment for age and sex.

The use of spot-tests for assaying faecal extracts for differential killing of *E. coli* WP2 and its triple repair-deficient partner CM871 (*uvrA recA lexA*) was discarded in favour of a test using liquid suspension and colony assay by Ferguson *et al.* (1985) because many of the ethanol extracts used in this study did not diffuse adequately through the agar. In this study, ethanol extracts from ether-extracted freeze-dried stools which had been incubated anaerobically at 22°C for 24 hours before extraction were prepared from 20 Caucasians, 11 Caucasians with bowel cancer, 9 Samoans, 9 Maoris and 18 Seventh-Day Adventists. A sample was considered positive if it gave an effect at two or more dose levels and gave a greater than fourfold difference in survival at both doses (Tweats *et al.*, 1984). The authors showed that faecal extracts had growth-enhancing properties which might have affected the interpretation of differential killing. However, there was no significant difference in growth-enhancement between faeces from the different study groups, and the use of the triple mutant minimized the possibility of poor growth in the repair-deficient strain (Tweats *et al.*, 1984). Positive results were obtained in 4/11 bowel-cancer patients, 8/20 controls, 2/9 Samoans, 2/9 Maoris, and 0/18 Seventh-Day Adventists. With the exception of the results for Seventh-Day Adventists, the differences in differential killing activity between faeces from the various groups were not significant ($p > 0.2$, Fisher's Exact test). The difference between Seventh-Day Adventists (who were presumably Caucasian) and the other Caucasian groups was highly significant ($p < 0.01$). The authors concluded that diet can reduce the level of ethanol-soluble mutagens in New Zealand Caucasians (Europeans), since the Seventh-Day Adventists were ovo-lacto-vegetarians, whereas all the other groups were omnivorous.

3. *The SOS Chromotest*

Another way of inferring DNA damage in bacteria is to monitor the induction of the 'SOS' system, which promotes DNA repair, mutagenesis and other functions. This system consists of a set of subordinate (damage-inducible (*din*)) genes which are repressed by a single repressor (*lexA* protein) and which are switched on (derepressed) by another protein (*recA*) in response to DNA damage (Kenyon, 1983). Fusion of the operator region of a *din* gene to the coding sequence of a gene whose product is more easily assayed (such as the *lac*Z beta-galactosidase gene) produces a bacterial strain which responds to DNA damage by switching on synthesis of beta-galactosidase to a level which is related to the amount of DNA damage and thus to the dose of the genotoxic agent. The SOS Chromotest (Quillardet *et al.*, 1982, 1985, Quillardet and Hofnung, 1985) is the best known and most extensively validated example of this type of test. It uses *E. coli* PQ37, which contains an operon-fusion between a *din* gene (*sfiA*) and the *lac*Z gene (beta-galactosidase). In addition, it is constitutive for alkaline phosphatase, and is DNA-repair deficient (*uvrA*). Graded doses of the test agent are added to broth cultures of the bacterium, and after 2 hours' incubation, beta-galactosidase and alkaline phosphatase activity are measured colorimetrically. The alkaline phosphatase measurement gives an indication of toxicity, (a decline in activity signalling a decline in general protein synthesis) and the level of beta-galactosidase activity represents the level of SOS induction, hence DNA damage. The test is rapid (< 1 day), the SOS response occurs in mass culture, and unlike mutation tests, does not require the survival of the treated bacteria to detect a positive response. Venitt and Bosworth (1986) and Bosworth and Venitt (1986) have explored the use of the SOS Chromotest for detecting genotoxic activity in aqueous faecal samples as an alternative to the fluctuation test.

In the study referred to in sections D3 and D4 (Venitt and Bosworth, 1986), in which six faecal samples were collected from one man over 5 months, none of the aqueous faecal extracts which had given positive results in fluctuation tests were positive in the SOS Chromotest. This was not due to interference by faecal constituents, since the reference mutagen 4-nitroquinoline-*N*-oxide (4NQO) gave similar results whether tested in the presence or absence of faecal extract. In continuing studies of stool samples from five other donors it has been found that of the many extracts which give positive results in fluctuation tests employing reverse mutation, none were positive in the SOS Chromotest (Venitt and Bosworth, 1986, unpublished data). These results suggest that the SOS Chromotest is less sensitive to the genotoxic effects of aqueous faecal extracts than the fluctuation test. Quillardet *et al.* (1985) showed that there is a quantitative relationship between potency in the SOS Chromotest and potency in the *Salmonella* test, for a wide range of mutagens and carcinogens. However, it is generally accepted that the fluctuation test is more sensitive than the standard *Salmonella* test, especially to weak mutagens. It is possible therefore that the amounts of faecal extracts assayed in the SOS Chromotest were too low to evoke a positive response, even though the highest doses tested were over 5 times the dose at which positive responses were evident in aerobic fluctuation tests. Another explanation might lie in the nature of the faecal mutagens detected by fluctuation tests. In the SOS Chromotest the occurrence of DNA damage is inferred by measuring the induction of the SOS response. Clearly, agents which, although mutagenic, do not provoke this repair pathway, will not be detected. For example, nitrous acid, which is a deaminating agent, or hydroxylamine, which specifically attacks the 4-amino group of cytosine, are unlikely to induce SOS repair. Perhaps the faecal mutagens detected in fluctuation assays are compounds of this type, rather than those which form adducts with DNA.

Further studies (Bosworth and Venitt, 1986) showed that faecal extracts contained levels of beta-galactosidase and alkaline phosphatase sufficient to compromise the SOS Chromotest. It was recommended, therefore, that when the Chromotest is applied to biological samples, the following precautions should be taken: (*i*) the test material should be assayed for endogenous alkaline phosphatase and beta-galactosidase activity, (*ii*) a washing step should be included to minimize the effects of endogenous enzyme activity, and (*iii*) account should be taken of the presence of adventitious enzyme activity when calculating and interpreting results of assays.

F. Studies using Chromosomal and Nuclear Damage

1. *Chromosomal Anomalies in Cultured Mammalian Cells*

Short-term tests using induction of chromosomal anomalies in cultured mammalian cells are firmly established as useful predictors of mutagenic and carcinogenic activity (Preston *et al.*, 1981; IARC 1986). The advantages and disadvantages of such tests are fully discussed in IARC (1986).

Stich and Kuhnlein (1979) used the induction of chromosomal damage in cultured Chinese hamster ovary cells (CHO cells) as an indicator of genotoxic activity of human faecal extracts. Chloroform/methanol extracts of aqueous faecal slurries obtained from three healthy donors were applied to CHO cells for 3 hours at 37°C. The medium was changed, and the cells were incubated for a further 20 hours. The frequency of metaphases which contained breaks, acentric fragments and exchanges was significantly increased in cells treated with these extracts. The extent of chromosomal damage was dose-related and varied between individuals and between stool samples from the same individual. Induction of chromosomal aberrations was enhanced by divalent copper or manganese ions, and inhibited by divalent or trivalent iron. Addition of catalase to the faecal extracts reduced the frequency of damage. The enhancement of damage by copper and manganese, and its reduction by iron and catalase, suggested to the authors that the genotoxic agents in faeces might be reducing agents, since it had been previously shown that cysteine and glutathione caused chromosomal aberrations in CHO cells in similar conditions.

Using the same cell-line and method of assay, Barnes and Powrie (1982) investigated the clastogenic effects of faecal extracts from four people on a Western diet. The extraction method used was based on procedures for isolating faecal steroids in a neutral/basic fraction and an acidic fraction after saponification with KDOH. The acid fraction was expected to contain acid steroids, pure samples of which were also assayed for clastogenic activity. The neutral/basic fraction was negative. Acid fractions from two of the four donors gave dose-related increases in exchanges and in percent of aberrant metaphases. Statistical analyses of the data were not reported. Addition of S9 did not enhance the clastogenic activity. The authors claimed that their data indicated the presence of a third category of faecal genotoxin (the other two being (*i*) the water-soluble clastogen reported by Stich and Kuhnlein and (*ii*) the ether-soluble bacterial mutagen originally discovered by Bruce and his co-workers in 1977). Of several bile acids tested, only ursodeoxycholic gave dose-related increases in chromosomal aberrations (including exchanges) even at non-toxic doses. Although S9 enhanced this activity, the authors concluded that this was due to a physical rather than to an enzymic effect.

2. *Nuclear Damage in Colonic Cells of Mice Treated* in vivo

Short-term tests conducted *in vivo* are much more time-consuming and expensive than *in-vitro* tests, and their use in the study of faecal genotoxicity has been limited to just one published study (Suzuki and Bruce, 1984). This employed the quantitative assessment of nuclear aberrations in the colonic epithelium of mice after intrarectal instillation administration of faecal extracts. Earlier studies (Wargovich *et al.*, 1983) with carcinogens specific for the mouse colon (such as 1,2-dimethylhydrazine, 2,2'-dioxo-di-*N*-propylnitrosamine, 3,2'-dimethyl-4-

aminobiphenyl) showed that oral intubation of mice with these compounds caused dose-related increases in nuclear aberrations, whereas non-carcinogenic structural analogues did not. Intrarectal instillation of *N*-nitroso-*N*-methylurea, a directly acting carcinogen, was also positive in this test. Nuclear anomalies scored included micronuclei, pyknosis and karyorrhexis.

Faecal extracts from 10 adult Caucasian donors on a Western diet were prepared by the method of Gupta *et al.* (1983) previously used for isolating fecapentaenes, but omitting the HPLC steps (see section C1). Groups of 10 male C57BL/6 mice were used for each faecal extract, which was given by intrarectal instillation; 24 hours after treatment the mice were killed and their colons were removed for histological preparation and enumeration of nuclear anomalies. Only the dichloromethane fraction proved to be active in this test, faeces from two of the 10 donors giving dose-related and statistically significant increases in nuclear aberrations. The authors suggested that the active samples contained colon carcinogens, on the basis that their previous work had shown that the test was reasonably specific for such agents. They also concluded that fecapentaenes were not responsible for the activity found in the nuclear anomaly test, since they did not detect the characteristic u.v. spectrum of fecapentaenes in HPLC analysis of active fractions.

G. Are Bile Acids Genotoxic?

Hill *et al.* (1971) speculated, on the basis of a study of the bacterial flora and steroid content of faeces from groups at different risk of colon cancer, that intestinal bacteria may be aetiologically related to cancer of the large bowel via bacterial steroid metabolism (see also Thompson (1982)). This raises the question: are bile acids genotoxic?

Several different studies in which a variety of bile acids were assayed in the *Salmonella* test have proved uniformly negative. Silverman and Andrews (1977) tested 30 different bile acids in eight strains of *S. typhimurium* using a dose of 500 micrograms per plate; none was positive. Macdonald *et al.* (1978) assayed a variety of saturated bile acids at doses of 10^{-3} M and 10^{-4} M, including cholate, deoxycholate, chenodeoxycholate and lithocholate, again with negative results. More recently, McKillop *et al.* (1983) showed that 20 C-24, C-22 and C-19 bile acid derivatives (many of which were unsaturated) were negative in the *Salmonella* test. Bile acids are toxic to *S. typhimurium* at doses above about 0.5 mg per plate. As described in secton D1 (*a*), the fluctuation test is much more sensitive to weak mutagens at non-toxic doses than the *Salmonella* test. For this reason, Watabe and Bernstein (1985) tested cholic acid, chenodeoxycholic acid, deoxycholic acid, ursodeoxycholic acid and lithocholic acid in fluctuation tests with *S. typhimurium* TA98 and TA100 in the absence of S9, and in the *Salmonella* test with and without S9. They obtained negative results in the *Salmonella* test at doses between 20 and 500 micrograms per plate, in agreement with earlier results. However, dose-related and statistically significant increases in the numbers of positive tubes were obtained with cholic acid, chenodeoxycholic acid, deoxycholic acid, and ursodeoxycholic acid, in TA98 and TA100 at doses between 10 and 50 micrograms per plate. The results suggested to the authors that on a molar basis, these bile acids were about one quarter as potent as methyl methanesulphonate, one of their positive-control mutagens. The authors point out that the mutagenicity of bile acids resembles that of the faecal extracts assayed by Kuhnlein *et al.* (1981) (see sections D2 and D3). They suggested that water soluble faecal mutagens consist mainly of bile acids and that these may be a major cause of colon cancer. These claims deserve close scrutiny, bearing in mind the ubiquity and quantity (mg per g dry-weight) of bile acids in human faeces.

The authors provide raw data for triplicate experiments, in separate tables (their Tables 1 and 2) for TA98 and TA100. There is very close agreement in the number of positive tubes between each experiment at each dose. The extent to which the proportions would be expected to agree in three replications of experiments which produce binominal data (positive or negative tubes in this case) can be assessed using the standard test for homogeneity of proportions (Breslow and Day, 1980). The test statistic is referred to the chi-squared distribution with 2 degrees of freedom (e.g., for the controls in Table 1 of Watabe and Bernstein, χ^2 = 0.872). If all 22 test statistics in Table 1 are summed, the resulting value 22.55 can be referred to the chi-squared distribution on 44 degrees of freedom (since the sum of independent chi-squared distributions is itself a chi-squared distribution). This value corresponds to the *lower* 0.3% point on the chi-squared distribution, that is, $p = 0.003$. Analysis of Table 2 of Watabe and Bernstein gives a summed chi-squared distribution of 16.8 with 44 degrees of freedom, p (lower tail) = 0.00007. Combining the data from both tables gives a value of 39.4 (88 degrees of freedom), p (lower tail) = 1.7×10^{-6}. In other words, there is significantly *too much* agreement between the proportions of positive tubes in each of the three independent assays than would be expected for binomially distributed data. Another striking feature of these data is that they were obtained in assays where an exogenous source of metabolic activation (rat-liver S9, for example) was not supplied. The bile acids claimed to be mutagenic by these authors are not electrophilic reagents, and it is very unlikely that the bacteria used in the test are capable of converting them to electrophiles. It is biologically implausible, therefore, that bile acids are directly-acting mutagens, except perhaps by a frameshift mechanism. However, this would not explain the positive results in the basepair-substitution mutant TA100. In view of the anomalous statistics and the lack of requirement for metabolic activation, the direct mutagenicity of cholic acid, chenodeoxycholic acid, deoxycholic acid and ursodeoxycholic acid claimed by Watabe and Bernstein requires independent confirmation before it can be accepted.

H. Summary and Conclusions

1. *Summary*

Genotoxic activity has been detected in faecal extracts prepared by a number of different methods from donors living under widely differing geographical, cultural and dietary conditions. Faecal extracts cause point mutations in bacteria. Strain-specificity suggests the presence of several different kinds of faecal mutagen, some reverting basepair-substitution mutants, other reverting frameshift mutants. Some act directly, others require metabolic activation. There is limited indirect evidence that faecal extracts induce DNA repair in bacteria. There are two small-scale studies showing that faecal extracts cause chromosomal damage in cultured mammalian cells. In one study, faecal extracts caused nuclear anomalies in mice treated *in vivo*.

There is wide variation in genotoxic activity between different stool samples from one person, and between different stool samples from different people. There is conflicting evidence for inhibition or enhancement of the mutagenicity of reference mutagens by faecal extracts. Claims have been made that faecal co-mutagenicity as well as mutagenic activity *per se* is relevant to colon cancer.

The use of different assay methods gives conflicting estimates of the proportion of people who excrete genotoxic faeces. In general, results from fluctuation tests suggest that most people excrete faecal mutagens, whereas the *Salmonella* test indicates that 20% to 30% of populations on Western diets produce mutagenic faeces. However, the fluctuation test is more susceptible than the *Salmonella* test to giving false-positive results when used for assaying faecal extracts. Tests performed under anaerobic conditions sometimes give results which are substantially different from those conducted aerobically.

Some studies suggest that the proportion of people excreting mutagenic faeces is higher in groups at high risk of large-bowel cancer than in groups at low risk. Comparisons of cancer patients with controls have revealed no differences in faecal genotoxicity between these two groups. Studies of dietary intervention (high and low meat, fibre and vitamin-supplementation) suggest that genotoxic activity of faeces can be altered by changes in diet. The claims that endogenously formed *N*-nitrosamines are detectable in human faeces have been withdrawn by their proponents.

A new class of mutagen – the fecapentaenes – has been isolated from organic-solvent extracts of human faeces and their structure has been elucidated. Fecapentaenes are glyceryl ether lipids containing a conjugated pentaene chain. The natural products occur as mixtures of highly labile isomers, with polyene chains of 12 or 14 carbon atoms, different donors producing different ratios of fecapentaene-12 and fecapentaene-14. The distribution of fecapentaenes in the general population is not known in detail, but there is evidence that some people produce high levels, and others produce very low levels. Natural fecapentaenes are potent, directly-acting bacterial mutagens. Fecapentaenes appear to be products of anaerobic metabolism of an unknown precursor by several species of *Bacteroides* commonly found in the human colon. Model studies suggest that the potent mutagenicity of fecapentaenes results from their alkylating activity following formation of strongly electrophilic carbonium ions. A more stable synthetic *all-trans* isomer of fecapentaene-12 has been synthesized which is a potent bacterial mutagen, and which, at low doses, induces DNA repair and point mutations in cultured mammalian cells. Studies with plasmid DNA suggest that fecapentaene-12 forms cross-links in DNA.

Mutagenic activity has been detected in both urine and faeces of volunteers fed fried beef known to contain mutagenic heterocyclic amines produced during cooking. Faecal mutagenic activity rose within a few hours of the meal, and declined to control levels 2 to 3 days after the meal. Clearance from urine was more rapid.

The possibility that bile acids are genotoxic has been raised. Ursodeoxycholic acid caused chromosomal damage in cultured mammalian cells. A variety of bile acids and derivatives have been tested in the *Salmonella* test in several different studies with negative results. In one study, lower doses were assayed in fluctuation tests, and cholic, ursodeoxycholic, deoxycholic and chenodeoxycholic acid were claimed to be directly acting mutagens. These results require independent confirmation.

2. Conclusions

That genotoxic agents exist in human faeces is no longer in doubt. There is now good evidence that ingestion of exogenous mutagens (heterocyclic amines from fried meat) can produce mutagenic activity in faeces, and that potent faecal mutagens (fecapentaenes) can be produced endogenously. What is less certain is the relevance of faecal genotoxicity to large-bowel cancer. The existing evidence that dietary practices or interventions which are thought to confer high or low bowel cancer risk are reflected in high or low levels of faecal genotoxicity is suggestive rather than conclusive. Many of the earlier studies did not take account of the many problems inherent in assaying material as complex as faeces for genotoxic activity with assays which were designed for screening pure chemicals. Moreover, until we have enough base-line information from long-term studies of healthy populations, using appropriate assay methods of sufficient sensitivity, it is impossible to obtain reliable estimates of the effect of dietary changes on faecal genotoxicity. Getting these data will not be easy. It is extremely difficult to persuade large numbers of volunteers to provide faecal samples for large-scale studies conducted over weeks or months. It is even more difficult to ask them to adopt and adhere rigorously to diets which may be unpalatable or, in the case of the flatus induced by high-fibre diets, anti-social. This will be true whether short-term mutagenicity assays or chemical methods (e.g., for detecting fecapentaenes) are used. Nevertheless, until such prospective studies are undertaken, it will not be possible to determine the relevance of faecal genotoxins to the aetiology of cancer of the large bowel.

Acknowledgment

The author thanks the Cancer Research Campaign and the Medical Research Council of the United Kingdom for financial support.

References

Alderson, M. R. (1984). Epidemiological aspects of precancerous states. *In*: "Precancerous States" (ed. R. L. Carter), pp. 1–41. Oxford University Press.

Ames, B. N., McCann, J. and Yamasaki, E. (1975). Methods for detecting carcinogens and mutagens with the Salmonella/mammalian-microsome mutagenicity test. *Mutat. Res.* **31**, 347–364.

Anonymous (1982). Faecal nitrosamines. *Fd Chem. Toxicol.*, **20**, 479–480.

Archer, M. C., Saul, R. L., Lee, L -J. and Bruce, W. R. (1981). Analysis of nitrate, nitrite, and nitrosamines in human feces. *In*: "Banbury Report 7. Gastrointestinal Cancer: Endogenous Factors" (eds W. R. Bruce, P. Correa, M. Lipkin, S. R. Tannenbaum and T. D. Wilkins), pp. 321–327. Cold Spring Harbor Laboratory, New York.

Armstrong, B. K. and Mann, J. I. (1985). Diet. *In*: "Cancer Risks and Prevention" (eds M. P. Vessey and M. Gray), pp. 68–98. Oxford University Press.

Askew, A. R., Ward, M., Green, M. K. and Reibelt, D. (1982). Faecal mutagenesis and colonic cancer. *Aust. N.Z. J. Surg.* **52**, 27–29.

Baker, R., Arlauskas, A., Bonin, A. and Angus, D. (1982). Detection of mutagenic activity in human urine following fried pork or bacon meals. *Cancer Lett.* **16**, 81–89.

Balmain, A. (1985). Transforming *ras* oncogenes and multistage carcinogenesis. *Br. J. Cancer,* **51**, 1–7.

Baptista, J., Bruce, W. R., Gupta, I., Krepinsky, J. J., Van Tassell, R. L. and Wilkins, T. D. (1984). On distribution of different fecapentaenes, the fecal mutagens, in the human population. *Cancer Lett.* **22**, 299–303.

Barnes, W. S. and Powrie, W. D. (1982). Clastogenic activity of bile acids and organic acid fractions of human feces. *Cancer Lett.* **15**, 317–327.

Berenblum, I. (1982). Sequential aspects of chemical carcinogenesis. *In*: "Cancer: A Comprehensive Treatise" (ed. F. F. Becker), pp. 451–484. Plenum Press, New York, London.

Bosworth, D. and Venitt, S. (1986). Testing human faecal extracts for genotoxic activity with the SOS Chromotest: the importance of controlling for faecal enzyme activity. *Mutagenesis* **2**, 143–149.

Boyle, P., Zaridze, D. G. and Smans, M. (1985). Descriptive epidemiology of colorectal cancer. *Int. J. Cancer* **36**, 9–18.

Breslow, N. E. and Day, N. E. (1980). "Statistical Methods in Cancer Research. Volume 1. The Analysis of Case-Control Studies" IARC Publications No. 32, p. 147. International Agency for Research on Cancer, Lyon.

Bruce, W. R., Baptista, J., Che, T., Furrer, R., Gingerich, J. S., Gupta, I., Krepinsky, J. J., Grey, A. A. and Yates, P. (1982). General structure of "fecapentaenes" – the mutagenic substances in human faeces. *Naturwiss.,* **69**, 557–558.

Bruce, W. R. and Dion, P. W. (1980). Studies relating to a fecal mutagen. *Amer. J. Clin. Nutr.* **33**, 2511–2512.

Bruce, W. R., Varghese, A. J., Wang, S. and Dion, P. (1979). The endogenous production of nitroso compounds in the colon and cancer at that site. *In*: "Naturally Occurring Carcinogens–Mutagens and Modulators of Carcinogenesis" (ed. E. C. Miller), pp. 221–228. Japan. Sci. Press, Tokyo; University Park Press, Baltimore.

Bruce, W. R., Varghese, A. J., Furrer, R. and Land, P. C. (1977). A mutagen in the feces of normal humans. *In*: "Origins of Human Cancer", Book C "Human Risk Assessment" (eds. H. H. Hiatt, J. D. Watson & J. A. Winsten), Cold Spring Harbor Conferences on Cell Proliferation Vol. 4, pp. 1641–1646. Cold Spring Harbor, New York.

Bruce, W. R., Varghese, A. J., Land, P. C. and Krepinsky, J. J. F. (1981) Properties of a Mutagen Isolated from Faeces. *In* "Banbury Report 7, Gastrointestinal Cancer: Endogenous Factors" (W. R. Bruce, P. Correa, M. Lipkin, S. R. Tannenbaum and T. D. Wilkins) pp. 227–239. Cold Spring Harbor Laboratory, New York.

Burkitt, D. P. (1980). Colon cancer: the emergence of a concept. *In*: "Medical Aspects of Dietary Fiber" (eds G. E. Spiller and R. McPherson Kay), pp. 75–81. Plenum Medical Book Company, New York and London.

Carter, R. L. (1984). Introduction. *In*: "Precancerous States" (ed. R.L. Carter), pp. xv–xviii. Oxford University Press.

Combes, R., Anderson, D., Brooks, T., Neale, S. and Venitt, S. (1984). The detection of mutagens in urine, faeces and body fluids. *In*: "Report of the UKEMS Sub-Committee on Guidelines for Mutagenicity Testing" (ed.

B.J. Dean), Part II, pp. 203–244. United Kingdom Environmental Mutagen Society, Swansea.

Correa, P. and Haenszel, W. (1978). The epidemiology of large-bowel cancer. *Adv. Cancer Res.* **26**, 1–141.

Cummings, J. H. (1985). Cancer of the large bowel. *In*: "Dietary Fibre, Fibre-Depleted Foods and Disease" (eds H. Trowell, D. Burkitt, K. Heaton), pp. 161–189. Academic Press, London.

deVet, H. C. W., Sharma, C. and Reddy, B. S. (1981). Effect of fried meat on fecal mutagenic and co-mutagenic activity in humans. *Nutr. Rep. Int.* **23**, 653–660.

Dion, P. W., Bright-See, E. B., Smith, C. C. and Bruce, W. R. (1982). The effect of dietary ascorbic acid and alpha-tocopherol on fecal mutagenicity. *Mutat. Res.* **102**, 27–37.

Dion, P. and Bruce, W. R. (1983). Mutagenicity of different fractions of extracts of human faeces. *Mutat. Res.* **119**, 151–160.

DHSS (1984). "On the State of the Public Health. The Annual Report of the Chief Medical Officer of the Department of Social Security for the Year 1983". Her Majesty's Stationery Office, London.

Doll, R. and Peto, R. (1981) The causes of cancer: quantitative estimates of avoidable risks of cancer in the United States today. *J. Natl. Cancer Inst.*, **66**, 1192–1308.

Dyrby, T. and Ingvardsen, P. (1983). Sensitivity of different *E. coli* and Salmonella strains in mutagenicity testing calculated on the basis of selected literature. *Mutat. Res.* **123**, 47–60.

Eide, T. J. (1986). Risk of colorectal cancer in adenoma-bearing individuals within a defined population. *Int. J. Cancer.* **38**, 173–176.

Eisenbrand, G., Spiegelhalder, B. and Preussman, R. (1981). Analysis of human biological specimens for nitrosamine contents. *In*: "Banbury Report 7. Gastrointestinal Cancer: Endogenous Factors" (eds W. R. Bruce, P. Correa, M. Lipkin, S. R. Tannenbaum and T. D. Wilkins), pp. 275–283. Cold Spring Harbor Laboratory, New York.

Ehrich, M., Aswell, J. E., Van Tassell, R. L., Walker, A. R. P., Richardson, N. J. and Wilkins, T. D. (1979). Mutagens in the feces of 3 South African populations at different levels of risk for colon cancer. *Mutat. Res.* **64**, 231–240.

Fang, W. -F. and Strobel, H. W. (1978). Activation of carcinogens and mutagens by rat colon mucosa. *Cancer Res.* **38**, 2939–2944.

Farber, E. (1982). Sequential events in chemical carcinogenesis. *In*: "Cancer: A Comprehensive Treatise" (ed. F. F. Becker) (second ed), pp. 485–506. Plenum Press, New York, London.

Ferguson, L. R. and Alley, P. G. (1982). Fecal mutagens from population groups within New Zealand at different risk of colorectal cancer. *In*: "Mutagens in Our Environment", pp. 423–429. Alan R. Liss, New York.

Ferguson, L. R., Alley, P. G. and Gribben, B. M. (1985). DNA-damaging activity of feces from New Zealand groups at varying risks of colorectal cancer. *Nutr. Cancer* **7**, 93–103.

Gatehouse, D. G. and Delow, G. F. (1979). The development of a microtitre fluctuation test for the detection of indirect mutagens, and its use in the evaluation of mixed-enzyme induction of the liver. *Mutat. Res.* **60**, 239–252.

Göggelman, W., Maier, F. K. and Pfaendler, H. R. (1986). Mutagenicity of

454   S. VENITT

synthetic racemic fecapentaene-12. *Mutat. Res.* **174**, 165–167.

Grasso, P. (1984). Carcinogens in food. *In*: "Chemical Carcinogens, Second Edition" (ed. C. E. Searle), Volume 2, ACS Monograph 182, pp. 1205–1239. American Chemical Society, Washington, DC.

Green, M. H. L. and Muriel, W. J. (1976). Mutagen testing using TRP[+] reversion in *Escherichia coli*. *Mutat. Res.* **38**, 3–32.

Green, M. H. L., Muriel, W. J. and Bridges, B. A. (1976). Use of a simplified fluctuation test to detect low levels of mutagens. *Mutat. Res.* **38**, 33–42.

Gunatilaka, A. A. L., Hirai, N. and Kingston, D. G. I. (1983). Synthesis of racemic fecapentaene-12, a potent mutagen from human feces, and its regioisomer. *Tetrahedron Lett.* **24**, 5457–5460.

Gupta, I., Baptista, J., Bruce, W. R., Che, C. T., Furrer, R., Gingerich, J. S., Grey, A. A., Marai, L., Yates, P. and Krepinsky, J. J. (1983). Structures of fecapentaenes, the mutagens of bacterial origin isolated from human feces. *Biochemistry*, **22**, 241–245.

Gupta, I., Suzuki, K., Bruce, W. R., Krepinsky, J. J. and Yates, P. (1984). A model study of fecapentaenes: mutagens of bacterial origin with alkylating properties. *Science,* **225**, 521–523.

Harris, C. C., Plummer, S. M., Yang, L., Curren, R. and Kakefuda, T. (1985). The cytotoxicity and mutagenicity of fecapentaene-12 in bacterial and human cells. *In*: "Abstracts: Fourth International Conference on Environmental Mutagens." Stockholm, June 24–28 1985, p. 330.

Hayatsu, H., Arimoto, S., Togawa, K. and Makita, M. (1981a). Inhibitory effect of the ether extract of human feces on activities of mutagens: inhibition by oleic and linoleic acids. *Mutat. Res.* **81**, 287–293.

Hayatsu, H., Inoue, K., Ohta, H., Namba, T., Togawa, K., Hayatsu, T., Makita, M. and Watya, Y. (1981b). Inhibition of the mutagenicity of cooked-beef basic fraction by its acidic fraction. *Mutat. Res.* **91**, 437–442.

Hayatsu, H., Haytsu, T., Wataya, Y. and Mower, H. F. (1985a). Fecal mutagenicity arising from ingestion of fried ground beef in the human. *Mutat. Res.* **143**, 207–211.

Hayatsu, H., Hayatsu, T. and Ohara, Y. (1985b). Mutagenicity of human urine caused by ingestion of fried ground beef. *Jpn J. Cancer Res. (Gann)*, **76**, 445–448.

Hill, M. J., Drasar, B. S., Aries, V., Crowther, J. S. and Williams, R. E. O. (1971). Bacteria and aetiology of cancer of the large bowel. *Lancet* **i**, 95–100.

Hirai, N., Kingston, D. G. I., Van Tassell, R. L. and Wilkins, T. D. (1982). Structure elucidation of a potent mutagen from human feces. *J. Am. Chem. Soc.* **104**, 6149–6150.

Hirai, N., Kingston, D. G. I., Van Tassell, R. L. and Wilkins, T. D. (1985). Isolation and structure elucidation of fecapentaenes-12, potent mutagens from human feces. *J. Natural Products*, **48**, 622–630.

Hoensch, H. P., Steinhardt, H. J. and Malchow, H. (1982). Metabolism of xenobiotics in human small intestinal mucosa: relationship to carcinogenic factors. *In*: "Colonic Carcinogenesis" (eds R. A. Malt and R. C. N. Williamson), Falk Symposium 31, pp. 83–90. MTP Press, Lancaster, Boston, The Hague.

Howe, G. R., Craib, K. J. P. and Miller, A. B. (1985). Age at first pregnancy and risk of colorectal cancer. *J. Natl Cancer Inst.*, **74**, 1155–1159.

IARC (1982). Report of the second IARC coordinated international collaborative study on diet and large bowel cancer in Denmark and Finland. *Nutr. Cancer*, **4**, 3–79.

IARC (1986). "Long-Term & Short-Term Assays for Carcinogens: a Critical Appraisal." (Eds R. Montesano, H. Bartsch, H. Vainio, J. Wilbourn, H. Yamasaki, R. A. Greisemer & S. Venitt) IARC Scientific Publications No 83. International Agency for Research on Cancer, Lyon.

Ikeda, M., Yoshimoto, K., Yoshimura, T., Kono, S., Kato, H. and Kuratsune, M. (1983). A cohort study on the possible association between broiled fish intake and cancer. *Gann* **74**, 640–648.

Kenyon, C. J. (1983). The bacterial response to DNA damage. *Trends Biochem. Sci.* March, 84–87.

Kingston, D. G. I., Wilkins, T. D., Van Tassell, R. L., MacFarlane, R. D. and McNeal, C. J. (1981). Structural studies on a mutagenic bacterial product from human faeces. *In*: "Banbury Report 7. Gastrointestinal Cancer: Endogenous Factors" (eds W. R. Bruce, P. Correa, M. Lipkin, S. R. Tannenbaum and T. D. Wilkins), pp. 215–223. Cold Spring Harbor Laboratory, New York.

Kinlen, L. J. (1983). Fat and cancer. *Br. Med. J.* **286**, 1081–1082.

Knize, M. G., Andresen, B. D., Healy, S. K., Shen, N. H., Lewis, P. R., Bjeldanes, L. F., Hatch, F. T. and Felton, J. S. (1985). Effects of temperature, patty thickness and fat content of the production of mutagens in fried ground beef. *Fd Chem. Toxicol.*, **23**, 1035–1040.

Knudson, A. G. (1982). Genetic influences in human tumors. *In*: "Cancer: A Comprehensive Treatise" (ed. F.F. Becker) (second edn), pp. 73–88. Plenum Press, New York, London.

Kuhnlein, U., Bergstrom, D. and Kuhnlein, H. (1981). Mutagens in feces from vegetarians and non-vegetarians. *Mutat. Res.* **85**, 1–12.

Kuhnlein, U., Gallagher, R. and Freeman, H. J. (1983). Effects of purified cellulose and pectin fiber diets on mutagenicity of feces and luminal contents of stomach, small and large bowel in rats. *Clin. Invest. Med.* **6**, 253–260.

Kuhnlein, H. V. and Kuhnlein, U. (1980). Mutagens in feces from subjects on controlled formula diets. *Nutr. Cancer* **2**, 119–124.

Kuhnlein, H. V., Kuhnlein, U. and Bell, P. A. (1983). The effect of short-term dietary modification on human fecal mutagenic activity. *Mutat. Res.* **113**, 1–12.

Land, H., Parada, L. F. and Weinberg, R. A. (1983). Cellular oncogenes and multistep carcinogenesis. *Science*, **222**, 771–778.

Lederman, M., Van Tassell, R., West, S. E. H., Ehrich, M. F. and Wilkins, T. D. (1980). *In vitro* production of human fecal mutagen. *Mutat. Res.* **79**, 115–124.

Lee, L.-j., Archer, M. C. and Bruce, W. R. (1981). Absence of volatile nitrosamines in human feces. *Cancer Res.* **41**, 3992–3994.

Leifer, Z., Kada, T., Mandel, M., Zeiger, E., Stafford, R. and Rosenkranz, H. S. (1981). An evaluation of tests using DNA repair-deficient bacteria for predicting genotoxicity and carcinogenicity. A report of the U.S. EPA's Gene-Tox Program. *Mutat. Res.* **87**, 211–297.

Levin, D. E., Hollstein, M., Christman, M. F., Schwiers, E. A. and Ames, B. N. (1982). A new *Salmonella* tester strain (TA102) with A.T base pairs at the site of mutation detects oxidative mutagens. *Proc. Natl. Acad. Sci. USA.* **79**, 7445–7449.

MacDonald, I. A., Singh, G., Mahony, D. E. and Meier, C. E. (1978). Effect of pH on bile salt degradation by mixed fecal cultures. *Steroids*, **32**, 245–256.

Maron, D. M. and Ames, B. N. (1983). Revised methods for the Salmonella mutagenicity test. *Mutat. Res.* **113**, 173–215.

Maskens, A. P. (1982). Multistep models of colorectal carcinogenesis. *In*: "Colonic Carcinogenesis" (eds R. A. Malt and R. C. N. Williamson), pp. 211–219. MTP Press, Lancaster, Boston.

McKillop, C. A., Owen, R. W., Bilton, R. F. and Haslam, E. A. (1983). Mutagenicity testing of steroids obtained from bile acids and cholesterol. *Carcinogenesis* **4**, 1179–1183.

Moolgavkar, S. H. and Knudson, A. G. (1981). Mutation and cancer: a model for human carcinogenesis. *J. Natl. Cancer Inst.* **66**, 1037–1052.

Morson, B. C., Bussey, H. J. R., Day, D. W. and Hill, M. J. (1983). Adenomas of large bowel. *Cancer Surveys* **2**, 451–477.

Mower, H. F., Ichinotsubo, D., Wang, L. W., Mandel, M., Stemmermann, G., Nomura, A., Heilbrun, L., Kamiyama, S. and Shimada, A. (1982). Fecal mutagens in two Japanese populations with different colon cancer risks. *Cancer Res.* **42**, 1164–1169.

Nader, C. J., Potter, J. D. and Weller, R. A. (1981). Diet and DNA-modifying activity in human fecal extracts. *Nutr. Rep. Int.* **23**, 113–117.

Nagao, M., Wakabayashi, K. and Sugimura, T. (1985). Mutagens in food and drinks, and their carcinogenicity. *In*: "Mutagenicity Testing in Environmental Pollution Control" (eds F. K. Zimmermann and R. E. Taylor-Mayer), pp. 69–85. Ellis Horwood, Chichester.

Nicolaou, K. C., Zipkin, R. and Tanner, D. (1984). Total synthesis of the potent mutagen (*S*)-3-(Dodeca-1,3,5,7,9-pentaenyloxy)propane-1,2-diol. *J. Chem. Soc., Chem. Commun.* 349–350.

Nilsson, L, Övervik, E., Fredholm, L., Levin, O., Nord, C -E. and Gustafsson, J. -Å (1986). Influence of frying fat on mutagenic activity in lean pork meat. *Mutat. Res.* **171**, 115–121.

O'Neil, I. K., Von Borstel, R. C., Miller, C. T., Long, J. and Bartsch, H. (1984). "*N*-Nitroso Compounds: Occurrence, Biological Effects and Relevance to Human Cancer", IARC Scientific Publications No. 57, International Agency for Research on Cancer, Lyon.

Övervik, E., Nilsson, L., Fredholm, L., Levin, O., Nord, C -E. and Gustafsson, J. -A. (1984). High mutagenic activity formed in pan-broiled pork. *Mutat. Res.* **135**, 149–157.

Pertel, R. (1985). Intestinal-microflora/host-diet interactions in the production of mutagens in the mini-pig. *In*: "Abstracts: Fourth International Conference on Environmental Mutagens", Stockholm, June 24–28 1985, p. 331.

Pfaendler, H. R., Maier, F. K. and Klar, S. (1986). Synthesis of crystalline (±)-fecapentaene. *J. Am. Chem. Soc.* **108**, 1338–1339.

Plummer, S. M., Grafstrom, R. C., Yang, L. L., Curren, R. D., Linnainmaa, K. and Harris, C. C. (1986). Fecapentaene-12 causes DNA damage and mutation in human cells. *Carcinogenesis* **7**, 1607–1609.

Potter, J. D. and McMichael, A. J. (1983). Large bowel cancer in women in relation to reproductive and hormonal factors: a case-control study. *J. Natl. Cancer Inst.* **71**, 703–709.

Preston, R. J., Au, W., Bender, M. A., Brewen, J. G., Carrano, A. V., Heddle, J. A., McFee, A. F., Wolff, S. and Wassom, J. S. (1981). Mammalian *in vivo* and *in vitro* cytogenetic assays. A report of the U.S. EPA'S Gene-Tox Program. *Mutat. Res.* **87**, 143–188.

Quillardet, P., de Bellecombe, C. and Hofnung, M. (1985). The SOS Chromotest, a colorimetric assay for genotoxins: validation study with 83 compounds, *Mutat. Res.* **147**, 79–95.

Quillardet, P. and Hofnung, M. (1985). The SOS Chromotest, a colorimetric assay for genotoxins: procedures, *Mutat. Res.* **147**, 65–78.

Quillardet, P., Huisman O., D'Ari, R. and Hofnung, M. (1982) SOS Chromotest, a direct assay of induction of an SOS function in *Escherichia coli* K-12 to measure genotoxicity, *Proc. Natl. Acad. Sci. USA.* **79**, 5971–5975.

Reddy, B. S. (1986). Fecal mutagens as a function of diet. *In*: "Genetic Toxicology of the Diet", *Prog. Clin. Biol. Res.*, Vol. 206, pp. 213–224. Alan R. Liss, New York.

Reddy, B. S., Sharma, C., Darby, L., Laakso, K. and Wynder, E. L. (1980a). Metabolic epidemiology of large-bowel cancer. Fecal mutagens in high- and low-risk population for colon cancer. A preliminary report. *Mutat. Res.* **72**, 511–522.

Reddy, B. S., Sharma, C. and Wynder, E. L. (1980b). Fecal factors which might modify the formation of fecal co-mutagens in high- and low-risk population for colon cancer. *Cancer Lett.* **10**, 123–132.

Reddy, B. S., Sharma, C., Mathews, L. and Engle, A. (1984). Fecal mutagens from subjects consuming a mixed western diet. *Mutat. Res.* **135**, 11–19.

Reddy, B. S., Sharma, C., Mathews, L., Engle, A., Laakso, K., Choi, K., Puska, P. and Korpella, R. (1985). Metabolic epidemiology of colon cancer: fecal mutagens in healthy subjects from rural Kuopio and urban Helsinki, Finland. *Mutat. Res.* **152**, 97–105.

Samelson, S. L., Nelson, R. L. and Nyhus, L. M. (1985). Protective role of faecal pH in experimental colon carcinogenesis. *J. Roy. Soc. Med.* **78**, 230–233.

Saul, R. L., Kabir, S. H., Cohen, Z., Bruce, W. R. and Archer, M. C. (1981). Reevaluation of nitrate and nitrite levels in the human intestine. *Cancer Res.* **41**, 2280–2283.

Shaw, R., Andrews, A. W. and Riggs, C. W. (1985). Assay of mutagens in aqueous faecal extracts with a modified Ames *Salmonella* test. *Teratog. Carcinogen. Mutagen.* **5**, 15–27.

Silverman, S. J. and Andrews, A. W. (1977). Bile acids; co-mutagenic activity in the *Salmonella*-mammalian microsome mutagenicity test. *J. Natl. Cancer Inst.* **59**, 1577–1559.

Silverman, S. H., Turnell, D. C., Youngs, D. J. and Keighley, M. R. B. (1986). What is the role of histidine in studies of faecal mutagenicity? *Mutat. Res.* **173**, 99–104.

Smith, A. H., Pearce, N. E. and Joseph, J. G. (1985). Major colorectal cancer aetiological hypotheses do not explain mortality trends among Maori and non-Maori New Zealanders. *Int. J. Epidemiol.* **14**, 79–85.

Sousa, J., Nath, J., Tucker, J. D. and Ong, T. M. (1985). Dietary factors affecting the urinary mutagenicity assay system. I. Detection of mutagenic activity in human urine following a fried beef meal. *Mutat. Res.* **149**, 365–374.

Strobel, H. W. and W -F. Fang (1981). Role of cytochrome P-450 in the response of the colon to xenobiotics. *In*: "Banbury Report 7. Gastrointestinal Cancer: Endogenous Factors" (eds W. R. Bruce, P. Correa, M. Lipkin, S. R. Tannenbaum and T. D. Wilkins), pp. 141–149. Cold Spring Harbor Laboratory, New York.

Stich, F. H. and Kuhnlein, U. (1979). Chromosome breaking activity of human feces and its enhancement by transition metals. *Int. J. Cancer* **24**, 284–287.

Sugimura, T. (1985). Carcinogenicity of mutagenic heterocyclic amines formed during the cooking process. *Mutat. Res.* **150**, 33–41.

Suzuki, K. and Bruce, W. R. (1984). Human faecal fractions can produce nuclear damage in the colonic epithelial cells of mice. *Mutat. Res.* **141**, 35–39.

Suzuki, K. and Mitsuoka, T. (1981). Increase in faecal nitrosamines in Japanese individuals given a Western diet. *Nature* **294**, 453–455.

Suzuki, K. and Mitsuoka, T. (1985). Reevaluation of volatile nitrosamines in human feces. *Environ. Toxicol. Chem.* **4**, 623–627.

Thompson, M. H. (1982). The role of diet in relation to faecal bile acid concentration and large bowel cancer. *In*: "Colonic Carcinogenesis" (eds R. A. Malt and R. C. N. Williamson), Falk Symposium 31, pp. 49–56, MTP Press, Lancaster, Boston, The Hague.

Tweats, D., Bootman, J., Combes, R., Green, M. and Watkins, P. (1984). Assays for DNA repair in bacteria. *In*: "Report of the UKEMS Sub-Committee on Guidelines for Mutagenicity Testing: Part II, Supplementary Tests; Mutagens in Food; Mutagens in Body Fluids and Excreta; Nitrosation Products" (ed. B. J. Dean), pp. 5–25. United Kingdom Environmental Mutagen Society, Swansea.

Van Tassell, R. L., MacDonald, D. K. and Wilkins, T. D. (1982a). Stimulation of mutagen production in human feces by bile and bile acids. *Mutat. Res.* **103**, 233–239.

Van Tassell, R. L., MacDonald, D. K. and Wilkins, T. D. (1982b). Production of a fecal mutagen by *Bacteroides* spp. *Infect. Immunol.* **37**, 975–980.

Varghese, A. J., Land, P. C., Furrer, R. and Bruce, W. R. (1978). Non-volatile *N*-nitroso compounds in human faeces. *In*: "Environmental Aspects of *N*-Nitroso Compounds (eds E.A. Walker, L. Griciute, M. Castegnaro, R. Lyle and W. Davis), IARC Scientific Publications No. 19, pp. 257–264. International Agency for Research on Cancer, Lyon.

Venitt, S. (1980). Bacterial mutation as an indicator of carcinogenicity. *Brit. Med. Bull.* **36**, 57–62.

Venitt, S. (1981). Faecal mutagens: their discovery and possible relevance to the aetiology of large-bowel cancer in man. *In*: "Progress in Mutation Research" (ed. A. Kappas), Vol. 2, pp. 3–10. Elsevier/North Holland Biomedical Press, Amsterdam, Oxford, New York.

Venitt, S. (1982a). Faecal mutagens in the aetiology of colonic cancer. *In*: "Colonic Carcinogenesis" (eds R.A. Malt and R.C.N. Williamson), Falk Symposium 31, pp. 59–72, MTP Press, Lancaster, Boston, The Hague.

Venitt, S. (1982b). Mutagens in human faeces: are they relevant to cancer of the large bowel? *Mutat. Res.* **98**, 265–286.

Venitt, S. and Bosworth, D. (1983). The development of anaerobic methods for bacterial mutation assays: aerobic and anaerobic fluctuation tests of human faecal extracts and reference mutagens. *Carcinogenesis* **4**, 339–345.

Venitt, S. and Bosworth, D. (1986). Further studies on the detection of mutagenic and genotoxic activity in human faeces: aerobic and anaerobic fluctuation tests with *S. typhimurium* and *E. coli*, and the SOS Chromotest. *Mutagenesis* **1**, 49–64.

Venitt, S., Bosworth, D. and Alldrick, A. J. (1986). Pilot study of the effect of diet on the mutagenicity of human faeces. *Mutagenesis* 1, 353–358.

Venitt, S., Crofton-Sleigh, C. and Forster, R. (1984). Bacterial mutation assays using reverse mutation. *In*: "Mutagenicity Testing: a Practical Approach" (eds S. Venitt and J. M. Perry), pp. 45–98, IRL Press, Oxford, Washington DC.

Walker, A. R. P., Walker, B. F. and Walker, A. J. (1986). Faecal pH, dietary fibre intake, and proneness to colon cancer in four South African populations. *Br. J. Cancer* **53**, 489–495.

Wang, T., Kakizoe, T., Dion, P., Furrer, R., Varghese, A. J. and Bruce, W. R. (1978). Volatile nitrosamines in normal human faeces. *Nature* **276**, 280–281.

Wargovich, M. J., Goldberg, M. T., Newmark, H. L. and Bruce, W. R. (1983). Nuclear aberrations as a short-term test for genotoxicity to the colon: evaluation of nineteen agents in mice. *J. Natl. Cancer Inst.* **71**, 133–137.

Watabe, J. and Bernstein, H. (1985). The mutagenicity of bile acids using a fluctuation test. *Mutat. Res.* **158**, 45–51.

Whitehead, R. (1984). Precancerous states of the large intestine. *In*: "Precancerous States" (ed. R. L. Carter), pp. 230–253, Oxford University Press.

Wilkins, T. D., Lederman, M., Van Tassell, R. L., Kingston, D. G. I. and Henion, J. (1980). Characterization of a mutagenic bacterial product in human feces. *Am. J. Clin. Nutr.* **33**, 2513–2520.

Wilkins, T. D., Lederman, M. and Van Tassell, R. L. (1981). Isolation of a mutagen produced in the human colon by bacterial action. *In*: "Banbury Report 7. Gastrointestinal Cancer: Endogenous Factors" (eds W. R. Bruce, P. Correa, M. Lipkin, S. R. Tannenbaum and T. D. Wilkins), pp. 205–212. Cold Spring Harbor Laboratory, New York.

Wilkins, T. D. and Van Tassell, R. L. (1983). *In*: "Human Intestinal Microflora in Health and Disease" (ed. D. J. Hentges), pp. 265–288. Academic Press, New York, London.

Zaridze, D. G. (1983). Environmental aetiology of large-bowel cancer. *J. Natl. Cancer Inst.* **70**, 389–400.

Zimmermann, F. K. and Taylor-Mayer, R. E. (1985). "Mutagenicity Testing in Environmental Pollution Control". Ellis Horwood, Chichester.

NOTE ADDED IN PROOF

Section **A**.2. Recent discoveries strengthen the evidence that point mutations and chromosomal rearrangements play an important part in the development of colon cancer. A high incidence of c-K-*ras* oncogenes with specific point mutations was found in tumours of the human colon (Bos *et al.* 1987; Forrester *et al.* 1987). 20% of sporadic colorectal adenocarcinomas were found to have lost one of a pair of alleles of a gene thought to be associated with the development of familial adenomatous polyposis (Solomon *et al.* 1987; Bodmer *et al.* 1987).

Section **B**.4. Reddy *et al.* (1987), using the *Salmonella* test, showed that of 15 subjects who produced mutagenic faeces, mutagenicity was markedly reduced in most of the subjects during the 4-week period when they ate additional whole-wheat fibre.

Section **C**.1. Krepinsky (1987) has reviewed the formation and biological effects of fecapentaenes.

Section **C**.1.(*e*) Synthetic fecapentaene-12 was found to display an unexpectedly high reactivity towards nucleophiles under anhydrous basic conditions (de Wit *et al.* (1986).

Section **C**.1.(*f*) In studies performed in rats *in vivo*, Hinzman *et al.* (1987) showed that surgical instillation of fecapentaene-12 into closed intestinal segments increased the proliferation of colonic mucosal cells and raised the levels of alkali-labile sites in DNA recovered from colonic mucosa. These authors also demonstrated a dose-related increase in alkali-labile sites in DNA treated *in vitro* with fecapentaene-12 under anaerobic conditions. Venitt and Bosworth (1987) showed that fecapentaene-12 was less mutagenic to the frameshift mutant TA98 under aerobic conditions than under anaerobic conditions. However, plate assays with *S. typhimurium* TA100 and *E. coli* WP2*uvr*ApKM101 and fluctuation tests using TA100 showed that the mutagenicity of fecapentaene-12 was significantly reduced when assayed anaerobically. Anaerobic conditions therefore appear to suppress the base-substitution activity but not the frameshift activity.
Section **G**. The three bile acids (cholic acid, chenodeoxycholic acid and deoxycholic acid) claimed by Watabe and Bernstein (1985) to be mutagenic were assayed for mutagenicity in fluctuation tests of the type used by these authors. At the doses tested there was no evidence of mutagenicity (Venitt *et al.* 1987).

Bodmer, W. F. *et al.* (1987) *Nature*, **328**, 614–616.
Bos, J. H. L. *et al.* (1987) *Nature*, **327**, 293–297.
de Wit, P. P. *et al.* (1986) *Tetrahedron Lett.* **27**, 6263–6266.
Forrester, K. *et al.* (1987) *Nature*, **327**, 298–303.
Hinzman, M. J. *et al.* (1987) *Carcinogenesis*, **8**, 1475–1479.
Krepinsky, J. J. (1987). *Progr. Biochem. Pharmacol.*, **22**, 1–10.
Reddy, B. S. *et al.* (1987) *Cancer Res.*, **47**, 644–648.
Schiffman, M. H. (1986). *Epidemiologic Reviews*, **8**, 92–105.
Solomon, E. (1987). *Nature*, **328**, 616–619.
Venitt, S. *et al.* (1987). *Mutat. Res.*, **190**, 191–196.
Venitt, S. and Bosworth, D. (1988). *Mutagenesis*, **3**, (in press).

18

Gut Flora and Cancer in Humans and Laboratory Animals

MICHAEL HILL

A. Introduction

In humans it has been estimated that 80–90% of cancers are caused by environmental agents. In laboratory animals, where the existence of inbred strains permits the importance of genetic factors to be more apparent, it is nevertheless clear that a high proportion of cancers have an environmental aetiology rather than an inherited genetic cause. Since all body surfaces are colonized by bacteria, the normal flora is in a unique position to mediate in the interaction between the host and its environment, either by degrading, releasing or forming genotoxic agents. It is extremely unlikely, when considered in that light, that the bacterial flora has *no* role in the causation of cancer, either in humans or in laboratory animals.

In this review I will begin by discussing the production of carcinogens, mutagens, etc. by the normal bacterial flora. This will be followed by examples of studies in laboratory animals where there is a clear and identifiable (though not necessarily identified) role for the normal flora in spontaneous carcinogenesis or in models of carcinogenesis using target organ specific carcinogens. Finally the evidence for a role for the normal flora in carcinogenesis in humans will be reviewed.

B. Production of Carcinogens by Gut Bacteria

Bacteria are able to produce carcinogens or tumour promoters from a variety of substrates which reach the gut either in the diet or in bile. The substrates to be considered here are dietary β-glucosides, biliary β-glucuronides, the amino acids methionine, tryptophan and tyrosine, the nitrosatable amines, the bile acids and cholesterol.

1. *Dietary β-glucosides*

There are numerous β-glucosides present in plants, some of which yield carcinogenic aglycones. The most widely studied such glucoside is cycasin, which is present in cycad nuts native to many Pacific islands and parts of south-east Asia. Cycasin is the β-glucoside of methylazoxymethanol and is highly hepatotoxic to rodents and to humans. When given orally to rodents at a dose insufficient to cause hepatotoxic death, a high proportion of the animals develop tumours of the intestinal tract. When administered intravenously, or to germ-free rats by any route, cycasin is non-toxic and non-carcinogenic. The carcinogenicity of cycasin was demonstrated by Laqueur *et al.* (1967) and was reviewed by Laqueur and Spatz (1968).

The dependence of the toxicity of cycasin on the presence of the gut bacterial flora is at first surprising. The mammalian intestinal mucosa has a β-glucosidase; however, it is highly substrate specific and has very low activity against the plant glucosides in general and against cycasin in particular. In contrast the β-glucosidase produced by the gut bacteria (Table 18.1) has a very much lower substrate specificity and cycasin is readily hydrolysed by the bacterial enzyme to yield the toxic and carcinogenic aglycone.

Although the hepatotoxicity of cycasin is well established in both man and laboratory animals, its carcinogenicity has only been demonstrated in animals. In the past cycads have been widely used in eastern Asia and the Pacific Islands as a starch source, but only after prior aqueous

Table 18.1. *Glycosidases produced by the human gut bacteria (data from Hawksworth* et al. *(1971))*

	Enzyme Activity (μmol degraded/h/10^8 cells)		
	β-glucuronidase	β-glucosidase	β-galactosidase
Escherichia coli	24.7 ± 2.1	5.8 ± 2.5	42.4 ± 3.4
Strep. faecalis	2.9 ± 0.6	192.7 ± 19.5	53.8 ± 6.0
Lactobacillus spp.	1.6 ± 0.2	26.0 ± 7.4	90.6 ± 10.7
Clostridium spp.	11.3 ± 2.3	22.1 ± 5.0	13.7 ± 2.7
Bacteroides fragilis	6.0 ± 3.5	35.1 ± 4.8	50.7 ± 4.9
Bifidobacterium spp.	29.3 ± 6.0	1.9 ± 0.8	39.1 ± 4.7

extraction of the cycasin. In recent times, following hurricane damage and during the resultant food shortages, isolated communities have eaten cycads but have neglected to extract the cycasin. Such communities have experienced the hepatotoxic effects and are being monitored by the National Cancer Institute; to date no excess risk of colorectal cancer has been detected in such persons and so the carcinogenicity of cycasin in humans has still to be demonstrated.

For many years it was not known whether cycasin was simply a well documented member of a (still to be discovered) family of carcinogenic glucosides produced by plants or whether it was unique. This question has still to be answered; however, the widespread use of the microbial mutagenesis assay system has revealed the existence of a large family of mutagenic compounds present in plants as their β-glucosides. In the assay of mutagens in plant products it is now routine to test such compounds both before and after treatment with bacterial β-glucosidase.

2. *Bacterial β-glucuronidase and the Enterohepatic Circulation of Carcinogens*

The polycyclic aromatic hydrocarbons (PAHs) form a family of carcinogens that are widely distributed in the environment. They are formed by the pyrolysis of organic matter and so are present in grilled, fried or roasted foods, in cigarette smoke, and in the vapours from combustion in the kitchen, from domestic fires and from motor exhausts. Such compounds are lipid-soluble, and so are passively absorbed from the gastro-intestinal tract and transported to the liver where they are hydroxylated and conjugated as their β-glucuronides. These conjugates (which have no carcinogenic activity) are then secreted in the bile for excretion in faeces. During transit through the intestine such conjugates may be hydrolysed by the bacterial β-glucuronidase (Table 18.1), and this releases the hydroxylated PAHs; these are non-carcinogenic but the parent carcinogen may be released by bacterial dehydroxylases (Renwick and Drasar, 1976) produced principally by the clostridia. In addition, Kinoshita and Gelboin (1978) showed that during hydrolysis with bacterial β-glucuronidase a high energy intermediate was released from PAH-glucuronides which is able to bind to DNA and is therefore potentially carcinogenic.

There is no clear evidence relating the products of hydrolysis of PAH glucuronides to the risk of cancer at any site, but it has been suggested by Renwick and Drasar (1976) that they may be of importance in colorectal carcinogenesis.

Table 18.2. *Evidence that tryptophan metabolites are carcinogenic, co-carcinogenic or mutagenic*

Metabolite	Assay	Indication
Tryptophan	Feeding to AAF-treated rats	Co-carcinogenic or tumour promoting action by metabolites
Indole	Feeding to AAF-treated rats	Indole (or its metabolites) is a co-carcinogen or tumour promoter
3-hydroxykynurenine	Bladder implantation test	Co-carcinogen
	Mammalian cell mutagenesis	Mutagen
3-hydroxyanthranilic acid	Bladder implantation	Co-carcinogen
	Mammalian cell mutagenesis	Mutagen
Quinaldic acid	Bladder implantation	Co-carcinogen
8-hydroxyquinaldic acid	Bladder implantation	Co-carcinogen
Xanthenuric acid	Bladder implantation	Co-carcinogen
Kynurenine	Bladder implantation	Co-carcinogen

3. Production of Ethionine from Methionine

Ethionine, the *S*-ethyl analogue of methionine, is a potent hepatotoxin in many animals and a powerful carcinogen in rodents (Farber, 1963). It was shown to be produced by a range of bacterial species including *E. coli* when grown in a medium containing mineral salts, sulphate, methionine and glucose (Fisher and Mallette, 1961). Interestingly, the ethionine remains extracellular to the bacteria and so does not induce mutation in the producer strains, but is available to cause toxicity and cancer in the host animal. Its mode of action remains unclear despite intensive study. Ethionine competes with methionine for the production of *S*-adenosyl analogues, resulting in the accumulation of adenosylethionine at the expense of adenosylmethionine; the latter is a general methylating agent involved in the methylation of t-RNA, DNA and r-RNA (this latter being important in the maturation of ribosomes).

Although the carcinogenicity of ethionine has been studied in animals there is little published work on its role in human carcinogenesis.

4. *Tryptophan Metabolism*

Tryptophan undergoes extensive metabolism by the gut bacterial flora. The most widely recognized pathway is via tryptophanase, which yields ammonia, indole and pyruvate. In addition, there are the simple deamination and decarboxylation reactions. In the context of carcinogenesis the most important pathway is via kynurenine (Fig. 18.1). Interest in tryptophan metabolism was first aroused by Dunning *et al.* (1950), who showed that rats fed 2-acetylaminofluorene (AAF) and tryptophan developed many more bladder tumours than did rats fed AAF alone. This work has been repeated and developed; the tryptophan could be replaced by indole or by indoleacetic acid.

A wide range of tryptophan metabolites has been assayed for their carcinogenic, promoting or mutagenic activity using a variety of assay systems (Table 18.2). The most widely used test, and the one that causes most controversy in its interpretation, is the bladder implantation test. In this test implants of the test compound mixed with cholesterol are introduced into the bladder wall and the number of bladder tumours compared with that obtained using implants of cholesterol alone.

All of the pathways in Fig. 18.1 are available to bacteria (indeed, they were discovered using bacteria) and many are also available to the liver

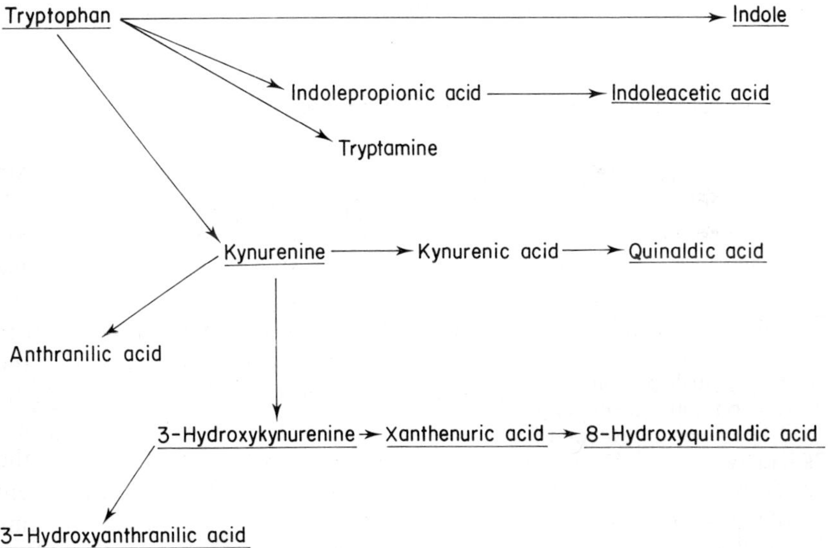

Fig 18.1 The metabolism of tryptophan by bacteria. The products underlined have been claimed to be tumour promoters.

as well. A role for the tryptophan metabolites in human bladder carcinogenesis was proposed by Bryan (1971); all of the metabolites in Fig. 18.1 are excreted in normal human urine.

5. *Tyrosine Metabolism*

Tyrosine is metabolized by the gut bacteria to a range of phenolic compounds, principally phenol and *p*-cresol, which are absorbed from the colon and excreted in urine as their sulphate or glucuronide conjugates. In normal western persons 50–100 mg of urinary volatile phenol (UVP) are excreted each day (Table 18.3) the amount being higher when a high protein diet is consumed or in patients with small bowel overgrowth, and lower in patients whose bowel flora has been disturbed either by preoperative bowel preparation or by total colectomy. Interestingly, left hemicolectomy has little effect on the daily UVP, suggesting that the site of their formation is the proximal colon.

Boutwell and Bosch (1959) showed that a wide range of phenolic compounds, including phenol and *p*-cresol, were promoters of tumours of the mouse skin initiated by dimethylbenzanthracene. Germ-free rats do not have UVP, and it has been hypothesized by Bakke and Midtvedt (1970) that the UVP synthesized in the liver and detoxified by the liver are the cause of the hepatomas which are common in conventional but rare in germ-free rats.

Table 18.3. *The daily urinary excretion of the volatile phenols in normal healthy persons and in various patient groups*

Patients	Urinary volatile phenols (mg/day)		
	Phenol	*p*-cresol	Total
Healthy British persons	11.3	56.8	68.1
Persons on 140 g protein/day			108.1
60 g protein/day			74.1
Patients with small bowel overgrowth	46.5	93.7	140.2
Patients with pre-operative bowel preparation	2.4	19.2	21.6
Patients with total colectomy	5.0	1.2	6.2
Patients with left hemi-colectomy	4.8	56.7	61.5

6. *N-nitroso Compounds*

N-nitroso compounds are formed by the action of nitrite on a suitable nitrogen compound, such as a secondary amine, an amide, a urea group etc. The *N*-nitroso compounds form a class of potent carcinogens, some of which are locally acting (e.g. *N*-nitrosamides, *N*-nitrosoureas) whilst others are target organ specific (e.g. *N*-nitrosamines). The *N*-nitrosation reaction can be catalysed by acid (with a pH-optimum dependent on the parent amino or amido group) or by bacteria at neutral pH values.

Some of the evidence that bacteria are able to catalyse the *N*-nitrosation reaction is summarized in Table 18.4, and began with the experiments of Sander (1968). Initially he regarded the reaction as enzymic, but later concluded that the bacteria generated nitrite and the acid needed to catalyse the reaction. Numerous studies since then have, in almost all cases, confirmed that bacteria catalyse the *N*-nitrosation reaction, but

Table 18.4. *The formation of N-nitroso compounds by the action of gut bacteria (for details and references see Hill, 1986)*

Reference	Observation
Sander (1968)	*N*-nitroso compounds are formed at neutral pH values in the presence of bacteria and not in their absence.
Hawksworth *et al.* (1971)	Confirmed the results of Sander (1968) and extended the number of strains tested. Only a proportion of *E. coli* strains stimulate the reaction and growing cultures are needed.
Klubes *et al.* (1972)	Repeated the above. Concluded that the reaction is partly enzymic and partly non-enzymic.
Brooks *et al.* (1972)	*N*-nitrosation *in vivo* in urine by *Proteus* spp.
Coloe and Heywood (1976)	Studied kinetics of the reaction. Confirmed the wide variation in the ability of bacteria to stimulate the reaction.
Tannenbaum *et al.* (1978)	Demonstrated *N*-nitrosation in saliva. Live bacteria needed.
Ruddell *et al.* (1978)	Demonstrated *N*-nitrosation in gastric juice by bacteria
Kunisaka and Hayashi (1979)	Concluded that *N*-nitrosation in *E. coli* is enzymic
Leach *et al.* (1985)	Confirmed bacterial nitrosation and studied the kinetics of the reaction.

have continually debated whether the catalysis is enzymic or non-enzymic. The main problems have been caused by the evolution of the assay techniques; as each successive method has been found to have shortcomings the number and type of controls needed has been realized, usually retrospectively. In 1985 Leach *et al.* published the results of a meticulous study designed to resolve this question, and concluded that the bacterial catalysis of the *N*-nitrosation of morpholine and similar secondary amines is enzymic. The enzymic activity is very much greater in denitrifying bacteria (e.g. *Pseudomonas* spp., some *Neisseria* spp.) than in non-denitrifying bacteria (e.g. *E. coli*) (Table 18.5), has a pH-optimum close to 7 and has first order kinetics with respect to both nitrite and nitrosatable amine. The characteristics of the reaction are summarized in Table 18.6.

Table 18.5. *The activity of N-nitrosation by various bacterial genera and species (data from Leach* et al. *(1985))*

Organisms	Class	Rate of nitrosation
Pseudomonas aeruginosa	Denitrifying	50 – 24000
Bacillus licheniformis	Denitrifying	340 – 2900
Neisseria spp.	Denitrifying	240 – 1900
Neisseria spp.	Non-denitrifying	0
Pseudomonas spp.	Non-denitrifying	0
E. coli	Non-denitrifying	0 – 90
Clostridium spp.	Non-denitrifying	0
Streptococcus spp.	Non-denitrifying	0
Veillonella spp.	Non-denitrifying	0

Table 18.6. *The characteristics of the N-nitrosation reaction when catalysed by bacteria*

Characteristic	Observation
pH-optimum	Between 6.5 and 8.5
Kinetics	First order with respect both to amine and nitrite concentration
	Rate depends on the pK_a of the amine
Enzyme location	Whole cells are needed for enzyme activity; disruption of the cells leaves both the cell debris and the supernatant without activity
Enzyme production	In some strains, related to aerobiosis and to nitrate concentration
	Induced in denitrifiers by nitrite

Bacterial nitrosation can occur at any site in the body where bacteria, nitrate or nitrite, and nitrosatable nitrogen compounds occur together. The reaction has been demonstrated in saliva, the hypochlorhydric stomach, the small bowel of patients with chronic renal failure, the infected urinary bladder, the colon and the vagina of women with *Trichomonas vaginalis* infection (Table 18.7).

Although nitrate is present in most body secretions, it is nitrite which is involved in *N*-nitrosation; the only source of nitrate reductase in the body that has been unambiguously demonstrated is the bacterial flora, amongst which the enzyme is widely distributed. Nitrosatable amino compounds in the body are mainly of endogenous origin and include alkylureas, secondary amines and amides. The secondary amines dimethyl-amine, piperidine and pyrrolidine are produced by bacterial action in

Table 18.7. *Sites in the body where N-nitrosation has been demonstrated or claimed*

Site	Special Conditions
Saliva	*in vitro*
Stomach	Normal (acid catalysed)
	Achlorhydric (bacterial catalysis?)
Urinary bladder	Bacterial infection
	Bilharzial infection
Colon	Normal
	In unreterosigmoidostomy
Cervix	*Trichomonas vaginalis* infection

the colon, from where they are absorbed, secreted in a wide range of body secretions (e.g. saliva, gastric juice) and finally excreted in the urine. Lecithin is hydrolysed by lecithinase C to release choline, which in turn is dealkylated to dimethylamine. Lysine is decarboxylated and the resultant diamine deaminated to yield an amino aldehyde which spontaneously cyclizes and hydrogenates to piperidine. Ornithine under-goes a similar series of microbial reactions to give pyrrolidine. Approximately 20–40 mg/day of dimethylamine, 1 mg/day piperidine and 0.5 mg/day pyrrolidine is synthesized in the human large bowel and excreted in the urine.

Thus bacteria are implicated in the endogenous production of *N*-nitroso compounds in (*i*) the synthesis of nitrosatable amines, (*ii*) reduction of nitrate to nitrite, and (*iii*) catalysis of the *N*-nitrosation reaction.

7. *Bile Acid Metabolites*

The bile acids synthesized by the liver are the taurine and glycine conjugates of cholic (3,7,12-trihydroxycholanic) and chenodeoxycholic (3,7-dihydroxycholanic) acids. These are metabolized by the gut bacteria via (*i*) cholanoylamide hydrolase, which releases the free bile acids from their conjugates; (*ii*) hydroxysteroid dehydrogenase active at the 3, 7 and 12 positions which convert the hydroxyl groups (as synthesized by the liver) to oxo groups with, in some cases, the reverse reaction – yielding hydroxyl groups; (*iii*) 7α-dehydroxylase which removes the 7α-hydroxyl group from cholic acid (to give deoxycholic acid) and from chenodeoxycholic acid (to give lithocholic acid); (*iv*) the nuclear dehydrogenation reactions that yield unsaturated bile acids and which include 4-dehydrogenase and aromatase. These are summarized in Table 18.8; the subject was reviewed by Hill (1975).

Although the liver of the human and some other animals is only able to hydroxylate at the 3,7 and 12 positions, other carbons are hydroxylated in some other species and this results in an extremely complex pattern of bile acid metabolites. Table 18.9 lists some of the bile acids produced by non-humans, together with their bacterial metabolites.

There is now a copious literature on the co-carcinogenicity or co-mutagenicity of the bile acids, and this is summarized in Table 18.10. In early studies the bile acids were injected in an oily vehicle now known to be a major source of phorbol esters (a potent group of co-carcinogens); these gave rise to subcutaneous tumours. In later animal studies the bile acids have been delivered per-rectum to animals treated with a known colon carcinogen; these studies will be discussed in more detail later. In addition, the bile acids have been tested by a wide array of *in vitro* tests of mutagenicity or co-mutagenicity. In a small number of cases bile acids

Table 18.8. *Bacterial enzymes which degrade the bile acids*

Enzyme	Substrate	Product
Cholanoylglycine hydrolase	Conjugated bile acids	Free bile acids
Hydroxysteroid oxido reductases	Hydroxy bile acids	Oxo bile acids
7α-dehydroxylase	Cholic acid	Deoxycholic acid
	Chenodeoxycholic acid	Lithocholic acid
4-dehydrogenase	3-oxo-5β-cholanoate	3-oxo-4-cholenoate
Aromatase	3-oxo-4-cholenoate	Bile acid with a phenolic A ring

Table 18.9. *Bile acids synthesized by various animal species*

Name	Position of hydroxyls	Animal species	Major bacterial metabolites
Cholic acid	3α, 7α, 12α	Humans and most mammals and birds	Deoxycholic acid 3α, 12α
Chenodeoxycholic acid	3α, 7α	Most mammals and birds	Lithocholic acid (3α)
Hyocholic acid	3α, 6α, 7α	Pigs	Hyodeoxycholic acid $(3\alpha, 6\alpha)$ 3β 6α dehydroxycholanic acid
α-muricholic acid	3α, 6β, 7α	Rats, mice	3α 6β dehydroxycholonic acid β-muricholic acid
β-muricholic acid	3α, 6β, 7β	Rats, mice	3α 6β dehydroxycholonic acid
7-hydroxy-3-oxo-4-cholonic acid	7α	Domestic fowl	3 oxo-4, 6-choladienoic acid
β-Lagodeoxycholic acid (allodeoxycholic acid)	3α, 12α	Rabbits	Probably itself a bacterial metabolite

Table 18.10. *Evidence that bile acids are carcinogens, co-carcinogens, mutagens or co-mutagens*

Test System	Active Bile Acids	Activity
Skin painting on rats	Deoxycholic acid	Co-carcinogen
Skin painting on mice	Apocholic acid Deoxycholic acid	Co-carcinogen
Bacterial mutagenicity	(*a*) Deoxycholic acid	Mutagen
	(*b*) Deoxycholic acid Lithocholic acid	Co-mutagen
Drosophila mutagenicity	Deoxycholic acid	Mutagen
Cell transformation test	Lithocholic acid	Transforming agent
MNNG or DMH-treated rats	Lithocholic acid Deoxycholic acid	Colon co-carcinogen

have been shown to be full mutagens and to possess cell transforming activity (Kelsey and Pienta, 1979; Demerec, 1948), but in general they have been shown to be tumour promoters in animal studies and mutagenicity promoters in the *in vitro* assays. Almost all of the work has been with deoxycholic and lithocholic acids or the primary bile acids from which they were derived. No study has yet shown unambiguously that the primary bile acids, as synthesized by the liver, have any mutagenicity, carcinogenicity, co-mutagenicity or co-carcinogenicity, and only the bile acid metabolites have proved to be active. In the small number of studies where positive results were obtained with primary bile acids there was clear evidence of bacterial metabolism. There has been one study of the structure–activity relationships in bile acid co-mutagenicity. Wilpart *et al.* (1985) used promotion of mutagenesis caused by dimethylhydrazine in the Ames *Salmonella* mutagenesis assay to show that (*i*) conjugated and primary bile acids were inactive; (*ii*) steroids with 3β hydroxyl groups were more active than those with 3α-hydroxyl groups, and (*iii*) the 5β-bile acids were more active than the 5α-bile acids. Thus the key enzymes in increasing the comutagenicity of the bile acids are the amide hydrolase and the 7α-dehydroxylase (the two major reactions carried out by bacteria on the bile acids), the 3-hydroxysteroid dehydrogenase (which inverts the 3-hydroxyl group) and the 3-oxo-4-dehydrogenase (necessary for the inversion of the 5 carbon atom).

8. Cholesterol Metabolism

Cholesterol is metabolized by the gut bacterial flora at two positions; the 5–6 double bond is hydrogenated and the 3-hydroxyl group may be oxidized or inverted (Table 18.11). By far the most important metabolite

Table 18.11. *The principal metabolites of cholesterol produced by the gut bacterial flora*

Metabolite	Bacterial enzymes used
Coprostanol	Reduction of the 5–6 bond to give a 5β steroid
Coprostanone	Reduction of the 5–6 bond and oxidation of the 3 hydroxyl group
Cholesterol	Inversion of the 3β hydroxyl group to give a 3 group
Cholestanol	Inversion of the 3β hydroxyl group and reduction of the 5–6 double bond

is coprostanol, although on occasions significant amounts of coprostanone may also be formed.

Much has been written about the possible carcinogenicity of cholesterol following the reports by Hieger (summarized in Hieger (1958)) that cholesterol, when injected subcutaneously in the rat, caused an increased incidence of tumours. This was studied in detail by a number of groups, and in his review of the evidence Bischoff (1969) concluded that the phenomenon observed was solid state carcinogenesis caused by the crystals of cholesterol formed after subcutaneous injection.

It is hard to believe that cholesterol, which is present in the tissues of all animals in large amounts, could be carcinogenic. However, if it is, then bacterial metabolism would be a protective process inactivating the carcinogen and also (since coprostanol is insoluble and does not readily form mixed micelles with fatty acids and bile acids) removes it from solution.

C. The Gut Flora and Cancer in Laboratory Animals

The role of the gut bacterial flora in carcinogenesis in laboratory animals can be studied at a number of levels. The overall risk of cancer in animals can be observed in germ-free compared with the conventional states. In this context 'conventional' means that the animals possess a normal bacterial flora of the gastro-intestinal tract. Alternatively, animals may be treated with target-organ-specific carcinogens and the effect of the flora determined by comparing germ-free with conventional animals or by removing the flora at the target site, etc. Alternatively, where a specific bacterial metabolite has been incriminated, germ-free animals may be compared with animals colonized only by organisms possessing the specific activity to be studied.

1. *Hepatic Neoplasma*

Roe and Grant (1970) studied the effect of germ-free status on the rate of development of liver tumours in C3H mice. The major part of the study involved treatment of the animals with dimethylbenzanthracene (DMBA). When conventional animals were treated with 30 g DMBA within 24 hours of birth 17 of 21 developed hepatic tumours and 10 of 21 developed lung tumours during the next 30 weeks; the comparable tumour rate for the germ-free animals was 3/23 with liver tumours and 1/23 with lung tumours (Table 18.12). In the untreated control animals,

Table 18.12. *The effect of germ-free status on the development of cancers in C3H mice (data from Roe and Grant (1970))*

Microbiological status of the mice	Treatment	Age at end of experiment (weeks)	Number of mice with tumours	
			Liver	Lung
Conventional	None	12	7/22	0/22
Germ-free	None	28–30	1/16	0/16
Conventional	30 μg DMBA at <24 hours	29–30	17/21	10/21
Germ-free	30 μg DMBA at <24 hours	30–31	3/23	1/23

which were followed for 40 weeks, none of the animals in either group developed lung tumours, but 7 of the 22 conventional mice developed hepatic tumours compared with only 1 of 16 in the germ-free mice. In addition, the authors noted that the female conventional mice developed more ovarian and uterine tumours than did their germ-free sisters, although the difference was not statistically significant.

Mizutani and Mitsuoka (1979) have developed the story further by introducing specific mixtures of organisms back into germ-free C3H male mice and noting the effect on the rate of development of hepatomas during a 48 week life span (Table 18.13). In the germ-free animals 39% developed hepatomas compared with 82% of conventional mice; of the mono-infected animals *Bacteroides multiacidus* gave tumours in 100% of the mice, *Cl. indolis* and *Bif. infantis* gave tumours in 70–80% and *E. coli*, *Strep. faecalis* and *Bif. adolescentis* gave tumours in 60–70%. When mixtures of strains were used, high rates of tumour production were observed with mixtures of *E. coli* + *Cl. perfringens*, *E. coli* + *S. faecalis* + *B. fragilis* or *E. coli* + *S. faecalis* + 4 strains of *Cl. paraputrificum* (Table 18.13). When as many as eight more strains were added to these mixtures there was no further enhancement of tumorigenesis, but when *L. acidophilus* was added the rate of tumour formation dramatically decreased. Unfortunately it was not possible to confirm the suppression of hepatic tumour formation by *L. acidophilus* because it was not possible to monocontaminate animals with that organism.

It was hypothesized by Bakke and Midtvedt (1970) that the spontaneous hepatic tumours in conventional C3H mice were caused, at least in part, by the tumour promoting effect of the volatile phenols produced by the gut flora and which would be transported to the liver via the portal blood system for detoxification. In accordance with this, it has been noted that

Table 18.13. *The incidence of hepatomas in C3H male mice either conventionally colonized, or germ-free or colonized with a single organism (data from Mizutani and Mitsuoka (1979))*

Colonic flora	Number of mice	Animals with hepatomas	Number of nodules/ mouse
Germ-free	49	19 (39%)	0.5
Conventional	17	14 (82%)	1.6
E. coli	13	8 (62%)	1.5
Bacteroides multiacidus	12	12 (100%)	1.5
Clostridium indolis	19	14 (74%)	1.4
Bif. infantis	19	15 (79%)	1.5
Bif. adolescentis	16	11 (69%)	1.0
Strep. faecalis	18	12 (67%)	1.0
E. coli + *Cl. perfringens*	16	14 (88%)	1.7
E. coli + *S. faecalis* + *B. fragilis*	20	16 (80%)	1.5
E. coli + *S. faecalis* + *Cl. paraputrificum*	20	19 (95%)	2.9
E. coli + *S. faecalis* + *B. fragilis* + *Cl. perfringens* + *L. acidophilus*	13	6 (46%)	0.9

the rate of hepatic tumour formation was increased by increased dietary protein.

2. *Intestinal Tumours*

Early studies on the effect of germ-free status on the rate of intestinal carcinogenesis were reported by Laqueur *et al.* (1967) who showed that cycasin (the glycoside of methylazoxymethanol) was a potent intestinal carcinogen in the intestine of conventional rodents, but caused no tumours or hepatotoxicity in germ-free rodents because of their lack of bacterial β-glucosidase (see section A1).

There are no other examples where a specific bacterial enzyme has been clearly incriminated in the causation of any tumours. Reddy *et al.* (1974, 1975) have studied the effect of the gut flora on the rate of intestinal carcinogenesis when various intestinal carcinogens were used as tumour initiators (Tables 18.14 and 18.15). In the first study (Reddy *et al.* 1974) the initiating agent was dimethylhydrazine (DMH) and the rate of tumour formation was much more rapid in conventional than in germ-free rats; at 20 weeks 17% of conventional rats had colon carcinomas compared with none of the germ-free animals with either an adenoma or

Table 18.14. *The effect of the gut flora on the rate of formation of intestinal tumours initiated by various carcinogens in Fischer rats (data from Reddy* et al. (1974))

Microbiological status of the rats	Initiating carcinogen	Age of the rats at the end of the experiment (weeks)	Tumour formation	
			Proportion of rats affected	Proportion with carcinoma
Germ-free	DMH	40	2/18 (11%)	0/18 (0%)
Conventional	DMH	40	6/24 (25%)	4/24 (17%)
Germ-free	DMH	20	0/12 (0%)	0/12 (0%)
Conventional	DMH	20	2/12 (17%)	2/12 (17%)
Germ-free	MNNG	50	24/24 (100%)	21/24 (88%)
Conventional	MNNG	50	23/23 (100%)	19/23 (83%)

Table 18.15. *The effect of the presence of an intestinal flora and the type of tumour initiation on the formation of tumours at various sites (data from Reddy* et al. (1975))

Microbiological status of the rats	Initiating carcinogen	Age at the end of the experiment (weeks)	Animals with tumours (%)			
			Ear	Kidney	Small intestine	Colon
Germ-free (28)	DMH	35	7	0	11	43
Conventional (28)	DMH	35	50	36	36	86
Germ-free (20)	AOM	35	30	10	55	100
Conventional (28)	AOM	35	25	18	46	60

a carcinoma. At 40 weeks a small proportion of germ-free rats had benign adenomas (although still none had carcinomas), but the proportion was much lower than that in conventional rats at 20 weeks; by 40 weeks the proportion of conventional rats with adenomas and carcinomas was 50% higher than at 20 weeks. Thus the gut flora had a tumour-promoting effect when DMH was the tumour initiator. When N-methyl-N-nitro-N-nitrosoguanidine (MNNG) was used as the initiator, in contrast, the rate of tumour formation was as high in the germ-free as in the conventional animals in terms of the proportion of rats affected. In a subsequent study (Reddy *et al.*, 1975) the effect of DMH was compared with that of azoxymethane in germ-free and conventional rats (Table 18.15). In the rats treated with DMH, germ-free status protected not only against colon cancers but also against the formation for tumours of the ear duct, kidney and small intestine. In contrast AOM caused more tumours at all sites (except the kidney) in germ-free than in conventional rats. Thus in conclusion the presence of an intestinal bacteria flora is associated with an increased risk of tumours from DMH but a decreased risk from AOM and MNNG.

Goldin and Gorbach have extended the studies of the role of the gut flora in DMH carcinogenesis; they showed that treatment with an antibiotic cocktail likely to suppress the intestinal flora also decreased the rate of tumour formation (Goldin and Gorbach, 1981). In another study, animals treated with DMH were fed dietary supplements of *Lactobacillus acidophilus*; this resulted in a decreased rate of tumour formation (Goldin and Gorbach, 1980) and a decreased activity of several faecal enzymes including β-glucuronidase, azoreductase and nitroreductase (Goldin and Gorbach, 1977). Beef, which increased the faecal enzyme activity, also increased the number of colonic tumours (Table 18.16). A similar pattern was seen with the small bowel tumours; the effects of the *L. acidophilus* supplements were only apparent at 20 weeks and were not seen at 36 weeks, indicating that the organisms affected the rate of development of tumours, not the final number.

Other groups have extended the studies on AOM induced intestinal tumours and here the evidence shows some inconsistencies. Whereas Reddy *et al.* (1975) showed that germ-free status had no effect on the rate of tumour formation, Campbell *et al.* (1975) showed that diversion of the faecal stream had a profound effect and resulted in a decrease in the number of tumours in the defunctionalized colon. Obviously the faecal stream contains more than simply bacteria, and so its diversion may have decreased the exposure of the defunctionalized colon remnant to something other than a bacterial metabolite. The rate of tumour

Table 18.16. *The effect of diet and the activity of various faecal enzymes on the rate of carcinoma formation in rats treated with DMH (data from Goldin and Gorbach (1980))*

| | | | | % of carcinomas | |
Diet	Enzyme level[a]	Induction period	Number of animals	Small bowel	Colon
Grain	Low	36	13	8	31
Beef	High	20	22	64	77
		36	12	67	83
Beef + *L.*	Moderate	20	20	45	40
acidophilus		36	11	73	73

[a] Enzymes were β-glucuronidase, nitroreductase and azoreductase.

formation could partially be restored by irrigating the colonic remnant with dilute faeces (Rainey *et al.*, 1983).

D. The Gut Flora and Cancer in Humans

A role for bacteria has been proposed in carcinogenesis at a number of sites, and the evidence has been reviewed in detail elsewhere (Hill, 1986). The reader is referred to that book for a more detailed discussion and for more detailed references. The sites to be discussed here are the stomach, the colon, the urinary bladder and the breast.

1. *Gastric Cancer*

Cancer of the stomach is very common in East Asia and the Andean countries of South and Central America and is relatively rare in North America and Australasia. In Europe the incidence of the disease is higher in the south and east than in the north and west; within the United Kingdom the incidence of the disease is much lower in the south and east than in the north and west. Despite these geographical variations the incidence of the disease appears to be decreasing in all countries for which reliable statistics are available.

Studies of migrants from Japan to the United States, or from Eastern Europe to the United States or Australia have shown that environmental factors early in life (i.e. in the first 15 years) are important determinants of gastric cancer risk. The incidence of the disease is inversely related to socio-economic status and it seems reasonable to assume that diet is an important risk factor. However, it has proved to be extremely difficult to demonstrate a strong correlation with any dietary component in case-control studies (Table 18.17). This is readily rationalized; usually the patient has gastric symptoms for some considerable time before the carcinoma is diagnosed and this results in diet modification to ameliorate the symptoms. In consequence it is necessary to utilize dietary recall even to determine the diet at the time of the onset of serious symptoms. Despite these difficulties, the strong correlations from the comparisons of populations and the prospective cohort study and the weaker correlations from the case-control studies give a reasonably coherent picture. This is that a mixed western diet containing milk (and other dairy products) and meat is associated with a relatively low risk of gastric cancer whilst a poor diet based on root vegetables or cereals is associated with a high risk of the disease. In addition to these observations on

Table 18.17 *The relationship between diet and gastric cancer incidence (for details and references see Hill, 1986)*

Type of study	Dietary item most strongly correlated	Reference
Comparison of Populations	Animal protein (protective) Animal fat (protective)	Gregor *et al.* (1979)
	Meat (protective fibre)	Armstrong and Doll (1975)
	Salt intake	Joossens and Geboers (1981)
	Vegetarian diet	Kinlen *et al.* (1983)
Case-control studies	No strong correlations. Weak correlations with root vegetables and cereals; protective effect of meat and salad vegetables	Haenszel (1958) Wynder *et al.* (1963) Graham *et al.* (1972) Terris (1963)
Cohort Study	Milk (protective), meat (protective)	Hirayama (1977)

macronutrients, a correlation with salt intake (Joossens and Geboers, 1981) and with nitrate exposure (Hill, 1981) has also been noted. The epidemiology of gastric cancer has been well reviewed by Correa (1985).

Lauren (1965) has identified two histological types of gastric cancer, namely the diffuse and the intestinal types; most pathologists also identify a third intermediate type. This classification has been of great value in epidemiological studies because it has been noted that the incidence of the diffuse type of gastric cancer shows little geographical or temporal variation and the large variations in the incidence of gastric cancer between countries and with time are largely due to variation in the incidence of the intestinal type. This suggested that the environmental and dietary factors found to correlate with gastric cancer incidence were risk factors for the intestinal type of disease. Furthermore, Lehtola (1978) showed that whereas the risk of gastric cancer in relatives of cases of intestinal-type gastric cancer had no excess risk of the disease, that in relatives of cases of diffuse-type disease was more than seven fold higher than the risk in the general population. This genetic factor could be associated only with the diffuse type whilst environmental factors were associated with the intestinal type of disease (Table 18.18). It is in this latter type of disease that we should search, therefore, for a bacterial role.

Table 18.18. *Diffuse and intestinal gastric cancer*

	Histological types	
	Diffuse	Intestinal
Sex ratio of cases	Approx. 1	>1
Relative age at onset	Younger	Older
Associated genetic factors	ABO blood groups	None
	Familial risk	
Predisposing diseases	None	Gastric atrophy
		Gastric surgery
Association with	Weak	Strong
environmental factors		
Prognosis	Poor	Better

Correa *et al.* (1975), based on a long and copious literature from many
countries, proposed a histopathological sequence in the causation of
intestinal type gastric cancer which is illustrated in Fig. 18.2. On this
hypothesis the first stage in the disease is atrophy of the gastric mucosa
with resultant decrease in acid secretion. This may be due to natural
ageing, but can occur in young people as a result of malnutrition, high
salt intake or virus infection. Atrophic gastritis is also associated with
Campylobacter pyloridis infection, and it has been suggested that the loss
of gastric acid secretion is a direct consequence of *C. pyloridis* infection
(Marshall *et al.*, 1985). Chronic atrophic gastritis is the next stage following
gastric atrophy, and this is followed by the development, within the
atrophic areas, of zones of intestinal metaplasia. The final stages are
increasingly severe dysplasia (from mild, through moderate to severe)
and finally carcinoma. Dysplasia can occur in areas of atrophic gastritis
but is much more likely to occur within intestinal metaplasia. Although
intestinal metaplasia usually occurs in large areas of atrophic gastritis, it
can often be detected in localized areas of atrophic gastritis and where
most of the gastric mucosa is still normal and secreting acid.

The histopathological sequence as described above is accepted by most
pathologists, but Correa *et al.* (1975) also proposed a possible mechanism
in which the development of a resident gastric bacterial flora played a
crucial role. In this hypothesis, the gut flora reduced nitrate to nitrite
and then catalysed the formation of *N*-nitroso compounds which were
responsible for the progression from atrophic gastritis through intestinal
metaplasia and increasingly severe dysplasia to carcinoma. If this
hypothesis is correct than (*i*) any condition which results in decreased
gastric acidity and the establishment of a resident bacterial flora should

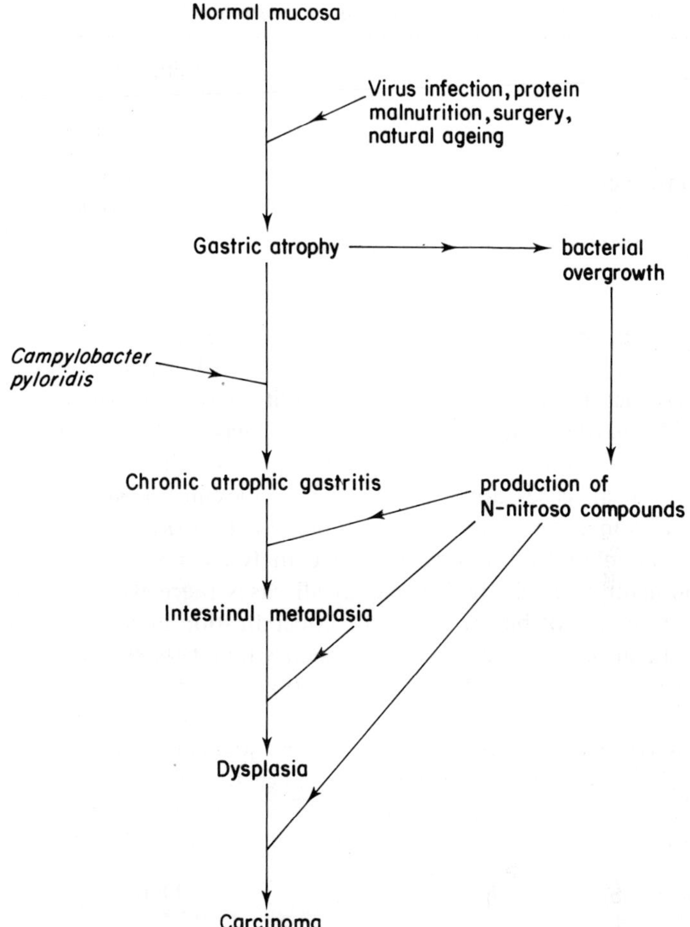

Fig 18.2 The histopathogenesis of gastric cancer.

predispose to gastric cancer; (*ii*) the rate of progression through the histopathological sequence should be correlated with the gastric juice nitrite concentration; (*iii*) this progression should also be correlated with the amount and type of *N*-nitroso compounds, and (*iv*) since some *N*-nitroso compounds are target-organ-specific and since a family of *N*-nitroso compounds is likely to be produced the conditions favouring *N*-nitroso compound formation should predispose to cancer at other sites as well as the stomach.

Table 18.19. *The relation between loss of gastric acidity and gastric cancer risk*

Gastric status	Magnitude of excess risk
Gastric atrophy	2–4–fold
Atrophic gastritis	4–fold
Intestinal metaplasia	4–6–fold
Pernicious anaemia	4–6–fold
Gastric surgery	4–6–fold after 20 year latency
Vagotomy	6–10–fold after 20 year latency

The evidence for each of these points varies considerably in strength and is good for (*i*), (*ii*) and (*iv*) but weak for (*iii*). Table 18.19 summarizes the evidence relating loss of gastric acidity with increased risk of gastric cancer; regardless of whether the loss of gastric acid is due to natural ageing, environmental factors, genetic predisposition or surgical action there is in all cases an increased risk of carcinogenesis in the stomach and this is in strong support of that part of the Correa hypothesis. There have been many studies of gastric juice analyses in patients with decreased gastric acidity (Table 18.20) and in all cases there was a great increase in the numbers of bacteria and the concentration of nitrite in the gastric juice. In all cases in which it has been studied there was a correlation between gastric juice nitrite concentration and the severity of epithelial

Table 18.20. *Gastric juice analyses in patients with decreased gastric acidity (for details and references see Hill, 1986)*

Patient Group	Reference	Effect of increased pH	
		Flora	Nitrite
Pernicious anaemia	Ruddell *et al.* (1978)	Increased	Increased
	Caygill *et al.* (1984)	Increased	Increased
	Stockbrugger *et al.* (1984)	Increased	Increased
	Hall *et al.* (1984)	Increased	Increased
	Reed *et al.* (1981)	Increased	Increased
	Watt *et al.* (1984)	Increased	Increased
	Jones *et al.* (1978)	–	Increased
Polya partial gastrectomy	Ruddell *et al.* (1976)	Increased	Increased
	Schlag *et al.* (1980)	Increased	Increased
	Redd *et al.* (1981)	Increased	Increased
	Watt *et al.* (1984)	Increased	Increased
	Kieghley *et al.* (1984)	Increased	Increased
	Caygill *et al.* (1984)	Increased	Increased
	Hall *et al.* (1984)	Increased	Increased

dysplasia or the presence of intestinal metaplasia (Table 18.21). There has, however, been considerable confusion in the literature on the relation between gastric juice pH and the concentration of N-nitroso compounds in gastric juice (Table 18.22), and this is due to differences in methodology which appear to have been resolved recently. Schlag *et al.* (1980) found a correlation between pH and N-nitroso compound concentration, and this was confirmed in a large study by Reed *et al.* (1981) and a smaller study by Stockbrugger *et al.* (1984); the two latter studies used the method of Walters *et al.* (1978). A number of other groups (for example Hall *et*

Table 18.21. *The relation between gastric juice analyses and the severity of epithelial dysplasia or the presence of intestinal metaplasia in gastric biopsies*

Patient Group	Reference	Observation
Polya partial gastrectomy	Jones *et al.* (1978)	Nitrite concentration correlated wtih severity of dysplasia
	Mortensen *et al.* (1984)	Bacterial flora and nitrite concentration correlated with dysplasia
	Hall *et al.* (1984)	Nitrite correlated to dysplasia
	Watt *et al.* (1984)	Bacterial flora and nitrite concentration correlated with dysplasia
Pernicious anaemia	Watt *et al.* (1984)	Bacterial flora and nitrite concentration correlated with dysplasia
	Hall *et al.* (1984)	Nitrite concentration correlated with dysplasia

Table 18.22. *N-nitroso compound concentration in gastric juice samples from various patient groups*

Patient Group	Reference	Observation
Polya partial gastrectomy	Schlag *et al.* (1980)	Higher than control value
	Reed *et al.* (1981)	Higher than control
	Hall *et al.* (1984)	No different from control
	Keighley *et al.* (1984)	No different from control
Pernicious anaemia	Reed *et al.* (1981)	Higher than control
	Stockbrugger *et al.* (1984)	Higher than control
	Hall *et al.* (1984)	No different from control

al. (1984) and Keighley *et al.* (1984)) used the method of Bavin *et al.* (1982) and observed either no correlation or an inverse relation with pH. Recent comparisons of the two methods by Massey *et al.* (1985) and by Pignatelli *et al.* (1987) have resulted in the emergence of new improved techniques for *N*-nitroso analysis which favour the Walters method and which are critical of a number of aspects of the method of Bavin *et al.* Crucially Pignatelli *et al.* showed a positive correlation between pH and total *N*-nitroso compound concentration and the consensus view must now be that this is the true result. Thus in all of the aspects in which it has been tested the hypothesis of Correa *et al.* (1975) has been confirmed; however it has still to be demonstrated that the *N*-nitroso compound concentration, like the nitrite concentration, correlates with the severity of epithelial dysplasia in the gastric mucosa.

The final available evidence of the Correa hypothesis is derived from studies of the risk of cancer at other sites. Caygill *et al.* (1984), in a small study of approximately 300 patients from York who had a Polya partial gastrectomy for peptic ulcer between 1940 and 1948, noted that, in addition to the excess risk of gastric cancer with a 20 year latency observed by others, there was an excess risk of cancer of the biliary tract and of the large bowel, also with a 20 year latency (Table 18.23). In addition, they showed an excess risk of gastric, colorectal and biliary tract cancer in a group of 1000 patients with pernicious anaemia. In a follow-up study of 5018 patients treated surgically for peptic ulcer the previous results were confirmed (Caygill *et al.*, 1985), and in addition an excess risk with the same 20 year latency was observed in cancer of the breast, oesophagus and pancreas (Table 18.24). These observations are consistent with the hypothesis that in the achlorhydric stomach the resident bacterial flora produces nitrate reductase to yield nitrite, and also catalyses the production

Table 18.23. *The risk of carcinogenesis in 300 York patients following gastric surgery and in patients with pernicious anaemia (data from Caygill* et al. *(1984)).*

Patient Group	Cancer Risk	Latency
300 patients from York General Hospital treated surgically for peptic ulcer	Excess risk of cancer of the stomach, colorectum and biliary tract	20 years for each site
1000 patients with pernicious anaemia	Excess risk of cancer of the stomach, colorectum and biliary tract	Not determinable

Table 18.24. *Cancer risk in 5018 patients treated surgically for peptic ulcer at St James Hospital, Balham (data from Caygill* et al. *(1985))*

| | Excess risk of cancer after gastric surgery | |
Site of cancer	0–20 years	More than 20 years
Stomach	None	4.5–fold (5.5–fold)[a]
Colorectum	None	1.6–fold (3.0–fold)
Biliary tract	None	8.6–fold (15.8–fold)
Oesophagus	None	2.3–fold (3.0–fold)
Breast	None	4.0–fold (4.0–fold)
Bladder	None	2.4–fold (2.5–fold)
Pancreas	None	3.8–fold (5.8–fold)
Lung	1.3–fold	3.9–fold (3.7–fold)

[a] Figures in brackets are for patients treated for gastric ulcer

of N-nitroso compounds that cause the production of local and of distant tumours.

2.   *Bacterial N-nitrosation and Other Cancers*

Since N-nitroso compounds produced by bacterial action in the stomach are responsible for the high risk of local cancers, a similar high risk of local cancer would be expected at other sites with a resident flora and where N-nitroso compound formation would be expected. Such sites include the chronically infected urinary bladder, the infected vagina, chronic small bowel overgrowth and the colon of persons with ureterocolic anastomosis (Table 18.25).

Although the urinary bladder is normally sterile, infections are far from rare; in a study by Sinclair and Tuxford (1971) in a rural general practice in England more than 20% of adults had a urinary tract infection (usually asymptomatic and of short duration) at some time during a year. There is no evidence that such infections carry any cancer risk, but chronic urinary tract infection is associated with an increased risk of bladder cancer (Radomski *et al.*, 1978); such chronic infections are usually simple and involve a single infecting organism. The risk of malignancy is much greater when the infection involves a mixed bacterial flora such as those associated with bilharzia of the bladder (Hicks *et al.*, 1977) or paraplegia (Hicks, 1982). In those situations the nitrate reductase activity of the flora is very high, as is the amount of N-nitroso compound formed.

Table 18.25. *The association between chronic bacterial infection, the demonstration of N-nitroso compound formation, and increased risk of carcinogenesis (for details and references see Hill, 1986)*

Site	Disease	N-nitroso compounds	Cancer risk
Urinary bladder	Chronic infection	+	Increased (Radomski *et al.*, 1978)
	Bilharzia	+	Increased (El-Sebai, 1977)
	Paraplegia	+	Increased (Melzak, 1966)
Vagina	*Trichomonas vaginalis* infection	+	Increased cervical cancer (Robertson *et al.*, 1971)
Duodenum	Overgrowth associated with chronic renal failure	+	Increased cancer risk in CRF (Matas *et al.*, 1975)

In general the upper small intestine is only sparsely populated (Borriello, 1986), but in patients with chronic renal failure there is a profuse flora in the duodenum and jejunum (Simenhoff *et al.*, 1978). In such patients the formation of *N*-nitroso compounds in the small bowel has been demonstrated (Simenhoff *et al.*, 1984); and this is associated with an increased risk of total cancers (Matas *et al.*, 1975). Because such patients do not have a long life expectancy and the number of patient years at risk for a given patient group is therefore small, it has not been possible, as yet, to specify the cancer sites carrying the greatest excess risk.

The normal human vagina carries a profuse resident flora (Table 18.26) which is dominated by the lactic acid bacteria (lactobacilli and streptococci), as would be expected in an environment which has a pH of approximately 5. In women with vaginitis associated with *Gardnerella vaginalis* infection, gonorrhoea, non-specific vaginitis or *Trichomonas vaginalis* infection, in contrast, there is a highly putrefactive flora rich in *Bacteroides* spp. and coliforms, and a vaginal pH close to neutral. The sequence of events which give rise to this set of conditions is unclear. It is possible that the initial events favour the development of a putrefactive flora which generates a neutral pH and impairs the colonization resistance of the flora to pathogens; alternatively the pathogens could generate a neutral pH which favours the growth of a putrefactive flora, etc. Regardless of the route, the end result is a flora rich in nitrate reductase, in contrast to the normal vaginal flora which has little nitrate reductase activity. It is likely that nitrate is present in vaginal secretions (since it appears to

Table 18.26. *The bacterial flora of the normal human vagina (expressed as frequency of isolation)*

Organisms	Hurley *et al.* (1974)	Gordon *et al.* (1966)
Lactobacillus spp.	82	81
Corynebacterium spp.	83	39
Streptococcus spp. – total	41	24
– faecal	41	
– β-haemolytic	9	
– non-haemolytic	4	
Coliforms		12
– *E. coli*	19	
– *Proteus* spp.	6	
– *Klebsiella* spp.	1	
Staphylococcus aureus	5	
– *S. epidermidis*	66	
Anaerobic organisms		21
Streptococci	22	
Bacteroides spp.	5	
Yeasts	24	
Candida spp.		10
Mycoplasma	11	15

be present in all other body secretions); the smell of the exudate from the infected vagina testifies to the high amine content and so the conditions in the infected vagina are favourable for N-nitrosation. In support of this the presence of N-nitroso compounds in the vaginal exudate of patients with *T. vaginalis* infection has been reported (Allsobrook *et al.*, 1975), and it has been proposed that this is the mechanism for the observed excess risk of cervical cancer in such patients (Harington *et al.*, 1973).

The urine is the major route of excretion of nitrate and of nitrosatable amino compounds; in patients in whom the urine is diverted into the sigmoid colon (ureterosigmoidostomy or ureterosigmoid anastomosis patients) the ideal conditions for the bacterial production of N-nitroso compounds would appear to be created. In such patients there is a very high risk of cancer at the anastomotic junction with a 20 year latency; the excess risk has been estimated to be 200-fold (Stewart *et al.*, 1981), although earlier estimates suggested an even higher risk. Although ureterocolic anastomosis was the operation of choice for urine diversion until the 1960s, it has been replaced first by the ileal loop and, more recently, by the colonic loop. A study of the bacterial flora of urine from the three types of diversion (Hill *et al.*, 1983) revealed that the ileal loop contained a highly complex flora whilst the colonic loop was usually either bacteriologically clear or contained a single contaminating organism. By analogy with the situation in those with bladder infection, it would be expected that the ureterocolic anastomosis (which has the most complex flora) would carry the highest cancer risk, colonic loops (with the simplest flora) would carry the lowest risk and ileal loops would carry an intermediate risk. Already there have been reports of cancers in ileal loops (Shousa *et al.*, 1978) but it is too early to assess the magnitude of the excess risk. It is also, of course, much too early to assess the risk of cancer in colonic loops.

3.   *The Colonic Flora and Human Colorectal Cancer*

Colorectal cancer is common in north and west Europe, North America and Australasia, and is relatively uncommon in Africa, Asia and the Andean countries of South and Central America. Within Europe the disease is much more common in the north and west than in the south and east; similarly within the British Isles it is much more common in the north (Scotland) and west (Ireland) than in the south and east (particularly south east England). The disease is more common in urban than in rural areas and is more common in the higher socio-economic groups within a country. The epidemiology of the disease has been reviewed recently by Correa (1978), Faivre *et al.* (1985) and Hill (1986), and is briefly summarized in Table 18.27.

Considerable effort has been expended on the study of the relation between colorectal cancer risk and diet (Table 18.28). In general, studies comparing populations have shown a strong correlation with the intake of dietary fat and meat. In populations with a high fat/meat intake there is an inverse correlation with dietary fibre, but in populations with a low fat/meat intake there is no relation with dietary fibre. Case control studies have usually failed to reveal strong correlations, and there are good reasons why this might be expected. All colorectal diseases are associated both with decreased food intake and with changed diet (in order to try to ameliorate the symptoms). In the case of colorectal cancer, there is usually an interval of many months between the onset of symptoms (e.g. faecal blood, abdominal pain, etc.) and the diagnosis of cancer; during this time the diet may undergo considerable change and this makes it particularly difficult to determine the diet corresponding to the time before the onset of symptoms. Because of these inherent problems it is hardly surprising, in retrospect, that almost any dietary item has been implicated as either a causal or protective factor by somebody at some

Table 18.27. *The epidemiology of large bowel cancer*

Characteristic	Observation
Geographical distribution	Incidence high in western Europe, North America, Australasia, River Plate area; low in Asia, Africa, Andean countries of South and Central America
Incidence in Europe	High in west and north, relatively low in south and east
Urban/rural differences	Incidence higher in urban than in rural areas
Social class correlations	Incidence higher in higher socio-economic groups
Sex ratio (M : F)	Ratio is 0.8–1.0 for colon cancer in most countries, and 1.2–1.6 for rectal cancer
Migrant studies	Migrants have the risk associated with their new homeland, not their country of origin, suggesting a key role for environmental factors
Studies of cultural groups	Studies of religious, racial or other cultural groups show that the physical environment (e.g. climate altitude, air pollution) are much less important than cultural factors (e.g. diet, use of drugs, etc.)
Associated diseases	Associated cancers – breast, endometrium, prostate Associated diseases – heart diseases, diabetes, chronic colitis, colorectal adenomas

Table 18.28. *Diet and the causation of colorectal cancer (for details and references see Hill (1986))*

Type of study	Observation
Comparison of populations	Strong correlation with fat and meat If high fat/meat, inverse correlation with fibre If low fat/meat, no relation with fibre
Case-control studies	Correlations with fat, meat, beer, fibre, Inverse correlations with fibre, vitamin C, vitamin A (but most studies show no correlations)
Cohort study	Correlation with meat and fat; Inverse relation to green-yellow vegetable

time. The most important study to consider is the large cohort study of more than 250 000 Japanese by Hirayama (1985); this has shown a causal relationship with meat and fat and a protective effect of green-yellow vegetables.

The initial searches for a mechanism for the relationship between diet and colorectal carcinogenesis centred on the search for a dietary carcinogen. The diet is a rich source of carcinogens, mutagens and tumour promoters; some of these are naturally occurring (e.g. cycasin in cycad nuts, alkylhydrazines in mushrooms), some are present as a result of food additives (e.g. nitrite giving *N*-nitrosos compounds, food colours, etc.), some are produced during the cooking process (e.g. polycyclic aromatic hydrocarbons, the wide range of pyrolysis products formed in grilled or fried foods) and some are the result of food spoilage (e.g. aflatoxin and other mycotoxins). Despite this wide array of ingested carcinogens, none has been found to correlate with the risk of colorectal cancer. Consequently in 1969 we proposed (Aries *et al.*, 1969) that the disease was caused by a metabolite produced *in situ* in the colon by bacterial action on some benign substrate. Most of the carcinogens/promoters/mutagens described earlier in this chapter are produced in the human colon and so are potential candidates. There have been two principal routes to the testing of this hypothesis, one concentrating on determining the nature of the substrate and the other concentrating on the bacteriological aspects.

In studies of the bacteriological aspects, the first reports were of the composition of the faecal bacterial flora of population living in areas with a high or a low risk of the disease (Table 18.29). After initial hopeful results (e.g. comparing Ugandans eating a diet of matoke bananas and people living in London on a mixed western-style diet (Aries *et al.*, 1969)), it rapidly emerged that this was not a fruitful field of study for a number of reasons. The faecal bacterial flora is extremely complex and so, when standard bacteriological methods are used, only gross differences can be recognized. Further, the site of bacterial metabolism is the proximal colon (Hill, 1982; Fadden *et al.*, 1985; Boyer *et al.*, 1984), but the faecal flora appears to bear little relation to the caecal flora (Fernandez *et al.*, 1984, 1985). In addition, the hypothesis to be tested concerns the production of a metabolite and this is as likely to be due to enzyme induction as to changes in the composition of the flora. For these reasons, the stress was transferred to the study of enzyme activity using a set of 'sentinel enzymes'; the enzymes chosen for study (for example, nitro reductase, β-glucosidase, β-glucuronidase, 7-cholanoyldehydroxylase) were selected because *in vitro* studies suggested that they might be implicated in carcinogen/mutagen formation or release. The assay of the 'sentinel enzymes' has been carried out in populations at varying risk of colorectal cancer and in groups following dietary manipulations thought, on epidemiological criteria, to be associated with altered risk of the disease. Such assays are much more precise than counts of bacteria and so should be able to detect smaller differences; this is probably the reason

Table 18.29. *The bacterial flora of faeces from six populations in relation to the incidence of colorectal cancer (data from Hill et al. (1971))*

	Populations studied					
	Uganda	Japan	India	USA	England	Scotland
Incidence of colorectal cancer	0.6	4.9	5.7	28.1	18.2	31.2
Number of samples analysed	48	17	51	34	68	23
Anaerobic bacteria						
Total	9.3	9.9		10.2	10.1	10.2
Bacteroides spp.	8.2	9.4	9.2	9.8	9.8	9.8
Bifidobacterium spp.	9.3	9.7	9.6	10.1	9.8	9.9
Clostridium spp.	5.2	5.7	5.9	5.3	5.8	5.7
Veillonella spp.	5.3	4.7	5.8	3.9	4.2	3.8
Sarcina spp.	5.2		4.6	–	–	–
Facutlative organisms						
Total	8.2	9.4	8.2	7.5	8.0	7.7
Enterobacteria	8.0	9.3	7.9	7.4	7.9	7.6
Streptococcus spp.	7.8	8.5	7.9	7.0	7.1	6.8
Faecal strep.	7.0	8.1	7.3	5.9	5.8	5.3
Bacillus spp.	4.5	4.4	4.9	3.7	3.7	3.3
Microaerophilic organisms						
Lactobacillus spp.	7.2	7.4	7.6	7.1	6.5	7.7

for the higher proportion of positive correlations observed in assays of sentinel enzymes. However, the assays are of *faecal* enzymes and there is no evidence to suggest that this reflects the activity in the caecum.

The next step was to focus more on particular enzymes implicated in bile acid metabolism, because of the strong association between bile acids and colorectal carcinogenesis (summarized in Table 18.30). Two enzyme activities have received particular attention, the cholanoyl 7α-dehyroxylase and 3-oxo-steroid 4-dehydrogenase. The 7α-dehydroxylase yields lithocholic acid (LA) and deoxycholic acid (DCA) from cholic acid (CA) and chenodeoxycholic acid (CDCA) respectively. These bile acid products are co-carcinogenic in the rodent colon (Narisawa *et al.*, 1974) and are co-mutagenic in bacterial mutagenesis assay systems (Wilpart *et al.*, 1985), whereas the substrates are not. In comparisons of populations the faecal bile acids are more extensively dehydroxylated in populations at high risk of the disease (Hill, 1971); in case-control studies the activity of the

Table 18.30. *Evidence implicating cholanoyl 7α-dehydroxylase and 3-oxo-steroid 4-dehydrogenase in the causation of colorectal cancer*

Enzyme	Evidence
Cholanoyl 7α-dehydroxylase	Bile acids are more extensively dehydroxylated in faeces of populations at high risk of the disease than in those at low risk In case-control studies enzyme activity is higher in the faeces of cases than of controls Products of 7-dehydroxylation are much more co-mutagenic and co-carcinogenic than are the parent substrates
3-oxo-steroid-4-dehydrogenase	Organisms possessing the enzyme are more commonly found in populations at high risk than in those at low risk of colorectal cancer In case-control studies the organisms possessing the enzyme are present in stools of a high proportion of cases and in a relatively low proportion of controls In adenoma patients, the proportion of cases carrying organisms possessing the enzyme increases with adenoma size

enzyme is much higher in the faeces of cases than of controls (Mastromarino *et al.*, 1976; Jivraj and Hill, 1979, unpublished results).

The 3-oxo-steroid 4-dehydrogenase yields steroids with a 3-oxo-4-en structure from 3-oxo-5α steroid substrates; the products can undergo reduction under intestinal conditions either back to the substrate or to steroids with a 3-oxo-5α configuration (the allo bile acids) (Kallner, 1967). The allo bile acids have higher co-mutagenic activity than their 5 isomers (Wilpart *et al.*, 1985). In comparisons of populations the enzyme is present in faeces of a high proportion of populations at high risk than in populations at low risk of the disease (Goddard *et al.*, 1975). In case-control studies they are present in faeces of a higher proportion of cases than of controls (Hill *et al.*, 1975; Blackwood *et al.*, 1978), the carriage rate correlating with adenoma size (Hill *et al.*, 1985). Production of the enzymes by gut bacteria is summarized in Table 18.31. Colorectal cancer has a multistage histopathogenesis. Most, if not all, colorectal cancers arise in pre-existing adenomas (Morson, 1974); the risk of malignancy in an adenoma is related to its size, villousness and severity of epithelial dysplasia (Morson *et al.*, 1983), as illustrated in Table 18.32. Thus, although the first stage in carcinogenesis is adenoma formation (Fig. 18.3), there are subsequent stages including adenoma growth and the increase in severity of dysplasia within adenoma.

Table 18.31. *Production of cholanoyl 7α-dehydroxylase and 3-oxo-steroid 4-dehydrogenase by gut bacteria*

Organisms	7α-dehydroxylase		4-dehydrogenase	
	Number tested	% with enzyme	Number tested	% with enzyme
Bacteroides spp.	54	40	100	0
Bifidobacterium spp.	194	15	75	0
Veillonella spp.	92	3	50	0
Clostridium spp.	130	20	695	24
Cl. perfringens			100	3
Cl. bifermentans			100	0
Cl. paraputrificum			112	93
Cl. indolis			49	31
Cl. tertium			20	90
E. coli	342	0	100	0
Faecal streptococci	252	6	100	0
Strep. viridans	134	0	50	0
Lactobacillus spp.	60	0	50	0
Bacillus spp.	50	0	50	0

Table 18.32. *The malignant potential of adenomas in relation to their size, villousness and severity of epithelial dysplasia*

	Percentage of adenomas with a malignant component
Adenoma size	
Less than 3 mm	0.1
3–10 mm	1.3
10–20 mm	9.5
More than 20 mm	46.0
Villousness	
Tubular	4.8
Tubulovillous	22.5
Villous	41
Severity of dysplasia	
Mild	5.7
Moderate	18.0
Severe	34.5

The relation between various bacterial metabolites and the risk of colorectal cancer has been studied in depth and has been reviewed in detail elsewhere (see, for example, Hill (1986)). The best evidence implicates bile acid metabolites and the steroid 4-dehydrogenase, but

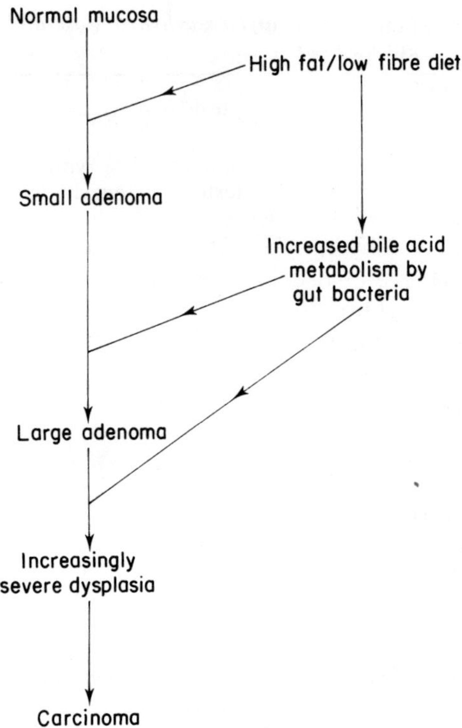

Fig 18.3 The postulated aetiology of colorectal cancer.

Table 18.33. *Evidence relating bile acid metabolites and the carriage of 3-oxo-steroid 4-dehydrogenase (nuclear dehydrogenase, NDH) in the stages of colorectal carcinogenesis*

Stage	Evidence
1. Adenoma formation	No relation between either FBA[a] or NDH[b] and either number or rate of formation of adenomas
2. Adenoma growth	Good correlation between adenoma size and both FBA and NDH
3. Increase in severity and dysplasia	Good correlation between severity of dysplasia and FBA but none with NDH

[a] FBA is faecal bile acid concentration
[b] NDH is carriage of strains producing nuclear dehydrogenase

these are not implicated in adenoma causation (Table 18.33). Neither are the organisms producing the 4-dehydrogenase implicated in the causation of increased epithelial dysplasia. The faecal bile acid concentration, however, is correlated both with adenoma size and with the severity of epithelial dysplasia, whilst the organisms producing the 4-dehydrogenase are correlated wih adenoma size (Hill *et al.*, 1985). In a separate study, Owen *et al.* (1986, 1987) have shown a relationship between the ratio of the products of 7-dehydroxylation (lithocholic to deoxycholic acid) and adenoma size; this ratio also discriminated well between colorectal cancer cases and controls (Owen *et al.*, 1985).

In conclusion, it has been hypothesized that bacterial metabolites of the bile acids are implicated in the causation of colorectal cancer, and there is evidence that the most important metabolites detected in faeces are the products of 7-dehydroxylation by gut bacteria of the primary bile acids synthesized by the liver. In addition, there is evidence that a further enzyme produced by the gut bacteria, the 3-oxo-steroid 4-dehydrogenase, may be of importance, although the products of its action have not been studied in detail in faeces.

4. *The Colonic Flora and Human Breast Cancer*

Cancer of the breast is highly correlated with colorectal cancer both in populations and in individuals. Geographically, both cancers have a high incidence in North America, western Europe and Australasia, and a relatively low incidence in Africa, Asia and the Andean countries of South and Central America. Within populations both cancers are more common in high than in low socio-economic groups. Within individuals, women who have been successfully treated for breast cancer have a risk of a subsequent colorectal cancer that is higher than that in the general population. In both cancers there is a strong correlation with dietary fat and meat. In view of the strong evidence of a role for bacteria in the causation of colorectal cancer there has been a lot of interest in their possible role in breast carcinogenesis.

Two types of investigation have been reported. The interrelation between the gut flora, oestrogen circulation and breast cancer has been reviewed recently by Gorbach (1984). There has also been interest in the relationship between bacteria, bile acids and breast cancer (Murray *et al.*, 1980; Papatestas *et al.*, 1982; Owen *et al.*, 1986).

There is a large body of evidence implicating oestrogens in human breast carcinogenesis, coming from studies of animal models of breast cancer, from the effects of surgery (such as ovariectomy, adrenalectomy, etc.) on slowing tumour growth, and from the effects of long-term oestrogen therapy (e.g. in long-term users of the contraceptive pill). Animal studies and some human observations suggest that the role of steroid oestrogens is far from simple and that, whilst there is good evidence that oestradiol is a potent tumour promoter, there is some evidence that oestradiol is an inhibitor of tumour growth. The steroid oestrogens undergo enterohepatic circulation, being conjugated by the liver to form the glucuronides and sulphates, secreted in bile, deconjugated in part by the gut bacterial flora and either (*i*) returned to the liver for further conjugation and resecretion in bile, (*ii*) conjugated by the intestinal mucosal enzymes and rapidly excreted in urine, or (*iii*) excreted in faeces. Retention of steroid oestrogens in the body, and the blood levels of such oestrogens, is determined in part, therefore, by the metabolic activities of the gut bacterial flora. Antibiotic therapy which affects the gut bacterial flora has a profound effect on oestrogen activity; it has been demonstrated that in women taking rifampicin for tuberculosis and also taking contraceptive pills there was a high proportion of failures in oral contraception and that in a group of 88 such women 5 became pregnant and 68 had menstrual cycle disorders. Gorbach has proposed that changes in the gut bacterial flora resulting from dietary changes might also have effects on oestrogen activity and that these could have important repercussions on the rate of growth of breast tumours. In a comparison of vegetarian and non-vegetarian women living in Boston they found much higher faecal oestrogen excretion in the vegetarians (who have a relatively low breast cancer incidence); levels of plasma oestrogens were inversely related to the faecal excretion rates. In addition, in the vegetarians there was a decreased activity of β-glucuronidase (Goldin *et al.*, 1982). In summary, it is known that oestrogens are important aetiological agents in breast carcinogenesis, and it is now established that the gut flora plays an important role in determining the rate of metabolism of oestrogens. It is proposed that the gut bacteria might play an important part in determining the interrelation between diet, oestrogens and breast carcinogenesis.

Papatestas *et al.* (1982) have taken a more literal line in studying the correlation between breast and colorectal carcinogenesis. If colorectal cancer is caused by bacterial metabolites of bile acids, and if breast and colorectal cancers are closely associated, perhaps bile acid metabolites might also be implicated in breast carcinogenesis. They studied 78 women with breast cancer and 71 controls and reported much higher faecal bile acid concentrations in postmenopausal breast cancer cases than in controls (but no differences between premenopausal cases and controls). In a follow-up paper (Miller *et al.*, 1983) they reported a study of the relation between faecal steroids and tumour stage. Whereas there was no difference in faecal primary bile acids, there was a strong association between tumour stage and faecal secondary bile acids. The authors cite this as evidence of a role for steroids as tumour promoters in breast carcinogenesis, the major role being for the bacterial metabolites (the secondary bile acids), and supporting evidence has come from similar studies by Murray *et al.* (1980) and by Owen *et al.* (1986).

E. Conclusions

It is recognized that a high proportion of human cancer is caused by environmental factors, particularly diet. Since the bacterial flora is in a uniquely favourable position to mediate the interaction between the gut contents and the host, it would be surprising if bacteria were *not* implicated in human carcinogenesis. The evidence that the metabolic activities of the gut bacteria *are* of importance is increasing, and comes from studies of animal models, *in vitro* experiments and observations on humans. It is hoped that our understanding of the role of the gut bacteria in human carcinogenesis will soon reach a level which will permit us to begin to act to prevent such cancers.

References

Allsobrook, A. J. R., Du Plessis, L. S., Harington, J. S., Nunn, A. J. and Nunn, J. R. (1975). Nitrosamines in the human vaginal vault. *In*: "*N*-nitroso compounds in the environment" (eds P. Bogovski and E.A. Walker), pp. 197–199. IARC, Lyon.

Aries, V. C., Crowther, J. S., Drasar, B. S. and Hill, M. J. (1969). Degradation of bile salts by human intestinal bacteria. *Gut* **10**, 575–7.

Bakke, O. M. and Midtvedt, T. (1970). Influence of germ-free status on the excretion of simple phenols of possible significance in tumour promotion. *Experientia* **26**, 519.

Bavin, P. M., Darkin, D. W. and Viney, N. J. (1982). Total nitroso compounds in gastric juice. *IARC Science Publications* No. 41, pp. 337–344. IARC, Lyon.

Bischoff, F. (1969). Carcinogenic effects of steroids. *Adv. Lipid Res.* **7**, 165–244.

Blackwood, A., Murray, W. R., Mackay, C. and Calman, K. (1978). Faecal bile acids and clostridia in the aetiology of colorectal cancer and breast cancer. *Br. J. Cancer* **38**, 175.

Borriello, S. P. (1986). Microbial flora of the gastrointestinal tract. *In*: "Microbial Metabolism in the Intestinal Tract" (ed. M.J. Hill), pp. 1–20. CRC Press, Boca Raton, FL.

Boutwell, R. K. and Bosch, D. K. (1959). The tumour-promoting action of phenol and related compounds on the mouse skin. *Cancer Res.* **19**, 413–427.

Boyer, J., Day, D.W. and Hill, M. J. (1984). Site of cholesterol degradation in the human gut. *Trans. Biochem. Soc.* **12**, 1104–1105.

Bryan, G. T. (1971). The role of urinary tryptophan metabolites in the aetiology of bladder cancer. *Am. J. Clin. Nutr.* **24**, 841–847.

Campbell, R. L., Singh, D. V. and Nigro, N. D. (1975). Importance of the fecal stream on the induction of colon tumours by azoxymethane in rats. *Cancer Res.* **35**, 1369–71.

Caygill, C. P. J., Hill, M., Craven, J. *et al.* (1984). Relevance of gastric achlorhydria to human carcinogenesis. *In*: "*N*-nitroso Compounds: Occurrence, Biological Effects and Relevance to Human Cancer" (eds I. O'Neill, R. C. Von Borstel, C. T. Miller, *et al.*), pp. 895–900. IARC, Lyon.

Caygill, C., Hill, M. J., Hall, N. *et al.* (1985). Gastric surgery as a risk factor in human carcinogenesis. *Gut* **26**, A553.

Coloe and Heywood (1976).

Correa, P. (1978). Epidemiology of polyps and cancer. *In*: "The Pathogenesis of Colorectal Cancer" (ed. B. C. Morson), pp. 126–152. Saunders, Philadelphia.

Correa, P. (1985). *In*: "Diet and Human Carcinogenesis" (eds J. Joossens, M. Hill and J. Geboers), Excerpta Medica, Amsterdam.

Correa, P., Haenszel, W., Chello, C., Tannenbakm, S. and Archer, M. (1975). A model for gastric cancer epidemiology. *Lancet* **ii**, 58–60.

Demerec, M. (1948). Mutations induced by carcinogens. *Br. J. Cancer* **2**, 114–117.

Dunning, W. F., Curtis, M. R. and Maun, M. E. (1950). The effect of added dietary tryptophane on the occurrence of 2-acetylaminofluorene-induced liver and bladder cancer in rats. *Cancer Res.* **10**, 454.

Fadden, K., Owen, R. W., Hill, M. J., Latymer, E., Low, G. and Mason, A. N. (1985). The use of multiply cannulated pigs to examine the effect of dietary fibre supplements on bile acid metabolism in the porcine hind gut. *In*: "Digestive Physiology in the Pig" (eds A. Just, H. Jorgensen and J. Fernandez), pp. 192–194. National Institute of Animal Science, Copenhagen.

Faivre, J., Boutron, M., Hillon, P., Bedonne, L. and Klepping, C. (1985). Epidemiology of Colorectal cancer. *In*: "Diet and Human Carcinogenesis" (eds J. Joossens, M. Hill and J. Geboers), pp. 123–136. Excerpta Medica, Amsterdam.

Farber, E. (1963). Ethionine carcinogenesis. *Adv. Cancer Res.* **7**, 383.

Fernandez, F., Kennedy, H., Hill, M. and Truelove, S. (1985). The effect of diet on the bacterial flora of ileostomy fluid. *Microbiol. Aliments Nutr.* **3**, 47–52.

Fernandez, F., Kennedy, H., Todd, E. *et al.* (1984). Diet and steroid composition in ileostomy fluid. *Trans. Biochem. Soc.* **12**, 1103–1104.

Fisher, J. F. and Mallette, M. F. (1961). The natural occurrence of ethionine in bacteria. *J. Gen. Physiol.* **45**, 1–13.

Goddard, P., Fernandez, F., West, B., Hill, M. J. and Barnes, P. (1975). The nuclear dehydrogenation of steroids by intestinal bacteria. *J. Med. Microbiol.* **8**, 429–435.

Goldin, B. R., Adlercreutz, H., Gorbach, S. L. *et al.* (1982). Estrogen excretion patterns and plasma levels in vegetarian and omnivorous women. *New Eng. J. Med.* **307**, 1542–7.

Goldin, B. R. and Gorbach, S.L. (1977). Alterations in fecal microflora enzymes related to diet, age, lactobacillus supplements and dimethylhydrazine. *Cancer*

40, 2421–6.

Goldin, B. R. and Gorbach, S. L. (1980). Effect of *L. acidophilus* dietary supplements on 1,2-dimethylhydrazine dihydrochloride induced intestinal cancer in rats. *J. Natl. Cancer Inst.* **64**, 263–5.

Goldin, B. R. and Gorbach, S. L. (1981). Effects of antibiotics on incidence of rat intestinal tumors induced by 1,2-dimethylhydrazine dichloride. *J. Natl Cancer Inst.* **67**, 877–880.

Gorbach, S. L. (1984). Estrogens, breast cancer and intestinal flora. *Rev. Infect. Dis.* **6**, S85–9.

Gordon, A. M., Hughes, H. E. and Barr, G. T. (1966). Bacterial flora in abnormalities in the female genital tract. *J. Clin. Path.* **19**, 429.

Graham *et al.* (1972).

Hall, C. N., Cook, A., Darkin, D. *et al.* (1984). Evaluation of the nitrosamine hypothesis of gastric carcinogenesis in man.

Harington, J. S., Nunn, J. R. and Irwig, L. (1973). Dimethylnitrosamine in the human vaginal vault. *Nature* **241**, 49–50.

Hawksworth, G. M., Drasar, B. S. and Hill, M. J. (1971). Intestinal bacteria and the hydrolysis of glycosidic bonds. *J. Med. Microbiol.* **4**, 451–459.

Hicks, R. M. (1982). Nitrosamines as possible etiological agents in bilharzial bladder cancer. *In*: "Nitrosamines and Human Cancer", Banbury Report 12 (ed. P. Magei), pp. 455–72. Cold Spring Harbor Laboratory, NY.

Hicks, R. M., Walters, C. L., Elsebai, I., El Aasser, A. -B., El Merzebani, M. and Gough, T. A. (1977). Demonstration of nitrosamines in human urine: Preliminary observations on a possible etiology for bladder cancer in association with chronic urinary tract infections. *Proc. Roy. Soc. Med.* **70**, 413–416.

Hieger, I. (1958). Cholesterol carcinogenesis. *Brit. Med. Bull.* **14**, 159–160.

Hill, M. J. (1971). The effect of some factors on the faecal concentration of acid steroids, neutral steroids and urobilins. *J. Path.* **104**, 239–245.

Hill, M. J. (1975). The role of colon anaerobes in the metabolism of bile acids and steroids and its relation to colon cancer. *Cancer* **36**, 2387–2400.

Hill, M. J. (1981). Nitrates and bacteriology. Are these important etiological factors in gastric carcinogenesis? *In*: "Gastric Cancer" (eds J. Fielding, C. Newman, C. Ford and B. Jones), pp. 35–46. Pergamon, Oxford.

Hill, M. J. (1982). Influence of nutrition on intestinal flora. *In*: "Colon and Nutrition" (eds H. Goebell and H. Kaspar). MTP, Lancaster.

Hill, M. J. (1986). "Microbes and Human Carcinogenesis". Edward Arnold, London.

Hill, M. J., Drasar, B. S., Williams, R. E. O., Meade, T. W., Cox, A. G., Simpson, J. E. P. and Morson, B. C. (1975). Faecal bile acids and clostridia in patients with cancer of the large bowel. *Lancet* **i**, 535–538.

Hill, M. J., Hudson, M. J. and Stewart, M. (1983). The urinary bacterial flora in patients with three types of urinary tract diversion. *J. Med. Microbiol.* **16**, 221–6.

Hill, M. J., Konishi, F., Morson, B. (1985). The role of bile acids in colorectal carcinogenesis. *Br. J. Surg.* **72** (suppl.), S123–4.

Hirayama, T. (1985). *In*: "Diet and Human Carcinogenesis" (eds J. Joossens, M. Hill and J. Geboers). Excerpta Medica, Amsterdam.

Hurley, R., Stanley, V., Leask, B. and DeLouvois, J. (1974). Microflora of the vagina during pregnancy. *In*: "The Normal Microbial Flora of Man" (eds E. Skinner and L. Carr), pp. 155–186. Academic Press, London.

Joossens, J. V. and Geboers, J. (1981). Nutrition and gastric cancer. *Nutr. Cancer* **2**, 251–261.

Kallner, A. (1967). The transformation of deoxycholic acid into allodeoxycholic acid in the rat. *Acta. Chem. Scand.* **21**, 87–92.

Kelsey, M. I. and Pienta, R. J. (1979). Transformation of hamster embryo cells by cholesterol-epoxide and lithocholic acid. *Cancer Lett.* **6**, 143–149.

Keighley, M., Youngs, D. and Poxon, V. *et al.* (1984). Intragastric *N*-nitrosation is unlikely to be responsible for gastric carcinoma developing after operations for duodenal ulcer. *Gut* **25**, 238–245.

Kinlen *et al.* (1983).

Kinoshita, N. and Gelboin, H. V. (1978). β-glucuronidase catalyzed hydrolysis of benzo[a]pyrene-3-glucuronide and binding to DNA. *Science* **199**, 307–310.

Lauren, P. (1965). The two histological main types of gastric carcinoma: diffuse and so-called intestinal type. *Acta. Path. Microbiol. Scand.* **64**, 31–49.

Laqueur, G., McDaniel, E. G. and Matsumoto, H. (1967). Tumour induction in germ free rats with methylazoxymethanol and synthetic MAM acetate. *J. Natl. Cancer Inst.* **39**, 355–71.

Laqueur, G. L. and Spatz, M. (1968). Toxicology of cycasin. *Cancer Res.* **28**, 2262–7.

Leach, S., Challis, B., Cook, A. R., Hill, M., Thompson, M. (1985). Bacterial catalysis of the *N*-nitrosation of secondary amines. *Trans. Biochem. Soc.* **13**, 380–381.

Lehtola, J. (1978). Family study of gastric carcinoma; with special reference to histological types. *Scand. J. Gastroenterol.* **13**, suppl. 50, 1–54.

Marshall, B. J., Armstrong, J. A., McGechie, D. B. *et al.* (1985). Attempts to fulfil Koch's postulates for pyloric campylobacter. *Med. J. Austr.* **142**, 436–439.

Massey, R. C., Key, P. E., McWeeny, D. J. and Knowles, M. (1985). The application of a chemical denitrosation and chemiluminescence detection procedure for estimation of the apparent concentration of total *N*-nitroso compounds in foods and beverages. *Food Add. Contam.* **1**, 11–16.

Mastromarino, A., Reddy, B. S. and Wynder, E. L. (1976). Metabolic epidemiology of colon cancer: Enzymic activity of the fecal flora. *Am. J. Clin. Nutr.* **29**, 1455–1460.

Matas, A. J., Simmond, R. L., Kjellstrand, C. M. *et al.* (1975). Increased incidence of malignancy during chronic renal failure. *Lancet* **i**, 883–6.

Melzak (1966).

Miller, S. R., Papatestas, A. E., Panveliwalla, D., Pertsemelidis, D. and Auses, A. H. (1983). Fecal steroid excretion and degradation and breast cancer stage. *J. Surgical Res.* **34**, 555–9.

Mizutani, T. and Mitsuoka, T. (1979). Effect of intestinal bacteria on incidence of liver tumors in gnotobiotic C3H/He male mice. *J. Natl. Cancer Inst.* **63**, 1365–1370.

Morson, B. C. (1974). The polyp-cancer sequence in the large bowel. *Proc. Roy. Soc. Med.* **67**, 451–457.

Morson, B. C., Bussey, H. J. R., Day, D. W. and Hill, M. J. (1983). Adenomas of large bowel. *Cancer Surveys* **2**, 451–478.

Mortensen *et al.* (1984).

Murray, W. R., Blackwood, A., Calman, K. C. and Mackay, C. (1980). Fecal bile acids and clostridia in patients with breast cancer. *Br. J. Cancer* **42**, 856–860.

Narisawa, T., Magadia, N., Weisburger, J. and Wynder, E. L. (1974). Promoting effect of bile acids on colon carcinogenesis after intrarectal instillation of *N*-methyl-*N*-nitro-*N*-nitrosoguaridine in rats. *J. Natl Cancer Inst.* **53**, 1093–1097.

Owen, R. W., Henly, P. J., Day, D. W., Thompson, M. H. and Hill, M. J. (1985). Fecal steroids and colorectal cancer: bile acid profiles in low and high risk groups. *In*: "Diet and Human Carcinogenesis" (eds J. Joossens, M. Hill and J. Geboers), pp. 165–170. Excerpta Medica, Amsterdam.

Owen, R. W., Henly, P. J., Thompson, M. H., Hill, M. J. (1986). Steroids and cancer: faecal bile acid screening for early detection of cancer risk. *J. Steroid Biochem.* **24**, 391–394.

Owen, R. W., Thompson, M. H., Hill, M. J., Wilpart, M., Mainguet, P. and Roberfroid, M. (1987). Importance of the ratio of lithocholic to deoxycholic acid in large bowel carcinogenesis. *Nutr. Cancer* **9**, 67–71.

Papatestas, A. E., Panvelliwalla, D., Tarttar, P. I., Miller, S., Pertsemlidis, D. and Aufses, A. (1982). Fecal steroid metabolite and breast cancer risk. *Cancer* **49**, 1201–1205.

Pignatelli, S., Richard, I., Bourgade, M. and Bartsch, H. (1987). An improved method for analysis of total *N*-nitroso compounds in gastric juice. *In*: "Ninth International Meeting on *N*-nitroso Compounds: Relevance to Human Cancer" (eds H. Bartsch and I. O'Neill). IARC, Lyon (in the press).

Radomski, J. L., Greenwald, D., Hearn, W. L., Block, N. L. and Woods, F. M. (1978). Nitrosamine formation in bladder infections and its role in the etiology of bladder cancer. *J. Urol.*, **120**, 48–56.

Rainey, J. B., Davies, P. W., Bristol, J. B. and Williamson, R. C. N. (1983). Adaptation and carcinogenesis in defunctioned rat colon: divergent effects of faeces and bile acids. *Br. J. Cancer* **48**, 477–484.

Reddy, B. S., Narisawa, T., Maronpot, R., Weisburger, J. and Wynder, E. L. (1975). Animal models for the study of dietary factors and cancer of the large bowel. *Cancer Res.* **35**, 3421–3426.

Reddy, B. S., Weisburger, J. H., Narisawa, T. and Wynder, E. L. (1974). Colon carcinogenesis in germ-free rats with dimethylhydrazine and *N*-methyl-*N*-nitro-*N*-nitrosoguanidine. *Cancer Res.* **34**, 2368–72.

Reed, P. I., Smith, P. L. R., Haines, K. *et al.* (1981). Gastric juice *N*-nitrosamines in health and gastroduodenal disease. *Lancet* **ii**, 550–2.

Renwick, A. G. and Drasar, B. S. (1976). Environmental carcinogens and large bowel cancer. *Nature* **263**, 234–235.

Roe, F. J. C. and Grant, G. A. (1970). Inhibition by germ-free status of development of liver and lung tumours in mice exposed neonatally to 7,12-dimethylbenzathracene: implications in relation to tests for carcinogenicity. *Int. J. Cancer* **6**, 133–144.

Sander, J. (1968). Nitrosaminsynthese durch Bakterien. *Z. Physiol. Chem.* **349**, 429–432.

Schlag, P. *et al.* (1978).

Schlag, P., Bockler, R., Ulrich, H., Peter, M., Merkle, P. and Herfarth, C. H. (1980). Are nitrite and N-nitroso compounds in gastric juice risk factors for carcinoma in the operated stomach? *Lancet* **i**, 727–729.

Shousa, S., Scott, J. and Polar, J. (1978). Ileal loop carcinoma after cystectomy for bladder extrophy. *Br. Med. J.* **2**, 397–8.

Simenhoff, M. L., Dunn, S. R. and Lele, P. S. (1984). Analysis for an intestinal metabolism of precursor nitroso compounds in normal subjects and in patients with chronic renal failure. *IARC Scientific Publication* No. 57, pp. 161–70.

IARC, Lyon.

Simenhoff, M. L., Saukkonen, J. J., Burke, J. F. *et al.* (1978). Bacterial populations of the small bowel in uremia. *Niphron* **22**, 460–4.

Sinclair, T. and Tuxford, A. F. (1971). The incidence of urinary tract infection and a symptomatic bacteriuria in a semi-rural practice. *Practitioner* **207**, 81–90.

Stewart, M., Hill, M. J., Pugh, R. C. B. and Williams, J. P. (1981). The role of *N*-nitrosamine in carcinogenesis at the ureterocolic anastomosis. *Br. J. Urol.* **53**, 115–8.

Stockbrugger, R., Cotton, P., Menon, G. *et al.* (1984). Pernicious anae.nia, intragastric bacterial overgrowth and possible consequences. *Scand. J. Gastroenterol.* **19**, 355–64.

Walters, C. L., Hill, M. J. and Uddell, W. S. J. (1978). *In*: "Environmental Aspects of *N*-nitroso Compounds" (eds Walker, E. A., Castagnero, M., Griciute, L. and Lyle, R. E.). IARC, Lyon.

Wilpart, M., Mainguet, P., Maskens, A. and Roberfroid, M. (1985). Structure-activity relationship amongst biliary acids showing co-mutagenicity towards 1,2-dimethylhydrazine. *Carcinogenesis* **4**, 1239–1241.

Index

of bile acids, 276–277
of faeces, 307
of mandelonitrile, 118–119
of nitropyrenes, 149–150
of rutin, 367
of steviol, 131–132
see also Faecal mutagens and large
     bowel cancer

Naphthalene metabolism, 93
Naphthaquinones, 119
Neomycin and cyclamate metabolism,
     190
Neoplasia and gastrectomy, 164
Neoplasma, hepatic, 473–475
Nephrocalcinosis and caecal
     enlargement, 392–393
Neurotoxicity of methylmercury, 208
     microflora elimination in, 213
Nitrate in drinking water
     and gastric cancer, 164
     and methaemoglobinamia, 160
Nitrate metabolism, 153–174
     formation *in vivo*, 154–156
     and pectin, 353
     pharmacokinetics, 157
     recirculation, 157
     reduction
          bacterial, 158–159
          biochemical, 159
          in colon, 54
     sources, 153
     toxic consequences of reduction
          methaemoglobinaemia, 159–160
          N-nitroso compounds, 160–166
Nitrite
     colonocyte stimulation, 54
     and methaemoglobinaemia, 159–160
Nitro compound metabolism, 145–152
     nitrobenzenes, 146–147
          and diet, 364
     nitropyrenes, 149–150
     nitrotoluenes, 147–148
     sources, 145
Nitrobenzene metabolism, 146–147
     and diet, 364
1-Nitropyrene metabolism, 149–150
Nitrogen compound metabolism,
     227–262
     amino acids, 232–236
     deamination, 233–235

decarboxylation, 235–236
ammonia, 236–247
     absorption, 243–245
     and encephalopathy, 246–247
     formation, bacterial, 236–239
     host metabolism, 245–246
     and lactulose, 291
     utilization, bacterial, 239–243
choline, 252
creatinine, 250–251
in hypochlorhydria, 350
proteins, 230–232
     Bacteroides in, 231
     colonic, 302–305
     fatty acids, short chain,, 232
     mucins, 231–232
     and saccharin, 179–182
urea, 247–250
     and lactulose, 29
     and renal failure, 249–250
     site, 248–249
     transamination, 245–246
     ureases, 248
uric acid, 251–252
see also Nitrate metabolism; Nitro
     compound metabolism; Nitrogen
     total Nitrogen, total, 228–230
forms of, 229–230
     and absorption, 230
in large intestine, 228–229
     and ileostomy, 228
Nitropropanol hydrolysis, 134–135
Nitropyrene metabolism, 149–150
Nitroreductase activity, and pectin,
     353, 363–364
Nitrosamines
in faeces, and mutagenicity,
     419–420
formation sites, 164–166
N-Nitrosation, and gnotobiotes, 16
N-Nitroso compounds
amino acid nitrosation, 162–164
     nitrosopeptides, 162, 164
     nitrosoproline, 162, 163
formation
     bacteria in, 467–469
     in vivo, 160–162
and gastric cancer, 483–485
nitrosamines
     in faeces, and mutagenicity,
          419–420
     formation sites, 164–166